A PRIMER OF **DRUG ACTION**

A concise, nontechnical guide to the actions, uses, and side effects of psychoactive drugs

Ninth Edition

Twenty–fifth Anniversary

ROBERT M. JULIEN M.D., PH.D.

St. Vincent Hospital and Medical Center

Portland, Oregon

WORTH PUBLISHERS

A Primer of Drug Action, Ninth Edition

© 2001 by Worth Publishers

Printed in the United States of America

First printing 2000

Library of Congress Cataloging-in-Publication Data

Julien, Robert M.
    A primer of drug action: a concise, nontechnical guide to the actions, uses, and side effects of psychoactive drugs / Robert M. Julien.—9th ed.
        p. cm.
    ISBN 0-7167-5109-7
    1. Psychotropic drugs. 2. Psychopharmacology. I. Title.

RM315 .J75 2000
615'.788—dc21   00-034080

Sponsoring Editor: Jessica Bayne
Marketing Manager: Renee Ortbals
Project Editor: Diane Cimino Davis
Art Director: Barbara Reingold
Cover Design: Ana Linneman
Production Manager: Sarah Segal
Compositor: TSI Graphics
Manufacturer: Quebecor World

Worth Publishers
41 Madison Avenue, New York, NY 10010
www.worthpublishers.com

Preface

Psychoactive drugs are substances that alter mood, thought processes, or behavior or that are used to manage neuropsychological illness. During the second half of the twentieth century we learned that drugs are effective treatment for disease, that drug dosage and drug responsiveness are related, that drugs act at specific sites of action, that *potency* and *efficacy* are different, and that specific drug receptors can be characterized. During that time, we identified certain "prototype" drugs that initiated the modern era of psychopharmacotherapy.

In the quarter century since the publication of the first edition of *A Primer of Drug Action*, there has been an explosion of knowledge about drugs, about the underlying disorders for which they are used, and about the receptor substrates upon which they act. This knowledge explosion is accelerating, and remarkable advances are occurring. Within the past five years, we have witnessed the introduction of totally new classes of drugs for treating schizophrenia, depression, and bipolar illness. We have come to recognize the chronic and disabling nature of persistent anxiety and dysthymia. We have watched the explosion in the diagnosis and treatment of psychological disorders of children and adolescents, and we have gained new understanding of the biochemical abnormalities in behavioral and psychological disorders. Currently, we can point to an exponential increase in the use of herbal medicines to treat psychological disorders (although they cannot be promoted for such use), and we struggle to understand the uses, efficacy, side effects, and limitations of these ancient products. Finally, as our knowledge of molecular biology increases, we are witnessing the identification, sequencing, and cloning of drug receptors, processes that will produce the psychotherapeutic drugs of the future.

In 1975, when the first edition of *A Primer of Drug Action* was published, we had few drugs to treat many of the psychological disorders discussed in this ninth edition. We had no idea of the structure or sources of drug receptors. Child and adolescent psychopharmacology was embryonic, and most of the drugs presented in this book had not even been conceived of. Even now, we are still in an embryonic period of psychopharmacology. As the twenty-first century progresses, we will describe the human genetic code and explore the mechanisms by which gene expression can be modified by drugs. We will develop new and better drug-delivery systems. We will develop remarkable new treatments for mental disorders; and we will see vast improvements in drug design, in drug delivery, and in the therapeutic uses of drugs as phenotype-specific agents. Drug abuse and dependence will undoubtedly continue to be problems; however, we will develop new medications to help people escape the ravages of drug dependency. Certainly we will develop new analgesic agents that are clinically efficacious yet devoid of reinforcing potential. I hope we will develop new treatments to prevent, delay, or ameliorate neurodegenerative disorders and to protect neurons after injury or insult.

To date, each edition of *A Primer of Drug Action* has managed to mirror and document scientific and clinical advances. *A Primer of Drug Action* discusses the general principles of each class of psychoactive drugs and provides specific information about each drug within that class. The book also addresses the mechanisms of action of each drug and drug class, current theories about the etiology of major psychological disorders and rationales for drug treatment, and the uses and limitations of psychopharmacology in patient care.

Drugs of compulsive abuse are again emphasized. Theories of drug-induced behavioral reinforcement, comorbidity of substance abuse with other psychological disorders, and the treatment of substance abuse are presented. In essence, the major changes that have occurred since the publication of the eighth edition in 1998 necessitate a complete revision of the book. More than 40 percent of the literature cited is from research published between 1998 and 2000.

The goal of the first edition was to provide pharmacological information that was concise, accurate, and timely. Information was presented in clear language and as free as possible of technical jargon so that it could be easily understood by readers with minimal background in the biological sciences. This philosophy continues, although recent advances in molecular biology necessitate a major change in presentation. For the first time in 25 years, this book is presented in two versions: (1) an "academic version" that contains in-depth discussion of drug mechanisms, and (2) a "trade version" that eliminates some of the more technical information. Here, in the academic version, current research into the mechanism of action of psychoactive drugs is fully discussed and referenced. This version is suggested for courses where emphasis is placed on drug mechanisms and where assistance is available to aid the student with some of the technical discussion.

The pharmacological and psychotherapeutic treatments of psychological disorders are integrated, and the interface between psychopharmacotherapy and the various professions of counseling, psychology,

Part 3
Drugs That Stimulate Brain Function: Psychostimulants 177

7 Cocaine, Amphetamines, and Other Behavioral Stimulants 178

Cocaine
Background / Forms of Cocaine / Pharmacokinetics / Mechanism of Action / Effects of Short-Term, Low-Dose Use / Toxic and Psychotic Effects of Long-Term, High-Dose Use / Comorbidity / Cocaine and Pregnancy / Pharmacological Treatment of Cocaine Dependency / Psychosocial Interventions

Amphetamines and Other Behavioral Stimulants
History / Mechanism of Action / Pharmacological Effects / Dependence and Tolerance / ICE: A Free-Base Form of Methamphetamine / Nonamphetamine Behavioral Stimulants / Pharmacologic Treatment of ADHD

8 Caffeine and Nicotine 220

Caffeine
Pharmacokinetics / Pharmacological Effects / Mechanism of Action / Reproductive Effects / Tolerance and Dependence

Nicotine
Pharmacokinetics / Pharmacological Effects / Mechanism of Action / Tolerance and Dependence / Toxicity / Therapy for Nicotine Dependence

Part 4
Drugs That Relieve Pain: Opioid and Nonopioid Analgesics 249

9 Opioid Analgesics 250
History / Terminology / Opioid Receptors / Classification of Opioid Analgesics / Morphine: A Pure Agonist Opioid / Other Pure Agonist Opioids / Partial Agonist Opioids / Mixed Agonist-Antagonist Opioids / Antagonist Opioids / Pharmacotherapy of Opioid Dependence

10 Nonnarcotic, Anti-inflammatory Analgesics 287
Nonselective Cyclooxygenase Inhibitors / Selective COX-2 Inhibitors

Contents

and psychotherapy is addressed. Professionals working with either people who are taking psychotropic medications or people who suffer from drug dependency disorders now must be knowledgeable about and conversant in the pharmacology of the drugs their patients may be taking. This has become even more important since the publication of clinical practice guidelines for the treatment of major psychological disorders. To this end, each chapter contains a brief discussion of the clinical interface between pharmacological and psychological treatments. Chapter 19, cowritten with Dr. Donald Lange, is devoted to this topic and includes listing and discussion of currently available practice guidelines.

FEATURES OF THE NINTH EDITION

In its first 25 years of publication, *A Primer of Drug Action* helped shape knowledge about psychopharmacology, drug abuse, and psychopharmacotherapy. In its ninth edition, *A Primer of Drug Action* is completely revised and updated with the aim of continuing its history as the most current, objective, and understandable introduction to the pharmacology of drugs that affect the mind and behavior. Each of the 20 chapters of the academic version has been completely rewritten and updated. Included in each presentation are not only the traditional and newly available drugs but discussions of both current and future directions in drug research (including new drugs that are on the horizon but not yet available for clinical use).

The academic version of the ninth edition of *A Primer of Drug Action* will, I hope, serve the needs of students who want a concise, clearly presented and comprehensive introduction to psychopharmacology, drug education, and psychopharmacotherapy. Each chapter includes study questions and extensive references. Also available is a *Test Bank* (ISBN 0-7167-5110-0) by Peter E. Simson of Miami University, Oxford, Ohio. This new *Test Bank* contains almost 800 items in multiple-choice, true-false, and short answer formats. Each question is keyed to the page where the answer is located.

Introduction to Psychopharmacology: How Drugs Interact with the Body and the Brain

This book begins with three chapters devoted to the fundamentals of drug action. Chapter 1 explores how the body reacts to the presence of a drug within it. Once a drug arrives in the stomach (if taken orally), how and why does it gain access to the bloodstream? Once in the bloodstream, how is it distributed throughout the body? Is it distributed evenly? How is this reflected in the actions of the drug? Finally, how does the body eventually get rid of the drug? The answers to all these questions fall under the general topic of pharmacokinetics, the aspect of pharmacology that explores how the body handles drugs and other foreign substances placed within it.

Chapter 2 explores the area of pharmacology called pharmacodynamics, the mechanisms through which drugs exert their biochemical or behavioral effects. The interaction between drugs and the receptors to which the drugs attach is examined, as well as how the attachment results in alterations in cell function and in behavior. Receptors are described both structurally and functionally, and how drugs alter receptor structure and function is discussed. Finally, the ways such actions underlie both the therapeutic and the side effects of drugs are illustrated.

Chapter 3 applies knowledge about basic pharmacology to the specifics of drug action on the brain and ultimately on behavior. This part of pharmacology is called psychopharmacology. Chapter 3 presents the structure and function of the neuron—the unit of nervous system function and the site of action of psychoactive drugs. By studying the process of synaptic transmission and specific neurotransmitters, we begin to understand the mode of action of psychoactive drugs as well as the complexity of brain functioning in both health and disease.

Pharmacokinetics: How Drugs Are Handled by the Body

When we have a headache, we take for granted that after taking some aspirin our headache will probably disappear within 15 to 30 minutes. We also take for granted that, unless we take more aspirin later, the headache may recur within 3 or 4 hours.

This familiar scenario illustrates four basic processes in the branch of pharmacology called *pharmacokinetics*, the study of the movement of drugs through the body. Using the aspirin example, the four processes are as follows:

1. *Absorption* of the aspirin into the body from the swallowed tablet.
2. *Distribution* of the aspirin throughout the body, including into a fetus, should a female patient be pregnant at the time the drug is taken.
3. *Metabolism* (detoxification or breakdown) of the drug. The aspirin that has exerted its analgesic effect is broken down into metabolites (by-products or waste products) that no longer exert any effect.
4. *Elimination* of the metabolic waste products, usually in urine excretion.

The goal of this chapter is to explore these processes of pharmacokinetics, concluding with discussion about how pharmacokinetcs can be used to determine the time course of action for drugs. The chapter also explores the steady-state maintenance of therapeutic blood levels of drugs in the body and the usefulness of therapeutic drug monitoring. Finally, the chapter discusses drug *tolerance* and drug *dependence*.

The understanding of pharmacokinetics, along with knowledge about the *dosage* taken, allows determination of the concentration of a drug at its sites of action (i.e., at its *receptors*) and the *intensity* of drug effect on the receptors as a function of time.[1]

Thus, pharmacokinetics in its simplest form describes the time course of a particular drug's actions—the time to onset and the duration of effect. Usually, the time course simply reflects the amount of *time* required for the rise and fall of the drug's concentration at the

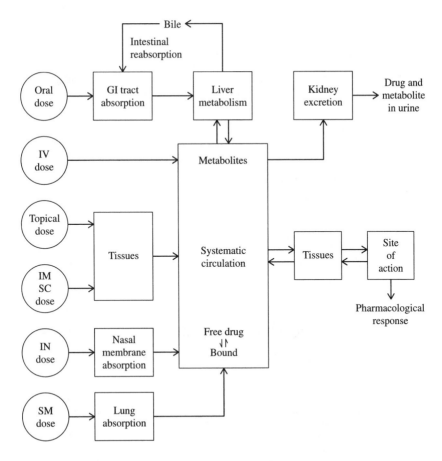

FIGURE 1.1 Schematic representation of the fate of a drug in the body. IM = intramuscular; IV = intravenous; IN = intranasal; SC = subcutaneous; SM = smoked.

target site. Figure 1.1 illustrates the complexity of drug movement through the body and its equilibrium at its site of action.

The root *kinetics* in the word *pharmacokinetics* implies movement and time. As each of the drugs in this book is discussed, the focus is first on the time course of the drug's movement through the body, particularly its half-life and any complications that arise from alterations in its rate of metabolism. Knowledge of movement and time offers significant insight into the action of a drug. At the very least, it helps distinguish a particular drug from other related drugs.

For example, the main difference between two benzodiazepines (Chapter 6), lorazepam (Ativan)* and triazolam (Halcion), is in their pharmacokinetics. Both these drugs depress the functioning of the brain, but the profile of lorazepam, which persists for at least 24 hours in the body, is very different from that of triazolam, which persists for only about 6 to 8 hours. If lorazepam is administered at bedtime for treatment of insomnia, daytime sedation the next day can be a problem, since lorazepam persists in the body through the next day. However, for longer, steady action (as might be useful in treating anxiety), lorazepam would be the superior agent to use. The kinetic differences between lorazepam and triazolam are illustrated in Figure 1.2, which shows three ranges: an ineffective range (where not enough drug is present to produce either sedative or antianxiety effects), a therapeuptic range, and a toxic range (where sedation becomes excessive). Triazolam reaches peak blood level rapidly and is of short duration. Lorazepam, on the other hand, reaches peak blood level later and persists longer in the therapeutic range. In essence, pharmacokinetic differences account for these results and allow two similar drugs to be used for quite different therapeutic goals.

Drug Absorption

The term "drug absorption" refers to processes and mechanisms by which drugs pass from the external world into the bloodstream. For any drug, a route of administration, a dose of the drug, and a dosage

---

*Most drugs used in medicine are known by two or even three names. The most complicated name for a drug is its *structural* name, which accurately describes its chemical structure in words. In this book, the chemical names for drugs are not used. The second name for a drug is its *generic* name, which is a somewhat easier-to-remember name given to the drug by its discoverer or manufacturer. After a drug's patent protection runs out (usually 17 years after the date of its patent registration by the manufacturer), any other generic drug manufacturer may legitimately sell the drug under this name. The third name is the drug's *trade* name, a unique name placed on the drug by its original patent holder. Only that manufacturer can ever sell the drug under that name, even after the patent runs out and others sell the drug. For example, many companies sell aspirin, a generic name for acetyl-salicylic acid, the structural name. However, only Bayer Pharmaceuticals (the original company that patented acetyl-salicylic acid) can call it Bayer Aspirin.

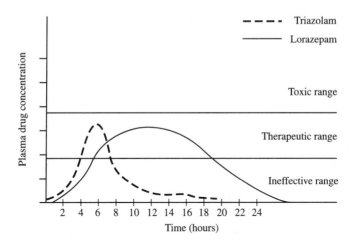

FIGURE 1.2 Theoretical blood levels of triazolam (a short-acting benzodiazepine) and lorazepam (a long-acting benzodiazepine) over time following oral administration. Approximations for ineffective, therapeutic, and toxic blood levels are shown. Solid line = lorazepam; dotted line = triazolam.

form (e.g., liquid, tablet, capsule, injection, patch, spray, or gum) must be selected that will both place the drug at its site of action in a pharmacologically effective concentration and maintain the concentration for an adequate period of time. Drugs are most commonly administered in one of six ways:

- Orally (swallowed when taken by mouth)
- Rectally (drug embedded in a suppository, which is placed in the rectum)
- Parenterally (given in liquid form by injection with a needle and syringe)
- Inhaled through the lungs as gases, as vapors, or as particles carried in smoke or in an aerosol
- Absorbed through the skin (usually as a drug-containing skin patch)
- Absorbed through mucous membranes (from "snorting" or sniffing drug, with the drug depositing on the oral or nasal mucosa)

Oral Administration

To be effective when administered orally, a drug must be soluble and stable in stomach fluid (not destroyed by gastric acids), enter the intestine, penetrate the lining of the intestine, and pass into the bloodstream. Because they are already in solution, drugs that are administered in liquid form tend to be absorbed more rapidly than those given in tablet or capsule form. When a drug is taken in solid form, both the rate at which it dissolves and its chemistry limit the rate of absorption.

After a tablet dissolves, the drug molecules contained within it are carried into the upper intestine, where they are absorbed across the intestinal mucosa by a process of *passive diffusion*. This process occurs at a rate that is determined by the ratio of water solubility to lipid solubility of the drug molecules.* As Figure 1.3 shows, once in solution, drugs exist as a mixture of two interchangeable forms: one that is water soluble (the *ionized*, or electrically charged, form) and one that is lipid soluble (the *nonionized*, or uncharged, form). When the drug molecule is in the water-soluble form, it does not readily cross cell membranes (it becomes "trapped" in this ionized form); in the lipid-soluble form, it can freely cross the membrane. Thus, the lipid-soluble form is in equilibrium across the gastric wall; absorption occurs because the ionized form of drug is trapped within plasma and cannot diffuse back into the stomach.

In general, most psychoactive drugs—the topic of this book—have sufficient lipid solubility to allow them to readily cross all cell membranes and enter the brain. Indeed, about 75 percent of the amount of an orally administered drug is absorbed within about two to three hours after administration.

Although oral administration of drugs is common, it does have disadvantages. First, it may lead to occasional vomiting and stomach distress. Second, although the amount of a drug that is put into a tablet or capsule can be calculated, how much of it will be absorbed into the bloodstream cannot always be accurately predicted because of genetic differences between individuals and because of differences in the manufacturing of the drugs.

Finally, some drugs, such as the local anesthetics and insulin, when administered orally, are destroyed by the acid in the stomach before they can be absorbed. To be effective, such drugs must be administered by injection.

---

*The proportion of a drug in the nonionized, more fat-soluble form depends on the *dissociation constant* (the pK_a) of the drug and on the *pH* of the fluid in which it is dissolved, a relationship shown by the *Henderson-Hasselbalch equation:*

$$pK_a = pH + \log \frac{[\text{nonionized acid}]}{[\text{ionized acid}]}$$

Most psychoactive drugs are weak acids. Therefore, at the pH of blood plasma (pH = 7.4) they are much more ionized when compared with the more acidic pH encountered in gastric and upper intestinal fluids. Figure 1.3 illustrates how this allows for absorption by passive diffusion, despite there being more drug in plasma than in the intestine (allowing rather complete absorption against a concentration gradient).

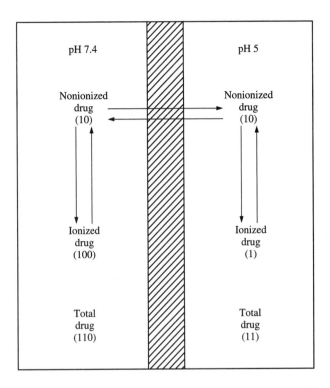

FIGURE 1.3 Distribution of a weakly acidic drug between upper intestinal fluid (pH = 5) and plasma (pH = 7.4). The solutions are separated by a cell membrane that is permeable only to the nonionized, lipid-soluble form of the drug. Note that different proportions of drug are ionized and nonionized in each of the two different pH compartments. Increased ionization traps drug in plasma. Concentrations at equilibrium are shown in brackets.

Rectal Administration

Although the primary route of drug administration is oral, some drugs are administered rectally (usually in suppository form) if the patient is vomiting, unconscious, or unable to swallow. However, absorption is often irregular, unpredictable, and incomplete, and many drugs irritate the membranes that line the rectum. In psychopharmacology, some phenothiazines (Chapter 17) are administered rectally to treat nausea and vomiting. Also, tetrahydrocannabinol derivatives (Chapter 11) prepared in suppository form are being tested for similar use (hopefully separating any "high" associated with smoking the drug in the form of a marijuana cigarette from any antiemetic action of the active ingredient).

Administration by Inhalation

In recreational drug misuse and abuse, inhalation of drugs is a popular method of administration. Examples of drugs taken by this route include nicotine in tobacco cigarettes and tetrahydrocannabinol in marijuana, as well as smoked heroin, crack cocaine, crank methamphetamine, and the various inhalants of abuse, all of which are discussed at length later in this book.

The popularity of inhalation as a route of administration follows from two observations:

1. Lung tissues have a large surface area through which large amounts of blood flow, allowing for easy and rapid exchange of drugs between lung and blood (often within seconds).

2. Drugs absorbed into pulmonary (lung) capillaries are carried in the pulmonary veins directly to the left side (arterial side) of the heart (Figure 1.4) and from there directly into the aorta and the arteries carrying blood to the brain.

As a result, drugs administered by inhalation may have an even faster onset of effect than drugs administered intravenously. If drugs administered in this fashion are behaviorally reinforcing, intoxicating, and subject to compulsive abuse, the rapid onset of effect can be intense, to say the least.

The various anesthetic gases (such as nitrous oxide) and vaporized liquids (such as halothane) are absorbed across lung membranes into the arterial circulation nearly as fast as they are inhaled, allowing for the rapid onset of anesthesia.

Administration Through Mucous Membranes

Occasionally, drugs are administered through the mucous membranes of the mouth or nose. A few examples:

-   A heart patient taking nitroglycerine places the tablet under the tongue, where the drug is absorbed into the bloodstream rapidly and directly into blood.

-   Cocaine powder, when sniffed, adheres to the membranes on the inside of the nose and is absorbed directly into the bloodstream. (Cocaine is discussed in Chapter 7.)

-   Nasal decongestants are sprayed directly onto mucous membranes from which they are both absorbed and also act locally to constrict mucous membranes, relieving nasal congestion.

-   Nicotine (Chapter 8) in snuff, nasal spray, or chewing-gum formulations (Chapter 6) is absorbed through the mucosal membranes directly into the bloodstream.

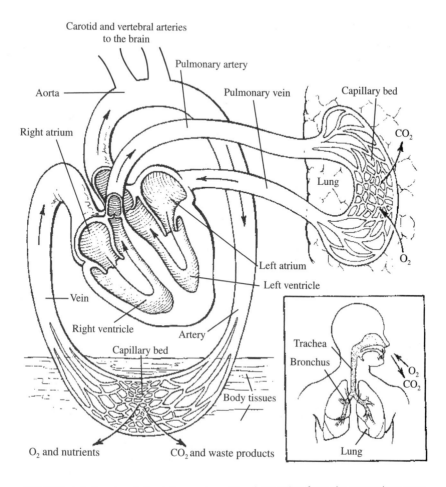

FIGURE 1.4 Heart and circulatory system. Blood returning from the systemic venous circulation to the heart enters the right atrium and flows into the right ventricle. With contraction of the heart, this blood is pumped into the pulmonary arteries leading to the lungs. Once in the pulmonary capillaries, carbon dioxide (CO_2) is lost and replaced by oxygen. This oxygenated blood returns to the heart in the pulmonary veins, which empty into the left atrium. With heart contraction, the oxygenated blood is pumped from the left ventricle into the aorta and is carried to the body tissues and brain, where oxygen and nutrients are exchanged in the systemic capillary beds. Oxygen and nutrients are supplied to the body tissues through the walls of the capillaries; CO_2 and other waste products are returned to the blood. The CO_2 is eliminated through the lungs, and the other waste products are metabolized in the liver and excreted in the urine.

- Caffeine (Chapter 8) became available in 1999 in chewing-gum form, the caffeine being rapidly absorbed as the gum is chewed.

- For use before and after surgery in children, the opioid narcotic fentanyl (Sublimase; Chapter 9) became available in 1998 in lollipop form, so this pain-relieving drug can be provided without subjecting a child to a painful injection. As the lollipop is sucked, the drug is released and absorbed through the mucous membranes of the mouth.

- Under investigation for use as a nasal spray is buprenorphine (Buprenex), a "weak" opioid ("narcotic") agonist, potentially effective and useful in narcotic detoxification and maintenance programs (Chapter 9).

Administration Through the Skin

In the 1990s, several prescribed medications were incorporated into *transdermal patches* that adhere to the skin.[2] This is a unique bandage-like therapeutic system that provides continuous, controlled release of a drug from a reservoir through a semipermeable membrane (Figure 1.5). The drug is slowly absorbed into the bloodstream at the area of contact. Some examples of drug-containing patches:

- Nicotine (used to deter smoking)
- Fentanyl (used to treat chronic, unrelenting pain)

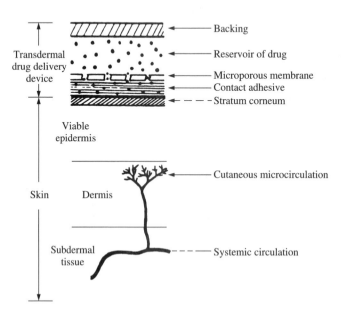

FIGURE 1.5 Diagrammatic representation of a transdermal fentanyl "patch" delivery system placed on the skin.

- Nitroglycerine (used to prevent the symptoms of angina pectoris in patients with coronary artery disease)
- Clonidine (used to treat hypertension)
- Estrogen (used to replace reduced hormones in postmenopausal women)
- Scopolamine (to prevent motion sickness)

In each case, the drug is slowly, predictably, and continuously released from the liquid in the patch and absorbed into the systemic circulation over a period of days, allowing the levels of drug in the plasma to remain relatively constant.

Administration by Injection

Administration of drugs by injection can be *intravenous* (directly into a vein), *intramuscular* (directly into a muscle), or *subcutaneous* (just under the skin). Each of these routes of administration has its advantages and disadvantages (Table 1.1), but some features are shared by all. In general, administration by injection produces a more prompt response than does oral administration because absorption is faster. Also, injection permits a more accurate dose because the unpredictable processes of absorption through the stomach and intestine are bypassed.

Administration of drugs by injection, however, has several drawbacks. First, the rapid rate of absorption leaves little time to respond to an unexpected drug reaction or accidental overdose. Second, administration by injection requires the use of sterile techniques. Hepatitis and AIDS are examples of diseases that can be transmitted as a drastic consequence of unsterile injection techniques. Third, once a drug is administered by injection, it cannot be recalled.

Intravenous Administration. In an intravenous injection, a drug is introduced directly into the bloodstream. This technique avoids all the variables related to oral absorption. The injection can be made slowly, and it can be stopped instantaneously if untoward effects develop. In addition, the dosage amount can be extremely precise, and the practitioner can dilute and administer in large volumes drugs that at higher concentrations would be irritants to the muscles or blood vessels.

The intravenous route is the most dangerous of all routes of administration, because it has the fastest speed of onset of pharmacological action. Too-rapid injection can be catastrophic, producing life-threatening reactions (such as collapse of respiration or of heart function). Also, allergic reactions, should they occur, may be extremely severe. Finally, drugs that are not completely solublized before injection cannot usually

TABLE 1.1 Some characteristics of drug administration by injection

Route	Absorption pattern	Special utility	Limitations and precautions
Intravenous	Absorption circumvented Potentially immediate effects	Valuable for emergency use Permits titration of dosage Can administer large volumes and irritating substances when diluted	Increased risk of adverse effects Must inject solutions slowly as a rule Not suitable for oily solutions or insoluble substances
Intramuscular	Prompt action from aqueous solution Slow and sustained action from repository preparations	Suitable for moderate volumes, oily vehicles, and some irritating substances	Precluded during anticoagulant medication May interfere with interpretation of certain diagnostic tests (e.g., creatine phosphokinase)
Subcutaneous	Prompt action from aqueous solution Slow and sustained action from repository preparations	Suitable for some insoluble suspensions and for implantation of solid pallets	Not suitable for large volumes Possible pain or necrosis from irritating substances

Modified from Benet, Mitchell, and Sheiner,[1] p. 6.

be given intravenously because of the danger of blood clots or emboli forming. Infection and transmission of infectious diseases are an ever present danger when sterile techniques are not employed.

Intramuscular Administration. Drugs that are injected into skeletal muscle (usually in the arm, thigh, or buttock) are generally absorbed fairly rapidly. Absorption of a drug from muscle is more rapid than absorption of the same drug from the stomach but slower than absorption of the drug administered intravenously. The absolute rate of absorption of a drug from muscle varies, depending on the rate of blood flow to the muscle, the solubility of the drug, the volume of the injection, and the solution in which the drug is dissolved and injected.

In general, most of the precautions that apply to intravenous administration also apply to intramuscular injection, but, as a rule, drugs that are intended for intramuscular administration are prepared in amounts much larger than those intended to be given intravenously. Accidental intravenous injection of doses intended for intramuscular use can be catastrophic.

Subcutaneous Administration. Absorption of drugs that have been injected under the skin (subcutaneously) is rapid. The exact rate depends mainly on the ease of blood vessel penetration and the rate of blood flow through the skin. Irritating drugs should not be injected subcutaneously, because they may cause severe pain and damage to local tissue. The usual precautions to maintain sterility apply.

Self-administration of any drug by injection is to be discouraged except when oral administration is not effective or when the drug is being taken therapeutically under the direction of a physician (injection of insulin by a diabetic is a prominent example). The risks associated with injection of a drug (infection, overdose, allergic responses, and transmission of the AIDS virus) are far greater than those associated with oral administration of the same drug.

Drug Distribution

Once absorbed into the bloodstream, a drug is distributed throughout the body by the circulating blood, passing across various barriers to reach its site of action (its receptors). At any given time, only a very small portion of the total amount of a drug that is in the body is actually in contact with its receptors (Figure 1.1). Most of the administered drug is found in areas of the body that are remote from the drug's site of action. For example, in the case of a psychoactive drug, most of the drug circulates outside the brain and therefore does not contribute directly to its pharmacological effect. This wide distribution often accounts for many of the side effects of a drug. *Side effects* are results that are different from the primary, or therapeutic, effect for which a drug is taken.

Action of the Bloodstream

In the average-size adult, the heart pumps every minute a volume of blood that is roughly equal to the total amount of blood within the circulatory system. Thus, the entire blood volume circulates in the body about once every minute, and once absorbed into the bloodstream, a drug is rapidly (usually within this 1-minute circulation time) distributed throughout the circulatory system.

A schematic diagram of the circulatory system is presented in Figure 1.4. Blood returning to the heart through the veins is first pumped into the pulmonary (lung) circulation system, where carbon dioxide is removed and replaced by oxygen. The oxygenated blood then returns to the heart and is pumped into the great artery (the aorta). From there blood flows into the smaller arteries and finally into the capillaries, where nutrients (and drugs) are exchanged between the blood and the cells of the body.

After blood passes through the capillaries, it is collected by the veins and returned to the heart to circulate again. Psychoactive drugs quite quickly become evenly distributed throughout the bloodstream, diluted not only by blood but also by the total amount of water contained in the body.

In addition to solubility, another factor often limits drug distribution: the reversible binding of drugs to proteins present in the blood plasma. A protein-bound drug exists in equilibrium with a free (unbound) drug, as shown in Figure 1.1. Because plasma proteins (albumin, for example) are quite large, they are unable to leave the bloodstream. Thus, the amount of drug that is bound to plasma proteins remains confined within the blood vessels, markedly affecting drug distribution.

How are drugs handled differently by the blood circulation as shown in Figure 1.4?

1. Taken orally, a drug passes through the cells lining the gastrointestinal (GI) tract. Occasionally, drug-metabolizing enzymes with those cells can markedly reduce the amount of drug absorbed into the bloodstream. Once in the venous system leading away from the GI tract, a drug flows toward the heart. Some passes through the liver, where another percentage of drug is taken up by liver cells and metabolized. These two mechanisms, which reduce the amount of orally administered drug that actually reaches the central circulation, are together called first-pass metabolism* and can significantly lower the blood level of certain drugs taken orally.

    An example may illustrate this point. Buspirone (BuSpar; Chapter 6) is an orally administered antianxiety drug. However, despite almost complete absorption after oral administration, only about 5 percent of the drug reaches the central circulation and is distributed to the brain. The reason for this is that 95 percent of the

---

*First-pass metabolism can be bothersome in clinical practice, as much more drug may have to be given orally than would be given by other routes (because much is metabolized before the drug reaches the central circulation).

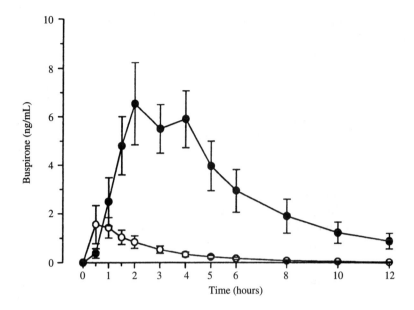

FIGURE 1.6 Plasma concentrations (mean and SEM) of buspirone (in nanograms per milliliter of plasma) in ten healthy volunteers after a single oral dose of 10 mg buspirone, after ingestion of 200 mL (about 7 oz) grapefruit juice (*solid circles*) or water (*open circles*) three times a day for 2 days, and on day 3 with buspirone administration 30 and 90 minutes later. [Data from Lilja et al.[3]]

absorbed drug is metabolized as it passes through the wall of the small intestine and the liver. Blocking such metabolism by drinking grapefruit juice[3] markedly increases the amount of drug in the bloodstream and improves its therapeutic action (Figure 1.6).

2. Injected (by whatever route), absorbed transdermally, or absorbed from mucous membranes, drug enters systemic veins and returns to the right side of the heart (usually with minimal amounts passing initially through the liver). Drug is then circulated through the pulmonary vessels, returns to the left side of the heart, and finally distributes through the aorta to the brain and the body.

3. Inhaled drugs absorbed from the lungs are carried in pulmonary veins directly to the left side of the heart and, from there, rapidly to the brain and the systemic circulation.

Body Membranes That Affect Drug Distribution

Four types of membranes in the body affect drug distribution: (1) the cell membranes, (2) the walls of the capillary vessels in the circulatory system, (3) the blood-brain barrier, and (4) the placental barrier.

Cell Membranes. To be absorbed from the intestine or to gain access to the interior of a cell, a drug must penetrate the cell membranes. What is known of the structure and properties of cell membranes that determines their permeability to drugs? In Figure 1.7, the two layers of circles represent the water-soluble head groups of complex lipid molecules called *phospholipids.* The phospholipid heads form a rather continuous layer on both the inside and the outside of the cell membrane. The wavy lines that extend from the heads into the membrane are the lipid chains of the phospholipid molecules. Therefore, for our present purposes, the interior of the cell membrane can be considered to consist of a sea of lipid in which large proteins are suspended.

Cell membranes, consisting of protein and fat, thus provide a physical barrier that is permeable to small, lipid-soluble drug molecules but is impermeable to large, lipid-insoluble drug molecules. Cell membranes (as barriers to the absorption and distribution of drugs) are

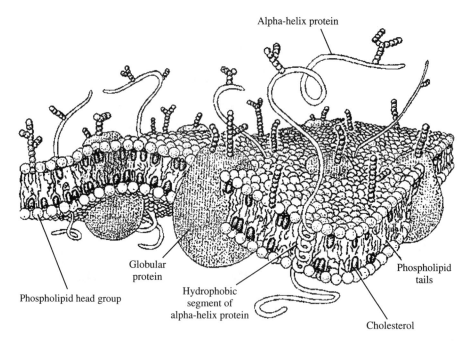

Alpha-helix protein

Globular
protein

Phospholipid
tails

Phospholipid head group

Hydrophobic
segment of
alpha-helix protein

Cholesterol

FIGURE 1.7 Diagrammatic representation of the cell membrane, a phospholipid bilayer in which cholesterol and protein molecules are embedded. Both globular and helical kinds of protein traverse the bilayer. Cholesterol molecules tend to keep the tails of the phospholipids relatively fixed and orderly in the regions closest to the hydrophilic phospholipid heads; the parts of the tails closer to the core of the membrane move about freely. [From M. S. Bretscher, "The Molecules of the Cell Membrane," *Scientific American* 253 (1985): 104.]

important for the passage of drugs (1) from the stomach and intestine into the bloodstream, (2) from the fluid that closely surrounds tissue cells into the interior of cells, (3) from the interior of cells back into the body water, and (4) from the kidneys back into the bloodstream.

Capillaries. Within a minute or so of entering the bloodstream, a drug is distributed fairly evenly throughout the entire blood volume. From there, drugs leave the bloodstream and are exchanged (in equilibrium) between blood capillaries and body tissues. Figure 1.8 is a cross-sectional diagram of a capillary. Capillaries are tiny, cylindrical blood vessels with walls that are formed by a thin, single layer of cells packed tightly together. Between the cells are small pores that allow passage of small molecules between blood and the body tissues. The diameter of these pores is between 90 and 150 angstroms, which is larger than most drug molecules. Thus, most drugs freely leave the blood through these pores in the capillary membranes, passing along their concentration gradient until equilibrium is established between the concentrations of drug in the blood and in body tissues and water.

The transport of drug molecules between plasma and body tissues is independent of lipid solubility, because the membrane pores are large enough for even fat-insoluble drug molecules to penetrate. However, the pores in the capillary membrane are not large enough to permit the red blood cells and the plasma proteins to leave the bloodstream. Thus,

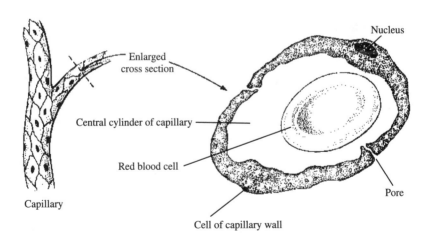

FIGURE 1.8 Cross section of a blood capillary. Within the capillary are the fluids, proteins, and cells of the blood, including the red blood cells. The capillary itself is made up of cells that completely surround and define the central cylinder (or lumen) of the capillary. Water-filled pores form channels, allowing free flow of blood plasma and extracellular fluid.

the only drugs that do not readily penetrate capillary pores are drugs that bind to plasma proteins.

The rate at which drug molecules enter specific body tissues depends on two factors: the rate of blood flow through the tissue and the ease with which drug molecules pass through the capillary membranes. Because blood flow is greatest to the brain and much less to the bones, joints, and fat deposits, drug distribution generally follows a similar pattern (Figure 1.9). However, some capillaries (such as those in the brain) have special structural properties that can further limit the diffusion of a drug into the brain.

Blood-Brain Barrier. The brain requires a protected environment in which to function normally, and a specialized structural barrier, called the blood-brain barrier, plays a key role in maintaining this environment. The *blood-brain barrier* involves specialized cells in the brain that affect nearly all its blood capillaries (Figure 1.10). In most of the rest of the body, the capillary membranes have pores; in the brain, however, the capillaries are tightly joined together and covered on the outside by a fatty barrier called the *glial sheath*, which arises from nearby astrocyte cells.

Thus, a drug leaving the capillaries in the brain has to traverse both the wall of the capillary itself (because there are no pores to pass through) and the membranes of the astrocyte cells in order to reach the cells in the brain. Therefore, as a general rule, the rate of passage of a drug into the brain is determined by the lipid (fat) solu-

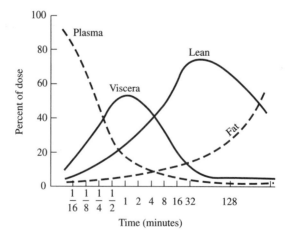

FIGURE 1.9 Diagrammatic representation of the distribution of a lipid-soluble drug (thiopental, a barbiturate discussed in Chapter 5) in blood plasma, body fat, lean body mass (muscle), and visceral tissues at various times after intravenous injection of the drug. Time scales (in minutes) progress geometrically.

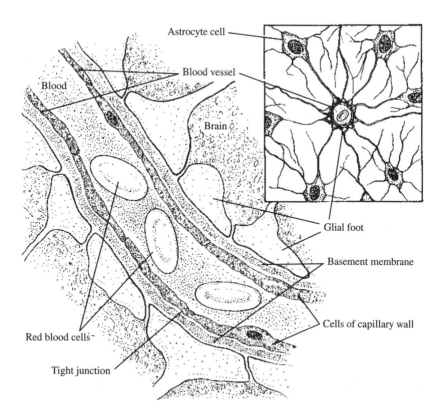

FIGURE 1.10 Blood-brain barrier. Blood and brain are separated by capillary cells packed tightly together and by a fatty barrier called the glial sheath, which is made up of extensions (glial feet) from nearby astrocyte cells (*inset*). A drug diffusing from blood to brain must move through the cells of the capillary wall because there are tight junctions rather than pores between the cells; the drug must then move through the fatty glial sheath.

bility of the particular drug. Highly ionized drugs (penicillin, for example) penetrate poorly, while fat-soluble drugs penetrate rapidly. Psychoactive drugs (those discussed in this book) are sufficiently lipid soluble to cross the blood-brain barrier, exerting their actions on neurons located within the brain. Drugs that cannot cross the blood-brain barrier are restricted in action to structures located outside the CNS. CNS actions are usually not of major significance. Penicillin is an example of such a drug. It does not cross the blood-brain barrier and is not of use in treating infections located in the CNS: its effectiveness as an antibiotic is restricted to infections located outside the brain.

Placental Barrier.   Among all the membrane systems of the body, the placenta membranes are unique, separating two distinct human beings with differing genetic compositions, and sensitivities to drugs. The fetus obtains essential nutrients and eliminates metabolic waste products through the placenta without depending on its own organs, many of which are not yet functioning. The dependence of the fetus on the mother places the fetus at the mercy of the placenta when foreign substances (such as drugs or toxins) appear in the mother's blood.[4] This is discussed further in the section "Role of the Liver in Drug Metabolism."

A schematic representation of the placental network, which transfers substances between the mother and the fetus, is shown in Figure 1.11. In general, the mature placenta consists of a network of vessels and pools of maternal blood into which protrude tree-like or finger-like villi (projections) that contain the blood capillaries of the fetus. Oxygen and nutrients travel from the mother's blood to that of the fetus, while carbon dioxide and other waste products travel from the blood of the fetus to the mother's blood.

The membranes that separate fetal blood from maternal blood in the intervillous space resemble, in their general permeability, the cell membranes that are found elsewhere in the body. In other words, drugs cross the placenta primarily by passive diffusion. Fat-soluble

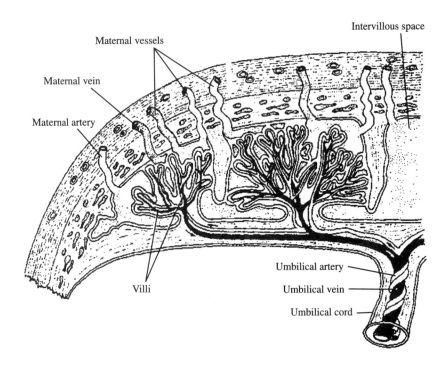

FIGURE 1.11 Placental network separating the blood of mother and fetus. Note the close relationship between fetal and maternal blood in the villus.

substances (including all psychoactive drugs) diffuse readily, rapidly, and without limitation:

> The view that the placenta is a barrier to drugs is inaccurate. A more appropriate approximation is that the fetus is to at least some extent exposed to essentially all drugs taken by the mother.[5]

As a general rule, any psychoactive drug will be present in the fetus at a concentration quite similar to that in the mother's bloodstream. This is not meant to imply that the presence of the drug in the fetus is necessarily detrimental to the fetus. Certainly some psychoactive drugs adversely affect the developing fetus, but most do not appear to be detrimental. Examples of drugs that can adversely affect a fetus include ethyl alcohol (Chapter 4) and several antiepileptic–mood-stabilizing drugs (Chapter 16). Garland[6] discusses in detail the transfer of drugs across the placenta.

Termination of Drug Action

Routes through which drugs can leave the body include (1) the kidneys, (2) the lungs, (3) the bile, and (4) the skin. Excretion through the lungs occurs only with highly volatile or gaseous agents, such as the general anesthetics and, in small amounts, alcohol ("alcohol breath"). Drugs that are passed through the bile and into the intestine are usually reabsorbed into the bloodstream from the intestine. Also, small amounts of a few drugs can pass through the skin and are excreted in sweat (perhaps 10 to 15 percent of the total amount of the drugs). However, most drugs leave the body in urine. More correctly, *the major route of drug elimination from the body is renal excretion of drug metabolites following the hepatic (liver) biodegradation of the drug into drug metabolites.*[*] These metabolites are more water-soluble, bulkier, less lipid-soluble, and (usually) less biologically active (even inactive) when compared with the parent molecule (the molecule that was originally ingested and absorbed).[†] Thus, in order for a

---

[*] This implies that, when evaluating urine for the presence of drugs of abuse, what is found in urine is inactive drug metabolites, rather than active drug. It is often unclear whether there is correlation between the presence of the metabolite in urine and active drug in plasma *at the time the urine sample was taken.*

[†] Some drugs are exceptions: administered drug may be metabolized into an "active" metabolite, which is at least as active and possibly more active, and may have a longer duration of action than the parent drug. Examples in psychopharmacology include diazepam (Valium; Chapter 6), which is metabolized to nordiazepam, and fluoxetine (Prozac; Chapter 15), which is metabolized to norfluoxetine. In both cases, the parent drug has an effect that lasts for two or three days, while the metabolite is active for over a week, until it is eventually biotransformed to an inactive compound that can be excreted.

lipid-soluble drug to be eliminated, it must be metabolically transformed (by enzymes located in the liver) into a form that can be excreted rapidly and reliably. Such biotransformation relieves the body of the burden of foreign chemicals and is essential to our survival. Such mechanisms are not new. Biotransformation of foreign substances probably originated millions of years ago when humans invented fire and began to eat the char of barbecued meat, ingesting and absorbing substances that were foreign and potentially toxic to the body.

Role of the Kidneys in Drug Elimination

Physiologically, our kidneys perform two major functions. First, they excrete most of the products of body metabolism; second, they closely regulate the levels of most of the substances found in body fluids. The kidneys are a pair of bean-shaped organs that lie at the rear of the abdominal cavity at the level of the lower ribs. The outer portion of the kidney is made up of more than a million functional units, called *nephrons* (Figure 1.12). Each nephron consists of a knot of capillaries (the *glomerulus*) through which blood flows from the renal artery to the renal vein. The glomerulus is surrounded by the opening of the nephron (*Bowman's capsule*), into which fluid flows as it filters out of the capillaries. Pressure of the blood in the glomerulus causes fluid to leave the capillaries and flow into the Bowman's capsule, from which it flows through the tubules of the nephrons and then into a duct that collects fluid from several nephrons. This fluid from the collecting ducts is eventually passed through the ureters and into the urinary bladder, which is emptied periodically.

In an adult, about 1 liter (1000 cubic centimeters) of plasma is filtered into the nephrons of the kidneys each minute. Left behind in the bloodstream are blood cells, plasma proteins, and the remaining plasma. As the filtered fluid (water) flows through the nephrons, most of it is reabsorbed into the plasma. By the time fluid reaches the collecting ducts and bladder, only 0.1 percent remains to be excreted. Because about 1 cubic centimeter per minute of urine is formed, 99.9 percent of filtered fluid is therefore reabsorbed.

Lipid-soluble drugs can easily cross the membranes of renal tubular cells, and they are reabsorbed along with the 99.9 percent of reabsorbed water. Drug reabsorption occurs passively, along a developing concentration gradient—the drug becomes concentrated inside the nephrons (as a result of water reabsorption), and the drugs are themselves reabsorbed with water back into plasma. Thus, the kidneys alone are not capable of eliminating psychoactive drugs from the body, and some other mechanism must overcome this process of passive renal reabsorption of the drug.

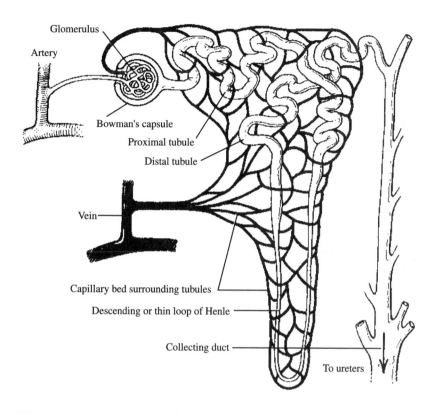

Glomerulus

Artery

Bowman's capsule

Proximal tubule

Distal tubule

Vein

Capillary bed surrounding tubules

Descending or thin loop of Henle

Collecting duct

To ureters

FIGURE 1.12 Nephron within a kidney. Note the complexity of the structure and the intimate relation between the blood supply and the nephron. Each kidney is composed of more than a million such nephrons.

Role of the Liver in Drug Metabolism

Since the kidneys are not capable of ridding the body of drugs, the reabsorbed drug is eventually picked up by liver cells (*hepatocytes*) and is enzymatically biotransformed (by enzymes located in these hepatocytes) into metabolites that are usually less fat soluble, less capable of being reabsorbed, and therefore capable of being excreted in urine. As the drug is carried to the liver (by blood flowing in the hepatic artery and portal vein), a portion is cleared from blood by the hepatocytes and metabolized to by-products that are then returned to the bloodstream (Figure 1.13). The metabolites are then carried in the bloodstream to the kidneys, filtered into the renal tubules, and are poorly reabsorbed, remaining in the urine for excretion. Mechanisms involved in drug metabolism by hepatocytes are complex, but they have gained increased importance in psychopharmacology because of recently described drug interactions involving certain antidepressant drugs (Chapter 15).[7]

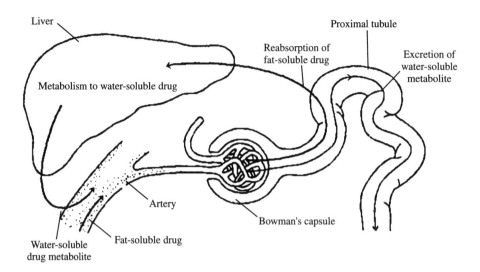

FIGURE 1.13 How the liver and kidneys interact to eliminate drugs from the body. Drugs may be filtered into the kidney, reabsorbed into the bloodstream, and carried to the liver for metabolic transformation to a more water-soluble compound that, having been filtered into the kidney, cannot be reabsorbed and is therefore excreted in urine.

The *cytochrome P450 enzyme family*, physically located in hepato-cytes (with a few located in the cells lining the GI tract), is the major system involved in drug metabolism. Originating more than 3.5 billion years ago, this gene family of enzymes has diversified to accomplish the metabolism (detoxification) of environmental chemicals, food toxins, and drugs—all foreign to our needs. Thus, the cytochrome P450 enzyme system (of which at least 12 different families exist in humans) can detoxify a chemically diverse group of foreign substances. Several of these families of P450 enzymes can be found within any given hepatocyte.

Of these 12 or more cytochrome P450 families, cytochrome families 1, 2, and 3 (designated as *CYP1, CYP2,* and *CYP3)* encode enzymes involved in most drug biotransformations. By definition, since these three families promote the breakdown of numerous drugs and toxins, enzyme specificity is low (i.e., they are nonspecific in action). Thus, the body is enzyme capable of metabolizing multiple different drugs.

CYP-3A4 (a subfamily of *CYP3*) catalyzes about 50 percent of drug biotransformations; and this variant is found not only in liver but in the GI tract. This is important, since drugs metabolized by CYP-3A4 in the GI tract may have limited absorption and reduced bioavailability. CYP-2D6 catalyzes about 25 percent of drugs, and CYP-2C catalyzes an additional 20 percent. CYP-1A2, CYP-2E1, and CYP-3A3/4 each catalyze about 5 percent of drug biotransformations.

Factors Affecting Drug Biotransformation

Several different factors can alter the rate at which drugs are metabolized, either increasing or decreasing the rate of drug elimination from the body. In general, *genetic, environmental,* and various *physiological factors* can be involved.

Increasing the activity of these CYP enzymes increases the rate at which the drugs are metabolized and eliminated. Thus, drug tolerance develops, and increasing doses of a drug must be administered to both maintain the same level of drug in the plasma and produce the same effect as previously administered smaller doses. *Carbamazepine* (Tegretol; Chapter 16) is particularly effective in stimulating the production of the drug-metabolizing enzyme CYP-3A3/4 within hepatocytes, inducing tolerance to both itself and other drugs metabolized by CYP-3A3/4. Carbamazepine markedly reduces the blood levels and subsequent therapeutic efficacy of many of the SSRI-type antidepressants discussed in Chapter 15. These include fluoxetine (Prozac), nefazodone (Serzone), and fluvoxamine (Luvox). The phenomenon of the association of tolerance to one drug with apparent tolerance to another is termed *cross-tolerance.*

Conversely, some psychoactive drugs inhibit the activity of the enzyme that metabolizes them and other drugs and increase the toxicity of all drugs metabolized by the same enzyme.[7-11] For example, certain antidepressants (again, the SSRI type; Chapter 15) inhibit enzymes CYP-1A2 and CYP-2C, increasing the toxicity of several other types of antidepressants, certain antiasthma drugs, certain antipsychotic drugs (Figure 1.14), and many heart medications. Such drug interactions are often severe and have been fatal. As Figure 1.6 illustrated, grapefruit juice is problematic since it can inhibit CYP-1A2 and CYP-3A4, raising blood levels of antidepressants and certain heart medications to toxic levels.[3,12-14] The substance in grapefruit juice responsible for inhibiting these drug-metabolizing enzymes has not been identified.[15]

Psychoactive drugs taken by a pregnant woman are easily distributed to the fetus through the placenta. Before delivery, psychoactive drugs are excreted through the umbilical cord back into the mother's bloodstream. The mother can then eliminate the drug through her liver and kidneys. After delivery, however, the newborn baby must get rid of the drug by itself. Unfortunately, the newborn (especially the premature infant) has few drug-metabolizing enzymes in its liver, and its kidneys may not yet be fully functional. Therefore, the infant has difficulty metabolizing and excreting drugs. If it has received a high concentration of depressants (anesthetics, narcotics, and so on) from the mother close to the time of delivery, the infant may be depressed for a prolonged period of time, occasionally necessitating medical intervention.

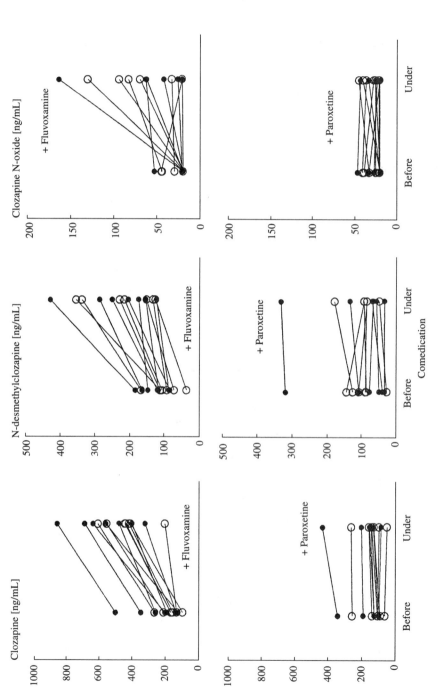

FIGURE 1.14 Blood level (in nanograms per milliliter plasma) of clozapine (Clozaril, an antipsychotic drug discussed in Chapter 17) and two of its metabolites (N-desmethylclozapine and N-oxide) before and one week after the start of coadministration of either fluvoxamine (Luvox) or paroxetine (Paxil) in patients with schizophrenia. Both fluvoxamine and paroxetine are newer SSRI-type antidepressants (Chapter 15). Note that fluvoxamine but not paroxetine increased clozapine blood levels, since paroxetine does not inhibit CYP enzymes to any significant degree.[11]

Other Routes of Drug Elimination

Other routes for excreting drugs include the air we exhale, bile, sweat, saliva, and breast milk. Many drugs and drug metabolites may be found in these secretions, but their concentrations are usually low, and these routes are not usually considered primary paths of drug elimination. Perhaps clinically significant, however, is the transfer of psychoactive drugs (such as nicotine) from mothers to their breast-fed babies.*

Time Course of Drug Distribution and Elimination: Concept of Drug Half-Life

Knowledge about the relationship between the time course of drug action in the body is essential for (1) predicting the optimal dosages and dose intervals needed to reach a therapeutic effect, (2) maintaining a therapeutic drug level for the desired period of time, and (3) determining the time needed to eliminate the drug. The relationship between the pharmacological response to a drug and its concentration in blood is fundamental to pharmacology. With psychoactive drugs, the level of drug in blood closely approximates the level of drug at the drug's site of action in the brain.

Figure 1.15 illustrates this time-concentration relationship. Note that after intravenous injection, the drug concentration in plasma peaked immediately, fell rapidly, and then declined more slowly. The rapid fall reflects the distribution of the drug out of the bloodstream (into which it was injected) into body tissues. This process of *redistribution* takes only minutes to spread a drug nearly equally throughout the major tissues of the body. The steeply sloped line in Figure 1.15 (tangent line A) represents this rapid-distribution phase, which is represented by a distribution half-life that indicates the time it takes for redistribution to reduce the initial peak level of the drug by 50 percent (here only 7.9 minutes).

The slower, prolonged decrease in the level of drug in the blood (tangent line B) represents the time required for the body to detoxify the drug by hepatic metabolism. The calculated elimination half-life is a measure of this process, and it allows the time course of drug action to be calculated.

Figure 1.15 shows that the peak levels of pain relief produced by the drug fentanyl (a narcotic analgesic) are reached within seconds after intravenous injection. Fentanyl is highly lipid soluble and is

---

*Moretti and co-workers[16] in 1999 reported that infants of breast-feeding mothers who were taking fluoxetine (Prozac) exhibited no significant differences in adverse neonatal effects or weight gain when they were compared with infants breast-fed by mothers who did not take fluoxetine.

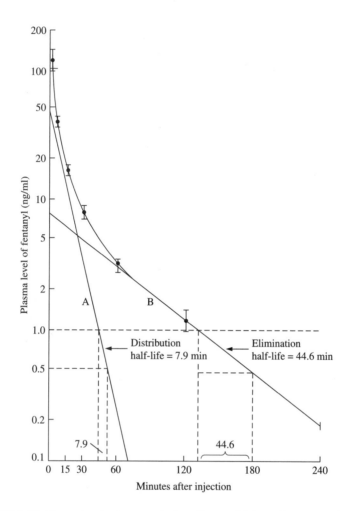

FIGURE 1.15 Plasma levels of a narcotic drug (fentanyl) injected intravenously into a rat. The elimination half-life is shown as 44.6 minutes. The horizontal line drawn at 1 nanogram per milliliter plasma concentration is the level needed for analgesic effect. Thus, analgesia would be lost about 130 minutes after drug injection. [Data from C. C. Hug, Jr., and M. R. Murphy, "Tissue Redistribution of Fentanyl and Termination of Its Effects in Rats," *Anesthesiology* 55 (1981): 369–375.]

rapidly redistributed to muscle and fat, reducing blood concentrations of the drug in the process. The elimination half-life is about 45 minutes.

As shown in Table 1.2, it takes four half-lives for 94 percent of a drug to be eliminated by the body and six half-lives for 98 percent of the drug to be eliminated. At that point, a person is, for most practical purposes, drug-free. It is important to remember that even though the blood level is reduced by 75 percent after two half-lives, the drug persists in the body at low levels for at least six half-lives. The so-called "drug hangover" is a result.

TABLE 1.2 Half-life calculations

	Amount of drug in the body	
Number of half-lives	Percent eliminated	Percent remaining
0	0	100
1	50	50
2	75	25
3	87.5	12.5
4	93.8	6.2
5	96.9	3.1
6	98.4	1.6

Throughout this book, drug half-lives are cited to describe the duration of action of psychoactive drugs in the body and allow comparisons between drugs with similar actions but differing half-lives. Most drug half-lives are measured in hours; others are measured in days, and recovery from the drug may take a week or more. For example, the elimination half-life of diazepam (Valium; Chapter 6) is more than two days in a healthy young adult (Figure 1.16). The half-life of its active

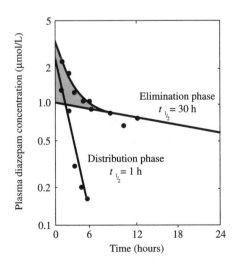

FIGURE 1.16 Plasma levels of diazepam (Valium, a benzodiazepine) following a single intravenous dose. The fast (distribution) phase has a half-life of about 1 hour. The slower, metabolic elimination phase shows a half-life of 30 hours. The long half-life of the active diazepam metabolite, nordiazepam, is not shown.

metabolite (nordiazepam, not illustrated in Figure 1.16) is even longer. The elderly exhibit even more prolongation of the half-lives of both diazepam and nordiazepam, implying a duration of action of one to two months.

Note that drug half-life is the *time* for the plasma level of drug to fall by 50 percent. Thus, half-life is independent of the absolute level of drug in blood: the level falls by 50 percent every half-life, regardless of how many molecules of drug were actually metabolized during that time. Therefore, a varying amount of drug is metabolized with each half-life (fewer actual molecules are metabolized per half-life as the plasma level of drug falls).

One of the rare exceptions to this concept is the metabolism of ethyl alcohol by the enzyme alcohol dehydrogenase. Here, a constant amount of alcohol is metabolized per hour, regardless of the absolute amount of alcohol present in blood,* and the blood level falls in a straight-line manner. (The metabolism of alcohol is discussed in Chapter 4.)

Drug Half-Life, Accumulation, and Steady State

The biological half-life of a drug is not only the time required for the drug concentration in blood to fall by one-half, but it is also the determinant of the length of time necessary to reach a steady state concentration (Figure 1.17). If a second full dose of drug is adminstered before the body has eliminated the first dose, the total amount of drug in the body and the peak level of the drug in the blood will be greater than the total amount and peak level produced by the first dose. For example, if 100 milligrams (mg) of a drug with a four-hour half-life were administered at 12 noon, 50 mg of drug would remain in the body at 4 P.M. If an additional 100 mg of the drug were then taken at 4 P.M., 75 mg of drug would remain in the body at 8 P.M. (25 mg of the first dose and 50 mg of the second). If this administration schedule were continued, the amount of drug in the body would continue to increase until a plateau (steady state) concentration was reached (Figure 1.17).

In general, the time to reach *steady-state concentration* (the level of drug achieved in blood with repeated, regular-interval dosing) is about six times the drug's elimination half-life and is independent of the actual dosage of the drug. The reason for this is as follows. In one half-life, a drug reaches 50 percent of the concentration that will eventually

---

*Usually, about 10 cc of absolute alcohol is metabolized per hour, regardless of blood level. The significance of this rate is discussed in Chapter 4.

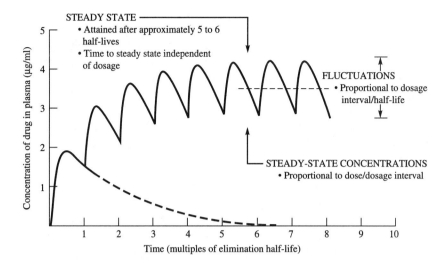

FIGURE 1.17 Plasma drug concentrations during repeated oral administration of a drug at intervals equal to its elimination half-life. The dashed line illustrates the elimination curve if only a single dose is given. Because only 50 percent of each dose is eliminated before the next dose is given, the drug accumulates, reaching steady-state concentration in five to six half-lives. The sinusoidal curve shows the maximal and minimal drug concentrations at the beginning and end of each dosage interval, respectively. The dotted line illustrates the average concentration achieved at steady state.

be achieved. After two half-lives, the drug achieves 75 percent concentration; at three half-lives, the drug achieves the initial 50 percent of the third dose, the next 25 percent from the second dose, plus half of the remaining 25 percent from the first dose. At 98.4 percent (the concentration achieved after six half-lives), the drug concentration is essentially at steady state. This is the rationale behind our general rule. The steady-state concentration is achieved when the amount administered per unit time equals the amount eliminated per unit time. The interdependent variables that determine the ultimate concentration (or steady-state blood level of drug) are the dose (which determines the blood level but not the time to steady state), the dose interval, the half-life of the drug, and other, more complex factors that can affect drug elimination.

In summary, steady, regular-interval dosing leads to a predictable accumulation, with a steady-state concentration reached after about six half-lives; the magnitude of the concentration is proportional to dose and dosage interval. Clinically, these factors guide drug therapy when blood levels of the drug are monitored and correlated with therapeutic results.

Therapeutic Drug Monitoring

Therapeutic drug monitoring (TDM) can aid a clinician in making critical decisions in therapeutic applications. Indeed, in psychopharmacology, TDM can dramatically improve the prognosis of psychological disorders, making previously difficult-to-treat disorders much more treatable.[17]

The basic principle underlying TDM is that a threshold plasma concentration of a drug is needed at the receptor site to initiate and maintain a pharmacological response. Critically important is that plasma concentrations of psychoactive drugs correlate well with tissue or receptor concentrations. Therefore, TDM is an indirect, although usually quite accurate, measurement of drug concentration at the receptor site. To make the correlation between TDM, dosage, and therapeutic response, large-scale clinical trials are performed, and blood samples are drawn at multiple time periods during both acute (short-term) and chronic (long-term) therapy. Statistical correlation is made between the level of drug in plasma and the degree of therapeutic response. A dosage regimen can then be designed to achieve the appropriate blood level of a drug.

The goals of TDM are many. One goal is to assess whether a patient is taking medication as prescribed; if plasma levels of the drug are below the therapeutic level because the patient has not been taking the required medication, therapeutic results will be poor. Another goal is to avoid toxicity; if plasma levels of the drug are above the therapeutic level, the dosage can be lowered, effectiveness maintained, and toxicity minimized. A third goal is to enhance therapeutic response by focusing not on the amount of drug taken but on the measured amount of drug in the plasma. Other goals include possible reductions in the cost of therapy (since a patient's illness is better controlled) and the substantiation of the need for unusually high doses in patients who require higher-than-normal intake of prescribed medication to maintain a therapeutic blood level of a drug.

Drug Tolerance and Dependence

Drug tolerance is defined as a state of progressively decreasing responsiveness to a drug. A person who develops tolerance requires a larger dose of the drug to achieve the effect originally obtained by a smaller dose. At least three mechanisms are involved in the development of drug tolerance—two are pharmacological mechanisms, and one is a behavioral mechanism.

Metabolic tolerance is the first of the two classically described types of pharmacological tolerance. As discussed earlier, the presence of a drug in blood perfusing the liver can induce the synthesis of hepatic cytochrome P450 drug-metabolizing enzymes. Thus, the drug is metabolized at a faster rate, and more drug must be administered to maintain the same level of drug in the body.

Cellular-adaptive or *pharmacodynamic tolerance* is the second type of pharmacological tolerance. Receptors in the brain adapt to the continued presence of the drug, with neurons adapting to excess drug either by reducing the number of receptors available to the drug or by reducing their sensitivity to the drug. Such reduction in numbers or sensitivity is termed *down regulation*, and higher levels of drug are necessary to maintain the same biological effect.

Behavioral conditioning processes are the third type of drug tolerance. The exposure of drugs to receptors does not account for the substantial degree of tolerance that many people acquire to opioids, barbiturates, ethyl alcohol, and other drugs. Instead, tolerance can be demonstrated when a drug is administered in the context of usual predrug cues but not in the context of alternative cues.[18] Poulos and Cappell[19] propose a *homeostatic theory* of drug tolerance. They found that, with morphine analgesia, testing in an environment in which tolerance had developed effected the manifestation of tolerance, and an environmental cue could maintain the tolerance. This *contingent tolerance* is pervasive and represents a general process underlying the development of all forms of systemic tolerance.

The environmental cues routinely paired with drug administration will become conditioned stimuli that elicit a conditioned response that is opposite in direction to, or compensation for, the direct effects of the drug. Over conditioning trials, the compensatory conditioned response grows in magnitude and counteracts the direct drug effects; that is, tolerance develops.

Physical dependence is an entirely different phenomenon from tolerance, even though the two are often associated temporally. A person who is physically dependent needs the drug to avoid withdrawal symptoms if the drug is not taken. The state is revealed by withdrawing the drug and noting the occurrence of physical and/or psychological changes (withdrawal symptoms). These changes are referred to as an *abstinence syndrome*. The symptoms of withdrawal can be relieved by readministering the drug.

Because physical dependence is often manifested following cessation of use of drugs of abuse such as alcohol and heroin, the term has been linked with "addiction," implying that withdrawal signs are "bad" and observed only with drugs of abuse. This is certainly far from the truth: rather severe withdrawal signs can follow cessation of such therapeutic drugs as the SSRI type of clinical antidepressants[*] (Chapter 15).[20-21] Therefore, the occurrence of withdrawal signs after drug removal is not a sign of drug "addiction" with "bad" drugs such as heroin. Rather, physical dependence is an indication that brain and body functions were altered by the presence of a drug and that a different homeostatic state must be initiated at drug withdrawal. It takes time (from a few days to about two weeks) for the brain and the body to adapt to this new state of equilibrium where drug is absent.

STUDY QUESTIONS

1. What is meant by the term *pharmacokinetics*? What does the term imply?

2. Why must a psychoactive drug be altered metabolically in the body before it can be excreted?

3. Discuss the advantages and disadvantages of the various methods of administering drugs.

4. List the various membrane barriers that may affect drug distribution.

5. Discuss the placental barrier as it affects the distribution of psychoactive drugs. What are the cautions for the use of psychotropic medication during pregnancy?

6. If a drug has an elimination half-life of 6 hours, how long does it take for the drug to be effectively eliminated from the body after administration of a single dose?

7. What is drug tolerance and why does it occur? Discuss three mechanisms underlying the development of tolerance.

8. What are the various routes through the body whereby a drug can be eliminated?

9. Define *half-life*. How does *half-life* apply to steady state?

10. What is meant by the term therapeutic drug monitoring? In what instances might it be of value?

---

[*]Removal of SSRI-type antidepressants is followed in many individuals by withdrawal signs that can be organized into five core somatic symptoms: (1) disequilibrium (dizziness, vertigo, ataxia), (2) GI symptoms (nausea, vomiting), (3) flu-like symptoms (fatigue, lethargy, myalgias, chills), (4) sensory disturbances (paresthesias, sensation of electric shocks), and (5) sleep disturbances (insomnia, vivid dreams).

REFERENCES

1. L. Z. Benet, "Introduction," in J. G. Hardman, L. E. Limbird, P. B. Molinoff, R. W. Ruddon, and A. G. Gilman, eds., *Goodman and Gilman's The Pharmacological Basis of Therapeutics*, 9th ed. (New York: McGraw-Hill, 1996), 1.
2. J. R. Varvel, S. I. Shafer, S. S. Hwang, et al., "Absorption Characteristics of Transdermally Administered Fentanyl," *Anesthesiology* 70 (1989), 928–934.
3. J. J. Lilja, K. T. Kivisto, et al., "Grapefruit Juice Substantially Increases Plasma Concentrations of Buspirone," *Clinical Pharmacology and Therapeutics* 64 (1998): 655–660.
4. L. C. Gilstrap and B. B. Little, *Drugs and Pregnancy*, 2nd ed. (New York: Chapman & Hall, 1998).
5. L. Z. Benet, D. L. Kroetz, and L. B. Sheiner, "Pharmacokinetics: The Dynamics of Drug Absorption, Distribution and Elimination," in J. G. Hardman, L. E. Limbird, P. B. Molinoff, R. W. Ruddon, and A. G. Gilman, eds., *Goodman and Gilman's The Pharmacological Basis of Therapeutics*, 9th ed. (New York: McGraw-Hill, 1996), 11.
6. M. Garland, "Pharmacology of Drug Transfer Across the Placenta," *Obstetrics and Gynecology Clinics of North America* 25 (1998): 21–42.
7. D. J. Greenblatt, L. L. von Moltke, J. S. Harmatz, and R. I. Shader, "Human Cytochromes and Some Newer Antidepressants: Kinetics, Metabolism, and Drug Interactions," *Journal of Clinical Psychopharmacology* 19, Suppl. 1 (1999): 23S–35S.
8. A. T. Harvey and S. H. Prescorn, "Cytochrome P450 Enzymes: Interpretation of Their Interactions with Selective Serotonin Reuptake Inhibitors. Part II." *Journal of Clinical Psychopharmacology* 16 (1996): 345–355.
9. A. Kashuba et al., "Effect of Fluvoxamine Therapy on the Activities of CYP-1A2, CYP-2D6, and CYP-3A as Determined by Phenotyping," *Clinical Pharmacology and Therapeutics* 64 (1998): 257–268.
10. V. Ozdemir et al., "The Extent and Determinants of Changes in CYP-2D6 and CYP-1A2 Activities with Therapeutic Doses of Sertraline," *Journal of Clinical Psychopharmacology* 18 (1998): 55–61.
11. H. Wetzel et al., "Pharmacokinetic Interactions of Clozapine with Selective Serotonin Reuptake Inhibitors: Differential Effects of Fluvoxamine and Paroxetine in a Prospective Study," *Journal of Clinical Psychopharmacology* 18 (1998): 2–9.
12. J. D. Spence, "Drug Interactions with Grapefruit: Whose Responsibility Is It to Warn the Public?" *Clinical Pharmacology and Therapeutics* 61 (1997): 395–400.
13. U. Fuhr, "Drug Interactions with Grapefruit Juice," *Drug Safety* 18 (1998): 251–272.
14. S. K. Garg et al., "Effect of Grapefruit Juice on Carbamazepine Bioavailability in Patients with Epilepsy," *Clinical Pharmacology and Therapeutics* 64 (1998): 286–288.
15. D. J. Edward et al., "6′,7′-Dihydroxybergamottin in Grapefruit Juice and Seville Orange Juice: Effects on Cyclosporin Disposition, Enterocyte CYP3A4, and P-Glycoprotein," *Clinical Pharmacology and Therapeutics* 65 (1999): 237–244.

16. M. E. Moretti et al., "Fluoxetine and Its Effects on the Nursing Infant: A Prospective Cohort Study," *Clinical Pharmacology and Therapeutics* 65 (1999): 141.

17. S. H. Preskorn, M. J. Burke, and G. A. Fast, "Therapeutic Drug Monitoring: Principles and Practice," *Psychiatric Clinics of North America* 16 (1993): 611–641.

18. S. Siegel, "Drug Anticipation and the Treatment of Dependence," in B. A. Ray, ed., *Learning Factors in Substance Abuse*, NIDA Research Monograph 84 (1988): 1–24.

19. C. X. Poulos and H. Cappell, "Homeostatic Theory of Drug Tolerance: A General Model of Physiological Adaptation," *Psychological Reviews* 98 (1991): 390–408.

20. J. Zajecka, K. A. Tracy, and S. Mitchell, "Discontinuation Symptoms After Treatment with Serotonin Reuptake Inhibitors: A Literature Review," *Journal of Clinical Psychiatry* 58 (1997), 291–297.

21. A. F. Schatzberg, ed., "Antidepressant Discontinuation Syndrome: Update on Serotonin Reuptake Inhibitors," *Journal of Clinical Psychiatry* 58, Suppl. 7 (1997).

Pharmacodynamics: How Drugs Act

While the body is trying to rid itself of an ingested psychoactive drug, the drug is exerting effects by attaching to receptors in cells in both the brain and the body. As a result of the interactions, the body experiences effects that are characteristic for the drug. *It is a basic principle of pharmacology that the pharmacological, physiological, or behavioral effects induced by a drug follow from their interaction with receptors.* The study of the interactions is termed *pharmacodynamics* and involves exploring the mechanisms of drug action that occur at the molecular level. It provides the basis for both the rational therapeutic use of a drug and the design of new and superior therapeutic agents.[1]

To produce an effect, a drug must bind to and interact with specialized receptors, usually located on cell membranes. In the case of psychoactive drugs, these receptors are usually located on the surface of neurons within the brain. The occupation of a receptor by a drug (*drug-receptor binding*) leads to a change in the functional properties of that neuron, resulting in the drug's characteristic pharmacological response.

In most instances, drug-receptor binding is both *ionic* and *reversible* in nature,[*] with positive and negative charges on various portions of the

---

[*] Reversible ionic binding is contrasted with the formation of a permanent, irreversible, covalent bond between a drug and a receptor. One of the rare instances in psychopharmacology where an irreversible covalent bond forms is between certain antidepressant drugs and the enzyme monoamine oxidase (Chapter 15).

drug molecule and the receptor protein attracting one to the other. The strength of ionic attachment is determined by the fit of the three-dimensional structure of the drug to the three-dimensional site on the receptor.

Receptors for Drug Action

Since drugs exert their effects by forming reversible ionic bonds with specific receptors, exactly what are receptors? A *receptor* is a fairly large molecule (usually a protein[*]) that is present on the surface of or within a cell that furnishes the site or sites where biologically active, naturally occurring, endogenous compounds (called *ligands,* or *neurotransmitters*) induce their normal biological effects. While literally hundreds of different types of ligand receptors are known (each a unique protein molecule), the ability to recognize one specific neurotransmitter characterizes each one.[2] Thus, only one neurotransmitter might be specific enough to fit or bind to a specific receptor protein. For example, if only serotonin binds to a specific protein receptor, that protein is called a serotonin receptor. But although that receptor is specific for serotonin, serotonin (as a neurotransmitter) also binds to other, structurally different receptors. To date, more than 15 different serotonin receptor proteins have been identified.[†] In pharmacology, such diversity makes it possible to develop closely related drugs, each with slightly different degrees of affinity for the different serotonin receptors. For example, a specific drug might have affinity for a serotonin-1 receptor but not for any of the other serotonin receptors. Until recently it was not possible to develop such a drug. However, with the understanding that drug receptors are proteins, it became possible to isolate a specific receptor protein from the rest of the brain, purify it, determine its amino acid sequence, isolate the portion of DNA responsible for making the protein, and clone the protein receptor to produce sufficient quantities of receptor against which drugs could be screened for affinity and activity. This is the pharmacology of the new millennium!

---

[*] A protein is a complex chain of various amino acids. Proteins are essential to life, functioning, among other things, as metabolic enzymes and receptors.

[†] Each receptor protein that binds serotonin, for example, has a slightly different amino acid composition; despite this, their three-dimensional structures are similar enough that serotonin, for example, still fits a "slot" (like a lock-and-key arrangement) and ionically binds to the protein. Pharmacologists have named these different protein receptors serotonin-1, serotonin-2, serotonin-3, and so on; in earlier years, multiple receptors for a single neurotransmitter were given more exotic names (e.g., muscarinic and nicotinic for acetylcholine receptors, alpha and beta for adrenergic receptors, and mu, delta, and kappa for opioid receptors).

It is now known that a given drug may be more specific for a given set of receptors than is the endogenous neurotransmitter. Serotonin, for example, attaches to all of the more than 15 different serotonin receptors (it has to, because it is the endogenous neurotransmitter at each receptor). However, a given drug might attach to only one receptor. For example, fluoxetine (Prozac) binds to and blocks the presynaptic serotonin reuptake receptor. Fluoxetine is therefore called a *serotonin-specific reuptake inhibitor* (SSRI) and is used clinically as an antidepressant. As far as we know, fluoxetine does not bind to any of the 15 or more postsynaptic serotonin receptors.

Another drug, buspirone (BuSpar) has no affinity for the presynaptic serotonin transporter; it attaches with great specificity to postsynaptic serotonin 1_A receptors, which results in an antianxiety action. This specificity implies that buspirone might not have the side effects of fluoxetine that follow from increased activity of serotonin at all postsynaptic receptors (Chapter 15).

Figures 2.1 through 2.4 demonstrate six important points about drug-receptor interactions:

1. A receptor is usually a membrane-spanning protein (Figure 2.1) that has binding sites for an endogenous neurotransmitter and appropriate drug molecules.

2. This membrane-spanning protein is not a simple globule (as suggested by Figure 2.1) but a continuous series of either 7 or 12

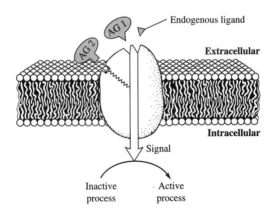

FIGURE 2.1 Diagrammatic representation of the classical concept of a receptor. One type of agonist (AG 1) fits the receptor site for an endogenous ligand and mimics the action of the ligand. Another type of agonist (AG 2) binds to an adjacent receptor site, thereby influencing (amplifying) signal transmission. Signal transmission activates intracellular processes that are inactive without receptor activation.

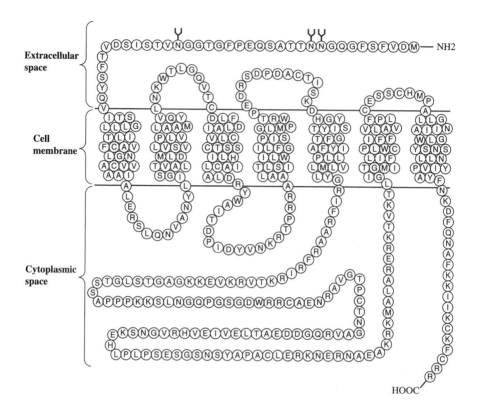

FIGURE 2.2 Schematic representation of the primary structure of the serotonin 1$_A$ postsynaptic receptor. Each circle represents an individual amino acid; the letter is the initial of the name of the amino acid. This receptor is one member of a large "family" of postsynaptic neurotransmitter receptors containing 7-transmembrane alpha-helical coils.

alpha-helical coils (loops of amino acids) embedded in the membrane (Figure 2.2).

3. The endogenous neurotransmitter (and presumably drugs also) attaches inside the space between these coils (Figure 2.3) and is held in place by ionic attractions.

4. This reversible ionic binding of the neurotransmitter specific for that receptor may activate the receptor, usually by changing the structure of the protein (Figure 2.4). This change allows a "signal," or "information," to be transmitted through the receptor to the inside of the cell.

5. The intensity of the resulting transmembrane signal is thought to be determined by the percentage of receptors that are occupied by molecules of neurotransmitter.

A

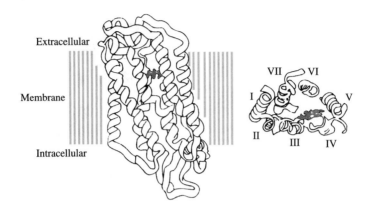

B

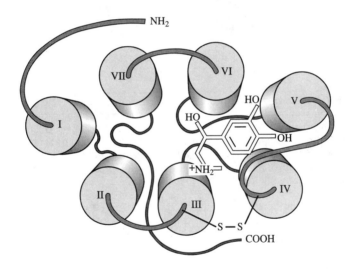

FIGURE 2.3 Schematic representation of a G-protein-coupled transmembrane receptor, with a molecule of neurotransmitter (norepinephrine) lying in its binding site. Note the arrangement of the 7-transmembrane helical coils and the site of transmitter attachment deep within the structure. The ionic interactions between the transmitter and particular amino acid side chains are not illustrated. In **A**, the membrane and continuous coils are shown. In **B**, the helical coils are represented as cylinders with the molecule of norepinephrine interacting with four of the coils.

6. A drug can affect the transmembrane signal by binding either to the receptor for the endogenous neurotransmitter or to a nearby site.

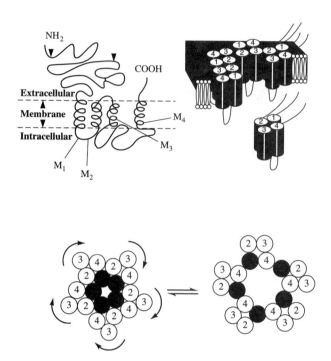

FIGURE 2.4 Presumed topology of the GABA$_A$ receptor. *Top left:* Single subunit with its large extracellular terminal part, and four transmembrane helical coils. *Top right:* Arrangement of the transmembrane domains of five subunits to form a central channel. *Bottom:* Transmembrane domain in a transverse section through the membrane when the channel is closed (*left*) and open (*right*). [From W. E. Haefley et al., "The Multiplicity of Actions of Benzodiazepine Receptor Ligands," *Canadian Journal of Psychiatry* 38, Suppl. 4 (1993): 5102–5107.]

Binding of a drug to a receptor results in one of three actions:

1. Binding to a receptor site normally occupied by the endogenous neurotransmitter can initiate a cellular response similar or identical to that exerted by the transmitter. The drug thus mimics the action of the transmitter. This is termed an *agonistic action* and the drug is termed an *agonist* for that transmitter.

2. Binding to a site near the binding site for the endogenous transmitter can facilitate transmitter binding. This is also an agonist action.

3. Binding to a receptor site normally occupied by a neurotransmitter but not initiating a transmitter-like action blocks access of the transmitter to its binding site, which inhibits the normal physiological action of the transmitter. This is called an *antagonistic action* and the drug is termed an *antagonist* for that neurotransmitter or receptor site.

Thus, directly binding to the receptor either blocks access of the transmitter to its receptor (an antagonist action) or else mimics or facilitates transmitter action (agonist actions).

Drugs do not create any unique effects; they merely modulate normal neuronal functioning, mimicking or antagonizing the actions of a specific neurotransmitter. Binding accompanied by drug-induced mimicry or facilitation of neurotransmitter action is an agonist action.* Drug occupation of a receptor that is not accompanied by neurotransmitter-like activation blocks the access of the neurotransmitter to the receptor and is an antagonist action.†

Receptor Structure

What does a receptor look like? As stated, most receptors are membrane-spanning proteins, each having 7 or 12 alpha-helical coils. Following are three different types of membrane-spanning proteins, as well as a fourth type of drug-receptor protein: enzymes.

The first type of membrane-spanning receptors are those that form an *ion channel*; the central portion of the receptor forms a pore, or channel, that enlarges in size when either an endogenous neurotransmitter or a specialized intracellular G-protein attaches to the receptor. The attachment allows flow of a specific *ion* (such as chloride ion) through the enlarged pore. A drug may also bind to this receptor, acting to either facilitate or block the action of the neurotransmitter. Figures 2.4 and 2.5 illustrate the neurotransmitter gamma-aminobutyric acid (GABA) and a drug (a benzodiazepine) opening a channel and allowing inward flow of chloride ions through an enlarged pore within a GABA-activated receptor.

Benzodiazepines (Chapter 6) serve as agonists at this site by binding to a site near the GABA-binding site and by facilitating the action of GABA. This action allows flow of chloride ions into the neuron, hyperpolarizing the neuron and inhibiting neuronal function. This action underlies the use of benzodiazepines as sedative, antianxiety, amnestic, and antiepileptic agents.

In contrast, the drug flumazenil (Romazecon) attaches to the benzodiazepine-binding site but does not facilitate the action of GABA. It does, however, compete with any benzodiazepine that is present,

---

* Example: Buspirone attaches to the serotonin 1_A receptor and activates it, mimicking serotonin action on the receptor, which results in an antianxiety action of clinical significance.

† Example: Fluoxetine competes with serotonin for the reuptake protein, blocking access of serotonin to the receptor and prolonging serotonin's presence in the synaptic cleft (Chapter 3). This allows more serotonin stimulation of postsynaptic receptors, eventually leading to down regulation in the number of serotonin receptors and relief of clinical depression (Chapter 15).

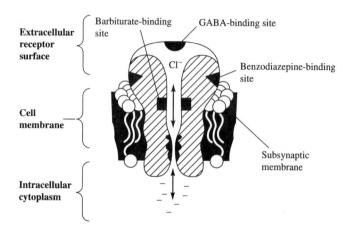

FIGURE 2.5 GABA$_A$ receptor in a perpendicular section through the membrane. The localization of the various binding sites is purely hypothetical. [From: W. E. Haefley et al., "The Multiplicity of Actions of Benzodiazepine Receptor Ligands," *Canadian Journal of Psychiatry* 38, Suppl. 4 (1993): 5102–5107.]

displacing the benzodiazepine from the receptor and reversing the actions of the benzodiazepine. Flumazenil is classified pharmacologically as a benzodiazepine reversal agent or benzodiazepine antagonist and is used clinically to treat benzodiazepine overdoses.*

Figure 2.6 illustrates the opening of a channel as a result of neurotransmitter attachment to an adjacent membrane-spanning receptor protein (a G-protein-coupled receptor). Receptor activation releases an intracellular G-protein that in turn activates other proteins that ultimately open an adjacent ion channel. Obviously, this can be quite confusing.

The second type of membrane-spanning receptor protein is a *carrier* (or *transport*) *protein*. This type of receptor transports small organic molecules (such as neurotransmitters) across cell membranes against concentration gradients. Important in psychopharmacology are the presynaptic carrier proteins that function to bind dopamine, norepinephrine, or serotonin in the synaptic cleft and transport them back into the presynaptic nerve terminal, terminating the synaptic transmitter action of these three neurotransmitters (Chapter 3).

---

*Also shown in Figure 2.5 is a barbiturate-binding site on the GABA-receptor complex. Barbiturates act like benzodiazepines in increasing the effect of GABA on the chloride channel within the GABA receptor. Thus, with a site and mechanism of action similar to that exerted by benzodiazepines, the two classes of drugs might be expected to demonstrate similar clinical and behavioral effects. In general, that is true (Chapters 5 and 6).

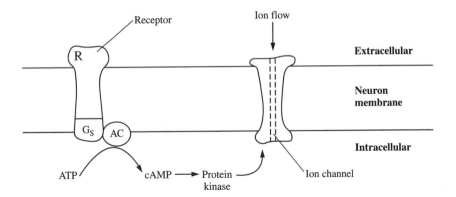

FIGURE 2.6 Hypothetical model of a G-protein-coupled receptor functioning to open an adjacent ion channel. A neurotransmitter binds to its receptor site (R). A conformational change results and a second-messenger enzyme, adenylate cyclase (AC), is activated through the action of a released G-protein (G_s). G_s forms cyclic adenosine monophosphate (cAMP), which activates a protein kinase (functioning as a second messenger), which ultimately acts on the ion channel to cause it to open, allowing a flow of ions into (or out of) the cell. This is but one model of an intracellular function being modulated by a G-protein-coupled transmembrane receptor activated by a neurotransmitter.

Cocaine and methylphenidate (Ritalin) (both covered in Chapter 7) block the carrier protein that is specific for transporting dopamine. Fluoxetine (Chapter 15) blocks the carrier protein that is specific for transporting serotonin. Imipramine (Tofranil) blocks the carrier protein that is specific for transporting norepinephrine. These molecular actions result in similar but still distinctly different effects.

Figure 2.7 illustrates the structure of the presynaptic transport receptor for dopamine. The presynaptic transport protein receptor is arranged as 12 helical arrays of amino acids, contrasted with the 7 helices present in postsynaptic serotonin (and other neurotransmitter) receptors, as shown in Figure 2.2.

A third type of membrane-spanning receptor protein is called a *G-protein-coupled receptor*. It is a postsynaptic receptor, activation of which induces the release of an attached intracellular protein (a *G-protein*) that, in turn, controls enzymatic function within the postsynaptic neuron. Figure 2.2 illustrates the structure of one of the more than 15 such receptors for serotonin (the serotonin 1_A receptor). Figure 2.8 illustrates some of the intracellular alterations that can be induced as a result of activation of this receptor.

G-protein-coupled receptors are discussed throughout this book because they are involved in the actions of many neurotransmitters, such as acetylcholine, norepinephrine, dopamine, serotonin, and opioid

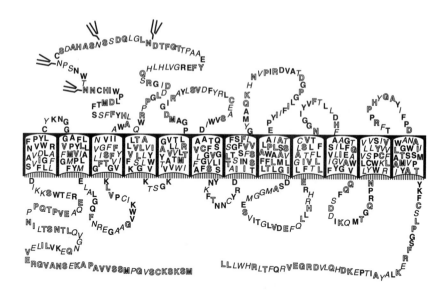

FIGURE 2.7 Schematic representation of the dopamine transporter showing proposed orientation in the presynaptic membranes [From S. Shimada et al., "Cloning and Expression of a Cocaine-Sensitive Dopamine Transporter Complimentary DNA," *Science* 254 (1991): 576–578.]

endorphins, all of which are sites of action of psychoactive drugs. The molecular structure of G-protein-coupled receptors (more than 50 have been identified, and more keep coming[3]) consists of a single protein chain of 400 to 500 amino acids possessing seven transmembrane alpha-helices (Figure 2.2). Both the extracellular and the intracellular terminal portions of the protein chain vary in length and in amino acid composition. G-protein-coupled receptors are the middlemen (the *second messenger**), able to communicate between the neurotransmitter-receptor complex and intracellular enzymes or adjacent ion channels (Figures 2.8 and 2.9). The protein consists of three functional subunits, which taken together have historically been called G-protein because they interact with guanine nucleotides within the cell. G-proteins control many cellular functions, among them control of ion channels, energy metabolism, cell division and differentiation, and neuronal excitability.[3] Simmonds[4] reviews the interaction between G-proteins and *adenylate cyclase*, a key intracellular regulatory enzyme.

---

* The endogenous neurotransmitter is the first messenger, carrying information between presynaptic and postsynaptic neurons across the synaptic cleft (Chapter 3).

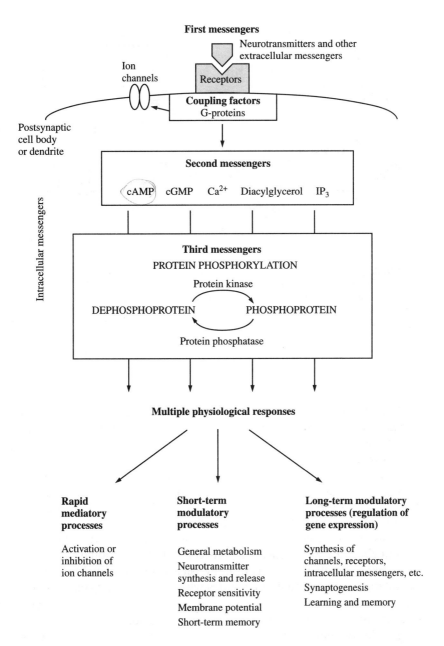

FIGURE 2.8 Schematic model of transmitter-receptor interaction and the resulting second messenger action. Second messengers are intracellular proteins, molecules, or ions that are regulated by transmitter-receptor activation. The neurotransmitter is the first messenger, and binding is a recognition action. Receptor alteration with G-protein release represents transduction of first messenger binding. As shown here, second messengers amplify the signal and serve to turn on or turn off numerous rapid and long-term physiological responses.

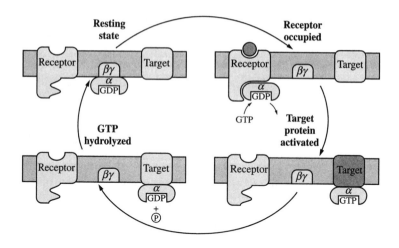

FIGURE 2.9 The function of the G-protein. The G-protein consists of three subunits, alpha, beta, and gamma, which function to anchor the G-protein to the transmembrane helical protein-receptor molecule. Coupling of the alpha subunit to an agonist-occupied receptor causes the bound GDP (guanine diphosphate) to exchange with intracellular GTP (guanine triphosphate); the alpha-GTP complex dissociates and interacts with adenylate cyclase. The original complex then regenerates through hydrolysis of the GTP. [From Rang et al.,[3] Figure 2.9.]

Finally, a fourth type of receptor protein for psychoactive drugs is *enzymes*, in particular enzymes that regulate the synaptic availability of certain neurotransmitters. These enzymes function to break down neurotransmitters, and their inhibition by drugs increases transmitter availability. Following are two examples, one of which has already been used: *acetylcholine esterase*, the enzyme that breaks down acetylcholine within the synaptic cleft (Chapter 3). The second example is *monoamine oxidase*, the enzyme that breaks down norepinephrine and dopamine within presynaptic nerve terminals, controlling the amount available for release (Chapters 3 and 15). Drugs known as irreversible acetylcholine esterase inhibitors form covalent bonds with the enzyme and are used as insecticides and as lethal "nerve gases." Drugs that reversibly inhibit acetylcholine esterase are used clinically as cognitive enhancers, delaying the onset of Alzheimer's disease.[5] Drugs that irreversibly inhibit monoamine oxidase are used primarily as antidepressants.

Drug-Receptor Specificity

As discussed, receptors exhibit high specificity both for one particular neurotransmitter and for certain drug molecules. Making only modest variations in the chemical structure of a drug may greatly alter the intensity of a receptor's response to it. For example, amphetamine and methamphetamine (Chapter 7) are both powerful psychostimulants. Although their chemical structures are very close, they differ by the simple addition of a methyl ($-CH_3$) group to amphetamine, forming methamphetamine. Methamphetamine produces much greater behavioral stimulation at the same milligram dosage. Both drugs attach to the same receptors in the brain, but methamphetamine exerts a much more powerful action on them, at least on a milligram basis. The drug molecule with the "best fit" to the receptor (methamphetamine, in this example) elicits the greatest response from the cell. In pharmacologic terms, methamphetamine is more *potent* than amphetamine, because a lower absolute dosage achieves the same level of response as a higher dose of amphetamine.

As a consequence of drug binding to a receptor, cellular function is altered, resulting in observable effects on physiological or psychological functioning. The total action of the drug in the body results from drug actions either (1) on one specific type of receptor or (2) at multiple different types of receptors. The use of drug for a given therapeutic (or recreational) effect also results in other effects, called *side effects*.

As an example of the side effects produced by the first mechanism, fluoxetine-induced blockade of presynaptic serotonin reuptake (an antagonist action) increases serotonin availability at all postsynaptic serotonin receptors. This single antagonist action results not only in relief of depression but in such side effects as anxiety, insomnia, and sexual dysfunction (Chapter 15).

As an example of the side effects produced by the second mechanism, certain other antidepressants (the so-called tricyclic antidepressants; Chapter 15) increase both serotonin and norepinephrine availability (reducing depression). They also produce sedation as a result of their blocking histamine receptors; dry mouth and blurred vision can result. A balance between wanted effects and inevitable but unwanted side effects is always desirable.

Dose-Response Relationships

One way of quantifying drug-receptor interactions is to use *dose-response curves*. In Figure 2.10, two different types of dose-response curves are illustrated. In graph A, the dose is plotted against the percentage of people (from a given population) who exhibit a characteristic effect at a given dosage. In graph B, the dose is plotted against the intensity, or magnitude, of the response in a single person. These curves indicate that a dose exists that is low enough to produce little or

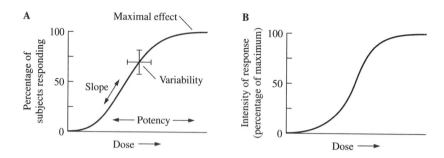

FIGURE 2.10 Two types of dose-response curves. **A.** Curve obtained by plotting the dose of drug against the percentage of subjects showing a given response at any given dose. **B.** Curve obtained by plotting the dose of drug against the intensity of response observed in any single individual at a given dose. The intensity of response is plotted as a percentage of the maximum obtainable response.

no effect; at the opposite extreme, a dose exists beyond which no greater response can be elicited. Dose-response curves demonstrate important characteristics (Figure 2.10):

1. *Potency* refers to the absolute number of molecules of drug required to elicit a response, a measurement of the dose required.

2. *Efficacy* refers to the maximum effect obtainable, with additional doses producing no more effect.

3. *Variability* and *slope* refer to individual differences in drug response, with some persons responding at very low doses and some requiring much more drug.

The location of the dose-response curve along the horizontal axis reflects the potency of the drug. If two drugs produce an equal degree of sedation, but one exerts this action at half the dose level of the other, the first drug is considered to be twice as potent as the second drug (Figure 2.11). Potency, however, is a relatively unimportant characteristic of a drug, because it makes little difference whether the effective dose of a drug is 1.0 milligram or 100 milligrams as long as the drug is administered in an appropriate dose with no undue toxicity. Thus, the more potent drug is not necessarily any "better."

Slope refers to the more or less linear central portion of the dose-response curve. A steep slope on a dose-response curve implies that there is only a small difference between the dose that produces a barely discernible effect and the dose that causes a maximal effect. The steeper the slope, the smaller the increase in dose that is required to go from a minimum response to a maximum effect. This can be good, as

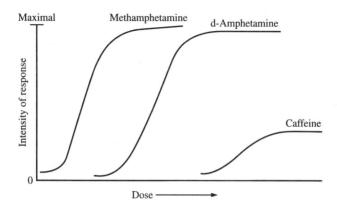

FIGURE 2.11 Theoretical dose-response curves for three psychostimulants to illustrate equal efficacy of methamphetamine and dextro-amphetamine; increased potency of methamphetamine; and reduced potency and efficacy of caffeine.

it may indicate that there is little biological variation in the response to the drug. Conversely, it may be a disadvantage if it indicates that untoward toxicity occurs with only minimal increases in dose.

The *peak* of the dose-response curve indicates the maximum effect, or efficacy, that can be produced by a drug, regardless of further increases in dose. Not all psychoactive drugs can exert the same level of effect. For example, caffeine, even in massive doses, cannot exert the same intensity of CNS stimulation as amphetamine (Figure 2.11). Similarly, aspirin can never achieve the maximum analgesic effect of morphine. Thus, the maximum effect is an inherent property of a drug and is one measure of a drug's efficacy.

Most psychoactive drugs are not used to the point of their maximum effect, because side effects and toxicities limit the upper range of dosage, regardless of whether the drug is administered for a therapeutic purpose or is taken for recreational use. Therefore, the usefulness of a compound is correspondingly limited, even though the drug may be inherently capable of producing a greater or more intense effect.

Drug Safety and Effectiveness

Variability in Drug Responsiveness

The dose of a drug that produces a specific response varies considerably between individuals. Interpatient variability can result from differences in rates of drug absorption and metabolism, previous experience with drug use, various physical, psychological, and emotional

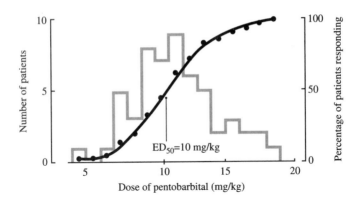

FIGURE 2.12 Example of biological variation. Histogram (left ordinate) and cumulative frequency histogram (right ordinate) following intravenous administration of pentobarbital, used to cause drowsiness in hospitalized patients. An ED_{50} of about 11 mg/kg body weight is shown. Note, however, that some patients exhibited sedation at about 4 mg/kg, while others required a dose of about 18 mg/kg The stair-step bars illustrate the data behind the dose-response curve.

states, and so on. Despite the etiology of the variability, any population of individuals will have a few subjects who are remarkably sensitive to the effects (and side effects) of a drug, while a few will exhibit remarkable drug tolerance, requiring quite large doses to produce therapeutic results. The variability, however, usually follows a predictable pattern, resembling a Gaussian distribution (Figure 2.12). In a few instances, however, a specific population of individuals (following a genetically predetermined pattern) will skew this distribution by exhibiting a unique pattern of responsiveness, usually due to genetic alterations in drug metabolism.

From Figure 2.12, it is obvious that, although the average dose required to elicit a given response can be calculated easily, some individuals respond at doses that are very much lower than the average and others respond only at doses that are very much higher. Thus, it is extremely important that the dose of all drugs be individualized. Generalizations about "average doses" are risky at best.

The dose of a drug that produces the desired effect in 50 percent of the subjects is called the ED_{50}, and the lethal dose for 50 percent of the subjects is called the LD_{50}. The LD_{50} is calculated in exactly the same way as the ED_{50}, except that the dose of the drug is plotted against the number of experimental animals that die after being administered various doses of the compound. Both the ED_{50} and the LD_{50} are determined in several species of animals to prevent accidental drug-induced toxicity in humans. The ratio of the LD_{50} to the ED_{50} is used as an index of the relative safety of the drug and is called the *therapeutic index.*

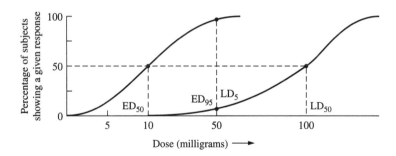

FIGURE 2.13 Two dose-response curves. *Left:* Dose of drug required to induce a given response. *Right:* Lethal dose of the compound. See text for discussion.

To illustrate, two dose-response curves are shown in Figure 2.13. The curve at the left illustrates the dose of drug necessary to induce sleep in a population of mice, and the one at the right illustrates the dose of drug necessary to kill a similar population. In this example, the $LD_{50}:ED_{50}$ ratio is seen to be 100:10, or 10. This may seem like a rather large margin, but note that at a dose of 50 milligrams, 95 percent of the mice sleep while 5 percent of the mice die. This overlap demonstrates both the difficulty in assessing the relative safety of drugs for use in large populations and the biological variation in individual responses to drugs. With this particular compound, a dose cannot be administered that will guarantee that 100 percent of the mice will sleep and none will die. Thus, a more useful indication of the margin of safety is a ratio of the lethal dose for 1 percent of the population to the effective dose for 99 percent of the population ($LD_1:ED_{99}$). A sedative drug with an $LD_1:ED_{99}$ of 1 would be a safer compound than the drug shown in Figure 2.13. Note that the clinical usefulness of indices obtained from laboratory animals is limited, because these indices do not reflect the occasional unexpected response (from the causes listed earlier) that can seriously harm a patient.

Drug variability is also intimately associated with drug toxicity. Therefore, the side effects that are invariably associated with a drug, as well as its more serious toxicities (including those that can be fatal), must always be considered.

Drug Interactions

The effects of one drug can be modified by the concurrent administration of another drug. This is particularly important in psychopharmacology.[6] For example, Chapter 1 explained how certain drugs may either increase or decrease the rate of hepatic metabolism of other drugs. Another mechanism of drug interaction involves drugs that can interact through an *additive mechanism,* where the effects of one drug potentiate the effects of another. For example, alcohol taken after a benzodiazepine tranquilizer has been ingested or after smoking marijuana, increases sedation and loss of coordination. This action may have little consequence if the doses of each drug are low, but higher doses of either or both drugs can be dangerous both to the user and to others. Even though a person may normally be able to ingest a limited amount of alcohol and still drive a car without significant loss of control or coordination, the concurrent use of tranquilizers or marijuana may profoundly impair driving performance, endangering the driver, passengers, and other motorists. Logan[7] reports the interaction between alcohol, marijuana, and methamphetamine on driving performance, noting additive impairments during both methamphetamine intoxication and withdrawal. Drug use was inconsistent with safe driving.

Drug Toxicity

All drugs can produce harmful effects as well as beneficial ones. The nature of these unwanted effects falls into two categories:

1. Effects that are related to the principal and predictable pharmacological actions of a drug (e.g., the sedation caused by drinking alcohol, or the dry mouth experienced while taking certain antidepressants)

2. Effects that are unrelated to the expected actions of a drug (e.g., a severe allergic reaction to a drug)

It is important to categorize harmful effects of drugs in terms of their severity and to distinguish between effects that cause a temporary inconvenience or discomfort and effects that can lead to organ damage, permanent disability, or even death.

Most drugs exert effects on several different body functions. To achieve the desired therapeutic effect or effects, some side effects often must be tolerated. This is possible if the side effects are minor, but if they are more serious, they may be a limiting factor in the use of the drug.

The distinction between therapeutic effects and side effects is relative and depends on the purpose for which the drug is administered: one person's side effect may be another person's desired therapeutic effect. For example, in one patient receiving morphine for its pain-relieving properties, the intestinal constipation that morphine induces may be an undesirable side effect that must be tolerated. For a second patient, however, morphine may be used to treat severe diarrhea, in which case the constipation induced is the desired therapeutic effect, and relief of pain is a side effect.

In addition to side effects that are merely irritating, some drugs may cause reactions that are very serious, including serious allergies, blood disorders, liver or kidney toxicity, or abnormalities in fetal development. Fortunately, the incidence of serious toxic effects is quite low.

Allergies to drugs may take many forms, from mild skin rashes to fatal shock. Allergies differ from normal side effects, which can often be eliminated or at least made tolerable by a simple reduction in dosage. However, a reduction in the dose of a drug may have no effect on a drug allergy, because exposure to any amount of the drug can be hazardous and possibly catastrophic for the patient.

Damage to the liver and kidneys results from their role in concentrating, metabolizing, and excreting toxic drugs. Examples of drug-induced liver damage include that caused either by alcohol or certain of the inhalants of abuse (Chapter 4). Certain of the major tranquilizers (e.g., the phenothiazines) may induce jaundice by increasing the viscosity of bile in the liver (Chapter 17).

The toxicity to a fetus of both socially abused and some therapeutic drugs should be mentioned. Data quite clearly show the adverse effects of nicotine and ethyl alcohol on the fetus. Similarly, the effects of cocaine abuse on the fetus have received much attention.[8] These three drugs are responsible for a majority of preventable fetal toxicities and are three of the major health hazards in the country today.

Placebo Effects

The term *placebo* refers to a pharmacologically inert substance that elicits a significant therapeutic response. Placebos work best on symptoms or diseases that vary (wax and wane) over time. Perhaps the most prominent examples are major depression and chronic pain.[9,10] Because the placebo action is independent of any chemical property of the drug, it arises largely because of what the patient or the prescriber expects or desires. A placebo response may result from a person's mental set or from the entire environmental setting in which the drug is taken. In certain predisposed persons, a placebo may produce extremely strong reactions with far-reaching consequences. Placebos can therapeutically empower patients to stimulate their psychophysiological self-regulation abilities. Possible mechanisms for the strength of placebo effect include conditioning, expectancy, and self-liberation of endogenous neurotransmitters, including endorphins and adrenaline-like catecholamines.

Swartzman and Burkell[11] discuss the influence of expectations on the response to placebo medication. Expectations guide the search for information and organize information obtained from the search. Both the patient and the prescriber may have expectations regarding anticipated benefits possibly resulting from drug administration. The biases and distortions that are inevitable consequences can influence both individual responses as well as the results of clinical drug trials.[12]

As discussed by Swartzman and Burkell, "Expectations play a role in the subjective and behavioral effects of a range of psychoactive substances including alcohol, caffeine, THC, and d-amphetamine."[11] In therapeutics, expectations of improvement at the start of drug therapy can predict subsequent therapeutic effectiveness and response. Perhaps the "feeling" of side effects serves to verify the expectation that the drug is "working."

Remarkably, placebos have been shown to evoke patterns of altered behavior that are similar to and as long-lasting as those observed when a pharmacologically active drug is ingested. Thus, in analyzing the pharmacology of a psychoactive agent, particular attention must be paid to the mental expectations, the social setting, and the predisposition of the subjects taking the placebo if the pharmacological effects of a drug are to be described accurately. Certainly the placebo effect is a powerful element in drug-induced responses.

STUDY QUESTIONS

1. What is meant by the term *pharmacodynamics*? What does the term imply?

2. What is a receptor? What is a drug receptor?

3. Discuss the structure of a drug receptor.

4. Distinguish between *agonist* and *antagonist* as they relate to drug-receptor interactions.

5. Compare and contrast a presynaptic receptor and a postsynaptic receptor.

6. List the four types of receptors discussed in this chapter.

7. Discuss drug-receptor specificity. Can a drug ever be more specific for a receptor than is the endogenous neurotransmitter? Explain.

8. What is meant by a dose-response relationship? Draw a hypothetical example of such a relationship.

9. Discuss the factors that influence the time course of drug action in the body.

10. Discuss how two drugs might interact with each other in the body.

11. Which factors contribute to the intensity of drug effects?

12. What are two important functions of neuronal receptors? How do drugs affect receptors?

REFERENCES

1. E. M. Ross, "Pharmacodynamics: Mechanisms of Drug Action and the Relationship Between Drug Concentration and Effect," in J. G. Hardman, L. E. Limbird, P. B. Molinoff, R. W. Ruddon, and A. G. Gilman, eds., *Goodman and Gilman's The Pharmacological Basis of Therapeutics*, 9th ed. (New York: McGraw-Hill, 1996), 29.

2. R. S. Feldman, J. S. Meyer, and L. F. Quenzer, *Principles of Neuropsychopharmacology* (Sunderland, Mass.: Sinauer, 1997), 13.

3. H. P. Rang, M. M. Dale, J. M. Ritter, and P. Gardner, *Pharmacology* (New York: Churchill Livingstone, 1995) 33–42.

4. W. F. Simmonds, "G-protein Regulation of Adenylate Cyclase," *Trends in Pharmacological Sciences*, 20 (1999), 66–73.

5. R. S. Feldman, J. S. Meyer, and L. F. Quenzer, *Principles of Neuropsychopharmacology* (Sunderland, Mass.: Sinauer, 1997), 887–909.

6. A. M. Callahan, M. Fava, and J. F. Rosenbaum, "Drug Interactions in Psychopharmacology," *Psychiatric Clinics of North America* 16 (1993): 647–671.

7. B. K. Logan, "Methamphetamine and Driving Impairment," *Journal of Forensic Sciences* 41 (1996): 457–464.

8. R. J. Konkol and G. D. Olsen, eds., *Prenatal Cocaine Exposure* (Boca Raton, Fla.: CRC Press, 1996).

9. E. D. Peselow, M. P. Sanfilipo, C. Difiglia, and R. R. Fieve, "Melancholic/Endogenous Depression and Response to Somatic Treatment and Placebo," *American Journal of Psychiatry* 149 (1992): 1324–1334.

10. C. Peck and G. Coleman, "Implications of Placebo Theory for Clinical Research and Practice in Pain Management," *Theoretical Medicine* 12 (1991): 247–270.

11. L. C. Swartzman and J. Burkell, "Expectations and the Placebo Effect in Clinical Drug Trials: Why We Should Not Turn a Blind Eye to Unblinding, and Other Cautionary Notes," *Clinical Pharmacology and Therapeutics* 64 (1998): 1–7.

12. F. M. Quitkin, "Placebos, Drug Effects, and Study Design: A Clinician's Guide," *American Journal of Psychiatry* 156 (1999): 829–836.

Chapter 3

The Neuron, Synaptic Transmission, and Neurotransmitters

All our thoughts, actions, memories, and behaviors result from biochemical interactions that take place between *neurons* located in our central nervous system (CNS). Drugs that affect these processes (*psychoactive drugs*) do so because they alter one or more biochemical processes either within or between neurons. Psychoactive drugs are chemicals that alter (mimic, potentiate, or inhibit) the normal neuronal processes associated with neuronal function or communication between neurons. To understand the actions of psychoactive drugs, it is necessary to have some idea of what a neuron is and how neurons interact with each other.

Overall Organization of the CNS

The human brain consists of perhaps 90 billion individual neurons located in the skull and the spinal canal. The *spinal cord* extends from the lower end of the medulla to the sacrum. The spinal cord consists of neurons and fiber tracts involved in the following:

- Carrying sensory information from the skin, muscles, joints, and internal body organs to the brain
- Organizing and modulating the motor outflow to the muscles (to produce coordinated muscle responses)

- Modulating sensory input (including pain impulses)
- Providing autonomic (involuntary) control of vital body functions

The lower part of the brain, attached to the upper part of the spinal cord, is the *brain stem* (Figure 3.1). It is divided into three parts: the *medulla*, the *pons*, and the *midbrain*. All impulses that are conducted in either direction between the spinal cord and the brain pass through the brain stem, which is also important in the regulation of vital body functions, such as respiration, blood pressure, heart rate, gastrointestinal functioning, and the states of sleep and wakefulness. The brain stem is also involved in behavioral alerting, attention, and arousal responses. Depressant drugs, such as the barbiturates (Chapter 5), depress the brain stem activating system; this action probably underlies much of their hypnotic action.

Behind the brain stem is a large bulbous structure—the *cerebellum*. A highly convoluted structure, the cerebellum is connected to the brain

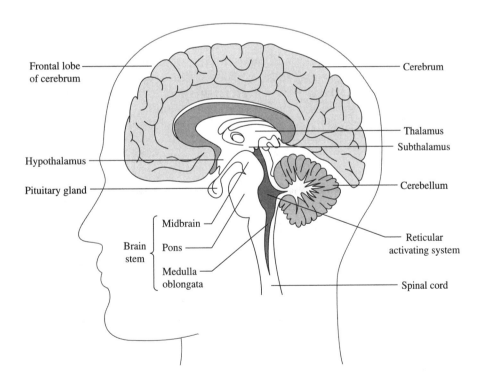

FIGURE 3.1 Midline section of the brain illustrating several structures lying below the cerebral cortex.

stem by large fiber tracts. The cerebellum is necessary for the proper integration of movement and posture. Drunkenness, which is characterized by ataxia (loss of coordination and balance, staggering, and other deficits), appears to be caused largely by an alcohol-induced depression of cerebellar function.

The area immediately above the brain stem and covered by the cerebral hemispheres is the *diencephalon*. This area includes the hypothalamus, pituitary gland, various fiber tracts (bundles of axons that travel as a group from one area to another), subthalamus, and thalamus. Three of these areas are discussed here: the subthalamus, the hypothalamus, and the limbic system.

The *subthalamus* is a small area underneath the thalamus and above the midbrain. It contains a variety of small structures that, together with the basal ganglia, constitute one of our motor systems, the *extrapyramidal system*. Patients who have Parkinson's disease (Chapter 18) have a deficiency of the neurotransmitter dopamine in the terminals of their nerve axons, which originate in cell bodies in the substantia nigra (one of the subthalamic structures).

The *hypothalamus* is a collection of neurons in the lower portion of the brain near the junction of the midbrain and the thalamus. It is located near the base of the skull, just above the pituitary gland (the function of which it largely modulates). The hypothalamus is the principal center in the brain responsible for the integration of our entire autonomic (involuntary or vegetative) nervous system. Thus, it helps control such vegetative functions as eating, drinking, sleeping, regulation of body temperature, sexual behavior, blood pressure, emotion, and water balance. In addition, the hypothalamus closely controls hormonal output of the pituitary gland. Neurons in the hypothalamus produce substances called *releasing factors*, which travel to the nearby pituitary gland, inducing the secretion of hormones that regulate fertility in females and sperm formation in males. The hypothalamus is a site of action for many psychoactive drugs, either as a site for the primary action of the drug or as a site responsible for side effects associated with the use of a drug.

Closely associated with the hypothalamus is the *limbic system*, the major components of which are the *amygdala* and the *hippocampus*. These structures exert primitive types of behavioral control; they integrate emotion, reward, and behavior with motor and autonomic functions. Because the limbic system and the hypothalamus interact to regulate emotion and emotional expression, these structures are logical sites for the study of psychoactive drugs that alter mood, affect, emotion, or responses to emotional experiences.

The hypothalamic and limbic areas contain structures important in psychopharmacology and the abuse potential of drugs. Included here are the dopamine-rich reward centers that involve the *ventral tegmental area*, the *median forebrain bundle*, and the *nucleus accumbens*. Throughout this text, this system is discussed as a site of the behavior-reinforcing action of psychoactive drugs that are subject to compulsive abuse.

Almost completely covering the brain stem and the diencephalon is the *cerebrum*. In humans the cerebrum is the largest part of the brain. It is separated into two distinct hemispheres, left and right, with numerous fiber tracts connecting the two. Because skull size is limited and the cerebrum is so large, the outer layer of the cerebrum, the *cerebral cortex*, is deeply convoluted and fissured. Like other parts of the brain, the cerebral cortex is divided by function; it contains centers for vision, hearing, speech, sensory perception, and emotion. The various regions of the cerebral cortex can be classified in several ways, among them, the type of function or sensation that is processed. Figure 3.2 illustrates some of this categorization.

The Neuron

The neuron is the basic component of the CNS, and each neuron shares common structural and functional characteristics (Figure 3.3).

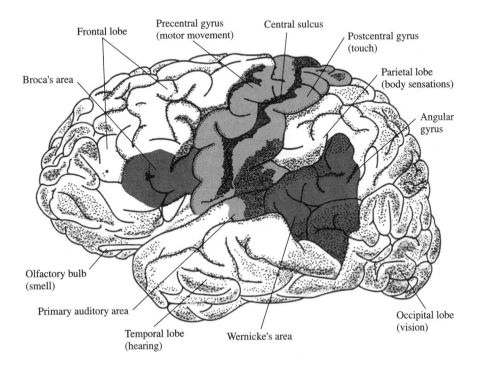

FIGURE 3.2 Surface structure of the brain showing major areas of the cerebral cortex.

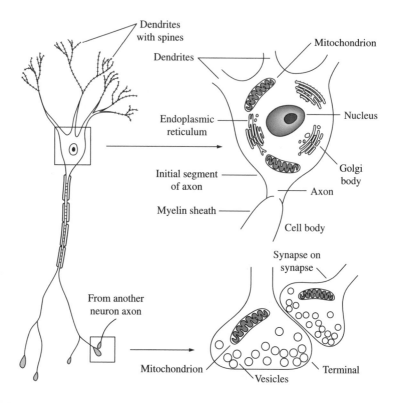

FIGURE 3.3 Major parts of a neuron. The genetic material (DNA) is contained in the nucleus, and several specialized organelles are present in the cytoplasm, the material of the cell outside the nucleus. The cell is covered by a thin wall, or membrane. Mitochondria are present in the cell body, the fibers, and the terminals. The terminals also contain small, round vesicles that contain neurotransmitter chemicals. Synaptic connections from the fibers of other neurons cover the cell body and dendrites. In many neurons the synapses on dendrites can be seen as little spines. The axon itself has no synapses on it except sometimes at its synaptic terminals, where other neuron axon terminals may form synapses on synapses. [From Thompson,[1] p. 31.]

A typical neuron has a *soma* (cell body), which contains the nucleus (within which is the genetic material of the cell). Extending from the soma in one direction are many short fibers, called *dendrites* (hundreds of widely branched extensions), that receive input from other neurons through *receptors* located on the dendritic membrane. On receipt of a signal from another cell, an electrical current is generated and travels down the dendrite to the soma. Extending in another direction from the soma is a single elongated process called an *axon*, which varies in length from as short as a few millimeters to as long as a meter (meter-length examples are the axons that run from the motor neurons of the spinal cord out to the muscles that they innervate). The axon, in essence, transmits electrical activity (in the form of *action potentials*) from the soma to other neurons or to muscles, organs, or glands of the body. Normally, the axon conducts impulses in only one direction—from the soma down the axon to a specialized structure that, together with one or more dendrites from another neuron, forms a complex microspace called a *synapse* (Figure 3.4).

> A given neuron in the brain may receive several thousand synaptic connections from other neurons. Hence if the human brain has 10^{11} neurons, then it has at least 10^{14} synapses, or many trillions. The number of possible different combinations of synaptic connections among the neurons in a single human brain is larger than the total number of atomic particles that make up the known universe. Hence the diversity of the interconnections in a human brain seems almost without limit.[1]

It had generally been thought that the brain has the maximal number of neurons at birth; once a neuron dies, it is not replaced. This basic principle is currently being questioned.[2,3] Certainly what continues to develop

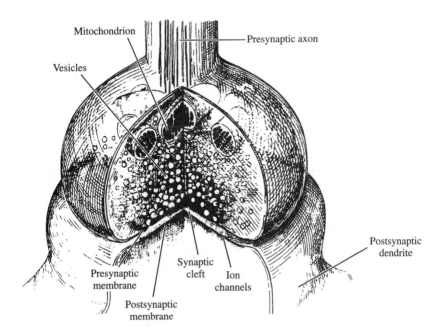

FIGURE 3.4 Three-dimensional drawing of a synapse. The axon terminal is the top knob-like structure, and the spine of the receiving neuron is the bottom one. Note that there is a space (synaptic cleft) between the presynaptic terminal membrane and the postsynaptic cell membrane.

during our lifetime is the number and pattern of synaptic connections, which are continually being reshaped, resynthesized, and "sculpted" by experience and appear to form the anatomical basis of memory.[4]

A synapse is the point of functional contact between an axon terminal and another cell (Figure 3.4). As defined here, a synapse consists of a minute space (the *synaptic cleft*) between the presynaptic membrane (which is the axon terminal) of one neuron and the postsynaptic membrane of the receiving neuron. The presynaptic terminal contains numerous structural elements, the most important of which (for our purposes) are the small synaptic vesicles, each of which contains several thousand molecules of neurotransmitter chemical. These vesicles store the transmitter, which is available for release (Figure 3.5). Through a process called *exocytosis*, and under the influence of calcium ions, vesicles fuse with the presynaptic membrane and molecules of transmitter are released into the synaptic cleft. The transmitter substance diffuses across the synaptic cleft and attaches to protein receptors (as was discussed in Chapter 2) on the postsynaptic membrane (e.g., located on dendrites of the next neuron), thereby transmitting information chemically from one neuron to another. Because the neurons do not physically touch each other, synaptic transmission is a chemical rather than an electrical process.

As a chemical process, it may sound as if synaptic transmission takes a rather long time, but the process can be remarkably fast and efficient.[5] In the case of the ligand-gated ion channel type of receptor, the entire process may occur over a time span as short as a millisecond for transmitter release (from presynaptic vesicles), diffusion (across the cleft), receptor attachment, channel opening, and ion influx.

The G-protein-coupled receptors (Chapter 2) are often termed slow-response receptors—they produce activation responses that may last from hundreds of milliseconds to perhaps many seconds. These responses are generally thought to be modulatory, with the neurotransmitter either dampening or enhancing intracellular enzymatic functions. Through release of the intracellular second messenger (Chapter 2), slow-response receptors trigger the cell's internal machinery, leading to effects as diverse as modulation of ion channel activity to protein transcription from genetic material (a process probably involved in mechanisms of long-term memory formation[4]). Thus, activation of these receptors can produce long-lasting, even permanent changes in the postsynaptic neuron.

Termination of Synaptic Transmission

As discussed, the arrival of an action potential at the synapse induces release of a neurotransmitter into the synaptic cleft, and the transmitter then reversibly binds to postsynaptic receptors. Certain mechanisms must be present to get rid of neurotransmitter; otherwise transmitter would remain in the synaptic cleft and continually bind to the

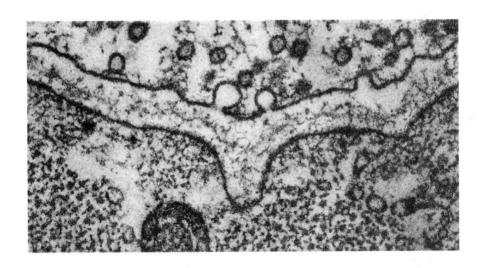

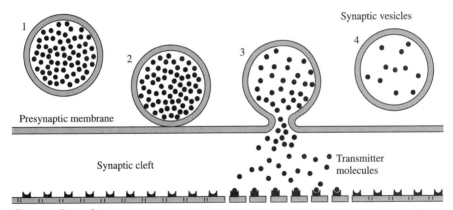

FIGURE 3.5 *Top:* Photomicrograph of a synapse in action taken with the electron microscope. Vesicles are releasing their transmitter chemical into the synaptic cleft. *Bottom:* Schematic of the process.

postsynaptic receptors. Every synapse is able to accomplish the removal of transmitter from the synaptic cleft. Transmitter removal occurs through either of two mechanisms:

1. An enzyme present in the synaptic cleft breaks down any neurotransmitter lingering within the synapse.
2. The transmitter is taken back into the presynaptic cell through the 12-helix reuptake transporter receptor present on the presynaptic membrane (see Figure 2.7).

The vast majority of neurotransmitters are removed by the second mechanism, reuptake. Examples:

- Norepinephrine, uptake of which is blocked by the *tricyclic antidepressants* (Chapter 15)
- Serotonin, uptake of which is blocked by the *serotonin-specific reuptake inhibitor* (SSRI) *antidepressants* (Chapter 15)
- Dopamine, uptake of which is blocked by *bupropion* (Welbutrin, Zyban; Chapters 8 and 15), *cocaine, amphetamine,* and *methylphenidate* (Ritalin; Chapter 7).

In the case of the neurotransmitter acetylcholine, the enzyme *acetylcholine esterase* breaks down the transmitter into acetate and choline, which are then taken up into the nerve terminal and the acetylcholine resynthesized.

Receptor Specificity

It would be nice to think that for each specific neurotransmitter there is a single receptor type. In reality, virtually every transmitter has at least two distinct receptor subtypes on which it acts. For example, as stated, the transmitters norepinephrine, serotonin, and dopamine act on (have affinity for) multiple postsynaptic receptors as well as a presynaptic transporter. On the postsynaptic membrane, a neurotransmitter may bind to both fast-response (ion channel) receptors and slow-response (G-protein-coupled) receptors. A transmitter may bind to different types of G-protein-coupled receptors, each initiating different intracellular processes. For example, for serotonin receptors, at least 18 different subtypes of receptors have been described. All this leads to immense opportunity for the development of drugs with incredible specificity—for example, for blocking one specific subtype of postsynaptic serotonin receptor, reducing or eliminating the side effects that limit the clinical usefulness of existing psychotherapeutic agents. Table 3.1 lists a few of the commonly recognized neurotransmitters, some of the receptor subtypes that have been identified, and some of the brain functions thought to be under the control of each transmitter.

The Soma

Present in all cells of the body (except red blood cells), the soma has a *nucleus* that contains the basic genetic material (the DNA) for the cell (Figure 3.3). Because the neuron is a specialized type of cell, its DNA expresses a subset of genes that encode the special structural and enzymatic proteins that endow the neuron with its size, shape, location, and other functional characteristics.[7] Also located in the soma are the

TABLE 3.1 Selected neurotransmitters in the CNS

Neurotransmitter	Receptors	Function[a]
Acetylcholine (ACh)	Muscarinic (M_1 through M_5) Nicotinic (N_N and N_M)	Memory function, sensory processing, motor coordination, neuromuscular junction neurotransmission, and ANS and PANS function
Norepinephrine (NE)	Alpha$_1$ and alpha$_2$; beta$_1$, beta$_2$, and beta$_3$.	CNS sensory processing, cerebellar function, sleep, mood, learning, memory, anxiety, and SANS
Dopamine (DA)	D_1 through D_5 in two families designated D-1 and D-2	Motor regulation, reinforcement, olfaction, mood, concentration, hormone control, and hypoxic drive
Serotonin (5HT)	Currently 18 receptors have been identified and broken into 8 families designated $5HT_1$ through $5HT_8$	Emotional processing, mood, appetite, sleep, pain processing, hallucinations, and reflex regulation
Glutamate (Glu)	NMDA, quisqualate, and kainate	Long-term potentiation, memory, major excitatory function within the CNS and PNS
Gamma-amino-butyric acid (GABA)	$GABA_A$ and $GABA_B$	Major inhibitory neurotransmitter in the CNS
Histamine (H)	H_1 and H_2	Sleep, sedation, and temperature regulation
Glycine (Gly)		Major inhibitory function within the spinal cord

[a]ANS = autonomic nervous system, PANS = parasympathetic autonomic nervous system, SANS = sympathetic autonomic nervous system
From Carvey[6], page 7, with permission.

mitochondria, which provide the biological energy for the neuron. This energy, in the form of *adenosine triphosphate* (ATP), is made available for all the various chemical reactions carried out in the cell (such as neurotransmitter synthesis, storage, release, and reuptake).

In response to stimuli (perhaps initiated by a second-messenger action), the DNA in the nucleus is transcribed into a second similar molecular form as strands of ribonucleic acid (RNA), which is then "edited" by several rapid steps and exported from the nucleus to the cytoplasm of the soma.[7] The edited RNA is called *messenger RNA*, and this nuclear material is then translated from the nucleic acid code of the RNA into the amino acid sequence of the protein that is to be expressed (Figure 3.6). Expression, or translation, occurs on the *endoplasmic reticulum*, where the neurotransmitters are synthesized and then "packaged" into vesicles that are then transported in specialized *microtubules* down the axon to the synaptic terminals, where they await release (Figure 3.7). Even the presynaptic receptors (such as the dopamine transporter) are made in the soma and carried down the axon, embedding in the cell membrane where they exert their synaptic functions.

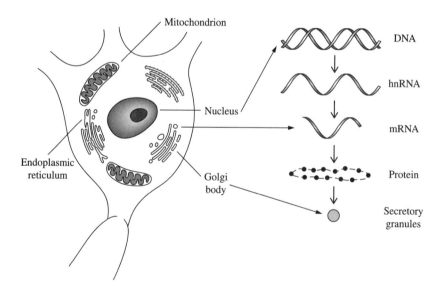

FIGURE 3.6 Formation of transmitter substances and "packaging" in vesicles from genetic material in the nucleus. DNA-encoded information is transcribed in the nucleus to a primary transcript form (hnRNA), which is edited and exported from the nucleus to the cytoplasm as messenger RNA (mRNA). The information is then translated from the genetic nucleic acid code of RNA into the amino acid sequence of the protein that is to be expressed. Within the Golgi body portion of the endoplasmic reticulum, the transmitter is packaged into secretory organelles for transport down the axon to the neuron terminals.

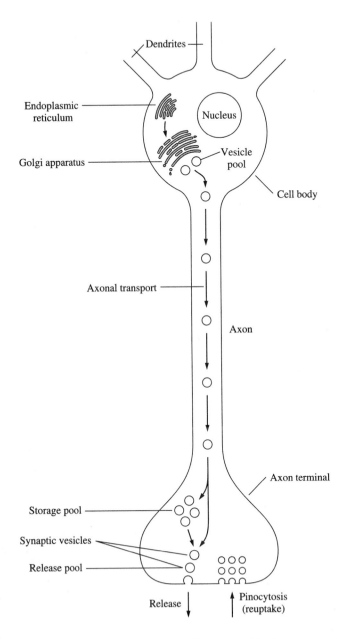

FIGURE 3.7 Axon transport. Chemicals travel from the cell body to the terminals. It is believed that they move along the axon in microtubules that fill the axon.

Summary

Neurotransmission is complex. Each nerve terminal releases many chemicals and perhaps even more than one transmitter; each neurotransmitter acts on many subtypes of receptors, some of which induce rapid and short-lived actions, others of which induce slow-onset, long-duration actions. Cellular responses are mediated by intracellular cascades ranging from ion fluxes to alteration in genetic expression. Despite this complexity, however, and the resulting difficulty in understanding brain function, mood, memory, cognition, thought processes, and behavior can be pharmacologically manipulated to an unprecedented degree. Soon psychological and memory processes may be able to be improved and dysfunctional thought and behavioral states alleviated to a degree never before known, perhaps even without necessarily inducing uncomfortable, debilitating, and limiting side effects and toxicities that complicate current therapies. The twenty-first century should see remarkable strides in pharmacotherapy.

Specific Neurotransmitters

Acetylcholine

Acetylcholine (ACh) was identified as a transmitter chemical first in the peripheral nervous system and later in brain tissue. Deficiencies in acetylcholine-secreting neurons have classically been associated with the dysfunctions seen in Alzheimer's disease. Certainly drugs that either potentiate or inhibit the central action of acetylcholine exert profound effects on memory. For example, scopolamine is a psychedelic drug (Chapter 12) that blocks central cholinergic receptors and as a result produces amnesia. Conversely, drugs that increase the amount of acetylcholine in the brain appear to improve memory function and are used to delay the onset of Alzheimer's disease.

ACh is synthesized in a one-step reaction from two precursors (choline and acetate) and then is stored within synaptic vesicles for later release. This reaction and the dynamics of ACh release, metabolism, and resynthesis are shown in Figure 3.8. Like other neurotransmitters, ACh is released into the synaptic cleft, rapidly diffuses across the cleft, and reversibly binds to postsynaptic receptors. Once ACh has exerted its effect on postsynaptic receptors, its action is terminated by *acetylcholine esterase* (AChE).

The enzymatic reaction that degrades ACh is important not only in the treatment of Alzheimer's disease but in agriculture and in the military. Drugs that inhibit the action of AChE are referred to as *AChE inhibitors* and are of three types: (1) reversible inhibitors, (2) irreversible inhibitors, and (3) "pseudo-irreversible" inhibitors.

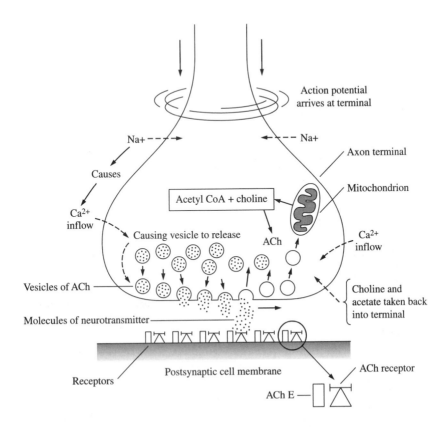

FIGURE 3.8 Chemical synapse. Acetylcholine (ACh) is used as the example. It is made in the axon terminal from acetyl coenzyme A (acetyl CoA) and choline, stored in vesicles, and released. When the action potential arrives at the terminal, closed calcium channels in the terminal are opened and Ca^{2+} rushes into the terminal, triggering vesicles to fuse with the membrane and release ACh molecules into the synaptic cleft. They attach to ACh receptors on the postsynaptic membrane and trigger the opening of Na^+ channels. ACh is immediately broken down at the receptors by acetylcholine esterase (AChE) into choline and acetate, which are taken back up by the terminal and reused. [From Thompson,[1] p. 77.]

Irreversible AChE inhibitors form a permanent covalent bond with the enzyme and totally inhibit enzyme function. Usually administered in "toxic" doses, the result is usually fatal. Some of these toxic drugs (such as *malathion* and *parathion*) are exploited in gardening and agriculture as insecticides, as they kill insects upon contact. Other irreversible AChe inhibitors (such as *Sarin* and *Soman*) are used in the military as lethal nerve gases.

Less toxic and shorter acting are the *reversible AChE inhibitors*. These are used to more modestly increase ACh levels in the brain. They increase ACh levels and clinically are used as cognitive enhancers, delaying the decline in cognitive function in patients with Alzheimer's disease. *Tacrine* (Cognex) and *donepezil* (Aricept) are the two reversible AChE inhibitors currently available for clinical use

Another AChE inhibitor, *rivastigmine* (Exelon), became clinically available in 1999. Rivastigmine is a longer-lasting drug; it forms a covalent bond with the enzyme, temporarily inactivating the enzyme. Slowly, the covalent bond is broken and enzymatic activity reestablished. The drug is therefore termed a "pseudo-irreversible" AChE inhibitor, with enzyme inhibition lasting much longer (about 10 hours) than the plasma half-life of the drug (about 1 hour).[8,9]

Two other AChE inhibitors are being evaluated for use in treating Alzheimer's disease. *Memantine*[10] is a neuroprotective agent; its action occurs because it is an antagonist of the NMDA type of glutamate receptor. Memantine is currently being studied for use in the treatment of the dementia of Alzheimer's disease.

Metrifonate is a "prodrug" (i.e., it has no activity of its own). It is enzymatically broken down to an active metabolite that forms a stable drug-enzyme complex with acetylcholine esterase, which results in long-lasting enzyme inhibition. Clinically, metrifonate has been shown to benefit the cognitive decline, behavior, and daily performance of patients with mild to moderate Alzheimer's disease.[11] Its clinical status is currently unclear.[12]

White and Levin[13] demonstrated that *nicotine skin patches* can produce sustained improvements in attentional behavior in Alzheimer's patients, although cognitive functioning was unchanged. Nicotine augments cholinergic (ACh) function, primarily in the frontal cortex, although effects on the hippocampus may also be involved.

Some 20 years ago the idea developed that symptoms of Alzheimer's disease are due to a deficiency of ACh in the brain. The activities of enzymes involved in the synthesis and degradation of acetylcholine were found to be reduced, and the deficiencies were associated with the severity of the disease. Pathological changes involve cholinergic neuronal pathways that project from the basal forebrain to the cerebral cortex and hippocampus. These pathways are known to be involved in memory, attention, learning, and other cognitive processes. The cholinergic deficiency hypothesis for Alzheimer's disease proposes that the cognitive deterioration is related to deficits in acetylcholine or cholinergic neurotransmission, and current medical treatments reflect this hypothesis.[14,15,16]

Recently, Davis and colleagues[17] challenged this cholinergic hypothesis by demonstrating that cholinergic deficits appear to be present only in patients in the late stages of Alzheimer's disease, not those in the early stages. What, then, might be the deficiency responsible for the early cognitive dysfunction seen in this disease? As stated by Davies[18] in an accompanying editorial:

Clinical symptoms appear to correlate with the spread of the disease from the hippocampus into the association areas of the neocortex. Disruption of hippocampal circuitry has been suggested as an explanation of the impairments of memory that are characteristic of Alzheimer's disease. Perhaps therapeutic efforts to treat the early cognitive decline in this disease will have to be directed toward restoration of these circuits, which, for the most part, use *glutamate* as the neurotransmitter.

ACh is distributed widely in the brain (Figure 3.9). The cell bodies of cholinergic neurons in the brain lie in two closely related regions. One involves the *septal nuclei* and the *nucleus basalis*. The axons of these neurons project to forebrain regions, particularly the hippocampus

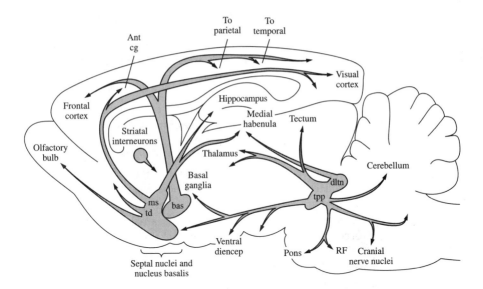

FIGURE 3.9 Representation of the cholinergic systems in the rat brain. As illustrated, central cholinergic neurons exhibit two basic organizational schemata: (1) local circuit cells (those that morphologically are arrayed wholly within the neural structure in which they are found) exemplified by the interneurons of the caudate-putamen nucleus; (2) projection neurons (those that connect two or more different regions). Of the cholinergic projection neurons that interconnect central structures, two major subconstellations have been identified: (1) the forebrain cholinergic complex composed of neurons in the medial septal nucleus (ms) and nucleus basalis (bas) and projecting to the entire nonstriatal telencephalon; (2) the pontomesencephalotegmental cholinergic complex, composed of cells in the pedunculopontine (tpp) and laterodorsal (dltn) tegmental nuclei and projecting ascendingly to the thalamus and other diencephalic loci and descendingly to the pontine and medullary reticular formation (RF), cerebellum, and cranial nerve nuclei. [Modified with permission from N. J. Woolf, "Cholinergic Systems in Mammalian Brain and Spinal Cord," *Progress in Neurobiology* 37 (1991), 475–524.]

and cerebral cortex. The second originates in the midbrain region and projects anteriorly to the thalamus, basal ganglia, and diencephalon and posteriorly to the reticular formation, pons, cerebellum, and cranial nerve nuclei. In addition to its generally agreed-on role in learning and memory, the diffuse distribution of ACh is consistent with suggestions that ACh is involved in circuits that modulate sensory reception; in mechanisms related to behavioral arousal, attention, energy conservation, and mood; and in REM activity during sleep.[19]

Catecholamine Neurotransmitters: Dopamine, Norepinephrine, and Epinephrine

The term catecholamine refers to compounds that contain a catechol nucleus (a benzene ring with two attached hydroxyl groups) to which is attached an amine group (Figure 3.10). In the CNS, the term usually refers to the transmitter dopamine (DA) and its metabolic product (in some neurons) norepinephrine (NE). In the peripheral nervous system, epinephrine ("adrenalin") is a third catecholamine transmitter. In the brain, a large number of psychoactive drugs (both licit and illicit) exert their effects by altering the synaptic action of NE and DA.

The chemical synthesis of DA is illustrated in Figure 3.10. NE is produced by an additional step that involves oxidation of the proximal carbon of the ethyl side chain. Biosynthesis of the catecholamines begins with the amino acid tyrosine and is an exceedingly complicated process involving genetic and enzymatic regulation. Following synthesis, the transmitter is stored in vesicles for release into the synaptic space. Interestingly, such release is tightly controlled (modulated) by *presynaptic receptors* (autoreceptors) that are activated not only by NE or DA but by such substances as ACh, prostaglandins, other amines, and possibly glutamate and/or endorphins. Such autoreceptors will probably become important targets of action for newly developed drugs, such as the antidepressant *mirtazapine* (Remeron; Chapter 15). In addition, drugs such as the amphetamines (Chapter 7) can induce the release of stored catecholamines.

Following release, NE and DA exert their characteristic postsynaptic effects. As discussed earlier, inactivation in the synaptic cleft occurs primarily by reuptake of the transmitter from the synaptic cleft back into the presynaptic nerve terminal. Within the nerve terminal, catecholamines can be inactivated by enzymes, such as monoamine oxidase (MAO). The products of inactivation are further metabolized and eliminated from the body through the urine. The class of antidepressants referred to as MAO inhibitors (Chapter 15) act by inhibiting MAO and thereby increasing the amounts of DA and NE available for synaptic release.

Postsynaptic Catecholamine Receptors.   Unlike transmitters such as ACh and GABA (Chapter 6), which affect ion channels, postsynaptic

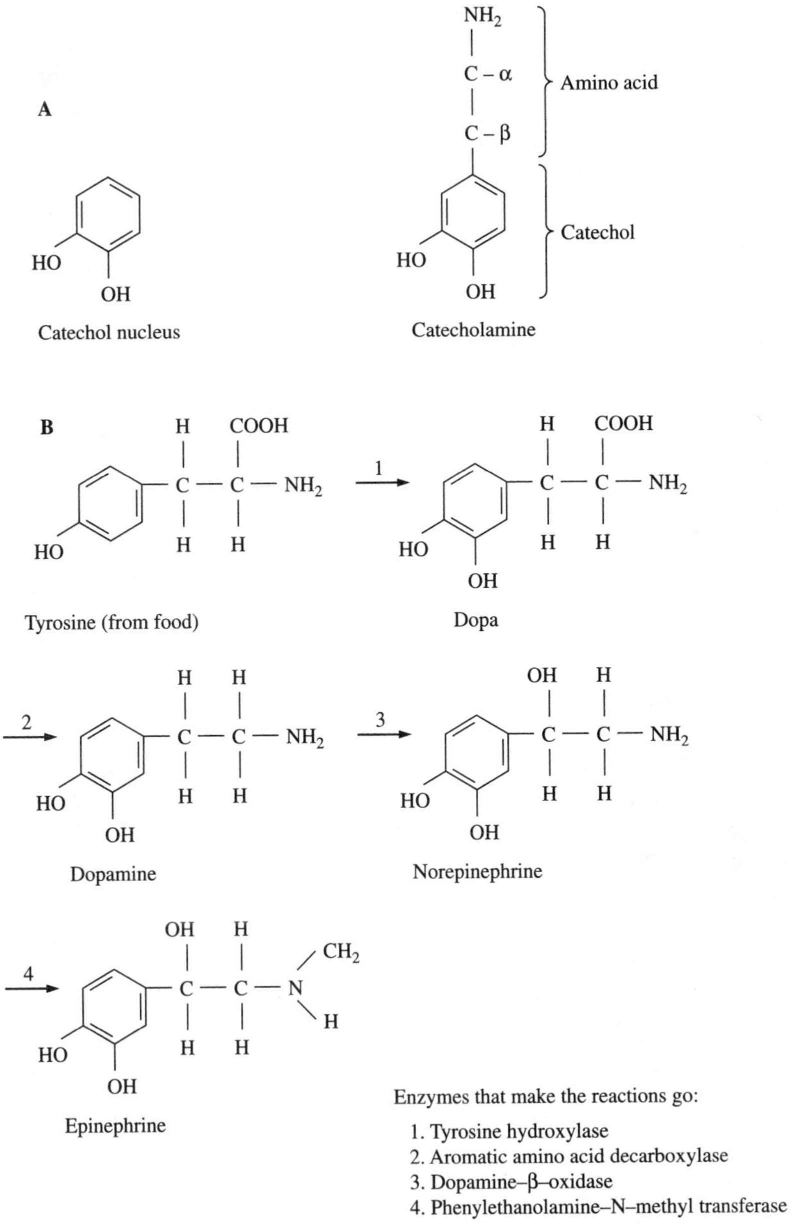

FIGURE 3.10 (A) Catechol and catecholamine structure. All catecholamines share the catechol nucleus, a benzene ring with two adjacent hydroxyl (OH) groups. **(B)** Structures and synthesis of the catecholamines. Tyrosine, an amino acid found in foods, is converted into dopa, then into dopamine, next into norepinephrine, and, finally (in the peripheral nervous system) into epinephrine, depending on which enzymes (1–4) are present in the cell.

binding of DA or NE triggers a sequence of chemical events within the postsynaptic cell membrane (Figure 2.8), eventually affecting either ion channels or intracellular metabolic activity. It is likely that the slow onset of action of antidepressant drugs (several weeks to achieve a therapeutic effect) follows the down regulation of postsynaptic catecholamine receptors as an adaptation to the presence of increased amounts of transmitter present in the synaptic cleft (because the reuptake elimination of the transmitter was blocked by the drug).

Each catecholamine transmitter exerts effects on a number of different postsynaptic receptors. Norepinephrine and epinephrine exert effects at two primary types of receptors (*alpha* and *beta*), each of which has at least two subtypes. Dopamine exerts postsynaptic effects on at least six receptors, divided into two families (D_1 and D_2). Confusingly, D_1 receptors are subdivided into two types: D_1 and D_5. There are four subtypes of D_2 receptors, termed D_{2A}, D_{2B}, D_3, and D_4. Postsynaptic dopamine receptors of the D_2 family are responsible for at least part of the antipsychotic activity of the drugs discussed in Chapter 17. Alterations in dopamine receptor function have been implicated in numerous disease and behavioral states including schizophrenia, Parkinsonism, Huntington's chorea, affective disorders, sexual activity, reward, ADHD, and others.

Norepinephrine Pathways.   The cell bodies of NE neurons are located in the brain stem, mainly in the *locus coeruleus* (Figure 3.11). From there, axons project widely throughout the brain to nerve terminals in the cerebral cortex, the limbic system, the hypothalamus, and the cerebellum. Axonal projections also travel to the dorsal horns of the spinal cord, where they exert an analgesic action (Chapter 9). The release of NE produces an alerting, focusing, orienting response, positive feelings of reward, and analgesia. NE release may also be involved in basic instinctual behaviors, such as hunger, thirst, emotion, and sex.

Dopamine Pathways.   Dopamine pathways in the brain originate in the brain stem, sending axons both rostral to the brain and caudal to the spinal cord. Three dopamine circuits are classically described (Figure 3.12):

1. Cell bodies in the hypothalamus send short axons to the pituitary gland. Such neurons are believed to function in the regulation of certain body hormones. Alterations in hormone function are commonly seen in people with schizophrenia taking phenothiazine antipsychotics, which block these dopamine receptors (Chapter 17).

2. Cell bodies in the brain stem structure called the substantia nigra project to the basal ganglia, playing a major role in the regulation of movement. Parkinsonism, its treatment with l-DOPA (Chapter 18),

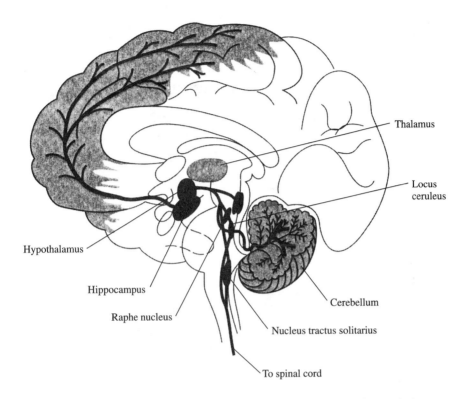

Thalamus

Locus
ceruleus

Hypothalamus

Hippocampus

Raphe nucleus

Cerebellum

Nucleus tractus solitarius

To spinal cord

FIGURE 3.11 NE projection system in the human brain. The cell bodies are in the locus coeruleus and adjacent regions of the brain stem and project widely to the forebrain and cerebellum and to the brain stem and spinal cord.

and antipsychotic-induced extrapyramidal side effects (Chapter 17) all involve this pathway.

3. Cell bodies in the midbrain (ventral tegmentum), near the substantia nigra, project to higher brain regions including the cerebral cortex (especially the frontal cortex) and the limbic system, including the limbic cortex, nucleus accumbens, amygdaloid complex, and the entorhinal cortex; the entorhinal cortex is the major source of neurons projecting to the hippocampus. Alterations in the development of this pathway may be involved in the pathogenesis of schizophrenia and its amelioration by neuroleptic drugs. In addition, this dopaminergic pathway involving the ventral tegmentum, nucleus accumbens, and frontal cortex appears to underlie our "central reward pathway" (Figure 3.13), augmentation of which appears necessary to induce compulsive abuse and sustain continued use of most drugs of abuse (discussed further in Chapter 7).

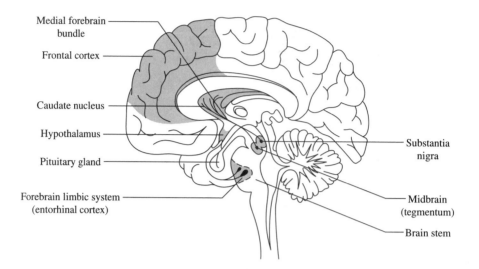

Medial forebrain bundle

Frontal cortex

Caudate nucleus

Hypothalamus

Pituitary gland

Forebrain limbic system (entorhinal cortex)

Substantia nigra

Midbrain (tegmentum)

Brain stem

FIGURE 3.12 The three dopamine systems in the brain. One is a local circuit in the hypothalamus; another is the pathway from the substantia nigra to the caudate nucleus of the basal ganglia, which is involved in motor functions and Parkinson's disease; the third consists of cell bodies in the brain stem and midbrain (tegmentum) that project widely to the cerebral cortex and forebrain limbic system (entorhinal cortex).

Serotonin (5-hydroxytryptamine, 5-HT)

Serotonin was first investigated as a CNS neurotransmitter in the 1950s when lysergic acid diethylamide (LSD) was found to structurally resemble serotonin and blocked the contractile effect of serotonin on the GI tract. At that time, it was hypothesized that LSD-induced hallucinations might be caused by alterations in the functioning of serotonin neurons and that serotonin might be involved in abnormal behavioral functioning. Today, drugs that potentiate the synaptic actions of serotonin are widely used as antidepressants and antianxiety agents against such disorders as obsessive compulsive disorder, panic disorder, and phobias. Most such drugs fall under the category of *serotonin-specific reuptake inhibitors* (SSRIs; Chapter 15). Serotonin plays a role in depression and other affective states, sleep, sex, and the regulation of body temperature; use of an SSRI to treat depression can be associated with such side effects as insomnia, anxiety, and loss of libido. Jacobs[20] edits a recent symposium on serotonin.

Significant amounts of serotonin are found in the upper brain stem, with a large collection in the pons and the medulla (areas that are collectively called the *raphe nuclei*). Rostral projections from the brain stem terminate diffusely throughout the cerebral cortex, hippocampus, hypothalamus, and limbic system (Figure 3.14). Serotonin

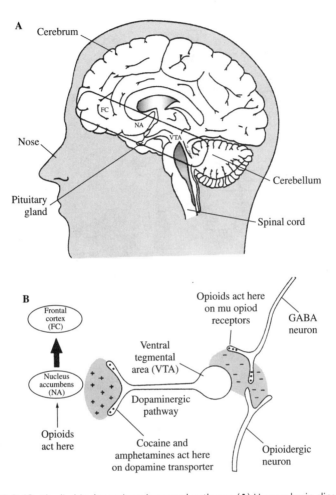

FIGURE 3.13 The limbic dopaminergic reward pathway. (**A**) Human brain sliced open lengthwise, showing the relevant midbrain and forebrain area, outlined by an oval, with ventral tegmental area (VTA), nucleus accumbens (NA), and frontal cortex (FC) labeled. (**B**) Diagram of the area outlined in (**A**). Heavy dots = stored neurotransmitter at nerve endings; + = excitatory neurotransmitter; − = inhibitory neurotransmitter.

projections largely parallel those of DA, although they are not as widespread. Serotonin seems to have an effect that is opposite that of DA, and altered serotonin function has been postulated to augment the behavioral stimulant actions of cocaine[21]; serotonin receptors have been postulated to "modulate the activity of dopaminergic reward pathways and thus the effects of various drugs of abuse."[22] Axons of serotonin neurons projecting to the spinal cord from cell bodies located in the raphe nuclei may be involved in the modulation of both pain (Chapter 9) and spinal reflexes.

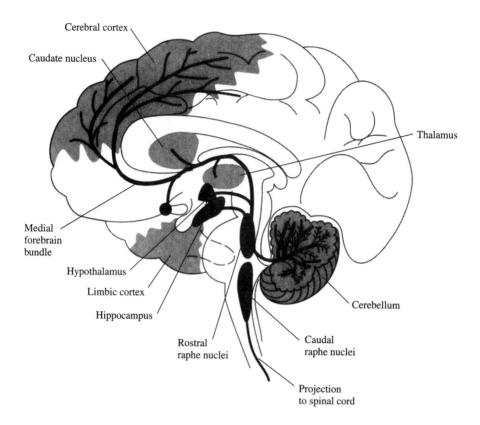

FIGURE 3.14 Serotonin pathways in the human brain. Cell bodies and fiber tracts (axonal projections) are shown in black. Serotonergic terminals are represented by the shaded areas.

In addition to the presynaptic serotonin transporter (blocked by SSRIs), more than 18 subtypes of postsynaptic serotonin (5-HT) receptors have been identified. They have been classified in terms of families (designated by a number) and subtypes within a family (designated by a letter). Note that this is a different type of designation than the one for dopamine. The four main families of 5-HT receptors are designated 5-HT_1, 5-HT_2, 5-HT_3, and 5-HT_4. The 5-HT_3 receptor is a ligand-gated ion channel; the others use a G-protein-coupled second-messenger system. Beyond this, receptor function becomes exceedingly complicated.[23]

Amino Acids as Neurotransmitters

The "classical" neurotransmitters (ACh, NE, DA, and serotonin), although important in behavioral regulation and in the actions of psychotropic drugs, are nevertheless used by only a small proportion of the neurons in the brain.[24] Amino acids are small molecules that serve as neurotransmitters for the remaining majority population of neurons. While some amino acids serve as precursor molecules for biosynthesis of other transmitters (e.g., tyrosine for catecholamines and tryptophan for serotonin), others act directly as neurotransmitters themselves.[24] These amino acid neurotransmitters are the main excitatory and inhibitory transmitters in the brain; they act to modulate a number of ion channels and G-protein-coupled receptors.

Glutamate (also called *glutamic acid* in its nonionized form) and *aspartate* (*aspartic acid*) are the principle excitatory transmitters for fast-responding excitatory signals. Of these two amino acids, glutamate is the better studied, especially in drug action.

Equal to glutamate and aspartate as excitatory neurotransmitters, inhibitory neurotransmission is vital to behavioral control mechanisms, and two amino acids function as universally inhibitory neurotransmitters. These two compounds are *gamma-aminobutyric acid* (GABA) and *glycine*. The following sections focus on glutamate and GABA as prototypes because they are currently more implicated in the action of psychoactive drugs than are aspartate and glycine.

Glutamate. Glutamate is a major excitatory neurotransmitter in the brain. Glutamate receptors are found on the surface of virtually all neurons. Interestingly, glutamate is also the precursor for the major inhibitory neurotransmitter GABA; GABA is formed from glutamate under control of the enzyme *glutamic acid decarboxylase*. Glutamate neurotransmission plays a critical role in cortical and hippocampal cognitive function, pyramidal and extrapyramidal motor function, cerebellar function, and sensory function.[25] Research is focusing on the importance of glutamate dysfunction in the pathogenesis of schizophrenia (especially the negative symptoms and the cognitive dysfunction associated with the disorder; discussed at length in Chapter 17).

Glutamate is a nonessential amino acid, meaning that it can be easily synthesized in the body and is not required in the diet. It can be synthesized by a number of different chemical reactions, among which is the normal breakdown of glucose. A second reaction is synthesis from glutamine. In this mechanism (which might be the more important for neuronal glutamate), there is a glutamine cycle in which synaptically inactive glutamine serves as a reservoir of glutamate. In this cycle, after glutamate is released from a neuron and exerts its excitatory effect, it is transported (taken up) into astrocytes (neighboring support cells in the brain) and converted to glutamine, which is stored in the astrocyte. Eventually, the glutamine diffuses out of the astrocytes and enters the presynaptic nerve terminals, where it is converted to glutamate, the active neurotransmitter. The cycle then repeats.[26]

Postsynaptic glutamate receptors may be *ionotropic* (directly coupled to membrane ion channels permeable to sodium and/or calcium) or *metabotropic* (coupled to G-proteins).[27] The ionotropic receptor subtypes are of three types: NMDA, kainate, and AMPA (alpha-amino-hydroxy-methyl-isoxazolepropionate; Figure 3.15). These receptors mediate rapid excitation of postsynaptic neurons. Certain antianxiety and antiepileptic drugs may act by blocking these receptors, thus reducing brain excitability, although Kamiya and colleagues[28] found that while barbiturate sedatives (Chapter 5)

> depressed the AMPA receptor-mediated currents significantly at clinically relevant concentrations, both the convulsant and depressant isomers (of barbiturates) reduced the currents. . . . These results indicate that AMPA receptor inhibition is not important for the hypnotic action of barbiturates.

Lerma and co-workers [29] and Deshpande[30] discuss the possible roles of kainate-type glutamate receptors in health and disease.

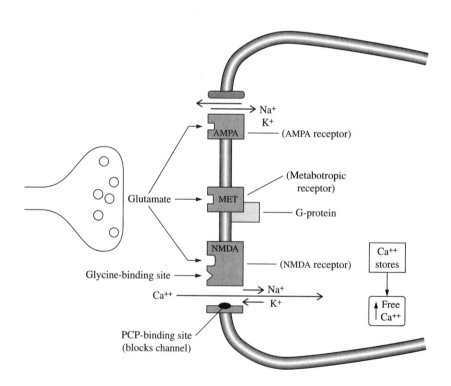

FIGURE 3.15 Glutamate receptor family. The AMPA receptor controls fast sodium and potassium channels; the NMDA receptor controls calcium channels; the metabotropic receptor controls a second-messenger system via a G-protein that acts on the intracellular machinery of the cell. (PCP is discussed in Chapter 12.)

The *N-methyl-D-aspartate* (NMDA) *receptor* is another glutamate ionotropic channel, primarily for calcium ions. NMDA receptors are widely distributed in the brain and spinal cord, with particularly high receptor densities in the hippocampus and cerebral cortex. These receptors appear also to be involved in the developmental plasticity of the brain and in processes of learning and memory.

NMDA receptors are selectively blocked by phencyclidine (PCP; Chapter 12), a psychedelic drug whose actions are characterized by analgesia, amnesia, and psychedelic effects. As discussed, they are also blocked by *memantine*. Besides being studied for use in Alzheimer's disease, memantine is marketed in Europe for the treatment of Parkinsonism. Overactivity of NMDA receptors may be involved in neurotoxicity following ischemia (lack of oxygen) or other types of brain injury.[30] In head injury, excess inflow of calcium ions leads to greatly increased postsynaptic neuronal transcription of messenger RNA with a complex series of events that stimulate gene expression and protein synthesis involving cellular destructive enzymes. NMDA antagonists such as memantine may aid in the protection of brain tissue following injury (such as after a stroke).[12]

As discussed, *metabotropic receptors* are the G-protein-coupled receptors activated by glutamate. They regulate both adjacent ion channels and intracellular enzymes, releasing second messengers.[31] Riedel[32] reviews the role of these receptors in learning and memory via second-messenger-induced alterations in synaptic plasticity that underlie memory formation. Conn and Pin[33] review the pharmacology of these receptors and their agonist and antagonist drugs, many of which have potential usefulness in treating a number of neurologic and psychologic disorders.

Modifinil (Provigil; Chapter 7) became available in 1999 for the treatment of narcolepsy. It appears to augment glutamine neurotransmission (and block GABA neurotransmission), although its exact receptor actions are still unclear. Modifinil theoretically has potential use as a cognitive enhancer, improving memory function in early Alzheimer's disease, a concept in agreement with the observation of Davies discussed earlier in this chapter. Interestingly, tetrahydrocannabinol (Chapter 11) inhibits the release of glutamate, which explains the cognitive inhibition and behavioral intoxication produced by this drug.

Gamma-Aminobutyric Acid (GABA).   GABA, a universally inhibitory transmitter, is found in high concentrations in the brain and spinal cord. Two different types of GABA receptors are described, $GABA_A$ and $GABA_B$. $GABA_A$ receptors are fast receptors, having four transmembrane helical complexes; five receptors join to form an ion channel receptor for chloride ions (Figure 3.16). Activation of this receptor by GABA opens the channel and leads to an influx of chloride into the cell, hyperpolarizing the cell and reducing its excitability. Barbiturate and benzodiazepine

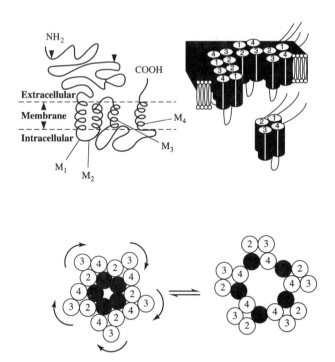

FIGURE 3.16 Presumed topology of the GABA$_A$ receptor. *Top left:* Single subunit with its large extracellular terminal part, and the four transmembrane domains (M1 to M4) with their intracellular connecting stretches. *Top right:* Arrangement of the transmembrane domains of five subunits to form a central channel. *Bottom:* The transmembrane domains in a transverse section through the membrane when the channel is closed (*left*) and (*right*). [Reprinted with permission from W. E. Haefley et al., "The Multiplicity of Actions of Benzodiazepine Receptor Ligands," *Canadian Journal of Psychiatry* 38, Suppl. 4 (1993): 5102–5107.]

binding to this receptor facilitates the action of GABA. Such action is associated with the anxiolytic, amnestic, and anesthetic effects of these sedative drugs.[34] These drugs are discussed at length in Chapters 5 and 6.

GABA$_A$ *receptors* are found in high density in the cerebral cortex, hippocampus, and cerebellum. GABA$_B$ *receptors* are slow-response receptors of the G-protein-coupled type. Activation of GABA$_B$ receptors in the amygdala is associated with the membrane-stabilizing, antiaggressive properties of valproic acid, a drug widely used to treat bipolar disorder (Chapter 16). Important for future pharmacologic research, about ten different subtypes of the GABA$_A$ receptor occur,[35] certainly allowing for the development of agonists and antagonists of specific GABA$_A$ receptor subtypes. Such drugs might be novel antianxiety agents, anticonvulsants, or cognitive enhancers. Wassef and colleagues[36] review the use of GABAergic drugs (especially *valproic acid*; Chapter 16) in the treatment of schizophrenia. Buggy and colleagues[37] reported that certain anesthetic drugs exert their sedative and amnestic actions by activating GABA$_A$ neurons that, in turn, reduce the functioning of glutamate neurons upon which they synapse.

Peptides.   Thirty years ago, only a few neurotransmitters, perhaps a dozen or so, were known, all of them small molecules such as ACh, DA, NE, serotonin, and the amino acids discussed. Now more than 50 (and perhaps hundreds) of neurotransmitters are recognized. Most of the newly identified ones are peptides, which are small proteins (chains of amino acid molecules attached in a specific order).

Peptide transmitters can be classified into several groups; one important group is the opioid-type peptides. Other groups include the hypothalamic releasing hormones, the pituitary hormones, and the so-called gut-brain peptides. Feldman, Meyer, and Quenzer[38] discuss these peptides and their possible implications in psychopharmacology.

In this book, the peptide transmitters of interest are those involved in the actions of the opioids, such as morphine. *Opioid peptides* include the *endorphins* (about 16 to 30 amino acids in length) and the shorter-chain *enkephalins* (5 amino acids in length). These substances are formed from a larger protein produced elsewhere in the body. The endorphins may be involved in a wide variety of emotional states, including pain perception, reward, emotional stability, energetic "highs," and acupuncture. Narcotics such as morphine, codeine, and heroin activate (are agonists at) receptors for endorphins and enkephalins (Chapter 9).

Opioid receptors are termed *mu, kappa,* and *sigma*; the mu receptor mediates most of the analgesic and reinforcing properties of morphine and other narcotics. These receptors are the usual 7-transmembrane-spanning proteins, consisting of about 370 to 400 amino acids. They are G-protein-coupled receptors; activation of the receptor by a neurotransmitter or an exogenous opioid serves to either activate adjacent ion channels (increasing potassium conductance or decreasing calcium conductance) or inhibit the intracellular function of the enzyme adenylate cyclase. From here, the intracellular consequences become quite complicated.

Another peptide transmitter of interest in this book is *substance P*, a *gut-brain peptide* (11 amino acids in length) that plays an important role as a sensory transmitter, especially for pain impulses that enter the spinal cord and brain from a peripheral site of tissue injury. Opioids, serotonin agonists, and norepinephrine agonists exert much of their analgesic effect by acting on substance P nerve terminals to limit the release of this pain-inducing peptide.

Receptors for substance P appears to be G-protein-coupled receptors; activation appears to result in inhibition of adjacent potassium channels and activation of intracellular second messengers (phospholipase C or adenylate cyclase). The role of substance P in pain transmission is discussed in Chapter 9.

STUDY QUESTIONS

1. Define a psychoactive drug.

2. What are some of the functions of the spinal cord?

3. What is a neuron? Describe the following parts of a neuron: dendrites, soma, axon, synaptic terminal.

4. What is a synapse? How does it function?

5. How is the synaptic transmitter action of a released chemical terminated? Give two examples.

6. Name a drug that blocks the action of acetylcholine as a neurotransmitter. What are the consequences of the blockade? Name a drug that potentiates the action of acetylcholine as a transmitter. What might such a drug be used for?

7. Name three catecholamine neurotransmitters. How is their neurotransmitter action terminated? What drugs block this process?

8. Describe the various types of serotonin receptors. What drugs might either stimulate or block them? How might these drugs be applied for therapeutic benefit?

9. Name two amino acid neurotransmitters. Describe any drugs that might potentiate or block the actions of each one. How might these drugs be used therapeutically?

10. What is substance P? How does it relate to neuropharmacology?

REFERENCES

1. R. F. Thompson, *The Brain: A Neuroscience Primer*, 2nd ed. (New York: W. H. Freeman and Company, 1993), 2–3.
2. C. M. Johansson et al., "Identification of a Neural Stem Cell in the Adult Mammalian Central Nervous System," *Cell* 96, (1999): 25–34.
3. G. Kempermann and F. H. Gage, "New Nerve Cells for the Adult Brain," *Scientific American*, May 1999: 48–53.
4. W. S. Sossin, "Mechanisms for the Generation of Synapse Specificity in Long-term Memory: The Implications of a Requirement for Transcription," *Trends in Neurosciences* 19 (1996): 215–218.
5. J. D. Clements, "Transmitter Timecourse in the Synaptic Cleft: Its Role in Central Synaptic Function," *Trends in Neurosciences* 19 (1996): 163–171.
6. P. M. Carvey, *Drug Action in the Central Nervous System* (Oxford: Oxford University Press, 1998), 7.
7. J. R. Cooper, F. E. Bloom, and R. H. Roth, *The Biochemical Basis of Neuropharmacology*, 7th ed. (New York: Oxford, 1996), 293–330.

8. M. Rosler, R. Anand, et al., "Efficacy and Safety of Rivastigmine in Patients with Alzheimer's Disease: International Randomized Controlled Trial," *British Medical Journal* 318 (1999): 633–640.

9. R. J. Polinsky, "Clinical Pharmacology of Rivastigmine: A New Generation Acetylcholinesterase Inhibitor for the Treatment of Alzheimer's Disease," *Clinical Therapeutics* 20 (1998): 634–647.

10. B. Winblad and N. Poritis, "Memantine in Severe Dementia: Results of the M-Best Study (Benefit and Efficacy in Severely Demented Patients During Treatment with Memantine)," *International Journal of Geriatric Psychiatry* 14 (1999): 135–136.

11. M. A. Raskind et al., "The Effects of Metrifonate on the Cognitive, Behavioral, and Functional Performance of Alzheimer's Disease Patients," *Journal of Clinical Psychiatry* 60 (1999): 318–325.

12. J. M. Ringman and J. L. Cummings, "Metrifonate: Update on a New Antidementia Agent," *Journal of Clinical Psychiatry* 60 (1999): 776–782.

13. H. K. White and E. D. Levin, "Four-Week Nicotine Skin Patch Treatment Effects on Cognitive Performance in Alzheimer's Disease," *Psychopharmacology* 143 (1999): 158–165.

14. G. W. Small et al., "Diagnosis and Treatment of Alzheimer's Disease and Related Disorders: Consensus Statement of the American Association for Geriatric Psychiatry, The Alzheimer's Association, and the American Geriatrics Society," *Journal of the American Medical Association* 278 (October 22/29, 1997): 1363–1371.

15. American Psychiatric Association, "Practice Guideline for Treatment of Patients with Alzheimer's Disease and Other Dementias of Late Life," *American Journal of Psychiatry* 154, no. 5, suppl. (May 1997).

16. R. Mayeux and M. Sano, "Treatment of Alzheimer's Disease," *New England Journal of Medicine* 341 (1999): 1670–1679.

17. K. L. Davis et al., "Cholinergic Markers in Elderly Patients with Early Signs of Alzheimer's Disease," *Journal of the American Medical Association* 281 (April 21, 1999): 1401–1406.

18. P. Davies, "Challenging the Cholinergic Hypothesis in Alzheimer's Disease," *Journal of the American Medical Association* 281 (April 21, 1999): 1433–1434.

19. J. L. Cummings, "Cholinesterase Inhibitors: A New Class of Psychotropic Compounds," *American Journal of Psychiatry* 157 (2000): 4–15.

20. B. L. Jacobs, "Special Supplement Issue: Serotonin 50th Anniversary," *Neuropsychopharmacology* 21, no. 25 (August 1999).

21. B. A. Rocha et al., "Cocaine Self-administration in Dopamine-transporter Knockout Mice," *Nature Neuroscience* 1 (1998): 132–137.

22. B. A. Rocha et al., "Increased Vulnerability to Cocaine in Mice Lacking the Serotonin-1B Receptor," *Nature* 393 (1998): 175–178.

23. R. S. Feldman, J. S. Meyer and L. F. Quenzer, *Principles of Neuropsychopharmacology* (Sunderland, Mass.: Sinauer, 1997).

24. R. S. Feldman, J. S. Meyer, and L. F. Quenzer, *Principles of Neuropsychopharmacology* (Sunderland, Mass.: Sinauer, 1997), 391.

25. J. T. Greenamyre and R. H. Porter, "Anatomy and Physiology of Glutamate in the CNS," *Neurology* 44 (1994): S7–S13.

26. R. S. Feldman, J. S. Meyer, and L. F. Quenzer, *Principles of Neuropsychopharmacology* (Sunderland, Mass.: Sinauer, 1997), 394.

27. R. J. Thomas, "Excitatory Amino Acids in Health and Disease," *Journal of the American Geriatrics Society*, 43 (1995): 1279–1289.
28. Y. Kamiya et al., "Comparison of the Effects of Convulsant and Depressant Barbiturate Stereoisomers on AMPA-type Glutamate Receptors," *Anesthesiology* 90 (1999): 1704–1713.
29. J. Lerma, M. Morales, M. A. Vicente, and O. Herreras, "Glutamate Receptors of the Kainate Type and Synaptic Transmission," *Trends in Neurosciences* 20 (1997): 9–12.
30. J. K. Deshpande, "Ischemic Brain Injury: An Update on Mechanisms and Treatment," *American Journal of Anesthesiology* 23 (1996): 206–211.
31. J. P. Pin and R. DuVoisin, "The Metabotropic Glutamate Receptors: Structure and Functions," *Neuropharmacology* 34 (1995): 1–26.
32. G. Riedel, "Function of Metabotropic Glutamate Receptors in Learning and Memory," *Trends in Neurosciences* 19 (1996): 219–224.
33. P. J. Conn and J.-P. Pin, "Pharmacology and Functions of Metabotropic Glutamate Receptors," *Annual Review of Pharmacology and Toxicology* 37 (1997): 205–237.
34. S. L. Tomlin et al., "Preparation of Barbiturate Optical Isomers and Their Effects on GABA$_A$ Receptors," *Anesthesiology* 90 (1999): 1714–1722.
35. R. M. McKernan and P. J. Whiting, "Which GABA$_A$-Receptor Subtypes Really Occur in the Brain?" *Trends in Neurosciences* 19 (1996): 139–143.
36. A. A. Wassef et al., "Critical Review of GABAergic Drugs in the Treatment of Schizophrenia," *Journal of Clinical Psychopharmacology* 19 (1999): 222–232.
37. D. J. Buggy et al., "Effects of Intravenous Anesthetic Agents on Glutamate Release: A Role for GABA$_A$ Receptor-Mediated Inhibition," *Anesthesiology* 92 (2000): 1067–1073.
38. R. S. Feldman, J. S. Meyer, and L. F. Quenzer, *Principles of Neuropsychopharmacology* (Sunderland, Mass.: Sinauer, 1997), 455–491.

PART 2

Drugs That Depress Brain Function: Sedative-Hypnotic Drugs

The CNS depressants are drugs that affect neurons so that the functioning of the brain is altered, resulting in a state of calm, relaxation, disinhibition, drowsiness, and sleep as doses of drug increase. What is observed is dose-related behavioral depression, resulting in relief from anxiety, release from inhibitions, sedation, sleep, unconsciousness, general anesthesia, coma, and, eventually, death from respiratory and cardiac depression.

Drugs that can produce this state include the barbiturates as well as several other sedative-hypnotics of diverse chemical structures, all of which are covered in Chapter 5. General anesthetics and the antiepileptic drugs are also covered in that chapter. Ethyl alcohol is covered in Chapter 4; its unique, nonmedical use in our culture necessitates separate discussion. Also included in that chapter are a variety of volatile inhaled substances (the inhalants of abuse).

Chapter 6 covers the benzodiazepines and several of the newer "second-generation" antianxiety and hypnotic drugs. The benzodiazepines have a somewhat lesser (compared to the older sedatives) capacity to produce deep and potentially fatal CNS depression. Because of this improved margin of safety, the benzodiazepines have largely replaced the older agents for the treatment of anxiety and insomnia and are finding use in the treatment of a wide variety of psychological disorders. Even the benzodiazepines, however, are not devoid of the potential for toxicity, dependency, or abuse. Therefore, the search continues for hypnotic and anxiolytic drugs with increased efficacy and possibly lower potential for toxicity and abuse.

Chapter 4

Ethyl Alcohol and the Inhalants of Abuse

The terms "sedative," "tranquilizer," "anxiolytic," and "hypnotic" can be applied to any CNS depressant, including alcohol, because all diminish environmental awareness, reduce response to sensory stimulation, depress cognitive functioning, decrease spontaneity, and reduce physical activity. Higher doses produce increasing drowsiness, lethargy, amnesia, antiepileptic effects, hypnosis, and anesthesia.

The uniformity of action of CNS depressants correctly implies that the effects of any CNS depressant potentiate the effects of any other CNS depressant. For example, alcohol exaggerates the depression induced by barbiturates, and barbiturates intensify the impairment of driving ability in a person who has been drinking alcohol.

The depressant effects of sedative drugs are frequently supra-additive. Thus, the depression that is observed in a person who has taken more than one drug is greater than would be predicted if the person had taken only one. Such intense depression is often unpredictable and unexpected, and it can lead to dangerous or even fatal consequences. Depressant drugs should not be used in combination, especially if one of the drugs is ethyl alcohol.

All the CNS sedative-hypnotic agents carry the risk of inducing physiological dependence, psychological dependence, and tolerance. *Physiological dependence* is characterized by the occurrence of withdrawal signs and symptoms when the drug is not taken. Signs and symptoms range from sleep disturbances to life-threatening withdrawal convulsions. *Psychological dependence* follows from the positive reinforcement effects of the drugs. *Tolerance* occurs as a result of the induction of drug-metabolizing enzymes in the liver and to the adaptation of cells in the brain. In addition, a remarkable degree of *cross-tolerance* may occur: tolerance to one drug results in a lessened response to another drug. *Cross-dependence* also may be exhibited, in which one drug can prevent the withdrawal symptoms that are associated with physical dependence on a different drug. This observation underlies the clinical use of benzodiazepines to help moderate the signs and symptoms associated with withdrawal from alcohol.

ETHYL ALCOHOL

The term *alcohol* means *ethyl alcohol* (ethanol)—a psychoactive drug that is similar in most respects to the sedative-hypnotic compounds that are discussed in Chapter 5. The main difference from the other depressants is that ethanol is used primarily for recreational rather than medical purposes. Because ethanol is the second most widely used psychoactive substance in the world (after caffeine), its use as a sedative and intoxicant has created special problems for both individual users and society in general.

Pharmacology of Alcohol

Pharmacokinetics

Absorption.   Ethyl alcohol is a simple two-carbon molecule (Figure 4.1). It is rarely drunk in its pure form; rather, it is found in 12 percent concentrations in wines, usually 3.5 to 5 percent in beers (as much as 7 to 10 percent in some "microbrews"*), and 40 to 50 percent in "hard" liquors. In the latter, concentration is usually expressed as alcohol "proof," which is twice the percent concentration (i.e., 80 proof = 40 percent ethanol).

Alcohol is soluble in both water and fat, and it diffuses easily across all biological membranes. Thus, after it is drunk, alcohol is rapidly and completely absorbed from the entire gastrointestinal tract, although most

---

*Micobrewed beers contain anywhere from 4.5 to 10 percent alcohol, depending on the product. Lighter brews contain about 4.5 to 6 percent; heavier bocks and porters may contain 7 to 9 percent alcohol; specialty products, triple beers, and barley wines may contain 10 percent or even more alcohol. Thus, some microbrewed beers may easily contain twice (or three times) as much alcohol as ordinary 3.5 percent beers. [From *The Associa*tion *of Brewers' 1999 Beer Style Guidelines,* American Association of Brewers, Institute of Brewing Studies, P.O Box 1679, Boulder, CO 80306–1679.]

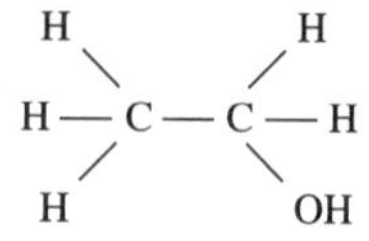

FIGURE 4.1 Structure of ethanol (CH_3CH_2OH).

is absorbed from the upper intestine because of its large surface area. The time from the last drink to maximal concentration in blood ranges from 30 to 90 minutes. In a person with an empty stomach, approximately 20 percent of a single dose of alcohol is absorbed directly from the stomach, usually quite rapidly. The remaining 80 percent is absorbed rapidly and completely from the upper intestine; the only limiting factor is the time it takes to empty the stomach. The importance of gastric emptying time will become apparent in the discussion of the metabolism of alcohol.

Distribution. After absorption, alcohol is evenly distributed through-out all body fluids and tissues. The blood-brain barrier is freely per-meable to alcohol. When alcohol appears in the blood and reaches a person's brain, it crosses the blood-brain barrier almost immediately. Alcohol is also freely distributed across the placenta and easily enters the brain of a developing fetus. Fetal blood alcohol levels are essentially the same as those of the drinking mother. Research on the impact of maternal alcohol consumption on human infants has demonstrated the occurrence of fetal alcohol syndrome, which consists of serious birth defects in 30 to 50 percent of all babies born to alcoholic mothers. Fetal alcohol syndrome was first described more than 20 years ago.[1]

Metabolism and Excretion. Approximately 95 percent of the alcohol a person ingests is enzymatically metabolized by the enzyme *alcohol dehydrogenase*. The other 5 percent is excreted unchanged, mainly through the lungs.* About 85 percent of the metabolism of alcohol oc-curs in the liver. Up to 15 percent of alcohol metabolism is carried out by a gastric alcohol dehydrogenase enzyme, located in the lining of the stomach, which can decrease the blood level of alcohol by about 15 percent, obviously attenuating alcohol's systemic toxicity. The metabo-lism of alcohol by gastric alcohol dehydrogenase is part of what was called *first-pass metabolism* in Chapter 1. Oneta and co-workers[2]

---

*Small amounts of alcohol are excreted from the body through the lungs; most of us are familiar with "alcohol breath." This excretion forms the basis for the breath analysis test, because alcohol equilibrates rapidly across the membranes of the lung. In the "breathalyzer" test, a ratio of 1:2300 exists between alcohol in exhaled air and in venous blood. The blood alcohol concentration is easily extrapolated from the alcohol concentration in the expired air.

demonstrated that rapid gastric emptying (as by drinking on an empty stomach) reduces the time that alcohol is susceptible to first-pass metabolism and results in increased blood levels. Drinking on a full stomach retains alcohol in the stomach, increases its exposure to gastric alcohol dehydrogenase, and reduces the resulting blood level of the drug. Ten years ago, Frezza and co-workers[3] reported that whenever women and men consume comparable amounts of alcohol (after correction for differences in body weight), women have higher blood ethanol concentrations than men (Figure 4.2). The reasons appear to be threefold:

- Women have about 50 percent less gastric metabolism of alcohol than men because women, whether alcoholic or nonalcoholic, have

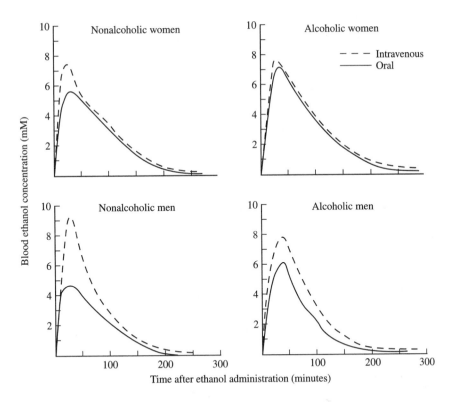

FIGURE 4.2 Effects of route of administration and gender on BAC. Ethanol was administered in a dose of 0.3 mg/kg body weight either by intravenous injection (dashed lines) or orally (solid lines) to nonalcoholic and alcoholic men and women. The higher BAC after oral alcohol intake by women compared with men shows that first-pass metabolism (in the stomach) is lower in women than in men. This is especially noticeable in alcoholic women compared with all other groups of men and women. [Modified from Frezza et al.[3]]

a lower level of gastric alcohol dehydrogenase enzyme. Since the gastric enzyme metabolizes about 15 percent of ingested alcohol, the BAC is increased by about 7 percent over that in a male drinking the same weight-adjusted amount of alcohol.

- Men may have a greater ratio of muscle to fat than do women. Men thus have a larger vascular compartment (fat has little blood supply). Therefore alcohol is somewhat more diluted in men, again increasing blood alcohol levels in women compared to men.

- Women, with a higher body fat than men (fat contains little alcohol), concentrate alcohol in plasma, drink for drink, more than men, raising the apparent blood level.*

The metabolism of alcohol by alcohol dehydrogenase is only the first step in a three-step metabolic process involved in the breakdown of alcohol (Figure 4.3):

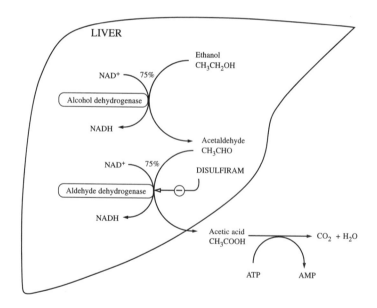

FIGURE 4.3 Metabolism of ethanol. Ethanol is oxidized by the enzyme alcohol dehydrogenase using NAD^+ as a cofactor to form acetaldehyde. A second oxidative step converts acetaldehyde to acetic acid, which, in turn, is broken down to carbon dioxide and water. The first step involving alcohol dehydrogenase is the rate-limiting step. The drug disulfiram (Antabuse) blocks the second step by blocking the activity of aldehyde dehydrogenase.

*These three factors may increase the vulnerability of some women to both acute intoxication and to the chronic complications of alcoholism.[3]

1. *Alcohol dehydrogenase* functions to convert alcohol to acetaldehyde. A coenzyme called *nicotinamide adenine dinucleotide* (NAD) is required for the activity of this enzyme. The availability of NAD is the rate-limiting step in this reaction; enough is present so that the maximum amount of alcohol that can be metabolized in 24 hours is about 170 grams.[4]

2. The enzyme *aldehyde dehydrogenase* converts acetaldehyde to acetic acid. The drug *disulfiram* (Antabuse) irreversibly inhibits this enzyme.

3. Acetic acid is broken down into carbon dioxide and water, thus releasing energy (calories).

The average person metabolizes 6 to 8 grams (about 8 to 10 milliliters) of 100 percent alcohol per hour (about 170 grams divided by 24 hours), independent of the blood level of alcohol. This rate is fairly constant for a given individual[4] and among individuals.* Thus, it would take an adult 1 hour to metabolize the amount of alcohol that is contained in a 1-ounce glass of 80-proof whiskey, a 4-ounce glass of wine, a 12-ounce bottle of 3.5 percent beer, and a 6-ounce glass of 7 percent microbrew. Consumption of 4 ounces of wine, 12 ounces of 3.5 percent beer, 6 ounces of microbrew, or 1 ounce of whiskey per hour would keep the blood levels of alcohol in a person fairly constant. If a person ingests more alcohol in any given hour than is metabolized, his or her blood concentrations increase. Consequently, there is a limit to the amount of alcohol that a person can consume in an hour without becoming drunk.

These kinetics permit not only estimation of blood alcohol concentration after drinking a known amount of alcoholic beverage but also estimation of the fall in blood concentration over time after drinking ceases. The following may serve to explain the relationship between the amount of alcohol consumed, the resulting blood levels of alcohol, and the impairment of motor and intellectual functioning (here, driving ability). Most states define a *blood alcohol concentration* (BAC) of 0.08 grams percent (g%)† as intoxication, and a person who drives with a BAC above this amount can be charged with driving while under the influence of alcohol. Thus, one might assume that a level of 0.07 g% is acceptable but a level of 0.09 g% is not. However, the behavioral effects

---

*In biochemical terms, this is called zero-order metabolism. Virtually all other drugs are metabolized by first-order metabolism, which means that the amount of drug metabolized per unit time depends on the amount (or concentration) of drug in blood (see Chapter 1). Perhaps zero-order metabolism occurs because the amount of enzyme (or a cofactor required for activity of the enzyme) is limited and becomes saturated with only small amounts of alcohol in the body.

†Grams percent is the number of grams of ethanol that would be contained in 100 milliliters of blood.

of alcohol are not all or none; alcohol (like all sedatives) progressively impairs a person's ability to function. Thus, the 0.08 g% blood level is only a legally established, arbitrary value. Driving ability is minimally impaired at a BAC of 0.01 g%, but at 0.05 to 0.08 g%, a driver has increasingly impaired judgment and reactions and becomes less inhibited. As a result, the risk of an accident quadruples. The deterioration of a person's driving ability continues at a BAC of 0.10 to 0.14 g%, leading to a sixfold to sevenfold increase in the risk of having an accident. At 0.15 g% and higher, a person is 25 times more likely to become involved in a serious accident.

Figure 4.4 illustrates the correlation between the number of drink equivalents imbibed, body weight, and the resulting blood alcohol concentration. To use this chart, first glance at the left margin and find the number that is closest to the body weight in pounds. Then look across the columns to the right and find the column that shows the number of drinks consumed. BAC is found by matching body weight with

Blood Alcohol Concentration—A Guide

Drinks   One drink equals 1 ounce of 80 proof alcohol; 12-ounce bottle of beer; 2 ounces of 20% wine; 3 ounces of 12% wine.

Weight (lb)	1	2	3	4	5	6	7	8	9	10
100	.029	.058	.088	.117	.146	.175	.204	.233	.262	.290
120	.024	.048	.073	.097	.121	.145	.170	.194	.219	.243
140	.021	.042	.063	.083	.104	.125	.146	.166	.187	.208
160	.019	.037	.055	.073	.091	.109	.128	.146	.164	.182
180	.017	.033	.049	.065	.081	.097	.113	.130	.146	.162
200	.015	.029	.044	.058	.073	.087	.102	.117	.131	.146
220	.014	.027	.040	.053	.067	.080	.093	.106	.119	.133
240	.012	.024	.037	.048	.061	.073	.085	.097	.109	.122
	CAUTION			DRIVING IMPAIRED			LEGALLY DRUNK			

Alcohol is "burned up" by the body at .015 g% per hour, as follows:

Number of hours since starting first drink	1	2	3	4	5	6
Percent alcohol burned up	.015	.030	.045	.060	.075	.090

Calculate BAC

Example:

180 lb. man — 8 drinks in 4 hours is .130 g% on chart.

Subtract .060 g% burned up in 4 hours. BAC equals .070 g% — DRIVING IMPAIRED.

FIGURE 4.4 Relation between blood alcohol concentration, body weight, and the number of drinks ingested. See text for details.

number of drinks ingested. From this number, subtract the amount of alcohol that has been metabolized (remember that approximately 1 drink equivalent is metabolized in 1 hour). The final figure is the approximate BAC. By calculating this number, the degree to which driving ability is impaired can be predicted.

The following examples illustrate how to use the chart. Consider a 160-pound man who takes 6 drinks in 2 hours. The chart value for the blood alcohol concentration is 0.109 g%. Subtract 0.030 g% for metabolism (0.015 g% in 2 hours). His resulting BAC is 0.079 g%, which is not legally intoxicating but is enough to impair his driving ability. Next consider a 120-pound woman who takes the same 6 drinks in the same 2 hours. The chart value is 0.145 g%. Subtract the same 0.030 g% for metabolism. Her resulting BAC is 0.115 g%, which is a legally intoxicating value.

Some agencies and organizations have even more stringent BAC standards than the states. For example, the Federal Department of Transportation regulations test and limit truck drivers from driving at 0.04 g% and airline pilots from flying at 0.02 g% after 24 hours of abstinence.

Factors that may alter the predictable rate of metabolism of alcohol are usually not clinically significant. With long-term use, however, alcohol can induce drug-metabolizing enzymes in the liver, thereby increasing the liver's rate of metabolizing alcohol (and so inducing *tolerance*) as well as its rate of metabolizing other compounds that are similar to alcohol (termed *cross-tolerance*).

Pharmacodynamics

Identifying the mechanism of the action of alcohol continues to be difficult. For many years, it was presumed that alcohol acted through a general depressant action on nerve membranes and synapses. Because it is both water soluble and lipid soluble, ethanol dissolves into all body tissues. This property led to a unitary hypothesis of action—that the drug dissolves in nerve membranes, distorting, disorganizing, or "perturbing" the membrane, similar to the action of general anesthetics (Chapter 5). The result is nonspecific and indirect depression of neuronal function.

Although this hypothesis may explain the high-dose, or anesthetic, properties of alcohol, experimental evidence is being gathered that alcohol may both disturb the synaptic activity of various neurotransmitters, especially major excitatory (glutamate) and inhibitory (GABA) systems, as well as various intracellular transduction processes. These processes include suppression of calcium ion currents,[5] alteration in intracellular cyclic AMP pathways,[6] and alteration in ATP-activated ion channels.[7]

Glutamate Receptors.   Ethanol is a potent inhibitor of the function of the NMDA-subtype of glutamate receptors.[8-10] Ethanol disrupts glutamatergic neurotransmission by depressing the responsiveness of NMDA receptors to released glutamate. Such attenuation of glutamate responsiveness may be exacerbated by its known enhancement of inhibitory GABA neurotransmission. With chronic alcohol intake and persistent glutamineric suppression, there is a compensatory up regulation of NMDA receptors. Thus, on removal of ethanol's inhibitory effect (as would occur during alcohol withdrawal), these excess excitatory receptors would result in withdrawal signs including seizures.

The drug *acamprosate*, a structural analogue of glutamate (Figure 4.5), is an anticraving drug used to maintain abstinence in alcohol-dependent individuals, an action postulated to be produced by interaction with glutaminergic NMDA receptors, attenuating neuronal hyperexcitability induced by chronic alcohol ingestion and withdrawal.[9,11]

GABA Receptors.   Ethanol activates the GABA-mediated increase in chloride ion flows, resulting in neuronal inhibition.[12] The behavioral results of this would include sedation, muscle relaxation, and inhibition of cognitive and motor skills. A GABAergic antianxiety effect was illustrated by Kushner and co-workers,[13] who demonstrated that low doses of ethanol act acutely to reduce both panic and the anxiety surrounding panic. This finding lends support to the view that drinking by those with panic disorder and anxiety is reinforced by this GABAergic agonist effect. Thus, the use of alcohol to self-medicate one's panic or anxiety disorder may contribute to the high rate at which alcohol-use disorders cooccur with anxiety and panic disorders.

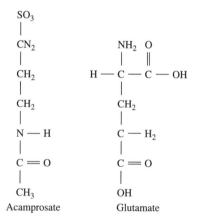

FIGURE 4.5 Structures of acamprosate and glutamate.

Drinking may be both promoted by the short-term anxiolytic effects of alcohol and inhibited by the long-term anxiogenic effects of alcohol. Further, it seems likely that subgroups of those with panic disorder may be more or less prone to escalate drinking aimed at the control of anxiety and panic. Variations in sensitivity to the anxiolytic properties of alcohol, personality dimensions, beliefs about alcohol, and availability of effective coping responses may all influence the likelihood that alcohol is used to control anxiety and panic.[13]

Ethanol binds to a different subunit on the $GABA_A$ receptor than do other GABA agonists.[14] A chronic adaptive effect seems to involve changes in intracellular mRNA, suggesting that chronic alcohol can affect gene expression.[15] As a result of the GABAergic agonist action, other transmitter systems, including the cholinergic (acetylcholine), the dopaminergic (dopamine), the opioid (endorphin), and the serotoninergic (serotonin) systems, are affected.

The GABA agonist action of ethanol has been linked to the positive reinforcing effects of the drug.[16] Indeed, the abuse potential of alcohol follows from an ultimate action to augment dopamine neurotransmitter systems, particularly the dopaminergic projection from the ventral tegmental area (VTA) to the nucleus accumbens and to the frontal cortex (Chapter 3). Whether such action is a direct effect exerted on dopamine-secreting neurons or an indirect effect is still unclear. These possible effects of ethanol are summarized in Figure 4.6.

Wand and co-workers[17] present data consistent with a dysfunctional brain opioid system as part of a neurocircuitry involved in heavy alcohol drinking and alcohol dependence. Alcohol-dependent individuals and their offspring may have a deficit in brain opioid activity; ethanol may induce opioid release; this, in turn, triggers dopamine release in the brain reward system. Administration of *naltrexone* (ReVia, Trexan) blocks opioid release and may reduce alcohol craving.

Serotonin.   There is a growing literature on the role of serotonin in the actions of alcohol. Chronic alcohol consumption results in augmentations in serotoninergic activity, and serotonin dysfunction may play a role in the pathogenesis of alcoholism. Today, emphasis is on the role of serotonin 5-HT_2 and 5-HT_3 receptors in the central effects of ethanol; these receptors are located on dopaminergic neurons in the nucleus accumbens. Antagonist drugs blocking these receptors reduce ethanol intake in animals, secondary to drug-induced increases in serotonin availability in the nucleus accumbens.[18] Consistent with this effect are the observations that serotonin reuptake-inhibiting antidepressants such as *fluoxetine* (Prozac) reduce alcohol craving. In addition, presynaptic serotonin transporter dysfunction can be correlated with predisposition to early-onset alcoholism.[19]

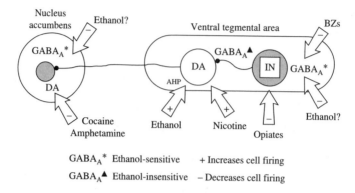

FIGURE 4.6 Putative substrates of pharmacological reinforcement. Schematic illustration of some of the ways in which drugs of abuse might interact with the ventral tegmental area/nucleus accumbens system. Cocaine and amphetamine are likely to act by potentiating dopamine (abbreviated DA) effects in nucleus accumbens, which would have a primarily depressant effect on cell firing, whereas nicotine appears to have a direct excitatory effect on DA neurons in the ventral tegmental area. Opiates, benzodiazepines (BZs), and ethanol may all act to inhibit the firing of inhibitory interneurons (IN) via effects on opiate receptors or on ethanol-sensitive GABA_A receptors. Alternatively, ethanol might have a direct excitatory effect upon the DA cells via a mechanism that does not involve a GABAergic receptor. [From Harris, Brodie, and Dunwiddie.[16]]

Pharmacological Effects

The graded, reversible depression of CNS function is the primary pharmacological effect of alcohol. Respiration, although transiently stimulated at low doses, becomes progressively depressed and, at very high blood concentrations of alcohol, is the cause of death. Alcohol is also anticonvulsant, although it is not clinically used for this purpose. On the other hand, withdrawal from alcohol ingestion is accompanied by a prolonged period of hyperexcitability, and seizures can occur; seizure activity peaks approximately 8 to 12 hours after the last drink.*

In the CNS, the effects of alcohol are additive with those of other sedative-hypnotic compounds, resulting in more sedation and greater impairment of motor and cognitive abilities. Other sedatives (especially the benzodiazepines) and marijuana are the drugs that are most frequently combined with alcohol, and they increase its deleterious effects on motor and intellectual skills (e.g., driving ability) as well as alertness. Patients suffering from insomnia find alcohol to be an effective hypnotic agent.[20]

---

*Ethanol withdrawal seizures may follow from chronic suppression of the NMDA subtype of glutamate receptors with up regulation of these receptors and unmasking of these increasingly sensitive receptors after ethanol ingestion is stopped and withdrawal begins.[8]

Alcohol also affects the circulation and the heart. Alcohol dilates the blood vessels in the skin, producing a warm flush and a decrease in body temperature. Thus, it is pointless and possibly dangerous to drink alcohol to keep warm when one is exposed to cold weather. Long-term use of alcohol is also associated with diseases of the heart muscle, which can result in heart failure. Several reports have noted that low doses of alcohol consumed daily (up to 2.5 ounces) may reduce the risk of coronary artery disease. This protective effect occurs because of an alcohol-induced increase in high-density lipoprotein in blood with a corresponding decrease in low-density lipoprotein. (The higher the concentration of high-density lipoprotein and the lower the concentration of low-density lipoprotein, the lower the incidence of coronary heart disease.) Unfortunately, the cardioprotective effect of low doses of alcohol is lost on people who also smoke cigarettes.

Interestingly, light to moderate doses of alcohol (about two drinks per day) have been shown to reduce the incidence of ischemic strokes (strokes due to loss of oxygen delivery to specific areas of the brain).[21,22] Higher amounts of alcohol (more than five drinks per day) were associated with an increased risk of stroke (Figure 4.7). These

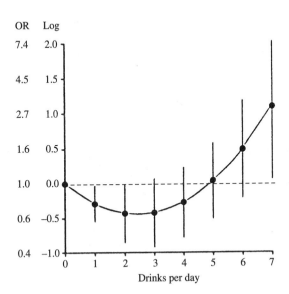

FIGURE 4.7 Relationship between alcohol and stroke. The reference group (indicated by the dashed horizontal line) is those not drinking during the past year. Analysis is matched for age, sex, and race/ethnicity and adjusted for hypertension, diabetes, heart disease, cigarette use, and education. OR = odds ratio for having a stroke. Log = logarithmic scale of stroke incidence. Vertical lines indicate 95 percent confidence intervals. [From Sacco et al.[22]]

levels of alcohol consumption have been shown to decrease the risk of coronary heart disease in patients with adult-onset diabetes.[23] The mechanisms responsible for the protective effect of low doses of alcohol on ischemic stroke appear to involve alcohol-induced increases in (protective) high-density cholesterol and an aspirin-like decrease in platelet aggregation.

Alcohol exerts a diuretic effect on the body by increasing the excretion of fluids as a result of its effects on renal function, by decreasing the secretion of an antidiuretic hormone, and by the diuretic action produced simply by ingesting large quantities of fluid. Alcohol, however, does not appear to harm either the structure or the function of the kidneys.

Alcohol (like all depressant drugs) is not an aphrodisiac. The behavioral disinhibition induced by low doses of alcohol may appear to cause some loss of restraint, but alcohol depresses body function and actually interferes with sexual performance. As Shakespeare says in *Macbeth:* "It provokes the desire, but it takes away the performance."

Psychological Effects

The short-term psychological and behavioral effects of alcohol are primarily restricted to the CNS, where a mixture of stimulant and depressant effects is seen after low doses of the drug. Figure 4.8 correlates the effects of alcohol with levels of the drug measured in the blood. The behavioral reaction to disinhibition, which occurs at low doses, is largely determined by the person,[24] his or her mental expectations, and the environment in which drinking occurs. In one setting a person may become relaxed and euphoric; in another he or she may become withdrawn or violent. Mental expectations and the physical setting become progressively less important at increasing doses, because the sedative effects increase and behavioral activity decreases. At lower doses, behavioral stimulation may involve "the mesolimbic ventral tegmental area to nucleus accumbens dopaminergic pathway . . . where GABA and glutamate have been found to play a role in altering the activity of this dopaminergic pathway."[25]

At low doses, a person may still function (although with less coordination) and attempt to drive or otherwise endanger self and others. Memory, concentration, and insight are progressively dulled and lost. Perceptual speed is an important component of task performance and is markedly impaired by ethanol.[26] As the BAC increases, the drinker becomes progressively incapacitated.

Alcohol intoxication, with its resulting disinhibition, plays a major role in a large percentage of violent crimes, including rape, sexual assault, and certain kinds of deviant behaviors. More than 50 percent of crimes and highway accidents are alcohol related, a number that has changed little in 20 years. More than 10 million individuals in the

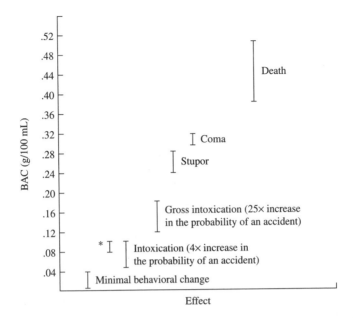

FIGURE 4.8 Correlation of the blood level of ethanol with degrees of intoxication. The legal level of intoxication (*) varies by state; the range of values is shown. BAC = blood alcohol concentration.

United States currently suffer the consequences of alcohol abuse, which include arrests, traffic accidents, occupational injuries, violence, and health and occupational losses. This number does not include the 10 million individuals considered to be alcohol dependent (with their own suffering of negative consequences). Thus, about 10 percent of our society is personally afflicted with (or suffers the consequences of) another's alcohol use.

Long-term effects of alcohol may involve many different organs of a person's body, depending on whether the drinking is moderate or heavy. Long-term ingestion of moderate amounts of alcohol seems to produce few physiological, psychological, or behavioral changes in a person. But long-term ingestion of larger amounts of alcohol leads to a variety of serious neurological, mental, and physical disorders. These disorders are described in the section on alcoholism.

As stated previously, alcohol is quite caloric but has little nutritional value; consumption of a high-alcohol diet (and little else!) slowly leads to vitamin deficiencies and nutritional diseases, which may result in physical deterioration. Indeed, alcohol abuse has been suggested as the most common cause of vitamin and trace element deficiencies in adults. Also, the interaction between ethanol and vitamin A has been implicated as a potential mechanism for the pathogenesis of fetal alcohol syndrome.[27]

Tolerance and Dependence

The patterns and mechanisms for the development of tolerance, physical dependence, and psychological dependence on alcohol are similar to those for other CNS depressants (Chapter 5). The extent of tolerance depends on the amount, pattern, and extent of alcohol ingestion. Persons who ingest alcohol only intermittently on sprees or more regularly but in moderation develop little or no tolerance; persons who regularly ingest large amounts of alcohol develop marked tolerance. The tolerance that does develop is of three types:

1. Metabolic tolerance, where the liver increases its amount of drug-metabolizing enzyme. This type of tolerance accounts for at most 25 percent of the tolerance that develops to alcohol.

2. Tissue, or functional, tolerance, where neurons in the brain adapt to the amount of drug present. Individuals who develop this type of tolerance characteristically display blood alcohol levels about twice those of a nontolerant individual at a similar level of behavioral intoxication.

3. Associative, contingent, or homeostatic tolerance. A variety of environmental manipulations can counter the effects of ethanol, and these counterresponses are a possible mechanism of tolerance.

The relationship of tolerance to the development of excessive drinking has yet to be determined. No evidence has been demonstrated that any degree of tolerance to the positive reinforcing effects of ethanol develops. Tolerance develops only to the motor-disrupting, hypothermic, sedative, anxiolytic, and anticonvulsant effects. Since many of the intoxicating effects of ethanol involve potentiation in $GABA_A$ function and antagonism of NMDA-type glutamate function, brain tolerance probably involves synaptic plasticity with intracellular enzymatic and translational alterations both during periods of intoxication and during the withdrawal process (see Chandler and co-workers[28] for a review).

When physical dependence develops, withdrawal of alcohol results, within several hours, in a period of rebound hyperexcitability that may eventually lead to convulsions. Alcohol abuse is one of the most common causes of adult-onset seizures; seizures occur in about 10 percent of adults during alcohol withdrawal. The period of seizure activity is relatively short, usually six hours or less in 85 percent of individuals between first and last seizure. D'Onofrio and colleagues[29] describe the efficacy of *lorazepam* (Ativan; Chapter 6) in successfully preventing recurrent alcohol-related seizures in patients with alcohol abuse who presented with a seizure.

Concomitant with hyperexcitability is a period of tremulousness, with hallucinations, psychomotor agitation, confusion and disorientation, sleep disorders, and a variety of associated discomforts—a syndrome that is sometimes referred to as *delirium tremens* (DTs). Fadda and Rossetti[30] review withdrawal as a sign of alcohol-induced neuroadaptation and the neurodegeneration that may play a role in the persistent cognitive deficits that result from alcohol dependence. Markianos and coworkers[31] assessed dopamine receptor responsiveness in alcoholic patients during their usual alcohol consumption and after detoxification. Detoxification was accompanied by a normalization of low responsiveness of dopamine receptors during alcohol abuse. The Markianos team postulated that the dopamine system is involved in alcohol dependence and withdrawal.

Side Effects and Toxicity

Many side effects and toxicities associated with alcohol have already been mentioned; following is a summary and expansion. In acute use, a *reversible drug-induced brain syndrome* is induced. This syndrome is manifested as a clouded sensorium with disorientation, impaired insight and judgment, antegrade amnesia (blackouts), and diminished intellectual capabilities. The person's affect may be labile, with emotional outbursts precipitated by otherwise innocuous events. With high doses of alcohol, delusions, hallucinations, and confabulations may occur. In social functioning, these alterations result in unpredictable states of disinhibition (drunkenness), alterations in driving performance, and uncoordinated motor behavior.

Liver damage is the most serious physiological long-term consequence of excessive alcohol consumption. Irreversible changes in both the structure and the function of the liver are common. For example, ethanol produces active oxidants during its metabolism by hepatocytes, which are reported to produce oxidative stress on liver cells.[32] The significance of alcohol-induced liver dysfunction is illustrated by the fact that 75 percent of all deaths attributed to alcoholism are caused by cirrhosis of the liver, and cirrhosis is the seventh most common cause of death in the United States.

Long-term alcohol ingestion may irreversibly cause the *destruction of nerve cells*, producing a permanent brain syndrome with dementia (Korsakoff's syndrome). More subtle cognitive deficits may be present whether Korsakoff's syndrome is present or not.[31]

The digestive system may also be affected. *Pancreatitis* (inflammation of the pancreas) and *chronic gastritis* (inflammation of the stomach), with the development of peptic ulcers, may occur.

A great deal of epidemiological evidence now shows that chronic excessive alcohol consumption is a major risk factor for *cancer* in humans.[33] Although ethanol alone may not be carcinogenic, it may be a cocarcinogen or a tumor promoter. The metabolism of ethanol leads to the generation of acetaldehyde and free radicals. Acetaldehyde has been shown to promote tumor growth, promoting cancers of the oral pharynx, stomach, and intestine.[34–36] Statistically, heavy drinking increases a person's risk of developing cancer of the tongue, mouth, throat, voice box, and liver. The risk of head and neck cancers for heavy drinkers who smoke is 6 to 15 times greater than for those who abstain from both. The risk of throat cancer is 44 times greater for heavy users of both alcohol and tobacco than for nonusers.

Although the finding is controversial, ethanol appears to increase the risk for breast cancer in women[37] by still unidentified means; it may produce free radicals that cause oxidative stress to cells in breast tissue.[38]

Besides the acetaldehyde and free-radical mechanisms, the cancer-promoting effect of ethanol might be explained by the role of alcohol in modifying the action of other cancer-causing agents, such as tobacco. Finally, as a fourth possible mechanism, alcohol has an immunosuppressive action and may promote tumor growth by reducing body defense mechanisms against tumor cells.[39]

Teratogenic Effects

Alcohol is both a physical and a behavioral teratogen;[40,41] drug-induced alterations occur in brain structure and/or function.[42] *Fetal alcohol syndrome* (FAS) is a devastating developmental disorder that occurs in the offspring of mothers who have high blood levels of alcohol during critical stages of fetal development; it affects as many as 30 to 50 percent of infants born to alcoholic women.[43] The rate of FAS is about 3 to 5 per 1000 live births, and this number appears to be increasing.

> Clearly, a relatively large number of otherwise biologically normal infants may be irreversibly damaged by maternal alcohol abuse during pregnancy, and such abuse during pregnancy appears to be the most frequent known teratogenic cause of mental retardation.[43]

Although the amount of alcohol that must be consumed to cause fetal injury is not known, it is generally accepted that more than 3 ounces of absolute alcohol daily, especially in conjunction with binge drinking, poses a special risk of FAS to the fetus.[44] Because subtle intellectual and behavioral effects of low-level alcohol consumption may go unnoticed, no safe level of alcohol intake during pregnancy has been established. Features of the fetal alcohol syndrome include the following:

- CNS dysfunction, including low intelligence and microcephaly (reduced cranial circumference), mental retardation, and behavioral abnormalities (often presenting as hyperactivity and difficulty with social integration)
- Retarded body growth rate (fetal growth retardation)
- Facial abnormalities (short palpebral fissures, short nose, wide-set eyes, and small cheekbones)
- Other anatomical abnormalities (for example, congenital heart defects and malformed eyes and ears)[44]

In the United States, an estimated 2.6 million infants are born annually following significant intrauterine alcohol exposure. While many display the full features of FAS, about 1 newborn out of every 100 live births may display a "lesser degree of damage, termed fetal alcohol effects,"[44] or perhaps more correctly termed *alcohol-related neurodevelopmental disorder* (ARND).[45] Taken together, the combined rate of FAS and ARND is estimated to be at least 9 per 1000 live births.[45] This would make alcohol ingestion the third leading cause of birth defects with associated mental retardation; it is the only one that is preventable. The impact of FAS and ARND is incalculable.

While the structural abnormalities and growth retardation of FAS are well described, the behavioral and cognitive effects of alcohol exposure are underappreciated. Affected and subject to deficits are intelligence (IQ), activity, attention, learning, memory, language, and motor and visiospatial activities in children prenatally exposed to varying amounts of alcohol.[46,47] Also noted are sensory problems involving ocular, auditory, vestibular, and speech and language development.[41]

Carmichael and co-workers[48] studied a cohort of 500 children, 250 of whom were infants of "heavier" drinkers who typically drank at "social drinking levels." The other 250 children were infants of infrequent drinkers and abstainers. There were significant alcohol-related differences in behavioral and learning difficulties during adolescence. Exposure to alcohol during pregnancy was associated "with a profile of adolescent antisocial behavior, school problems, and self-perceived learning difficulties." Thus, brain function can be markedly affected in offspring of alcohol-drinking mothers in the absence of the structural abnormalities.[47]

The mechanisms responsible for the production of FAS and ARND are unclear. One interesting hypothesis involves the interaction of ethanol and Vitamin A.[27] However, it seems unlikely that this one simple etiology underlies the entire etiology of FAS and ARND. Another hypothesis involves ethanol-induced production of reactive oxygen species that can induce lipid peroxidation in embryos, possibly inducing fetal damage.[49] Ikonomidou and co-workers[50] reported that ethanol-treated rats had reduced neuronal densities in their developing forebrain; the effects occurring during the time-period of synaptogenesis. The authors postulated that such neurodegeneration followed both from NMDA receptor blockade and from positive GABA$_A$ receptor activation.

The prevention of FAS and ARND obviously involves abstinence from alcohol by women who are, plan to, or are capable of becoming pregnant. Screening questionnaires may be effective in helping to protect not only the unborn infant but also the long-term health of the mother.[51] Because it can effectively identify women and infants at risk; it is recommended that alcohol screening be performed during prenatal visits.[52]

Alcoholism and Its Pharmacological Treatment

The recognition of alcoholism as a multifaceted disease and behavioral process is relatively recent. In 1935, Alcoholics Anonymous was founded based on a *moral model* of alcoholism; it offered a spiritual and behavioral framework for understanding, accepting, and recovering from the compulsion to use alcohol. In the late 1950s, the American Medical Association recognized the syndrome of alcoholism as an illness. In the mid-1970s, alcoholism was redefined as a *chronic, progressive, and potentially fatal disease*. In 1992, the description was expanded as follows:

> Alcoholism is a primary, chronic disease with genetic, psychosocial, and environmental factors influencing its development and manifestations. The disease is often progressive and fatal. It is characterized by impaired control over drinking, preoccupation with the drug alcohol, use of alcohol despite adverse consequences, and distortions in thinking, most notably denial. Each of these symptoms may be continuous or periodic.[53]

In this definition, "adverse consequences" involve impairments in such areas as physical health, psychological functioning, interpersonal functioning, and occupational functioning, as well as legal, financial, and spiritual problems. "Denial" refers broadly to a range of psychological maneuvers that decrease awareness of the fact that alcohol use is the cause of a person's problems rather than a solution to those problems. Denial becomes an integral part of the disease and is nearly always a major obstacle to recovery. Feldman and colleagues[54] discussed a *behavioral model* of alcoholism:

- Alcohol consumption ranges from complete abstention to levels that induce chronic intoxication, and individuals can move up and down the continuum of intoxication as a function of varying circumstances.

- The consequences of alcohol ingestion (at least in the short term) are behaviorally reinforcing.
- Alcohol drinking is subject to the same control mechanisms that govern other reinforced behaviors.
- Alcoholism is a learned but maladaptive behavior pattern.
- This behavior pattern can be altered by appropriate reinforcement contingencies, allowing for the possibility of controlled drinking in former alcoholics.

To this behavioral model, one must add inherent genetic factors that confer heightened vulnerability to alcoholism in some people. Prescott and Kendler[55] provide data and review the evidence for the strong role of genetic factors in the development of alcoholism among males; environmental factors seem to be much less important.

In many cases, alcohol may (at least at first) be ingested in an attempt at *self-medication* of psychological distress. A person who, before alcohol, experiences anxiety, depression, bipolar, or other responsive psychological disorders may find the symptomatology alleviated by ethanol. This then leads to unregulated and unmonitored drug ingestion (i.e., the drug is not taken under a physician's supervision). The person then becomes trapped by either the positive reinforcing effects of the drug or else drinks to avoid the unpleasantness of withdrawal. In support of this concept, Goodwin[56] stated:

> A good deal of evidence now indicates that many, and perhaps most, alcoholics do *not* have primary alcoholism. Their alcoholism *is* associated with other psychopathology, including addiction to other drugs, depression, manic-depressive illness, anxiety disorder, or antisocial personality.

Goodwin further states that 30 to 50 percent of alcoholics meet criteria for major depression; 33 percent have a coexisting anxiety disorder; many have antisocial personalities; some are schizophrenic; and many (36 percent) are addicted to other drugs. Some, if not many, alcoholics may have first used alcohol and become psychologically dependent on the drug as a self-prescribed medication to treat their primary disorder. Therefore, *dual diagnosis* (or *comorbid illness*) must always be presumed (until proven otherwise). Kushner and co-workers[57] demonstrate in a college-age population that

> cross-sectionally, the odds of having either an anxiety disorder or an alcohol use disorder were two- to fivefold greater when the other condition was present. . . . Alcohol use disorders (especially alcohol

dependence) and anxiety disorders demonstrate a reciprocal causal relationship over time, with anxiety disorders leading to alcohol dependence and vice versa.

Further, Lejoyeux and colleagues[58] noted that 38 percent of their alcohol-dependent patients presented with a diagnosable impulse-control problem. The cooccurrence of pathologic gambling (one type of impulse-control disorder) was associated with a younger age of onset of alcohol dependence, a higher number of detoxifications, and a longer duration of dependence. Both alcohol dependence and pathologic gambling are pleasure-seeking dependencies, and alcohol use may provide much the same reinforcement as gambling.

Whatever the etiology of excessive drinking, alcoholism is a major public health problem. Of the 160 million Americans who are old enough to drink legally, 112 million do so. As many as 14 million Americans may have serious alcohol problems, and about half that number (7 million) are considered to be alcoholic. Alcoholism costs about 100,000 Americans lives each year and in excess of $166 billion annually in direct and indirect health and societal costs. Older people who drink are at risk for their own set of problems. In 1996 the American Medical Association published "Alcohol in the Elderly,"[59] an update on alcohol use in this population.

Long-term alcoholism may lead to malnutrition and chronic physiological degeneration. Although this state of chronic degeneration is not present in the majority of alcoholics who receive adequate nutrition, nutrition alone does not fully protect the brain, the liver, or the digestive tract from damage.

Pharmacotherapies for Alcohol Abuse and Dependence

Because alcoholism involves the ingestion of alcohol, eliminating the taking of alcohol is an obvious therapeutic strategy. Achieving success, however, is an extremely difficult task. Vaillant[60] points to the poor long-term outlook of alcoholism treatment, whether pharmacologic or behavioral. Vaillant performed a 50-year follow-up of two cohorts of men who abused alcohol at an early age. One group consisted of university undergraduates and the second consisted of nondelinquent inner-city adolescents. By 60 years of age, 18 percent of the college alcohol abusers had died, 11 percent were abstinent, 11 percent were controlled drinkers, and 60 percent were still abusing alcohol. By 60 years of age, 28 percent of the inner-city alcohol abusers had died, 30 percent were abstinent, 12 percent were controlled drinkers, and 30 percent were still abusing alcohol. As alcohol abuse after age 60 can be devastating, the greater levels of abuse by college-educated males certainly need to be addressed.[59]

Goals of Pharmacotherapy for Alcohol Dependence and Abuse

The goals of pharmacotherapy for alcohol abuse or dependence include the following:

- Reversal of the acute pharmacologic effects of alcohol
- Treatment and prevention of withdrawal symptoms and complications
- Maintenance of abstinence and prevention of relapse with agents that decrease craving for alcohol or the loss of control over drinking or make it unpleasant to ingest alcohol
- Treatment of coexisting psychiatric disorders that complicate recovery.[61]

This section addresses each goal and discusses the extent (or lack thereof) to which each goal can be met. First, at this time, no agent that can reverse the acute pharmacologic effects of alcohol is available. Some feel that caffeine can antagonize alcohol intoxication and increase alertness. This is not true, as a behavioral stimulant can only increase activity and cannot reverse the motor, cognitive, or other dysfunctions induced by alcohol. Therefore, acute alcohol intoxication is usually treated with supportive care (Table 4.1) in order to protect both the intoxicated person as well as others whom he/she places at risk of injury.

Pharmacotherapies are available for the treatment and prevention of withdrawal symptoms and complications in alcohol-dependent people who are decreasing or discontinuing alcohol. The goals of these therapies were recently summarized by Saitz and O'Malley[61] and are shown in Table 4.2. Medication can effectively prevent and treat the symptoms, seizures, and DTs associated with withdrawal. The impact of pharmacologic management on other manifestations of the alcohol withdrawal syndrome remains less clear.

Pharmacotherapies for Alcohol Withdrawal

Today, the *benzodiazepines* (Chapter 6) are the drugs of choice for the treatment of acute alcohol withdrawal; they ameliorate the symptoms and also prevent seizures and DTs.[61] It may not seem logical to replace one potentially addictive drug (benzodiazepine) for another (ethanol). An explanation follows. The short duration of the action of alcohol and its narrow range of safety make it an extremely dangerous drug from which to withdraw. When alcohol ingestion is stopped, the remaining alcohol in the body is rapidly metabolized, and withdrawal symptoms occur within a few hours. Substituting a long-acting drug prevents or suppresses the withdrawal symptoms. The longer-acting benzodiazepine

TABLE 4.1 Pharmacological treatment of acute alcohol intoxication and withdrawal symptoms

State	Medication used	Comments
Intoxication	None	Supportive care only. Drug treatment not appropriate.
Alcohol withdrawal syndrome	Long-acting benzodiazepine (e.g., diazepam or chlordiazepoxide)	Loading dose technique is effective, simple, and tolerated, and it lowers the duration of treatment and total dose. Drugs of choice other than in the elderly or in severe liver disease
	Lorazepam	Drugs of choice in the elderly or in severe liver disease. Good parenterally.
	Clonidine	Superior to placebo, but inconsistent compared with benzodiazepines
	Atenolol (a beta-blocker)	Superior to placebo, but additional evidence not available
	Carbamazepine	Probably efficacious, but adverse effects limit routine use. Poorly effective against delirium.
	Chlormethiazole	Less effective and less well tolerated than benzodiazepines
	Barbiturates	Good evidence of efficacy; however, narrow safety margin limits use. Benzodiazepines are superior and preferred.
	Chlorpromazine (an antipsychotic)	Alleviates delirium and hallucinations, lowers seizure threshold and can intensify withdrawal convulsions

---

TABLE 4.2 Goals of pharmacotherapy for alcohol withdrawal

Goals for which substantial evidence of effectiveness exists
    Treatment of alcohol withdrawal symptoms
    Prevention of initial and recurrent seizures
    Prevention and treatment of delirium tremens
Other goals with less evidence of efficacy
    Prevention of medical and psychiatric complications of alcohol withdrawal
    Prevention of kindling effect
    Prevention of Korsakoff's psychosis
    Improvement in the likelihood of abstinence
    Minimization of adverse drug effects
    Entry into ongoing medical and addictions treatment
    Cost-effective treatment

[From Saitz and O'Malley.[61]]

is then either maintained at a level low enough to allow the person to function or is withdrawn gradually. Preferred drugs are the benzodiazepines with long-acting active metabolites—chlordiazepoxide (Librium) or diazepam (Valium)—while acute seizure activity is well controlled with the faster-onset, shorter-acting benzodiazepine lorazepam.[30] The pharmacology of the benzodiazepines is discussed in Chapter 6.

Treatment strategies[62] for management of alcohol withdrawal recommend benzodiazepines as first-line therapy and other drugs (beta-blockers, clonidine, carbamazepine, and antipsychotics) only as adjunctive therapy. Historically, barbiturates and phenytoin were used, but both have been replaced by the benzodiazepines. Beta-blockers and clonidine are drugs that block the functioning of the sympathetic nervous system; they help ameliorate some of the autonomic signs and symptoms of withdrawal. Their use is not without problems. Carbamazepine (Tegretol) is an anticonvulsant that has been used in place of benzodiazepines. However, it is less effective in alleviating delirium, and it is considered to be generally less effective than benzodiazepines. Antipsychotic drugs (Chapter 17) can alleviate delirium and hallucinosis, but they lower the seizure threshold and can increase the propensity for withdrawal seizures. Finally, vitamins such as thiamine and magnesium have a role in treating withdrawal. These treatments are well described in recent reviews.[61–63]

Drugs to Help Maintain Abstinence

Numerous drugs to decrease consumption and prevent clinical relapse have been tried; many of these are listed in Table 4.3. Some have been successful and many are of limited use.

Alcohol-sensitizing drugs, including *disulfiram* (Antabuse) and *calcium carbimide* (Temposil, available in Canada only), are used to deter a patient from drinking alcohol by producing an aversive reaction if the patient drinks. These drugs alter the metabolism of alcohol, allowing acetaldehyde to accumulate. If the patient ingests alcohol within several days of taking the aversive drug, the accumulation results in an acetaldehyde syndrome, characterized by flushing, throbbing headache, nausea, vomiting, chest pain, and other severe symptoms. It is felt that calcium carbimide has fewer side effects than does disulfiram.

If taken daily, aversive agents can result in total abstinence in many patients. However, controlled trials of disulfiram therapy to reduce alcohol consumption demonstrate that the drug fares little better than placebo treatment.[64,65]

The opioid antagonist *naltrexone* (ReVia, Trexan) was approved by the FDA in 1994 for use in the treatment of alcohol dependence to reduce the craving for alcohol. The hypothesis of action is that the reinforcing properties of alcohol involve the opioid system; blockade of that system by naltrexone should reduce craving by reducing the positive reinforcement associated with alcohol use. Initial studies with naltrexone were encouraging; however, more recent studies[66,67] have been less than optimistic. Under less-than-laboratory conditions, with less control over compliance, naltrexone showed only modest efficacy over placebo therapy. Therefore, the efficacy and the long-term place of naltrexone in reducing the craving for alcohol in withdrawn alcoholics is in question, although Garbutt and colleagues[64] consider it to be effective therapy.

Mason and co-workers[68] discuss the limitations to naltroxone therapy, including potentially serious hepatic side effects. They studied a related drug, *nalmefene* (Revex), that is devoid of adverse effects on the liver. In 105 adults with alcohol dependence, nalmefene was effective in preventing relapse to heavy drinking compared with placebo therapy (Figure 4.9); no medically serious side effects were observed. The pharmacology of nalmefene and other opioid antagonists is discussed further in Chapter 9.

Acamprosate (calcium acetylhomotaurinate) is approved for use as an anticraving drug in many European countries (marketed under the trade name Aotal), but not yet in the United States. It is the first pharmacologic agent specifically designed to maintain abstinence in ethanol-dependent people after detoxification. Acamprosate is thought to exert both a GABA-agonist action at GABA receptors and an inhibitory action at glutaminergic NMDA receptors; actions similar to

TABLE 4.3 Drugs used to decrease alcohol consumption, reduce craving, maintain abstinence, or prevent relapse in alcohol-dependent individuals*

Drug	Mechanism	Comments
Disulfiram	Inhibits aldehyde dehydrogenase to allow acetaldehyde accumulation	Clinical efficacy in question as a result of controlled trials. Effective in special situations.
Calcium carbimide	Same as disulfiram	May have fewer side effects than disulfiram. Available in Canada, not in USA.
Naltrexone	Endogenous opioid antagonist	FDA approved for treating alcohol dependence. Reduces consumption in heavy drinkers.
Acamprosate	NMDA and GABA$_A$ receptor modulator	Reduces unpleasant effects of alcohol abstinence, reduces craving. May have adverse fetal effects. Approved in Europe, not in USA.
Fluoxetine and other serotonin antidepressants	SSRI-type serotonin agonist	Reduces depression and anxiety occurring comorbid with alcohol dependency.
Buspirone	Serotonin 5-HT-IA agonist	Little demonstrable efficacy may be due to inadequate amounts in blood.
Ondansetron, Ritanserin	Serotonin 5-HT-3 antagonists	May reduce craving. Poorly demonstrated efficacy.
Carbamazepine	Mood stabilizer, anticonvulsant	Can reduce unpleasant withdrawal effects.
Gamma-hydroxy-butyrate (GHB)	NMDA antagonist	Sedative-euphoriant. Can alleviate withdrawal symptoms. Subject to abuse.
Bromocriptine	Dopamine agonist	Can reduce craving. Little documented efficacy in reducing relapse.

*Data tabulated from references 62, 64, 65.

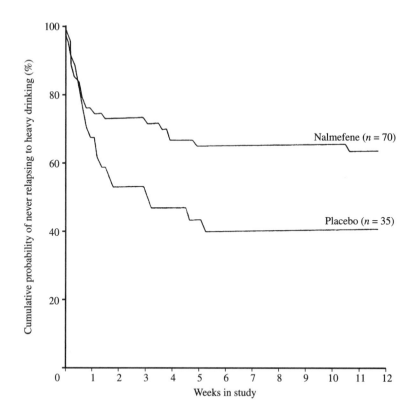

FIGURE 4.9 Rates of never relapsing to heavy drinking from randomization (week 0) through the end of double-blind treatment. [From Mason et al.[68]]

those exerted by ethanol, decreasing the need to drink alcohol. Acamprosate is well tolerated; diarrhea is the main side effect. In animals, acamprosate reduces alcohol consumption; in human studies, it is about three times as effective as placebo, with drinking frequency reduced by 30 to 50 percent. To date, there have been no reports of abuse of acamprosate. While much remains to be learned about acamprosate, early results are promising.[69,70]

Dopaminergic drugs have theoretical use in maintaining abstinence because (1) the positive reinforcement associated with alcohol attractiveness appears to involve the dopaminergic reward system; (2) withdrawal may be accompanied by hypofunction of this reward system[31]; and (3) depression is often comorbid with alcohol dependency and some dopaminergic drugs are antidepressant in action (e.g., *buproprion*, Chapter 15). It would appear that further study in this area is warranted.

Serotoninergic drugs have been quite well studied as agents to treat alcohol dependence. Several classes of such agents have been evaluated: (1) the serotonin-specific reuptake inhibitors (SSRIs) such as *fluoxetine* (Prozac); (2) a serotonin 5-HT$_{1A}$ agonist, *buspirone* (BuSpar); and (3) the serotonin 5-HT$_3$ antagonist *ondansetron* (Zofran). Currently, the SSRIs are FDA approved for treating depression and anxiety disorders (Chapter 15), buspirone for treating anxiety (Chapter 6), and ondansetron for treating nausea. Recently, these drugs have been evaluated for treating alcohol dependence, especially when patients exhibit comorbid mood or anxiety disorders.[64] In general, the results have been disappointing.[71] Major depressive disorder predisposed persons with alcoholism to more rapid relapse,[72] and fluoxetine is effective in reducing both depression and alcohol consumption in depressed alcoholics.[73] It is unknown whether or not fluoxetine or other SSRIs will reduce alcohol consumption in nondepressed alcoholics.

Buspirone has been shown to be effective in improving comorbid anxiety in alcoholics, but it is much less effective in reducing alcohol consumption.[74] Blood level correlations with efficacy have not been performed. Recall from Chapter 1 that buspirone is poorly absorbed (95 percent destroyed by first-pass metabolism) and that grapefruit juice greatly improves gastric absorption by reducing gastric metabolism. It would be interesting to see if buspirone administered with grapefruit juice might fare more favorably as an anticraving drug.

Finally, ondansetron and another 5-HT$_3$ agonist, ritanserin, have not been very effective in humans, although initial results in animals were encouraging.[75]

Many other drugs have been studied in attempts to pharmacologically treat alcoholism. In most cases, initial optimism was not verified. For example, *gamma-hydroxybutyrate* (GHB) can suppress alcohol withdrawal symptoms, but abuse and withdrawal from GHB also occur.[76]

INHALANTS OF ABUSE

Inhalant abuse is the intentional inhalation of a volatile substance for the purpose of achieving a euphoric state. It is also known as solvent abuse, volatile substance abuse, glue sniffing, sniffing, and huffing. Beginning with children as young as 6 years of age, it is an underrecognized form of substance abuse with a significant morbidity and mortality.[77]

The inhalants of abuse consist of a variety of organic solvents and other chemicals that are volatile at room temperature (they readily vaporize from the liquid state when exposed to air). When inhaled, they produce euphoria, delirium, intoxication, and alterations in mental status, resembling alcohol intoxication or a "light" state of general anesthesia. Inhaled substances include the following:

- Anesthetics, especially nitrous oxide and halothane
- Industrial or household solvents, including paint thinners or solvents, degreasers, and solvents in glues
- Art and office supply solvents, including typewriter correction fluid and marker pen solvents
- Gases used in household or commercial products, including butane lighters, aerosol cream dispensers, and propane tanks
- Household aerosol propellants, including paint, hair spray, and fabric protector sprays
- Aliphatic nitrites and organic solvents, including amyl nitrite capsules

Some of the substances found in these different products are listed in Table 4.4. Abused inhalants are rarely, if ever, administered by routes other than inhalation.

Why Inhalants Are Abused and Who Abuses Them

Why are inhalants used for recreational or abuse purposes, what is their attraction, and why do they have the potential for abuse? Yavich and co-workers [78] investigated in rats the behavior-reinforcing properties of glue vapors (which are a mixture of four organic solvents— toluene, benzene, ethyl acetate, and methyl chloride). At low to moderate concentrations of vapor, the motor activity of the rats increased, as did their rates of self-stimulation in the lateral hypothalamus. Increasing the vapor concentration suppressed the activation of brain reward systems and concomitantly brought on behavioral depression. These effects were similar to those produced by ether, nitrous oxide, chloroform, and other general anesthetics, all of which have been abused since their introduction into medicine over 100 years ago.

The extent of the problem of solvent abuse is greater than most people acknowledge. Currently, inhalant abuse is one of the most pervasive yet least recognized drug problems.[79] In the United States, the prevalence of inhalant abuse among adolescent youths is exceeded only by the use of marijuana, alcohol, and tobacco.[80] The peak of inhalant abuse occurs in youths aged 14 to 15 years, with onset occurring in some youths as young as 6 to 8 years; however, some users continue

TABLE 4.4 Chemicals commonly found in inhalants

	Inhalant	Chemical
Adhesives	Airplane glue	Toluene, ethyl acetate
	Other glues	Hexane, toluene, methyl chloride, acetone, methyl ethyl ketone, methyl butyl ketone
	Special cements	Trichloroethylene, tetrachloroethylene
Aerosols	Spray paint	Butane, propane (U.S.), fluorocarbons, toluene, hydrocarbons, "Texas shoe shine" (a spray containing toluene)
	Hair spray	Butane, propane (U.S.), CFCs
	Deodorant, air freshner	Butane, propane (U.S.), CFCs
	Analgesic spray	Chlorofluorocarbons (CFCs)
	Asthma spray	Chlorofluorocarbons (CFCs)
	Fabric spray	Butane, trichloroethane
	PC cleaner	Dimethyl ether, hydrofluorocarbons
Anesthetics	Gas	Nitrous oxide
	Liquid	Halothane, enflurane
	Local	Ethyl chloride
Cleaning agents	Dry cleaning	Tetrachloroethylene, trichloroethane
	Spot remover	Xylene, petroleum distillates, chlorohydrocarbons
	Degreaser	Tetrachloroethylene, trichloroethane, trichloroethylene
Solvents and Gases	Nail polish remover	Acetone, ethyl acetate
	Paint remover	Toluene, methyl chloride, methanol acetone, ethyl acetate
	Paint thinner	Petroleum distillates, esters, acetone
	Correction fluid and thinner	Trichloroethylene, trichloroethane
	Fuel gas	Butane, isopropane
	Lighter	Butane, isopropane
	Fire extinguisher	Bromochlorodifluoromethane
Whipped cream	Whipped cream	Nitrous oxide
	Whippets	Nitrous oxide
"Room odorizers"	Locker Room, Rush, poppers	Isoamyl, isobutyl, isopropyl or butyl nitrate (now illegal), cyclohexyl

into adulthood (Figure 4.10).[81] Patterns of abuse resemble patterns seen in abuse of other types of substances: there are experimenters, intermittent users, and chronic inhalant abusers. Although injuries are associated with the frequency of use, the so-called sudden sniffing death syndrome can occur in first-time users.[77] About 20 percent of youths have experience with inhalant abuse by the end of the eighth grade. Brown and co-workers[82] reviewed deaths from inhalant abuse in

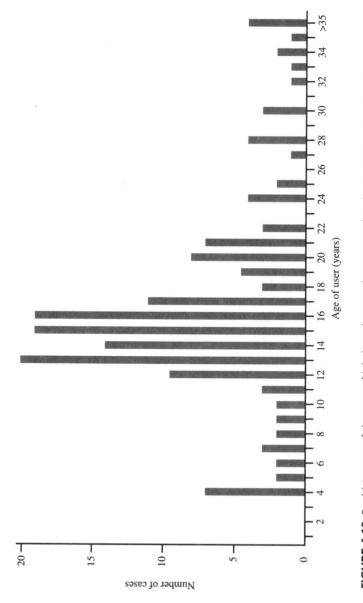

FIGURE 4.10 Bar histogram of the ages of inhalant abusers who presented to the emergency room (total number = 165). The youngest inhalant abusers were age 4 years. The peak incidence was at 12 to 16 years. [From Spiller and Krenzelok.[81]]

the state of Virginia over the ten-year period 1987–1996. The 39 deaths accounted for 0.3 percent of all deaths in males aged 13 to 22 years. Age of death ranged from 13 to 42 years; 70 percent of deaths occurred at 22 years of age or younger. Ninety-five percent of the deaths occurred in males. Gas fuels accounted for 46 percent of the fatalities.

Acute Intoxication and Chronic Effects

As noted in Table 4.4, a variety of volatile substances are abused by inhalation, each with its own pharmacology and toxicology.[83] In general, however, most inhaled vapors produce rapid onset of a state of intoxication (or "drunkenness") that resembles alcohol intoxication: the continuum of sedation with anxiolysis, disinhibition, drowsiness, lightheadedness, and euphoria. With increasing intoxication, the user experiences ataxia (staggering), dizziness, delirium, and disorientation. With severe intoxication, there is muscle weakness, lethargy, and signs of light to moderate general anesthesia. With lack of oxygen (hypoxia), hallucinations and behavior changes may occur.

Mechanistically,[84] very little is known about the cellular basis of the effects of volatile chemicals and gases that lead to their abuse by inhalation:

- With some agents (particularly the *nitrites*), vasodilation and muscle relaxant effects appear to underlie use.

- With anesthetics, such as *nitrous oxide*, a state of light general anesthesia is induced.

- With the *volatile solvents* and *fuels*, conclusions are difficult to draw, but "their profile of acute behavioral and pharmacological effects is in turn very similar to that observed with subanesthetic concentrations of clinically used volatile anesthetics. This common profile of effects seen with abused solvents and anesthetics is also very similar to the profile of acute effects produced by classical CNS depressants and alcohol."[84]

Although death is relatively rare during acute intoxication, when it does occur, it usually follows from lack of oxygen to the brain (anoxia), cardiac arrhythmias, aspiration of vomitus, or trauma. In Great Britain, sudden sniffing death syndrome is said to account for over 50 percent of fatalities from acute intoxication.[77] Volatile hydrocarbons sensitize the heart to serious arrhythmias when a person is startled or becomes excited during intoxication. The sudden surge of adrenalin acts on the sensitized heart to set off serious and life-threatening arrhythmias. This kind of episode can occur during initial experimentation or during any episode of abuse.

With *chronic abuse* of solvents, serious complications can include peripheral and central nervous system dysfunction (e.g., peripheral neuropathies and encephalopathy), liver and/or kidney failure, dementia, loss of cognitive and other higher functions, gait disturbances, and loss of coordination. Specific agents cause other specific morbidities.

Little and colleagues[85] and Jones and Balster[80] describe a fetal solvent syndrome characterized by "prenatal growth retardation (low birth weight, microcephaly), facial dysmorphism (resembling FAS), and digital malformations (short phalanges, nail hypoplasia).[85]

Treatment of acute solvent intoxication is primarily supportive with the administration of supplemental oxygen. Treatment of chronic solvent abuse is much more difficult. Misra and colleagues[86] describe one individual successfully treated with risperidone (Chapter 17).

STUDY QUESTIONS

1. Pharmacologically, what is ethyl alcohol?

2. Describe the metabolism of alcohol. What enzymes are involved? What drug blocks one of these enzymes?

3. How do women and men differ in their metabolism of alcohol?

4. How does the kinetics of alcohol metabolism differ from that of most other drugs?

5. How long does it take for an adult to metabolize the alcohol in a 1-ounce glass of 80-proof whiskey? A 4-ounce glass of wine? A 12-ounce bottle of beer? A pint of 7 percent microbrew?

6. What BAC is defined in most states as "intoxication"?

7. Describe how alcohol exerts its effects on the CNS.

8. If one has developed a physical dependence on alcohol, why might he or she be treated with a benzodiazepine as a substitute for the alcohol?

9. Summarize some of the drugs and techniques used in treating alcoholism. What medications might be used to ameliorate alcohol withdrawal? Differentiate alcohol withdrawal from alcoholism.

10. Describe the disease concept of alcoholism. Discuss the comorbidity of alcohol dependence with other psychological disorders.

11. Summarize some of the problems associated with inhalant abuse.

12. Describe some of the fetal effects of alcohol. Is there a "safe" level of drinking during pregnancy?

REFERENCES

1. J. W. Hanson, K. L. Jones, and D. W. Smith, "Fetal Alcohol Syndrome," *Journal of the American Medical Association* 235 (1976): 1458–1460.
2. C. M. Oneta et al., "First-pass Metabolism of Ethanol Is Strikingly Influenced by the Speed of Gastric Emptying," *Gut* 43 (1998): 612–619.
3. M. Frezza et al., "High Blood Alcohol Levels in Women: The Role of Decreased Gastric Alcohol Dehydrogenase Activity and First-pass Metabolism," *New England Journal of Medicine* 322 (1990): 95–99.
4. R. S. Feldman, J. S. Meyer, and L. F. Quenzer, *Principles of Neuropsychopharmacology* (Sunderland, Mass.: Sinauer, 1997), 627.
5. H. H. Kertschbaum and A. Hermann, "Ethanol Suppresses Neuronal Ca_2^+ Currents by Effects on Intracellular Signal Transduction," *Brain Research* 765 (1997): 30–36.
6. S. C. Pandey, "Neuronal Signaling Systems and Ethanol Dependence," *Molecular Neurobiology* 17 (1998): 1–15.
7. C. Li, R. W. Peoples, and F. F. Weight, "Ethanol-induced Inhibition of a Neuronal P_2X Purinoceptor by an Allosteric Mechanism," *British Journal of Pharmacology* 123 (1998): 1–3.
8. P. L. Hoffman and B. Tabakoff, "Ethanol, Sedative-hypnotics, and Glutamate Receptor Function in Brain and Cultured Cells," *Alcohol and Alcoholism*, Suppl. 2 (1993): 345–351.
9. G. E. Tsai et al., "Increased Glutamatergic Neurotransmission and Oxidative Stress After Alcohol Withdrawal," *American Journal of Psychiatry* 155 (1998): 726–732.
10. G. E. Tsai et al., "The Glutamatergic Basis of Human Alcoholism," *American Journal of Psychiatry* 152 (1995): 332–340.
11. M. al Qatari, O. Bouchenafa, and J. Littleton, "Mechanism of Action of Acamprosate. Part II: Ethanol Dependence Modifies Effects of Acamprosate on NMDA Receptor Binding in Membranes from Rat Cerebral Cortex," *Alcoholism: Clinical and Experimental Research* 22 (1998): 810–814.
12. R. S. Feldman, J. S. Meyer, and L. F. Quenzer, *Principles of Neuropsychopharmacology* (Sunderland, Mass.: Sinauer, 1997), 637.
13. M. G. Kushner, T. B. Mackenzie, J. Fiszdon, D. P. Valentiner, E. Foa, N. Anderson, and D. Wangensteen, "The Effects of Alcohol Consumption on Laboratory-induced Panic and State Anxiety," *Archives of General Psychiatry* 53 (1996): 264–270.
14. F.-J. Wan, F. Berton, S. G. Madamba, W. Francesconi, and G. R. Siggins, "Low Ethanol Concentrations Enhance GABAergic Inhibitory Postsynaptic Potentials in Hippocampal Pyramidal Neurons Only After Block of $GABA_B$ Receptors," *Proceedings of the National Academy of Sciences* 93 (1996): 5049–5054.
15. P. Montpied et al., "Prolonged Ethanol Inhalation Decreases $GABA_A$ Receptor Alpha Subunit mRNAs in the Rat Cerebral Cortex," *Molecular Pharmacology* 39 (1991): 157–163.
16. R. A. Harris, M. S. Brodie, and T. V. Dunwiddie, "Possible Substrates of Ethanol Reinforcement: GABA and Dopamine," *Annals of the New York Academy of Sciences* 654 (1992): 61–69.

17. G. S. Wand et al., "Family History of Alcoholism and Hypothalamic Opioidergic Activity," *Archives of General Psychiatry* 55 (1998): 1114–1119.
18. R. M. Swift et al., "Ondansetron Alters Human Alcohol Intoxication," *Biological Psychiatry* 40 (1996): 514–521.
19. A. Heinz et al., "In Vivo Association Between Alcohol Intoxication, Aggression, and Serotonin Transporter Availability in Nonhuman Primates," *American Journal of Psychiatry* 155 (1998): 1023–1028.
20. T. Roehrs, K. Papineau, L. Rosenthal, and T. Roth, "Ethanol as a Hypnotic in Insomniacs: Self-administration and Effects on Sleep and Mood," *Neuropsychopharmacology* 20 (1999): 279–286.
21. K. Berger et al., "Light to Moderate Alcohol Consumption and the Risk of Stroke Among U.S. Male Physicians," *New England Journal of Medicine* 341 (1999): 1557–1564.
22. R. L. Sacco et al., "The Protective Effect of Moderate Alcohol Consumption on Ischemic Stroke," *Journal of the American Medical Association* 281 (1999): 53–60.
23. C. T. Valmadrid et al., "Alcohol Intake and the Risk of Coronary Heart Disease Mortality in Persons with Older-onset Diabetes Mellitus," *Journal of the American Medical Association* 282 (1999): 239–246.
24. L. Holdstock and H. de Wit, "Individual Differences in the Biphasic Effect of Ethanol," *Alcoholism: Clinical and Experimental Research* 22 (1998): 1903–1911.
25. T. J. Phillips and E. H. Shen, "Neurochemical Bases of Locomotion and Ethanol Stimulant effects," *International Review of Neurobiology* 39 (1996): 243–282.
26. M. B. Jones, J. L. Chronister, and R. S. Kennedy, "Effects of Alcohol on Perceptual Speed," *Perceptual and Motor Skills* 87 (1998): 1247–1255.
27. R. D. Zachman and M. A. Grummer, "The Interaction of Ethanol and Vitamin A as a Potential Mechanism for the Pathogenesis of Fetal Alcohol Syndrome," *Alcoholism: Clinical and Experimental Research* 22 (1998): 1544–1556.
28. L. J. Chandler, R. A. Harris and F. T. Crews, "Ethanol Tolerance and Synaptic Plasticity," *Trends in Pharmacological Sciences* 19 (1998): 491–495.
29. G. D'Onofrio et al., "Lorazepam for the Prevention of Recurrent Seizures Related to Alcohol," *New England Journal of Medicine* 340 (1999): 915–919.
30. F. Fadda and Z. L. Rossetti, "Chronic Ethanol Consumption: From Neuroadaptation to Neurodegeneration," *Progress in Neurobiology* 56 (1998): 385–431.
31. M. Markianos, G. Moussas, L. Lykouras, and J. Hatzimanolis, "Dopamine Receptor Responsivity in Alcoholic Patients Before and After Detoxification," *Drug and Alcohol Dependence* 57 (2000): 261–265.
32. I. Kurose et al., "Ethanol-induced Oxidative Stress in the Liver," *Alcoholism: Clinical and Experimental Research* 20, 1 Suppl. (1996): 77A–85A.
33. H. K. Seitz, G. Poschi, and U. A. Simanowski, "Alcohol and Cancer," *Recent Developments in Alcoholism* 14 (1998): 67–95.
34. T. Koivisto and M. Salaspuro, "Acetaldehyde Alters Proliferation, Differentiation and Adhesion Properties of Human Colon Adenocarcinoma Cell Line Caco-2," *Carcinogenesis* 19 (1998): 2031–2036.

35. A. Yokoyama et al., "Alcohol-related Cancers and Aldehyde Dehydrogenase-2 in Japanese Alcoholics," *Carcinogenesis* 19 (1998): 1383–1387.

36. L. C. Harty et al., "Alcohol Dehydrogenase 3 Genotype and Risk of Oral Cavity and Pharyngeal Cancers," *Journal of the National Cancer Institute* 89 (1997): 1698–1705.

37. K. Singletary, "Ethanol and Experimental Breast Cancer: A Review," *Alcoholism: Clinical and Experimental Research* 21 (1997): 334–339.

38. R. M. Wright, J. L. McManaman, and J. E. Repine, "Alcohol-induced Breast Cancer: A Proposed Mechanism," *Free Radical Biology and Medicine* 26 (1999): 3–4.

39. S. I. Mufti, H. R. Darban, and R. R. Watson, "Alcohol, Cancer, and Immunomodulation," *Critical Reviews in Oncology/Hematology* 9 (1989): 243–261.

40. National Institute on Alcohol and Alcoholism, *Alcohol and Birth Defects: The Fetal Alcohol Syndrome and Related Disorders*, U.S. Department of Health and Human Services Publication ADM 87–1531 (Washington, D.C.: U.S. Government Printing Office, 1987), 6–10.

41. M. W. Church and E. L. Abel, "Fetal Alcohol Syndrome: Hearing, Speech, Language, and Vestibular Disorders," *Obstetrics and Gynecology Clinic of North America* 25 (1998): 85–97.

42. T. M. Roebuck, S. N. Mattson ,and E. P. Riley, "A Review of the Neuroanatomical Findings in Children with Fetal Alcohol Syndrome or Prenatal Exposure to Alcohol," *Alcoholism: Clinical and Experimental Research* 22 (1998): 339–344.

43. B. B. Little, T. T. VanBeveren, and L. C. Gilstrap, "Alcohol Use During Pregnancy and Maternal Alcoholism," in L. C. Gilstrap and B. B. Little, eds., *Drugs and Pregnancy*, 2nd ed. (New York: Chapman & Hall, 1998), 395–404.

44. L. P. Finnegan and S. R. Kandall, "Maternal and Neonatal Effects of Alcohol and Drugs," in J. H. Lowinson, P. Ruiz, R. B. Millman, and J. G. Langrod, eds., *Substance Abuse: A Comprehensive Textbook*, 3rd ed. (Baltimore: Williams & Wilkins, 1997), 528–529.

45. P. D. Sampson et al., "Incidence of Fetal Alcohol Syndrome and Prevalence of Alcohol-Related Neurodevelopmental Disorder," *Teratology* 56 (1997): 317–326.

46. S. N. Mattson and E. P. Riley, "A Review of the Neurobehavioral Deficits in Children with Fetal Alcohol Syndrome or Prenatal Exposure to Alcohol," *Alcoholism: Clinical and Experimental Research* 22 (1998): 279–294.

47. N. Z. Weinberg, "Cognitive and Behavioral Deficits Associated with Parental Alcohol Use," *Journal of the American Academy of Child and Adolescent Psychiatry* 36 (1997): 1177–1186.

48. H. Carmichael et al., "Association of Prenatal Alcohol Exposure with Behavioral and Learning Problems in Early Adolescence," *Journal of the American Academy of Child and Adolescent Psychiatry* 36 (1997): 1187–1194.

49. J. R. Woods, M. A. Plessinger, and A. Fantel, "An Introduction to Reactive Oxygen Species and Their Possible Roles in Substance Abuse," *Obstetrics and Gynecology Clinic of North America* 25 (1998): 219–236.

50. C. Ikonomidou et al., "Ethanol-Induced Apoptotic Neurodegeneration and Fetal Alcohol Syndrome," *Science* 287 (2000): 1056–1060.
51. K. A. Bradley et al., "Alcohol Screening Questionnaires in Women: A Critical Review," *Journal of the American Medical Association* 280 (1998): 166–171.
52. G. Chan et al., "Pregnant Women with Negative Alcohol Screens Do Drink Less. A Prospective Study," *American Journal of the Addictions* 7 (1998): 299–304.
53. R. M. Morse and D. K. Flavin, "The Definition of Alcoholism," *Journal of the American Medical Association* 268 (1992): 1012–1014.
54. R. S. Feldman, J. S. Meyer, and L. F. Quenzer, *Principles of Neuropsychopharmacology* (Sunderland, Mass.: Sinauer, 1997), 651.
55. C. A. Prescott and K. S. Kendler, "Genetic and Environmental Contributions to Alcohol Abuse and Dependence on a Population-based Sample of Male Twins," *American Journal of Psychiatry* 156 (1999): 34–40.
56. D. W. Goodwin and W. F. Gabrielli, "Alcohol: Clinical Aspects," in J. H. Lowinson, P. Ruiz, R. B. Millman, and J. G. Langrod, eds., *Substance Abuse: A Comprehensive Textbook*, 3rd ed. (Baltimore: Williams & Wilkins, 1997), 142–148.
57. M. G. Kushner, K. J. Sher, and D. J. Erickson, "Prospective Analysis Between DSM-III Anxiety Disorders and Alcohol Use Disorders," *American Journal of Psychiatry* 156 (1999): 723–732.
58. M. Lejoyeux, et al., "Study of Impulse-control Disorders Among Alcohol-dependent Patients," *Journal of Clinical Psychiatry* 60 (1999): 302–305.
59. Council on Scientific Affairs, American Medical Association, "Alcoholism in the Elderly," *Journal of the American Medical Association* 275 (1996): 797–801.
60. G. E. Vaillant, "A Long-term Follow-up of Male Alcohol Abuse," *Archives of General Psychiatry* 53 (1996): 243–249.
61. R. Saitz and S. S. O'Malley, "Pharmacotherapies for Alcohol Abuse: Withdrawal and Treatment," *Medical Clinics of North America* 81 (1997): 881–907.
62. A. Schaffer and C. A. Naranjo, "Recommended Drug Treatment Strategies for the Alcoholic Patient," *Drugs* 56 (1998): 571–585.
63. M. F. Mayo-Smith, "Pharmacological Management of Alcohol Withdrawal: A Meta-analysis and Evidence-based Practice Guidelines," *Journal of the American Medical Association* 278: (1997): 144–151.
64. J. C. Garbutt et al., "Pharmacological Treatment of Alcohol Dependence: A Review of the Evidence," *Journal of the American Medical Association* 281 (1999): 1318–1325.
65. R. M. Swift, "Drug Therapy for Alcohol Dependence," *New England Journal of Medicine* 340 (1999): 1482–1490.
66. J. R. Volpicelli et al., "Naltrexone and Alcohol Dependence: Role of Subject Compliance," *Archives of General Psychiatry* 54 (1997): 737–742.
67. D. Oslin et al., "Tolerability of Naltrexone in Treating Older, Alcohol-dependent Patients," *American Journal of the Addictions* 6 (1997): 266–270.
68. B. J. Mason et al., "A Double-blind, Placebo-controlled Study of Oral Nalmefene for Alcohol Dependence," *Archives of General Psychiatry* 56 (1999): 719–724.

69. R. Spanagel and W. Zieglgansberger, "Anticraving Compounds for Ethanol: New Pharmacological Tools to Study Addictive Processes," *Trends in Neurosciences* 18 (1997): 54–59.

70. M. I. Wilde and A. J. Wagstaff, "Acamprosate. A Review of Its Pharmacology and Clinical Potential in the Management of Alcohol Dependence After Detoxification," *Drugs* 53 (1997): 1038–1053.

71. J. A. Tinsley, R. E. Finlayson, and R. M. Morse, "Developments in the Treatment of Alcoholism," *Mayo Clinic Proceedings* 73 (1998): 857–863.

72. S. F. Greenfield et al., "The Effect of Depression in Return to Drinking," *Archives of General Psychiatry* 55 (1998): 259–265.

73. J. R. Cornelius et al., "Fluoxetine in Depressed Alcoholics," *Archives of General Psychiatry* 54 (1997): 700–705.

74. E. Malec et al., "Buspirone in the Treatment of Alcohol Dependence: A Placebo-controlled Trial," *Alcoholism: Clinical and Experimental Research* 20 (1996): 307–312.

75. B. A. Johnson et al., "Ritanserin in the Treatment of Alcohol Dependence," *Psychopharmacology* 128 (1996): 206–215.

76. G. Addolorato et al., "A Case of Gamma-hydroxybutyric Acid Withdrawal Syndrome During Alcohol Addiction Treatment: Utility of Diazepam Administration," *Clinical Neuropharmacology* 22 (1999): 60–62.

77. American Academy of Pediatrics, Committee on Substance Abuse and Committee on Native American Child Health, "Inhalant Abuse," *Pediatrics* 97 (1996): 420–423.

78. L. Yavich, N. Patkina, and E. Zvartau, "Experimental Estimation of Addictive Potential of a Mixture of Organic Solvents," *European Neuropsychopharmacology* 4 (1994): 111–118.

79. R. L. Balster, "College on Problems of Drug Dependence Presidential Address 1966: Inhalant Abuse, a Forgotten Drug Abuse Problem," *NIDA Research Monograph* 174 (1997): 3–8.

80. H. E. Jones and R. L. Balster, "Inhalant Abuse in Pregnancy," *Obstetrics and Gynecology Clinics of North America* 25 (1998): 153–167.

81. H. A. Spiller and E. P. Krenzelok, "Epidemiology of Inhalant Abuse Reported to Two Regional Poison Centers," *Journal of Toxicology—Clinical Toxicology* 35 (1997): 167–173.

82. S. E. Brown, J. Daniel, and R. L. Balster, "Deaths Associated with Inhalant Abuse in Virginia from 1987 to 1996," *Drug and Alcohol Dependence* 53 (1999): 239–245.

83. C. W. Sharp and N. L. Rosenberg, "Inhalants," in J. H. Lowinson, P. Ruiz, R. B. Millman, and J. G. Langrod, eds., *Substance Abuse: A Comprehensive Textbook*, 3rd ed. (Baltimore: Williams & Wilkins, 1997), 246–264.

84. R. L. Balster, "Neural Basis of Inhalant Abuse," *Drug and Alcohol Dependence* 51 (1998): 207–214.

85. B. B. Little, T. T. VanBeveren, and L. C. Gilstrap, "Inhalant (Organic Solvent) Abuse During Pregnancy," in L. C. Gilstrap and B. B. Little, eds., *Drugs and Pregnancy*, 2nd ed. (New York: Chapman & Hall, 1998), 457–461.

86. L. K. Misra, L. Kofoed and W. Fuller, "Treatment of Inhalant Abuse with Risperidone," *Journal of Clinical Psychiatry* 60 (1999): 620.

Chapter 5

Barbiturates, General Anesthetics, and Antiepileptic Drugs

Discussion of drugs that depress the functioning of the CNS began in Chapter 4 with the pharmacology of ethyl alcohol. This chapter continues coverage of CNS depressants by introducing the barbiturates, a structurally defined class of sedatives first introduced into medicine in 1912, and several older nonbarbiturate sedatives, as well as sedatives used in the treatment of epilepsy. This chapter is therefore important as a historical introduction to the treatment of anxiety, insomnia, and epilepsy. Chapter 6 covers the most widely used anxiolytics: the benzodiazepines and the newer second-generation anxiolytics.

Historical Background

From time immemorial, human beings have sought ways and means of achieving release from distressing and disabling anxiety and of inducing sleep to counteract debilitating insomnia. *Alcohol* is certainly the oldest of the sedative-hypnotic agents, having been used for thousands of years. It is ingested to ease anxiety, tension, and agitation and to induce a soporific state. The *opium alkaloids* (such as *morphine*) have similarly been used historically to induce a somnolent stupor for relief from anxiety and to bring on sleep. The addiction potential of the opioids, as well as their lethal potential, have limited their (usually illicit) use as antianxiety agents to relatively small groups.

128

In the middle of the nineteenth century, *bromide* and *chloral hydrate* became available as safer, more reliable alternatives to alcohol and opium as sedative agents. Then, in 1912, *phenobarbital* was introduced into medicine as a sedative drug, the first of the structurally classified group of drugs called *barbiturates* (Figure 5.1). Between 1912 and 1950, hundreds of barbiturates were tested and approximately 50 were marketed commercially. The barbiturates so dominated the stage that few structurally different sedatives were successfully marketed before 1960, when *chlordiazepoxide* (Librium) became the first available *benzodiazepine* tranquilizer, heralding a new era in the treatment of anxiety and insomnia.

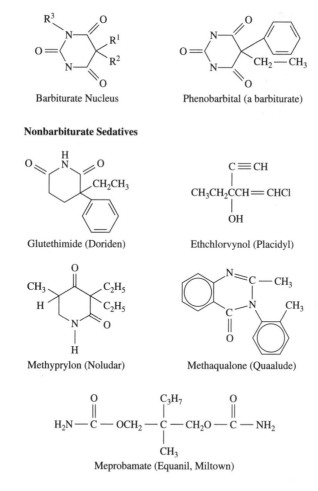

FIGURE 5.1 Chemical structures of classical sedatives. Barbiturates are defined by containing the barbiturate nucleus. Nonbarbiturate sedatives do not have this basic structure.

Between 1960 and 1990, about 15 benzodiazepines were marketed, differing from each other primarily in their pharmacokinetic properties (Chapter 6). The benzodizepines appeared to have a ceiling effect on CNS depression: overdoses were much less likely to result in a fatal outcome. Because of this, the benzodiazepines replaced the barbiturates for the treatment of anxiety and insomnia. Now, at the beginning of the twenty-first century, newer agents (the second-generation anxiolytics) are greatly reducing even the use of the benzodiazepines (Chapter 6). Undoubtedly, the twenty-first century will be accompanied by continued progress in the development of potentially superior sedative and hypnotic agents.

Sites and Mechanisms of Action

Historically, the sedative and hypnotic actions of the barbiturates and other sedatives have been perceived to result from a unique sensitivity of neurons within the CNS to nonselective neuronal depression that follows administration of these drugs. These compounds were presumed to depress polysynaptic, diffuse brain-stem neuronal pathways both in the brain-stem and in the cerebral cortex. Brain-stem depression would continue as dosage was increased, accounting for the deep coma and death that can follow drug overdosage.

Today, the mechanisms involved in the behavioral depressant action of the barbiturates are recognized as both complex and controversial. Few still invoke the classical concept of a nonselective depressant action affecting all neurons. Certainly barbiturates and other sedatives reduce electrical and metabolic activity of the brain, and the reductions are accompanied by decreases in whole brain glucose metabolism.[1] The reductions may follow from either reduction of excitatory activity or augmentation in inhibitory activity. As discussed in Chapter 3, *glutamate* is the predominant excitatory neurotransmitter in the brain, while *GABA* is the predominant inhibitory neurotransmitter.

Kamiya and colleagues[2] reported the effects of barbiturates on AMPA-type glutamate receptors (Chapter 3) and concluded that action on these receptors was probably not involved in the hypnotic action of these drugs. These results were verified by Joo and co-workers.[3] On the other hand, Zhu and colleagues[4] demonstrated that coma-producing doses of a barbiturate attenuated glutamate, providing a degree of "brain protection" following something like head injury. Implications for mechanisms of sedation were not addressed. Jetovic and co-workers[5] reported that the anesthetic gas *nitrous oxide* functions as an antagonist at glutamate NMDA-receptors, as does the psychedelic anesthetic *phencyclidine* (Chapter 12). It is thus likely that the amnestic properties of sedative drugs may result from glutamate antagonism (all these drugs have amnestic properties); while the sedative-hypnotic effect lies elsewhere.

That elsewhere now appears to involve augmentation of GABA neurotransmission. Recalling the discussion of the GABA$_A$ receptor in Chapter 2, barbiturates and benzodiazepines bind to this receptor, each at its own specific site, serving to facilitate binding of GABA to its receptor. Tomlin and colleagues[6] reported the effects of three barbiturates on GABA$_A$ receptors and concluded:

> There seems to be little doubt that the barbiturates exert their effects by binding to specific sites on the GABA$_A$ receptor, and that these effects play a major role in the anesthetic properties of these agents.

The same authors[7] reported a similar action on the GABA$_A$ receptor for the anesthetic drug *etomidate* (Amidate), although the location of the binding site on the receptor was not elucidated. Examining general anesthetics, Jenkins, Franks, and Lieb[8] reported that several *volatile anesthetic agents* (halothane, sevoflurane, isoflurane, and methoxyflurane) bind directly to the GABA$_A$ receptor and that the binding "plays an important role in general anesthesia." Davies and colleagues[9] demonstrated that the anesthetic-amnestic drug *propofol* (Diprovan) modulates the GABA$_A$ receptor complex, as do the barbiturates and volatile anesthetics. Thus, binding to GABA$_A$ receptors facilitates GABA-induced neurotransmission (channel opening with increased influx of chloride ions, and cellular hyperpolarization) and accounts for the sedative-hypnotic and anesthetic actions of barbiturates, benzodiazepines, anesthetics, and similar "depressant" drugs.

While barbiturates bind to the GABA$_A$ receptor and facilitate GABA binding, barbiturates are also capable of opening the chloride channel in the absence of GABA. This independent action accounts for the increased toxicity of barbiturates when compared with the relative lack of overdose toxicity seen with the benzodiazepines. The benzodiazepines have a ceiling effect on CNS depression since they enhance only the effects of GABA; they do not open chloride ion channels independently of GABA availability.

Uses

Use of barbiturates has declined rapidly in recent years for several reasons:

- They are lethal in overdose.
- They have a narrow therapeutic-to-toxic range.
- They have a high potential for inducing tolerance, dependence, and abuse.
- They interact dangerously with many other drugs.

Despite these disadvantages, the barbiturates are useful as anticonvulsants, as intravenous anesthetics, as death-inducing agents (they are the basic ingredient in cocktails used for suicides), to provide "brain protection" after head injury, and, in psychiatry, to sedate for an "Amytal interview."

Sedative-Induced Brain Dysfunction

Chapter 4 introduced the concept of a blackout that results from high levels of ethyl alcohol in the blood. A blackout is a state of antegrade amnesia, resulting in loss of memory for current events or actions at a certain blood level of alcohol that persists until the level of alcohol drops again below the amnestic level. More correctly, ethyl alcohol blackout is a manifestation of a *drug-induced, reversible, organic brain syndrome* that can follow use of any sedative. In other words, all sedatives can produce amnesia similar to that seen in such disorders as Alzheimer's disease (Chapter 3).

All dementias (drug-induced or organic) produce characteristic behavioral, intellectual, and cognitive patterns. One way to diagnose drug-induced dementia is to perform a *mental status examination* that evaluates 12 areas of mental functioning (Table 5.1). When a person's

---

TABLE 5.1 Mental status examination: Twelve areas
of mental functioning

---

1. General appearance
* 2. Sensorium
    a. Orientation to time, place, and person
    b. Clear vs. clouded thinking
3. Behavior and mannerisms
4. Stream of talk
5. Cooperativeness
6. Mood (inner feelings)
* 7. Affect (surface expression of feelings)
8. Perception
    a. Illusions (misperception of reality)
    b. Hallucinations (not present in reality)
9. Thought processes: logical vs. strange or bizarre
* 10. Mental content (fund of knowledge)
* 11. Intellectual function (ability to reason and interpret)
* 12. Insight and judgment

---

* Characteristically altered in both organic dementia and reversible, drug-induced dementia.

neurons are reversibly depressed by a depressant or when neurons are irreversibly destroyed (as in dementia), 5 of the 12 components of the mental status examination are particularly altered (sensorium, affect, mental content, intellectual function, and insight and judgment). The sensorium becomes clouded, which causes disorientation in time and place; memory becomes impaired, which is manifested by forgetfulness and loss of short-term memory (the blackout); the intellect becomes depressed; judgment is altered. Affect becomes shallow and labile, that is, the person becomes extremely vulnerable to external stimuli and may be sullen and moody at one moment and exhibit mock anger or rage at the next. This kind of mental status is diagnosed as a brain syndrome caused by depressed nerve cell function.

Certain people (such as the elderly) who already have some natural loss of nerve cell function are adversely affected by these drugs, experiencing increased disorientation and further clouding of consciousness. Frequently these people exhibit a state of drug-induced paradoxical excitement, which is characterized by a labile personality with marked anger, delusions, hallucinations, and confabulations, all part of the brain syndrome. Treating such a drug-induced dementia requires that administration of the sedative drug be stopped.

SPECIFIC CNS DEPRESSANTS

Barbiturates

The various barbiturates were the mainstays in treating anxiety and insomnia from 1912 to about 1960. During this period, they were associated with thousands of suicides, deaths from accidental ingestion, wide dependency and abuse, and many serious interactions with other drugs and alcohol. As we have discussed, however, they remain the classic prototype of sedative-hypnotic drugs against which newer drugs are compared.

Pharmacokinetics

Barbiturates are classified according to their pharmacokinetics. As shown in Table 5.2, their half-lives can be quite short (3-minute redistribution half-life for thiopental), longer (up to 48-hour elimination half-life for amobarbital, pentobarbital, and secobarbital), or very long (24- to 120-hour elimination half-life for phenobarbital). The hypnotic action of ultrashort-acting barbiturates (such as thiopental) is terminated by redistribution, while the action of other barbiturates is determined by their rate of hepatic metabolism followed by renal excretion of the metabolites.

TABLE 5.2 Half-lives and uses of some barbiturates

Drug name					Drug name		Uses		
Trade	Generic	R_1[a]	R_2[a]	R_3[a]	Distribution (min)	Elimination (h)	Insomnia	Anesthesia	Epilepsy
Amytal	Amobarbital	Ethyl	Isopentyl	H		10–40	X		
Alurate	Aprobarbital	Allyl	Isopentyl	H		12–34	X		
Butisol	Butabarbital	Athyl	sec-Butyl	H		34–42	X		
Mebaral	Mephobarbital	Ethyl	Phenyl	CH_3		50–120			X
Brevital	Methohexital	Allyl	1-Methyl, 2-Pentynyl	CH_3		1–2		X	
Nembural	Pentobarbital	Ethyl	Methyl butyl	H		15–50	X		
Luminal	Phenobarbital	Ethyl	Phenyl	H		24–120	X		X
Seconal	Secobarbital	Allyl	Methyl butyl	H		15–40	X		
Lotusate	Talbutal	Allyl	sec-Butyl	H			X		
Surital	Thiamylal	Allyl	Methyl butyl	H				X	
Pentothal	Thiopental	Ethyl	Methyl butyl	H	3	3–6		X	

[a] Symbols R_1, R_2, and R_3 refer to chemical substitution at these positions on the barbiturate nucleus shown in Figure 5.1.

Taken orally, barbiturates are rapidly and completely absorbed and are well distributed to most body tissues. The ultrashort-acting barbiturates are exceedingly lipid soluble, cross the blood-brain barrier rapidly, and induce sleep within seconds. Because the longer-acting barbiturates are more water soluble, they are slower to penetrate the CNS. Sleep induction with these compounds, therefore, is delayed for 20 to 30 minutes and residual hangover is prominent (since the plasma half-lives of most barbiturates vary from 10 to more than 48 hours).

Urinalysis is used to screen for the presence of barbiturates as well as other psychoactive drugs of abuse. Depending on the specific barbiturate, tests will be positive for as short as 30 hours or as long as several weeks after the drug is ingested. When urinalysis is positive for barbiturates, more specific confirmation is needed to determine the exact drug that was taken.

Pharmacological Effects

The barbiturates have a low degree of selectivity and therapeutic index: it is not possible to achieve anxiolysis without evidence of sedation. Barbiturates are not analgesic; they cannot be relied on to produce sedation or sleep in the presence of even moderate pain.

Sleep patterns are markedly affected by barbiturates, with rapid eye movement (REM) sleep being markedly suppressed. Because dreaming occurs during REM sleep, barbiturates suppress dreaming. During drug withdrawal, dreaming becomes vivid and excessive. Such rebound increase in dreaming during withdrawal (termed **REM rebound**) is one example of a withdrawal effect following prolonged periods of barbiturate ingestion. The vivid nature of the dreams can lead to insomnia, which can be clinically relieved by restarting the drug and thus negating the attempt at withdrawal.

Since barbiturates are sedatives and depress memory functioning, they are *cognitive inhibitors*. Drowsiness and more subtle alterations of judgment, cognitive functioning, motor skills, and behavior may persist for hours or days until the barbiturate is completely metabolized and eliminated.

Sedative doses of barbiturates have minimal effect on respiration, but overdoses (or combinations of barbiturates and alcohol) can result in death. Barbiturate-alcohol combinations have been responsible for both accidental and intentional suicides. Barbiturates exert few significant effects on the cardiovascular system, the gastrointestinal tract, the kidneys, or other organs until toxic doses are reached. In the liver, barbiturates stimulate the synthesis of enzymes that metabolize barbiturates as well as other drugs, an effect that produces significant tolerance to such drugs.

Psychological Effects

The behavioral depression and the motor and cognitive inhibition caused by barbiturates are similar to those caused by alcohol-induced inebriation and may even be indistinguishable from it. A person may respond to low doses either with relief from anxiety (the expected effect) or with withdrawal, emotional depression, or aggressive and violent behavior. Higher doses lead to more general behavioral depression and sleep. Mental set and physical or social setting can determine whether relief from anxiety, mental depression, aggression, or another unexpected or unpredictable response is experienced. Driving skills, judgment, insight, and memory all become severely impaired during the period of intoxication.

Adverse Reactions

Side Effects and Toxicity. Drowsiness is one of the primary effects induced by barbiturates and is an inescapable accompaniment to the anxiolytic effect. Drowsiness is often the effect sought if the drug is intended to produce either daytime sedation or nighttime sleep. Barbiturates significantly impair motor and intellectual performance and judgment:

> A person need not be rendered staggering drunk before his motor performance and, probably more important, his judgment are significantly impaired. The most common offending agent in this regard is alcohol. . . . At this time it should be emphasized that all sedatives are equivalent to alcohol in their effects; that all are additive in their effects with alcohol; and that their effects persist longer than might be predicted.[10]

There are no specific antidotes to the serious effects of barbiturate overdosage. Treatment of overdosage is aimed at supporting the respiratory and cardiovascular system until the drug is metabolized and eliminated.

Tolerance. The barbiturates can induce tolerance by either of two mechanisms: (1) the induction of drug-metabolizing enzymes in the liver and (2) the adaptation of neurons in the brain to the presence of the drug. With the latter mechanism, tolerance develops primarily to the sedative effects, much less to the brain-stem depressant effects on respiration. Thus, the margin of safety for the person who uses the drug decreases.

Physical Dependence. Normal clinical doses of barbiturates can induce a degree of physical dependence, usually manifested by sleep difficulties during attempts at withdrawal. Withdrawal from high doses of barbiturates may result in hallucinations, restlessness, disorientation, and even life-threatening convulsions.

Psychological Dependence.   Psychological dependence refers to a compulsion to use a drug for a pleasurable effect. All CNS depressants, including barbiturates, are subject to such an effect and are known to be abused compulsively. Because they can relieve anxiety, induce sedation, and produce a state of euphoria, these drugs may be used to achieve a variety of pleasurable psychological states in a variety of abuse situations.

Effects in Pregnancy.   Barbiturates, like all psychoactive drugs, are freely distributed to the fetus. Data are limited on whether deleterious fetal abnormalities occur as a result of a pregnant woman taking barbiturates, although there is a suggestion that developmental abnormalities occur. This can be a concern for pregnant females who are epileptic and must take a barbiturate to prevent seizures. As reviewed by Ramin and colleagues,[11]

> The risk for the pregnant woman treated with phenobarbital and other antiseizure medications of having an infant with congenital malformations is two to three times greater than that of the general population. It is not entirely clear whether this increased risk is secondary to the anticonvulsants, genetic factors, the seizure disorder itself, or possibly a combination of these factors, although . . . evidence exists for the implication of anticonvulsants as the etiology.

Other large epidemiological studies have failed to confirm this impression. Some studies report reduced Wechsler IQ scores in adult males whose mothers used phenobarbital, leading to a conclusion that barbiturate exposure during pregnancy can have long-term deleterious cognitive effects on offspring.[11] Studies on other anticonvulsant barbiturates have largely failed to confirm a teratogenic potential. A conservative conclusion might be that barbiturates have the potential to result in adverse neonatal outcomes in offspring of mothers taking these drugs. It would be best to avoid taking them while pregnant, but they do not appear to be contraindicated (necessarily avoided) during pregnancy should they be medically necessary, for example to prevent seizures in the mother (seizures that might also harm the fetus).

Miscellaneous Nonbarbiturate Sedative-Hypnotic Drugs

In the early 1950s, three "nonbarbiturate" sedatives, *glutethimide* (Doriden), *ethchlorvynol* (Placidyl), and *methyprylon* (Noludar) were introduced as anxiolytics, daytime sedatives, and hypnotics. They structurally resembled the barbiturates (Figure 5.1), but legally they did not have the exact barbiturate nucleus and were structurally not barbiturates, despite being pharmacologically interchangeable. These drugs offered no advantages over the barbiturates. Now considered obsolete, they are occasionally encountered as drugs of abuse.

Methaqualone (Quaalude) was another nonbarbiturate sedative that had little to justify its widespread use. During the late 1970s and early 1980s, its popularity rivaled that of marijuana and alcohol in its level of abuse. Such attention was due to an undeserved reputation as an aphrodisiac (as a sedative, it was actually an *an*aphrodisiac, much like alcohol). Extensive illicit use and numerous deaths led to its ban from sale in the United States in 1984, although illicit supplies occasionally emerge as a drug of abuse. Far from being a "love drug," methaqualone was merely one of several nonselective depressants that were thought to affect the user favorably when they were taken in the right setting and with a particular set of expectations. There are no reports associating the use of methaqualone during pregnancy with congenital malformations.[11]

Meprobamate (Equanil, Miltown), now largely of historical interest, was marketed in 1955 as another alternative to the barbiturates for daytime sedation and anxiolysis. Around it developed the term "tranquilizer" in a marketing attempt to distinguish it from the barbiturates, a distinction that was not borne out in reality. Like the barbiturates, meprobamate produces long-lasting daytime sedation, mild euphoria, and relief from anxiety. Meprobamate is not as potent a respiratory depressant as the barbiturates; attempted suicides from overdosage are seldom successful. Despite a continuing reduction in clinical use, abuse and dependency continue and are difficult to treat. There is a possibility that use of meprobamate during pregnancy may be associated with an increased frequency of congenital malformations.[11]

Chloral hydrate (Noctec) is yet another drug of largely historical interest, having been available clinically since the late 1800s. It is rapidly metabolized to *trichlorethanol* (a derivative of ethyl alcohol), which is a nonselective CNS depressant and the active form of chloral hydrate. The drug appears to be a relatively safe and effective sedative-hypnotic, with a plasma half-life of about 4 to 8 hours. Next-day hangover is less likely to occur than with compounds having longer half-lives. Its liability in producing tolerance and dependence is similar to that of the barbiturates. Withdrawal of the drug may be associated with disrupted sleep and intense nightmares. Occasionally, chloral hydrate is utilized as a bedtime sedative for elderly patients, because of its short half-life. One interesting aside is that the combination of chloral hydrate with alcohol can produce increased intoxication, stupor, and amnesia. This mixture was called a Mickey Finn and was an early example of a "date rape" drug or drug combination.

Teratogenicity of chloral hydrate in offspring of women taking the drug has not been demonstrated, although withdrawal signs may be seen in newborns of such females.

Paraldehyde, introduced into medicine before the barbiturates, is a polymer of acetaldehyde, an intermediate by-product in the body's metabolism of ethyl alcohol. Administered either rectally or orally, paraldehyde is occasionally used to treat delirium tremens (DTs) in hospitalized patients undergoing withdrawal from alcohol (detoxification). The drug is rapidly absorbed (from both rectal and oral routes), sleep ensues within 10 to 15 minutes after hypnotic doses, and the drug is metabolized in the liver to acetaldehyde and eventually to carbon dioxide and water. Some paraldehyde is eliminated through the lungs, producing a characteristic breath odor. People dependent on paraldehyde (usually people who received paraldehyde as a treatment for alcoholism) suffer a variety of toxicities, primarily to the stomach, liver, and kidneys.

GENERAL ANESTHETICS

General anesthetics are potent CNS depressants that produce a loss of sensation accompanied by unconsciousness. General anesthesia is therefore the most severe state of intentional drug-induced CNS depression. The agents that are used as general anesthetics are of two types: (1) those that are administered by inhalation through the lungs and (2) those that are injected directly into a vein to produce unconsciousness.

The inhalation anesthetics in current use include one gas (nitrous oxide) and five volatile liquids (isoflurane, halothane, desflurane, enflurane, and sevoflurane), whose vapors are delivered into the patient's lungs by means of an anesthesia machine. These drugs produce a dose-related depression of all functions of the CNS—an initial period of sedation followed by the onset of sleep. As anesthesia deepens, the patient's reflexes become progressively depressed and both amnesia and unconsciousness are induced. Adding an opioid narcotic to a volatile anesthetic induces a state of unconsciousness and analgesia, a state that Glass[12] defines as "general anesthesia":

> General anesthesia is a process requiring a state of unconsciousness of the brain (produced primarily by the volatile anesthetic or propofol). If only unconsciousness is achieved, a noxious (painful) stimulus will cause arousal/awakening as a result of the intensity of the stimulus. To prevent arousal, the noxious stimulus needs to be inhibited from reaching higher centers. This is achieved by the action of the opiate at opiate receptors within the spinal cord. Thus, general anesthesia consists of

producing both loss of consciousness through the action of drugs we administer on the brain, and the inhibition of noxious stimuli reaching the brain through the action of drugs we administer on the spinal cord.[*]

Prominent scientists have studied the possible mechanisms of action of the inhaled general anesthetics for more than 100 years.[13] Perhaps, the most plausible explanation for the action of anesthetics involves alteration in the physiochemical processes of nerve membranes. This action follows from the linear correlation (Figure 5.2) between the potency of various drugs as general anesthetic agents and their solubility in lipid. As anesthetics dissolve in the nerve membranes, the structure of the lipid matrix of the membranes becomes distorted, thereby "perturbing" the function of the ion channels and the membrane proteins.

Occasionally, the inhaled anesthetic agents are subject to misuse. *Nitrous oxide*, a gas of low anesthetic potency, is an example. Currently

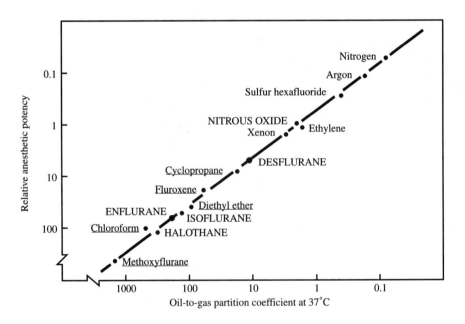

FIGURE 5.2 Correlation of anesthetic potency with the oil-to-gas coefficient. The correlation is shown for a number of general anesthetic agents and for other inert gases that are not usually used for anesthesia. Note the excellent correlation over a very wide range of fat solubilities and potencies. Agents that are used today in anesthesia are shown in boldface capital letters. Agents that were historically used as anesthetics are underscored.

---

[*]The actions of opioids (opiates) on the spinal cord are discussed in Chapter 9.

used not only in anesthesia but as a carrier gas in cans of whipped cream (e.g., Whippets), nitrous oxide induces a state of behavioral disinhibition, analgesia, and mild euphoria. Since the inhalation of nitrous oxide dilutes the air that a person is breathing, extreme caution must be exercised in order to prevent hypoxia. If the nitrous oxide were mixed only with room air, hypoxia would result, which could produce irreversible brain damage. Other inhaled anesthetics are similarly abused, presuming that the drug abuser can find a supply of the agents. Inhaled as vapors, these drugs produce intoxication, delirium, and eventually unconsciousness. Other forms of inhalant abuse were discussed in Chapter 4.

Several injectable anesthetics are available. *Thiopental* (Pentothal) and *methohexital* (Brevital) are ultrashort-acting barbiturates. *Propofol* (Diprovan) and *etomidate* (Amidate) are structurally unique; propofol structurally resembles the neurotransmitter GABA (Figure 5.3). The mechanism of action of all these anesthetics probably involves intense CNS

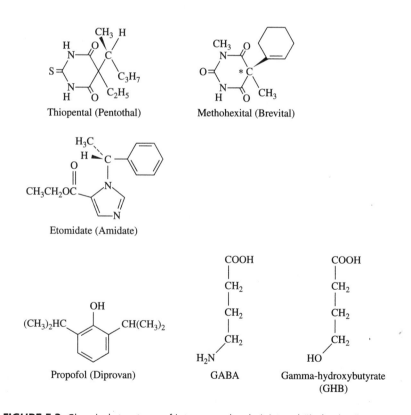

FIGURE 5.3 Chemical structures of intravenously administered "induction" anesthetics. Illustrated are two barbiturates (thiopental and methohexital) and two newer agents. Also illustrated are the structure of GABA and GHB. Propofol is structurally similar to GABA, as is GHB.

depression produced secondary both to facilitation of GABA$_A$-receptor activity and to depression of excitatory glutamate synaptic transmission.

Finally, *gamma-hydroxybutyric acid* (*gamma-hydroxybutyrate*, GHB) is a potent CNS depressant, used in some countries (but not the United States) as a general anesthetic. GHB is a naturally occurring 4-carbon molecule (Figure 5.3) with a structure similar to GABA. It is an endogenous constituent of mammalian brains, synthesized locally from GABA; it may play a role as a "central neuromodulator."[14] It freely crosses the blood-brain barrier and has been used in anesthesia, sleep disorders, and alcohol and opioid dependence. It can also be classified as a euphoriant; it is gaining increasing recognition and attention among substance abusers and athletes. Besides use as a general anesthetic, it is widely available illicitly and has been used as a body-building aid (as a "growth hormone stimulator"), as a euphoriant, and for sexual enhancement. It has been available from foreign sources through a variety of venues and can be made at home. It has been called "Nature's Quaalude," among a variety of other names. GHB has been widely implicated as a "date rape" drug, similar to the older drug chloral hydrate. There is no evidence that it aids body building or sexual performance: it is a potent sedative and depressant. Like any depressant, it can produce a state of disinhibition, excitement, drunkenness, and amnesia. It has been reported that GHB increases dopamine levels in the brain, perhaps activating the central dopaminergic reward system by increasing the expression of dopamine-receptor mRNA (a cocaine-like action).[15]

GHB overdoses are characterized by stupor, delirium, unconsciousness, and coma. Seizures, respiratory depression, and vomiting are common. There are no antidotes for treating overdoses: treatment is "supportive" until the drug is eliminated. The drug's half-life is about 1 hour. Several articles detail the pharmacology and abuse problems with GHB.[16–19]

ANTIEPILEPTIC DRUGS

Seizures are manifestations of electrical disturbances in the brain. The term *epilepsy* refers to CNS disorders characterized by relatively brief, chronically recurring seizures that have a rapid onset. Epileptic seizures are often associated with focal (or localized) lesions within the brain. Drugs suppress epileptic seizures by one of two mechanisms:[20]

1. Limiting the repetitive firing of neurons by blocking the transmembrane channels (Figure 5.4) through which sodium ions flow, thereby blocking the depolarizing action of sodium ions on the cell (repetitive discharge is thought to initiate or sustain a seizure)

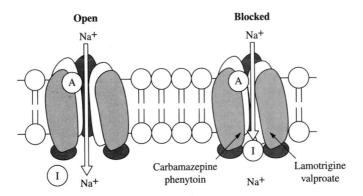

FIGURE 5.4 Antiseizure drug-enhanced sodium ion (Na^+) channel blockade. Some antiseizure drugs block Na^+ channels, thereby reducing the ability of neurons to fire at high frequencies. [Modified from McNamara.[20]]

2. Enhancing GABA-mediated synaptic inhibition[21] by reducing the metabolism of GABA, enhancing the influx of chloride ions, or facilitating GABA release from presynaptic nerve terminals

In laboratory animals, epileptic seizures can be induced by a variety of techniques, including "kindling" (repeated low-voltage electrical stimulation of the amygdala or hippocampus to increase the sensitivity of neurons therein). Post and Weiss[22] associate kindling not only with antiepileptic drug action but also with the treatment of bipolar disorders. Indeed, over the past ten years, antiepileptic drugs have become a mainstay for the treatment of bipolar disorder (Chapter 16). While the mechanisms involved in the genesis of epilepsy and bipolar disorder are far from being elucidated, the correlation is intriguing. Perhaps GABA-augmenting mechanisms occur at both $GABA_A$ and $GABA_B$ receptors. In addition to this overlap between bipolar disorder and epilepsy, other investigators have reported efficacy of antiepileptic drugs in treating a variety of explosive psychological disorders.[2] The observation that a drug may be sedative, anxiolytic, antiepileptic, and antimanic encourages the notion that epilepsy, mania, and explosive psychological disorders can be treated with CNS depressants that "stabilize" neuronal membranes either by facilitating inhibition or by limiting excitation.

Relationships Between Structure and Activity

Traditional antiepileptic drugs belong to one of two chemically similar classes, barbiturates or *hydantoins* (Figure 5.5). Older and structurally similar antiepileptic drugs still in use include *ethosuximide*

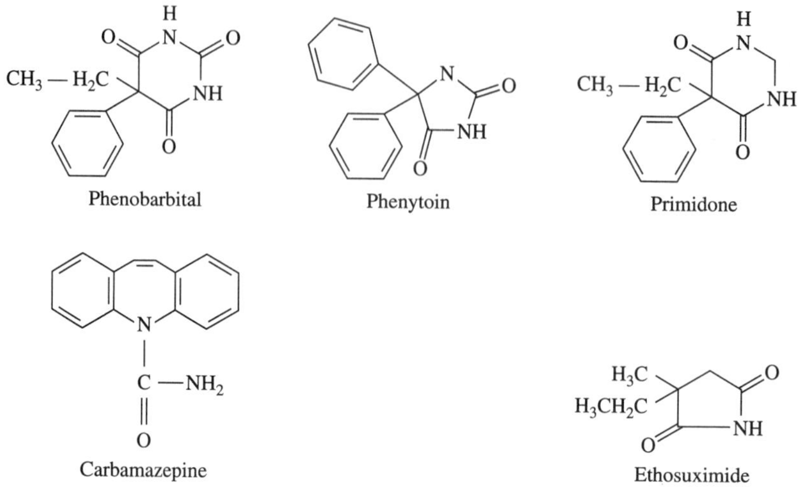

FIGURE 5.5 Chemical structures of several classic drugs used to treat epilepsy.

and *primidone*. *Carbamazepine* (Tegretol) structurally resembles both the tricyclic antidepressants (Chapter 15) and phenytoin (Dilantin).

More recently introduced drugs do not bear structural resemblance to classic drugs; rather, they were developed for antiepileptic potential because they either resembled GABA (Figure 5.6) or acted on GABA receptors to potentiate GABA neurotransmission. Development began in 1978 with the introduction of valproic acid (Depakine) and has continued through the 1990s with the introductions of felbamate (Felbatol), gabapentin (Neurontin), lamotrigine (Lamictal), topiramate (Topamax), and tiagabine (Gabitril). All these GABAergic drugs are effective antiepileptic agents, and most are also reported effective in the treatment of bipolar disorder (Chapter 16).

Felbamate[24] (Felbatol) structurally resembles meprobamate, an anxiolytic discussed earlier (Figure 5.6). To date, nonepileptic, psychological uses of felbamate have not been reported, although the structural resemblance to meprobamate implies an anxiolytic effect. At first thought to be free of serious side effects, felbamate's use was drastically curtailed in late 1994 because of serious hematological reactions. Felbamate is currently used only when the drug is absolutely necessary

---

*Overlapping uses of antiepileptic drugs began about 25 years ago, when phenytoin (Dilantin) was advocated to treat uncontrolled bouts of mania, panic, and aggression.[23] Other antiepileptic drugs are now widely used to treat not only bipolar disorder but also unipolar depression, schizoaffective disorder, dyscontrol syndromes, intermittent explosive disorder, posttraumatic stress disorder, and atypical psychosis.

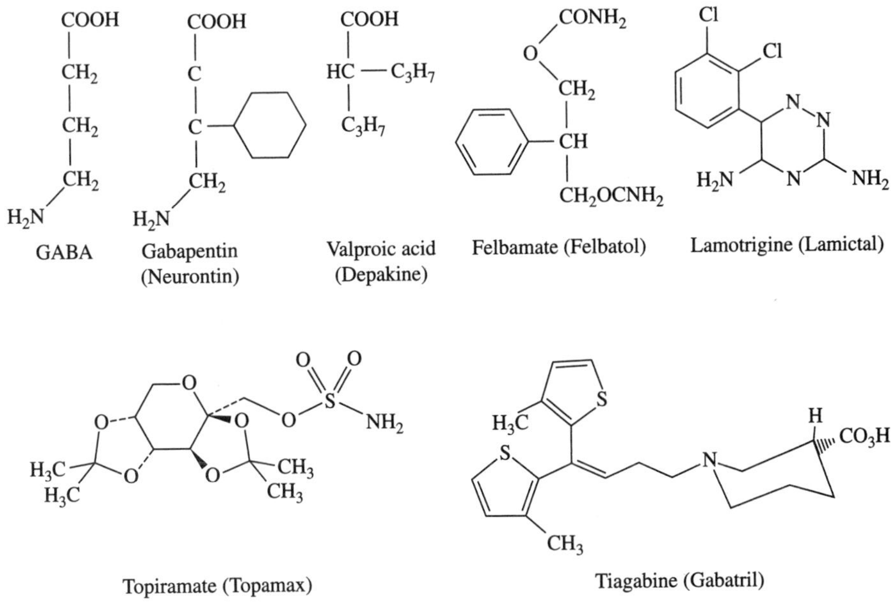

FIGURE 5.6 Chemical structures of several "GABA-ergic" drugs used to treat epilepsy. Most are also effective in treating bipolar disorder.

and irreplaceable as an antiepileptic. Recently, a practice advisory offering guidelines for the safe use of felbamate was published.[25]

Gabapentin, a structural analogue of GABA (Figure 5.6), was synthesized as a specific GABA-mimetic antiepileptic drug. In 1995, gabapentin was reported effective in treating both an anxiety disorder (phobia) and pain (reflex sympathetic dystrophy) in one female patient. Since then, gabapentin has been tried in a variety of psychiatric disorders, including bipolar disorder, and in the demented elderly to treat agitation and aggressive behavior. Gabapentin acts by promoting the release of GABA from presynaptic nerve terminals. Today, gabapentin is finding increasing use as an alternative to lithium and other anticonvulsants in the treatment of bipolar disorder[26] (Chapter 16).

Lamotrigine (introduced in 1995) acts by inhibiting ion fluxes through sodium channels, thereby stabilizing neuronal membranes and inhibiting the presynaptic release of neurotransmitters, principally glutamate.[27] It has thus found use as an antiepileptic drug, and it was reported in 1997 to improve mood, alertness, and social interactions in some epilepsy patients.[28] Since then, many case reports have attested to an antidepressant and antimanic action. The first double-blind,

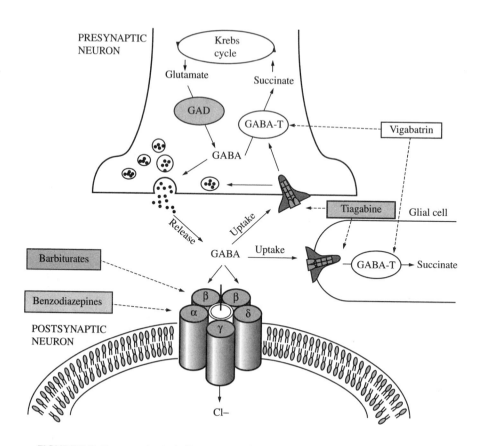

FIGURE 5.7 Pharmacological effects of tiagabine and other antiepileptic drugs at the GABA$_A$ receptor. GAD = glutamic acid decarboxylase. GABA-T = GABA-transaminase. Barbiturates bind to the beta-subunit of GABA$_A$ receptor to potentiate action of endogenous agonist GABA and prolong opening time of chloride ion channel. Benzodiazepines bind to alpha-subunit of GABA$_A$ to potentiate action of GABA and increase frequency of opening of chloride ion channel. Vigabatrin irreversibly binds to GABA-transaminase to inhibit degradation of inhibitory transmitter GABA. Tiagabine blocks uptake of synaptically released GABA into both pre-synaptic neurons and glial cells, allowing GABA to remain at site of action for longer periods. [From Leach and Brodie[32] p. 204].

placebo-controlled multicenter report of therapeutic efficacy in treating bipolar depression appeared in 1997.[29] Lamotrigine will probably achieve a place as another anticonvulsant used in the treatment of bipolar illness, although comparative studies remain to be published.

Interestingly, in the treatment of head injury, release of glutamate has been associated with permanent neuronal damage. Lamotrigine has been reported to inhibit hypoxia-induced or ischemia-induced release of glutamate; perhaps the drug may be clinically useful in providing brain protection in individuals suffering such injury.[27]

Among the *barbiturates, Phenobarbital,* the first widely effective antiepileptic drug, replaced the more toxic agent, *bromide,* which had been used during the nineteenth century. Two other barbiturates are also used occasionally for treating epilepsy—*mephobarbital* (Mebaral) and *metharbital* (Gemonil). Because of their efficacy in reducing seizures, barbiturates are still used occasionally, even though more effective, more specific, and less sedating antiepileptic agents are now the drugs of choice. Epileptic children given barbiturates can display adverse neuropsychological reactions (behavioral hyperactivity and interference with learning ability). *Primidone* (Mysoline), an antiepileptic agent structurally similar to phenobarbital, is metabolized to phenobarbital, which might well be the major active form of the drug.

Phenytoin (Dilantin) remains a commonly used *hydantoin* anticonvulsant, perhaps producing less sedation than do the barbiturates. Phenytoin has a half-life of about 24 hours; thus, daytime sedation can be minimized if the patient takes the full daily dose at bedtime.

All *benzodiazepines* (Chapter 6) possess antiepileptic properties. Two of them, *clonazepam* (Klonopin) and *clorazepate* (Tranxene), are promoted as anticonvulsants, among other uses. When used in children, drug-induced personality changes and learning disabilities must be carefully monitored. Both drugs have psychiatric applications that include the treatment of acute mania and other agitated psychotic conditions, usually in combination with other "mood stabilizers" (see Chapter 16).

Carbamazepine (Tegretol) is an antiepileptic drug with a sedative effect that is perhaps less intense than that of the other antiepileptic agents. The primary limitations of carbamazepine include rare but potentially serious alterations in the cellular composition of blood (reduced numbers of white blood cells), presumably secondary to a depressant effect on bone marrow. For nonepileptic, psychiatric use, carbamazepine is used in the treatment of bipolar disorder[30] and in certain chronic pain syndromes.

Valproic acid (Depakene, Depakote, Depacon, Divalproex, Valproate) is effective and widely used in treating seizure disorders in children. It acts by augmenting the postsynaptic action of GABA, probably by inhibiting the GABA-destroying enzyme GABA transaminase that normally functions to end the transmitter action of GABA. Valproic acid has a short half-life (about 6 to 12 hours); it must be administered several times a day. About 75 percent of epileptic patients receiving valproic acid respond favorably. Serious side effects from valproic acid are rare, but liver failure has been reported.

Like several of these newer anticonvulsants, valproic acid possesses both antiepileptic action and GABAergic actions, so it is not surprising that the drug is highly effective in individuals with bipolar disorder (Chapter 16).[31] Besides use as an anticonvulsant and antimanic drug, valproate has been reported useful in treating such disorders as pathologic aggression[32] and schizophrenia.[33]

Tiagabine (Gabitril) was released in 1998 as a new antiepileptic drug. The drug acts by inhibiting neuronal and glial uptake of GABA, secondary to its irreversibly inhibiting one of the GABA reuptake transporters located on the presynaptic nerve terminals of GABA-releasing neurons (Figure 5.7). This action serves to prolong GABA's synaptic action.[34,35] Tiagabine has also been reported to be useful in treating bipolar disorder.[36]

Finally, another new antiepileptic drug, *topiramate* (Topamax), has also found use in the treatment of bipolar disorder.[37] No comparative studies of efficacy of one of these newer antiepileptic-antimanic drugs have yet been reported.

Several novel classes of drugs are being evaluated for clinical usefulness as antiepileptic agents. Of particular interest are several steroid derivatives, referred to as epalons. *Epalons* are neuroactive endogenous or synthetic steroids that are devoid of hormonal action but that exert anxiolytic, sedative, and anticonvulsant effects by binding to a specific steroid-sensitive site on the $GABA_A$ receptor, facilitating GABA activity.[38] One such agent, *ganaxolone*, is in final clinical trials and offers promise as an antiepileptic agent.[39,40] Other epalons are being developed as nonsedating antianxiety agents. The plasma half-lives and therapeutic blood levels of available antiepileptic drugs are listed in Table 5.3.

Antiepileptic Drugs in Pregnancy

Rates of stillbirth and infant mortality are higher for mothers with epilepsy. Children of epileptic mothers who received antiseizure medication during the early months of pregnancy have an increased incidence of a variety of birth defects. The risk is approximately 7 percent, compared with 2 to 3 percent for the general population.[41] Pitting this fact against the obvious necessity to control seizures is a therapeutic dilemma in treating pregnant women who have epilepsy. In general, women with epilepsy of childbearing age should be advised of teratogenic potential. Prior to becoming pregnant, it should be determined whether drugs can be tapered off and discontinued. If termination cannot be done safely, one approach is to use a single medication at the lowest possible dose that will control seizures. Divided daily doses may decrease the peak levels in plasma while maintaining an adequate steady-state level of the drug in the blood. Cantrell and colleagues[42] recently reviewed the teratogenicity of antiepileptic drugs. They concluded: "With proper management, 90 percent of women with epilepsy can anticipate uneventful pregnancies and normal children." The neonatal complications of antiepileptic drugs used in the treatment of bipolar illness are discussed in Chapter 16.

TABLE 5.3 Antiepileptic drugs available in the United States

Year introduced	Generic name	Trade name	Half-life (hours)	Therapeutic blood level (mcg/mL) [a]
1912	Phenobarbital	Luminal	50+	15–40
1935	Mephobarbital	Mebaral	—[b]	—
1938	Phenytoin	Dilantin	18+	5–20
1946	Trimethadione	Tridione	6–13	>700
1947	Mephenytoin	Mesantoin	95	—
1949	Paramethadione	Paradione	—	—
1951	Phenacemide	Phenurone	—	—
1952	Metharbital	Gemonil	—	—
1953	Phensuximide	Milontin	8	—
1954	Primidone	Mysoline	5–20	5–40
1957	Methsuximide	Celontin	2–40	—
1957	Ethotoin	Peganone	4–9	15–50
1960	Ethosuximide	Zarontin	30+	40–400
1968	Diazepam	Valium	20–50	—
1974	Carbamazepine	Tegretol	18–50	4–12
1975	Clonazepam	Klonopin	18–60	20–80
1978	Valproic acid	Depakene	5–20	50–150
1981	Clorazepate	Tranxene	30–100	—
1981	Lorazepam	Ativan		
1993	Felbamate	Felbatol	22	—
1994	Gabapentin	Neurontin	5–7	—
1995	Lamotrigine	Lamictal	33	—
1998	Topiramate	Topamax	19–23	—
1998	Tiagabine	Gabatril	6–9	—

a mcg/mL = micrograms of drug per milliliter of blood
b — = data not available

STUDY QUESTIONS

1. List the various classes of nonselective CNS depressants and give examples of each class. What are common terms for CNS depressants?

2. What are the consequences of the drug blockade of glutamate receptors? Of GABA receptors?

3. Describe the gradation of action that occurs in a person as a result of taking progressively increasing doses of a nonselective CNS depressant.

4. What is meant by cross-tolerance of CNS depressant? Of cross-dependence?

5. Describe what is meant by "supra-additive CNS depression." How does potentiation work?

6. What is meant by the term "drug-induced, reversible brain syndrome"?

7. What mechanisms are responsible for the differing durations of action of various barbiturates?

8. What are the oldest CNS depressant? The newest?

9. Describe the effects of barbiturates on sleep patterns both acutely and during drug withdrawal.

10. Compare the effects of barbiturates and chloral hydrate on the elderly.

11. How does paraldehyde resemble ethyl alcohol?

12. What are the particular dangers of use of CNS depressants in the elderly? In the young?

13. Which antiepileptic drugs are also used in the treatment of bipolar disorder? Why might they work?

14. Why might antiepileptic drugs be considered for use in non-epileptic, psychological disorders?

REFERENCES

1. M. T. Alkire et al., "Functional Brain Imaging During Anesthesia in Humans: Effects of Halothane on Global and Regional Cerebral Glucose Metabolism," *Anesthesiology* 90 (1999): 701–709.
2. Y. Kamiya et al., "Comparison of the Effects of Convulsant and Depressant Barbiturate Stereoisomers on AMPA-type Glutamate Receptors," *Anesthesiology* 90 (1999): 1704–1713.
3. D. T. Joo et al., "Blockade of Glutamate Receptors and Barbiturate Anesthesia: Increased Sensitivity to Pentobarbital-induced Anesthesia Despite Reduced Inhibition of AMPA Receptors in GluR2 Null Mutant Mice," *Anesthesiology* 91 (1999): 1329–1341.
4. H. Zhu, J. E. Cottrell, and I. S. Kass, "The Effect of Thiopental and Propofol on NMDA- and AMPA-mediated Glutamate Excitotoxicity," *Anesthesiology* 87 (1997): 944–951.
5. V. Jevtovic-Todorovic et al., "Nitrous Oxide (Laughing Gas) Is an NMDA Antagonist, Neuroprotectant and Neurotoxin," *Nature Medicine* 4 (1998): 460–463.
6. S. L. Tomlin et al., "Preparation of Barbiturate Optical Isomers and Their Effects on GABA$_A$ Receptors," *Anesthesiology* 90 (1999): 1714–1722.

7. S. L. Tomlin et al., "Stereoselective Effects of Etomidate Optical Isomers on Gamma-aminobutyric Acid Type A Receptors and Animals," *Anesthesiology* 88 (1998): 708–717.

8. A. Jenkins, N. P. Franks, and W. R. Lied, "Effects of Temperature and Volatile Anesthetics on GABA$_A$ Receptors," *Anesthesiology* 90 (1999): 484–491.

9. M. Davies, R. P. Thuynsma, and S. M. J. Dunn, "Effects of Propofol and Pentobarbital on Ligand Binding to GABA$_A$ Receptors Suggest a Similar Mechanism of Action," *Canadian Journal of Physiology and Pharmacology* 76 (1998): 46–52.

10. H. Meyers, E. Jawetz, and A. Goldfien, *Review of Medical Pharmacology*, 3rd ed. (Los Altos, Calif.: Lange Medical Publications, 1972), 219.

11. S. M. Ramin, L. C. Gilstrap, and B. B. Little, "Psychotropics in Pregnancy," in L. C. Gilstrap and B. B. Little, eds., *Drugs and Pregnancy*, 2nd ed. (New York: Chapman & Hall, 1998), 172–175.

12. P. S. A. Glass, "Anesthetic Drug Interactions: An Insight into General Anesthesia—Its Mechanism and Dosing," *Anesthesiology* 88: (1998): 5–6.

13. J. H. Tinker, "Voices from the Past: From Ice Crystals to Fruit Flies in the Quest for a Molecular Mechanism of Anesthetic Action," *Anesthesia and Analgesia* 77 (1993): 1–3.

14. R. Bernasconi, P. Mathivet, S. Bischoff, and C. Marescaux, "Gamma-hydroxybutyric Acid: An Endogenous Neuromodulator with Abuse Potential," *Trends in Pharmacological Sciences* 20 (1999): 135–141.

15. C. Schmidt-Mutter et al., "Gamma-hydroxybutyrate and Cocaine Administration Increases mRNA Expression of Dopamine D$_1$ and D$_2$ Receptors in Rat Brain," *Neuropsychopharmacology* 21 (1999): 662–669.

16. R. L. Chin et al., "Clinical Course of Gamma-hydroxybutyrate Overdose," *Annals of Emergency Medicine* 31 (1998): 716–722.

17. J. Li, S. A. Stokes, and A. Woeckener, "A Tale of Novel Intoxication: A Review of the Effects of Gamma-hydroxybutyric Acid with Recommendations for Management," *Annals of Emergency Medicine* 31 (1998): 729–736.

18. M. B. Scharf et al., "Pharmacokinetics of Gamma-hydroxybutyrate (GHB) in Narcoleptic Patients," *Sleep* 21 (1998): 507–514.

19. V. R. Sanguineti, A. Angelo, and M. R. Frank, "GHB: A Home Brew," *American Journal of Drug and Alcohol Abuse* 23 (1997): 637–642.

20. J. O. McNamara, "Drugs Effective in the Therapy of the Epilepsies," in: J. G. Hardman, L. E. Limbird, P. B. Molinoff, R. W. Ruddon, and A. G. Gilman, eds., *Goodman and Gilman's The Pharmacological Basis of Therapeutics*, 9th ed. (New York: McGraw-Hill, 1996), 461–486.

21. P. Granger, B. Biton, C. Faure, X. Vige, H. Depoortere, D. Graham, S. Z. Langer, B. Scatton, and P. Avonet, "Modulation of the Gamma-aminobutyric Acid Type A Receptor by the Antiepileptic Drugs Carbamazepine and Phenytoin," *Molecular Pharmacology* 47 (1995): 1189–1196.

22. R. M. Post and S. R. B. Weiss, "Sensitization, Kindling, and Anticonvulsants in Mania," *Journal of Clinical Psychiatry* 50, Suppl. 12 (1989): 23–30.

23. J. Dryfus, *The Lion of Wall Street* (Washington D.C.: Regnery, 1996).

24. K. J. Palmer and D. McTavish, "Felbamate: A Review of Its Pharmacodynamic and Pharmacokinetic Properties, and Therapeutic Efficacy in Epilepsy," *Drugs* 46 (1993): 1041–1065.

25 J. French et al., "Practice Advisory: The Use of Felbamate in Treatment of Patients with Intractable Epilepsy: Report of the Quality Standards Subcommittee of the American Academy of Neurology and the American Epilepsy Society," *Neurology* 52 (1999): 1540–1545.

26. I. N. Ferrier, "Lamotrigine and Gabapentin: Alternatives in the Treatment of Bipolar Disorder," *Neuropsychobiology* 38 (1998): 192–197.

27. B. P. Conroy et al., "Lamotrigine Attenuates Cortical Glutamate Release During Global Cerebral Ischemia in Pigs on Cardiopulmonary Bypass," *Anesthesiology* 90 (1999): 844–854.

28. R. M. Post et al., "Drug-induced Switching in Bipolar Disorder: Epidemiology and Therapeutic Implications," *CNS Drugs* 8 (1997): 352–365.

29. J. R. Calabrese et al., "A Double-blind Placebo-controlled Study of Lamotrigine Monotherapy in Outpatients with Bipolar I Depression," *Journal of Clinical Psychiatry* 60 (1999): 79–88.

30. N. Coxhead, T. Silverstone, and J. Cookson, "Carbamazepine versus Lithium in the Prophylaxis of Bipolar Affective Disorder," *Acta Psychiatrica Scandinavia* 85 (1992): 14–118.

31. D. A. Soloman et al., "Lithium plus Valproate as Maintenance Polypharmacy for Patients with Bipolar I Disorder: A Review," *Journal of Clinical Psychopharmacology* 18 (1998): 38–49.

32. M. Fava, "Psychopharmacologic treatment of Pathologic Aggression," *Psychiatric Clinics of North America* 20 (1997): 427–451.

33. A. A. Wassef et al., "Critical Review of GABAergic Drugs in the Treatment of Schizophrenia," *Journal of Clinical Psychopharmacology* 19 (1999): 222–232.

34. J. P. Leach and M. J. Brodie, "Tiagabine," *Lancet* 351 (1998): 203–207.

35. *The Medical Letter,* "Tiagabine for Epilepsy," *The Medical Letter* 40 (April 10, 1998): 45–46.

36. K. R. Kaufman, "Adjunctive Tiagabine Treatment of Psychiatric Disorders: Three Cases," *Annals of Clinical Psychiatry* 10 (1998): 181–184.

37. D. Marcotte, "Use of Topiramate, a New Anti-epileptic, as a Mood Stabilizer," *Journal of Affective Disorders* 50 (1998): 245–251.

38. M. Gasior et al., "Anticonvulsant and Behavioral Effects of Neuroactive Steroids Alone and in Combination with Diazepam," *Journal of Pharmacology and Experimental Therapeutics* 282 (1997): 543–553.

39. E. P. Monaghan et al., "Initial Human Experience with Ganaxolone, a Neuroactive Steroid with Antiepileptic Activity," *Epilepsia* 38 (1997): 1026–1031.

40. O. C. Snead, "Ganaxolone, a Selective, High-affinity Steroid Modulator of the Gamma-aminobutyric Acid-A Receptor, Exacerbates Seizures in Animal Models of Absence," *Annals of Neurology* 44 (1998): 688–691.

41. D. Lindhout and J. G. Omtzigt, "Teratogenic Effects of Antiepileptic Drugs: Implications for the Management of Epilepsy in Women of Childbearing Age," *Epilepsia* 35, Suppl. 4 (1994): S19–S28.

42. D. T. C. Cantrell, L. C. Gilstrap, and B. B. Little, "Anticonvulsant Drugs During Pregnancy," in L. C. Gilstrap and B. B. Little, eds., *Drugs and Pregnancy*, 2nd ed. (New York: Chapman & Hall, 1998), 137–147.

Chapter 6

Benzodiazepines and Second-Generation Anxiolytics

BENZODIAZEPINES

Introduced in the 1960s, benzodiazepines have anxiolytic, sedative, anticonvulsant, amnestic, and relaxant properties. Because of these actions, they rapidly became the most widely used class of drugs. Even today, their use continues, although the antidepressant drugs (Chapter 15) are replacing the benzodiazepines for the treatment of many of the anxiety disorders.

The benzodiazepines are agonists of the GABA-benzodiazepine-chloride receptor complex; they facilitate the binding of GABA (Figure 6.1). That action, in turn, facilitates influx of chloride ions, causing hyperpolarization of the postsynaptic neuron, depressing its excitability. Benzodiazepines exert their anxiolytic properties by acting at limbic centers. Their actions at other regions (e.g., cerebral cortex and brain stem) produce side effects such as sedation, increased seizure threshold, and muscle relaxation.

Today, the term *anxiolytic* has become nearly synonymous with the benzodiazepines, because these compounds have been for almost 40 years the drugs of choice for the short-term pharmacological treatment of stress-related anxiety and insomnia: they are easy to use, and they have relatively low toxicity and tremendous effectiveness in relieving anxiety. The benzodiazepines relieve the psychological distress and the dysphoria associated with anxiety.

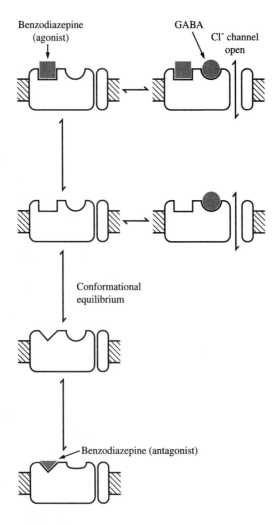

FIGURE 6.1 Benzodiazepine-GABA receptor interaction. BZD agonists (e.g., diazepam) and antagonists (e.g., flumazenil) bind to a site on the GABA receptor that is distinct from the GABA-binding site. A conformational equilibrium exists between states in which the BZD receptor exists in its agonist-binding conformation (*top*) and its antagonist-binding conformation (*bottom*). In the latter state, the GABA receptor has a much reduced affinity for GABA, so the chloride channel remains closed. [Modified from Rang and Dale,[11] Figure 25.6.]

However, their adverse effects and their potential for producing dependency is generally conceded to limit their therapeutic use to relatively short periods of time, perhaps three to four weeks, and only for conditions where short-term therapy is beneficial.[1] For longer-term treatment of such disorders as insomnia, generalized anxiety, phobias, panic disorder, and posttraumatic stress disorder, behavioral treatments and antidepressant drugs are preferred over benzodiazepine therapy (Figure 6.2).[2]

Benzodiazepines are generally not utilized for chronic anxiety disorders or for treating depression. They should be avoided in situations requiring fine motor or cognitive skills or mental alertness or in situations where alcohol or other central nervous system (CNS) depressants are used. They should be used only with great caution in the elderly, in children or adolescents, or in individuals prone to drug misuse. Despite these limitations, some feel that strong attitudes against the use of these drugs may be depriving many anxious patients of appropriate treatment. As Salzman[3] states:

> Benzodiazepines are neither a panacea nor a curse. Indiscriminate prescription of these medications is inappropriate and unwise for patients of any age. It is unfortunate that legitimate therapeutic use is sometimes obscured by controversy over issues of safety and dependence. Despite adverse effects, dependence, and inappropriate use, benzodiazepines remain appropriate pharmacological treatment for anxiety, one of the most prevalent forms of human suffering.

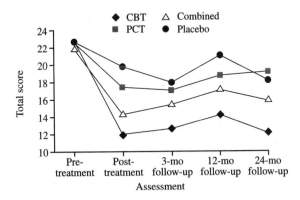

FIGURE 6.2 Effects of cognitive-behavioral therapy (CBT), pharmacotherapy (PCT), combination of CBT and PCT, and a placebo condition on late-life insomnia (as measured by changes in total score for the patient version of the Sleep Impairment Index) in 78 adults ages 65 years or older with chronic and primary insomnia. PCT consisted of a benzodiazepine—temazepan (Restoril)—administered in a dose of 7.5 to 30 mg 1 hour before bedtime. Pretreatment, posttreatment, and 3-, 12-, and 24-month follow-up assessments are illustrated. CBT was most effective, followed by combination treatment, PCT alone, and placebo. [Data from Morin et al.[2]]

Mechanism of Action:
The Benzodiazepine-GABA Receptor

Neuroanatomically, the *amygdala, orbitofrontal cortex,* and *insula* are associated with the production of behavioral responses to fearful stimuli and the central mediation of anxiety and panic. Electrical stimulation of these structures evokes behavioral and physiological responses that are associated with fear and anxiety. Electrical lesions of the amygdala in animals result in an anxiolytic effect. PET scanning of the brain demonstrates increased amygdala blood flow concomitant with anxiety responses; and MRI scanning of the brain demonstrates amygdala abnormalities in panic disorder patients. Also, patients with panic disorder (compared with matched controls) have a global decrease in benzodiazepine binding; the largest decreases occur in the orbitofrontal cortex and insula. This is consistent with the notion that anxiety and panic disorders may be due to "defective brain inhibition that leads to or allows paroxysmal elevations in anxiety during panic attacks."[4]

Blockade of GABAergic function can elicit anxiogenic-like effects, with both behavioral and physiologic alterations similar to symptoms of human anxiety states. Saunders and colleagues[5] "primed" or "kindled" the amygdala of rats by chronically blocking $GABA_A$-receptor function. Results indicated that increased activity of amygdala function (with lowered GABAergic inhibition of function) produced anxiogenic responses as measured both in animal models of anxiety and by increases in heart rate and blood pressure. Thus, hypofunctional $GABA_A$-receptor activity may sensitize the amygdala to anxiogenic responses to what might otherwise be considered nondistressing stimuli. This could be one potential mechanism for developing pathological emotional responses, such as chronic, high levels of anxiety. The benzodiazepines may reset the threshold of the amygdala to a more normal level of responsiveness. While it is widely presumed that this action is exerted at $GABA_A$ receptors, other GABA subtypes may be involved. Indeed, there may be five or more types of GABA receptors; $GABA_A$ and $GABA_B$ receptors are the most studied. Kerr and Ong[6] and Johnston[7] review respectively the physiology and pharmacology of $GABA_B$ and $GABA_C$ receptors. Hobbs and coworkers[8] detail the molecular biology of the interaction between benzodiazepines and $GABA_A$ receptor function.

---

*One benzodizepine (estazolam) that is not approved for use in the United States has been found in an herbal product called Sleeping Buddha. Not surprisingly, this product is promoted for insomnia and restlessness and is sold as an herbal alternative to sedatives.

Pharmacokinetics

Fifteen benzodiazepine derivatives are currently available in the United States (Table 6.1) and still more are available in other countries.* These agents are marketed for use as sedatives, anxiolytics, muscle relaxants, intravenous anesthetics, and anticonvulsants. They differ from each other mainly in their pharmacokinetic parameters, which include rates

TABLE 6.1 Benzodiazepines

| Drug name | | Dosage form | | Active metab-olite | Active compounds in blood | Mean elimination half-life in hours (range) |
Trade	Generic	Oral	Parent-eral			
LONG-ACTING AGENTS						
Valium	Diazepam	X	X	Yes	Diazepam	24 (20–50)
					Nordiazepam	60 (50–100)
Librium	Chlordiazepoxide	X		Yes	Chlordiaze-poxide	10 (8–24)
					Nordiazepam	60 (50–100)
Dalmane	Flurazepam	X		Yes	Desalkylflura-zepam	80 (70–160)
Paxipam	Halazepam	X		Yes	Halazepam	14 (10–20)
					Nordiazepam	60 (50–100)
Centrax	Prazepam	X		Yes	Nordiazepam	60 (50–100)
Tranxene	Chlorazepate	X		Yes	Nordiazepam	60 (50–100)
INTERMEDIATE-ACTING AGENTS						
Ativan	Lorazepam	X	X	No	Lorazepam	15 (10–24)
Klonopin	Clonazepam	X		No	Clonazepam	30 (18–50)
Dormalin	Quazepam	X		Yes	Quazepam	35 (25–50)
					Desalkylflura-zepam	80 (70–160)
ProSom	Estazolam	X		Yes	Hydroxyesta-zolam	18 (13–35)
SHORT-ACTING AGENTS						
Versed	Midazolam		X	No	Midazolam	2.5 (1.5–4.5)
Serax	Oxazepam	X		No	Oxazepam	8 (5–15)
Restoril	Temazepam	X		No	Temazepam	12 (8–35)
Halcion	Triazolam	X		No	Triazolam	2.5 (1.5–5)
Xanax	Alprazolam	X		No	Alprazolam	12 (11–18)

of metabolism to pharmacologically active intermediates and plasma half-lives of both the parent drug and any active metabolites. Of the benzodiazepines commercially available in the United States, 14 are available in a dosage form for oral ingestion, and 3 (diazepam, lorazepam, and midazolam) are also available for parenteral use.

Like the barbiturates (Chapter 5), all benzodiazepines have the basic benzodiazepine structure (Figure 6.3). Thus, derivatives differ from each other only in their substituent groups.[*]

General structure

Chlordiazepoxide (Librium)

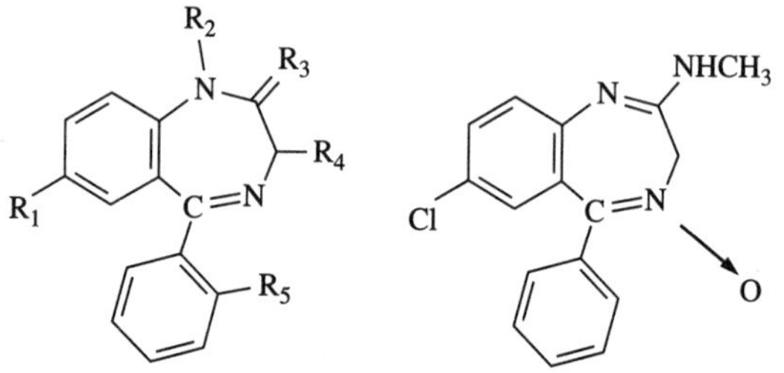

Drug	R_1	R_2	R_3	R_4	R_5
Diazepam	Cl	CH_3	$=O$	H_2	H
Nitrazepam	NO_2	H	$=O$	H_2	H
Flurazepam	Cl	$(CH_2)_2N(C_2H_5)_2$	$=O$	H_2	H
Flunitrazepam	NO_2	H	$=O$	H_2	F
Oxazepam	Cl	H	$=O$	OH	H
Temazepam	Cl	CH_3	$=O$	H_2	H
Clonazepam	NO_2	H	$=O$	H_2	Cl
Lorazepam	Cl	H	$=O$	OH	Cl
Clorazepate	Cl	H	$=O$	COOH	H
Nordiazepam	Cl	H	$=O$	H_2	H

FIGURE 6.3 Structures of some benzodiazepines. The basic "benzodiazepine" nucleus, which structurally defines this class of drugs, is shown on the left; chlordiazepoxide (the first marketed benzodiazepine) is shown on the right. Variations to the basic structure are located at the R_1–R_5 positions on the basic structure.

[*]Historically, drugs were often categorized by their chemical structure and given clinical effect. Drug manufacturers would make slight modifications to the structure in order to market competing and possibly better drugs either by changing side-chain substituents (making a different compound of the same class) or slightly modifying the basic structure (creating a different chemical class, but leaving the same biological action). Today, drugs are usually named by the receptors that they affect or that underlie their major clinical action (e.g., SSRI, a serotonin-1A agonist, a serotonin-3 antagonist, etc.). If discovered today, benzodiazepines probably would be known not by that name but as $GABA_A$ agonists.

Absorption and Distribution

Benzodiazepines are well absorbed when they are taken orally; peak plasma concentrations are achieved in about one hour. Some (e.g., oxazepam and lorazepam) are absorbed more slowly, while others (e.g., triazolam) are absorbed more rapidly. Clorazepate is metabolized in gastric juice to an active metabolite (nordiazepam) which is completely absorbed.[8]

Metabolism and Excretion

Usually, psychoactive drugs are metabolized to pharmacologically inactive, water-soluble products, which are then excreted in urine (Chapter 1). While this holds true for some benzodiazepines, several are first biotransformed to intermediate, pharmacologically active, products; these, in turn, are detoxified by further metabolism before they are excreted (Figure 6.4). As can be seen from Table 6.1 and Figure 6.4, several long-acting compounds are biotransformed into long-lasting pharmacologically active metabolites, primarily nordiazepam, the half-life of which is about 60 hours. Figure 6.5 demonstrates the buildup and slow metabolism of nordiazepam in a human volunteer who was given diazepam (Valium) daily for 14 days. Thus, the long-acting benzodiazepines are so because of the long half-lives of both the parent (original) drug and its pharmacologically active, long-half-life metabolite. In contrast, the short-acting benzodiazepines are short-acting because they are metabolized directly into inactive products. As Hobbs and colleagues[8] state:

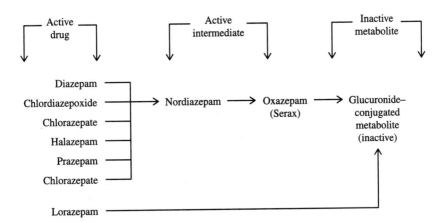

FIGURE 6.4 Metabolism of benzodiazepines. The intermediate metabolite nordiazepam is formed from many agents. Oxazepam (Serax) is comercially available and is also an active metabolite in the metabolism of nordiazepam to its inactive products.

A

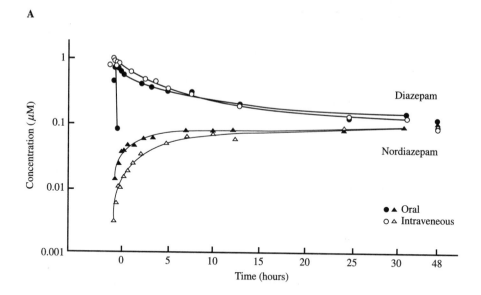

B

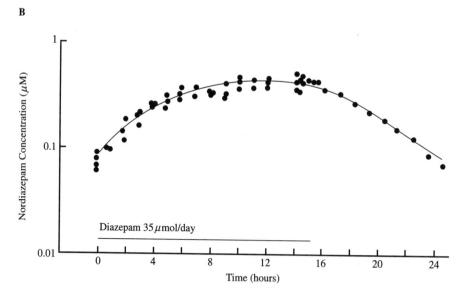

FIGURE 6.5 Pharmacokinetics of diazepam in humans. **A.** Concentrations of diazepam and its active metabolite, nordiazepam, following a single oral or intravenous dose. Note the negligible disappearance of both diazepam and noridiazepam after the first 20 hours. **B.** The accumulation of nordiazepam during two weeks of daily administration of diazepam is followed by a slow decline (half-life about 3 days) after the cessation of diazepam administration. [From Rang and Dale,[11] Figure 25.8.]

Because active metabolites are generated that are biotransformed more slowly than the parent compound, the duration of action of many benzodiazepines bears little relationship to the half-time of elimination of the drug that has been [originally] administered. . . . Conversely, the rate of biotransformation of those agents that are inactivated by the initial reaction is an important determinant of their duration of action; these agents include oxazepam, lorazepam, temazepam, triazolam, and midazolam.

The elderly have a reduced ability to metabolize long-acting benzodiazepines and their active metabolites. In this population, the elimination half-life for diazepam and its active metabolite is about seven to ten days. Since it takes about six half-lives to rid the body completely of a drug (Chapter 1), it may take an elderly patient one month or longer to become completely drug-free after even a single dose of the drug. With short-acting benzodiazepines, such as midazolam, pharmacokinetics are not so drastically altered, but the dose necessary to achieve effect is reduced by about 50 percent (Figure 6.6)[9]. Because all benzodiazepines can produce cognitive dysfunction, elderly patients can become clinically demented as a result.[10] In general, benzodiazepines should be used only with great caution (if at all) for the elderly. Rang and Dale[11] state:

> At the age of 91, the grandmother of one of the authors was growing increasingly forgetful and mildly dotty, having been taking nitrazepam for insomnia regularly for years. To the author's lasting shame, it took a canny general practitioner to diagnose the problem. Cancellation of the nitrazepam prescription produced a dramatic improvement.*

Pharmacological Effects

The clinical and behavioral effects of the benzodiazepines occur as a result of facilitation of GABA-induced neuronal inhibition at the various locations of GABA$_A$ receptors throughout the CNS. All benzodiazepines that exert actions similar to those exerted by diazepam are termed *complete agonists* because they faithfully facilitate GABA binding. Low doses of complete-agonist benzodiazepines alleviate anxiety, agitation, and fear by their actions on receptors located in the amygdala, orbitofrontal cortex, and insula. Mental confusion and amnesia follow action on GABA neurons located in the cerebral cortex and the

---

*My own 85-year-old grandmother experienced the identical problem with diazepam. Two months after discontinuation of the drug, her dementia disappeared and she remained lucid until her death ten years later.

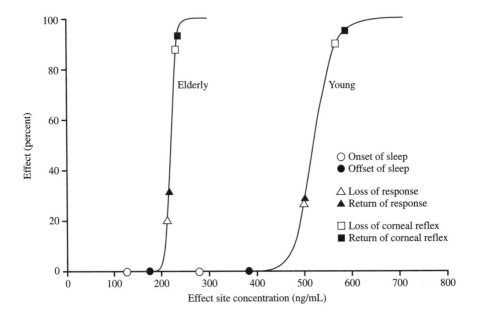

FIGURE 6.6 Concentration (effective dose-response) curve and clinical end points for young (24 to 28 years old) and elderly (67 to 81 years old) male volunteers receiving continuous infusion of midazolam (Versed) until the desired end points were attained. Plasma concentrations of drug were measured at the time of attainment of each clinical end point. In general, younger subjects required an effective site concentration about double that required in the elderly subjects. [From Albrecht et al.,[9] Figure 4.]

hippocampus. The mild muscle-relaxant effects of the benzodiazepines are probably caused both by their anxiolytic actions and by effects on GABA receptors located in the spinal cord, cerebellum, and brain stem. The antiepileptic actions seem to follow from actions on GABA receptors located in the cerebellum and the hippocampus. The behavioral rewarding effects and thus abuse potential and psychological dependency probably result from actions on GABA receptors that modulate the discharge of neurons located in the ventral tegmentum and the nucleus accumbens (see Figure 3.13).

Given a number of subgroups of $GABA_A$ receptors, benzodiazepine derivatives may be found that bind to various substituents of different types of $GABA_A$ receptors, perhaps with less than complete agonist action. Such drugs would be called *partial agonists*, and, hopefully, some might have specificity of action (e.g., anxiolysis without sedation). One such drug is clinically available: *zolpidem* (Ambien), marketed in the mid-1990s, is structurally not a benzodiazepine, but it binds to the $GABA_{1A}$ receptor and exhibits primarily a hypnotic effect rather than an anxiolytic one.

Uses

The major indication for benzodiazepine therapy is anxiety that is so debilitating that the patient's lifestyle, work, and interpersonal relationships are severely hampered. A benzodiazepine may alleviate the symptoms of nervousness, dysphoria, and psychological distress without necessarily blocking the physiological correlates accompanying the state of anxiety. Usually, resolution of the psychological distress is accompanied by amelioration of the physiological symptoms.

As sedatives, the benzodiazepines possess many of the characteristics of the barbiturates. Thus, they are effectively used as hypnotics for the treatment of insomnia. Here, agents with rapid onset, a 2- to 3-hour half-life, and no active metabolites may be preferred to minimize daytime sedation. However, when daytime sedation or next-day anxiolysis is desired, the long-acting drugs with active metabolites might be preferred.

Because increased GABA activity inhibits neuronal function, the benzodiazepines have been used as muscle relaxants, both to directly reduce states associated with increased muscle tension and to reduce the psychological distress that can predispose to muscle tension.

Benzodiazepines produce antegrade amnesia (amnesia that starts at the time of drug administration and ends when the blood level of drug has decreased to a point where memory function is regained). For this use, either of two injectable benzodiazepines is perhaps most reliable—lorazepam, when long-lasting amnesia is desirable, and midazolam, when shorter periods of amnesia are desirable. An example of a situation where amnesia might be a therapeutic goal is surgery, either during or before surgical procedures. Occasionally, an amnestic effect may be undesirable. For example, recently much concern has been expressed about an illegally imported "date rape" drug, which turned out to be a benzodiazepine that is commercially marketed outside the United States. This drug, *flunitrazepam* (Rohypnol), is very similar to *triazolam* (Halcion; Table 6.1), producing anxiolysis, sedation, and amnesia, especially when taken with alcohol. When so ingested by an unknowing victim, the effect closely resembles a Mickey Finn (chloral hydrate in alcohol) or GHB.

Panic attacks and phobias can be treated with benzodiazepines such as *alprazolam* (Xanax). Here, however, the efficacy of benzodiazepines may be less than that of the serotonin-type antidepressants, which may be "more-specific anxiolytics"[12] (Chapter 15). Davidson[13] reviewed the use of benzodiazepines, noting their advantages of rapid onset, anxiolysis, low-level side effects, and good patient acceptance. Disadvantages noted include impaired psychomotor performance and alertness and the potential for dependence and abuse. Treatment efficacy is therefore controversial.

Because benzodiazepines can substitute for alcohol, they are used both in treating acute alcohol withdrawal and in long-term therapy to reduce the rate of relapse to previous drinking habits (Chapter 4). All benzodiazepines exert antiepileptic actions because they raise the threshold for generating seizures. In general, however, benzodiazepines are used as secondary drugs or as adjuvants to other, more specific anticonvulsants.

Side Effects and Toxicity

Common acute side effects associated with benzodiazepine therapy are usually dose-related extensions of the intended actions. These include sedation, drowsiness, ataxia, lethargy, mental confusion, motor and cognitive impairments, disorientation, slurred speech, amnesia, and induction or extension of the symptoms of dementia. At higher doses, mental and psychomotor dysfunction progress to hypnosis.

Use of the benzodiazepine *triazolam* (Halcion) for the treatment of insomnia has been especially controversial; drug use has been associated with an increased incidence of paradoxical agitation (anxiety, aggression, hostility, behavioral disinhibition, and hallucinogenic reactions).[14] Rothschild and co-workers[15] dispute this statement, concluding that "alprazolam does not possess unique disinhibitory activity, and disinhibition may not be an important clinical problem associated with benzodiazepine use."

Respiration is not seriously depressed, even at high doses. Indeed, attempted suicides by overdose are rarely successful unless the benzodiazepine is taken along with another CNS depressant, such as alcohol. This combination can cause a serious and potentially fatal drug interaction. Sleep patterns can be altered markedly. When short-acting agents are taken at bedtime, both early-morning wakening and rebound insomnia for the next night are common. When long-acting agents (or agents with active metabolites) are taken at bedtime, daytime sedation can be a problem. Impairment of motor abilities—especially a person's ability to drive an automobile—is common.[16] This impairment is compounded by the drug-induced suppression of one's ability to assess his or her own level of physical and mental impairment.

The cognitive deficits associated with benzodiazepine use are significant. In both children and adults, benzodiazepines can significantly interfere with learning behaviors, academic performance, and psychomotor functioning. Cognitive and generalized intellectual impairments can persist even long after the benzodiazepine is discontinued, although cognitive improvements after discontinuation are the norm.

> Patients who had evidence of impaired cognitive functions while on long-term benzodiazepine therapy did improve in these functions

when therapy was discontinued. . . . Further, . . . patients who were able to discontinue their benzodiazepine intake after many years of use became more alert, more relaxed, and less anxious, and this change was accompanied by improved psychomotor functions.[17]

Tolerance and Dependence

Although benzodiazepines have a reputation for causing only a low incidence of abuse and dependence, the possibility of this adverse complication of chronic use must not be overlooked.[8] When benzodiazepines are taken for prolonged periods of time, a pattern of dependence can develop, even following only therapeutic dosages. Early withdrawal signs include a return (and possible intensification) of the anxiety state for which the drug was originally given. Rebound increases in insomnia, restlessness, agitation, irritability, and unpleasant dreams gradually appear. In rare instances, hallucinations, psychoses, and seizures have been reported. Most of these withdrawal symptoms subside within one to four weeks.

Regarding compulsive abuse of the benzodiazepines:

> Patients who have histories of drug or alcohol abuse are most apt to use these agents inappropriately, and abuse of benzodiazepines usually occurs as part of a pattern of abuse of multiple drugs.[8]

Rickels and co-workers[18] discuss strategies for discontinuing benzodiazepines in individuals who have developed dependence on them.

Effects in Pregnancy

During pregnancy, benzodiazepines and their metabolites freely cross the placenta and accumulate in the fetal circulation, concentrating there even more than in the maternal circulation.[19] While controversial, benzodiazepines administered during the first trimester of pregnancy have been reported to cause fetal abnormalities, although the risk is probably very small. Near the time of delivery, should a mother be on high doses of benzodiazepines, a fetus can develop benzodiazepine dependence, or even a "floppy-infant syndrome," followed after delivery by signs of withdrawal. Because benzodiazepines are excreted in breast milk and because they can accumulate in nursing infants, taking benzodiazepines while breast feeding is not recommended.[15]

Flumazenil: A GABA$_A$ Antagonist

Flumazenil (Romazicon) is a benzodiazepine that binds with high affinity to benzodiazepine receptors on the GABA$_A$ complex (see

Figure 6.1), but after binding, it exhibits no intrinsic activity. As a consequence, it competitively blocks the access of pharmacologically active benzodiazepines to the receptor, effectively reversing the anti-anxiety and sedative effects of any benzodiazepines administered before flumazenil.

Flumazenil is metabolized quite rapidly in the liver and has a short half-life (about 1 hour). Because this half-life is much shorter than that of most benzodiazepines, the benzodiazepine effects can reappear as flumazenil is lost, thus necessitating reinjection. Flumazenil is utilized as an antidote whenever benzodiazepine ingestion is suspected. Kantor[20] reviews the pharmacology and use of flumazenil.

SECOND-GENERATION ANXIOLYTICS

Zolpidem

Zolpidem (Ambien; Figure 6.7) is a nonbenzodiazepine that was marketed in 1993 for the short-term treatment of insomnia. Although structurally unrelated to the benzodiazepines, zolpidem acts similarly, binding to a specific subtype (type 1) of the $GABA_A$ receptor.[21] It displays most of the actions of all other benzodiazepine agonists: it is primarily a sedative rather than an anxiolytic, and its sedative actions overwhelm any anxiolytic effects. With a half-life of about 2 to 2.5 hours, zolpidem is often compared to triazolam (Halcion), a benzodiazapine

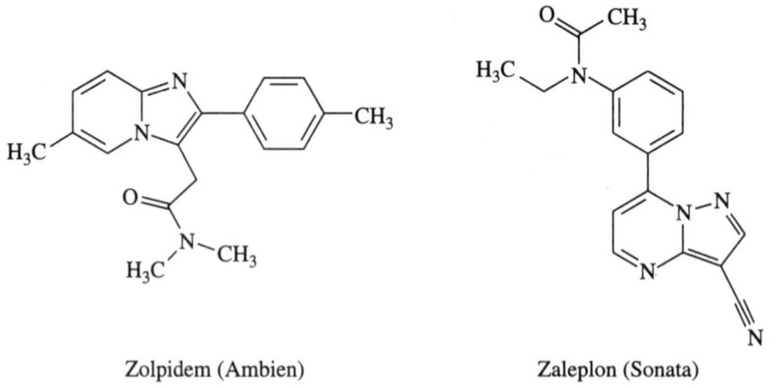

Zolpidem (Ambien)   Zaleplon (Sonata)

FIGURE 6.7 Structural formulas of zolpidem (Ambien) and zaleplon (Sonata). Note the close (but dissimilar) relationship of their basic three-ring structures to the benzodiazepine nucleus (Figure 6.3); thus, these two compounds are nonbenzodiazepines despite similar GABAergic actions and clinical effects.

with similar pharmacokinetics; at comparable doses, there appears to be little to differentiate the two drugs.[22]

Pharmacokinetics

Zolpidem is rapidly absorbed from the gastrointestinal tract after oral administration, with about 75 percent of the administered drug reaching the plasma. Only a small amount (about 20 percent) is metabolized by first-pass metabolism. Peak plasma levels are reached in about one hour. Following metabolism in the liver, the products are excreted by the kidneys. The calculated half-life is prolonged in the elderly.

Pharmacodynamics

At doses of 5 to 10 milligrams, zolpidem produces sedation and promotes a physiological pattern of sleep in the absence of anxiolytic, anticonvulsant, or muscle-relaxant effects. Memory is affected as it is by benzodiazepines. Wesensten and colleagues[23] reported that flumazenil effectively reverses any memory impairments or overdosages induced by zolpidem. They also reported that flumazenil tended to improve learning and memory function above levels seen with a placebo, denoting a possible role of some sort of endogenous benzodiazepines in modulating memory function. The clinical importance of this finding is unclear.

Adverse Effects

Dose-related adverse effects of zolpidem include drowsiness, dizziness, and nausea. In the elderly taking 20 milligrams or more, confusion, falls, memory loss, and psychotic reactions have been reported. A high-dose incidence of nausea and vomiting may tend to limit overdosage, such as in suicide attempts. Overdoses to 400 milligrams (20 times the high-dose therapeutic amount) have not been fatal.

In conclusion, zolpidem is an effective nonbenzodiazepine hypnotic that binds to benzodiazepine receptors in the brain. While structurally a nonbenzodiazepine, its actions are only minimally different; it produces similar levels of daytime sedation and cognitive impairment as would triazolam, one of the shortest half-life benzodiazepines. The potential for the drug to induce tolerance or be abused remains to be determined.

Zaleplon and Zopiclone

Zaleplon (Sonata; Figure 6.7) is another nonbenzodiazepine agonist at $GABA_{A1}$ receptors that exerts actions similar to those of the benzodiazepines.[24] It was released in late 1999 for clinical use as a hypnotic agent. Zaleplon is unique among these drugs in that its half-life is very short (about 1 hour) and only about 30 percent of an orally administered dose reaches the bloodstream; most undergoes first-pass metabolism. Orally, it is half as potent as zolpidem; perhaps this difference would disappear should zaleplon be taken with grapefruit juice. Sleep quality appears to improve without rebound insomnia. Dependence is unlikely to develop because of the short half-life: by morning the drug is metabolized. In essence, a person taking the drug withdraws daily, and drug does not persist in the body.[25]

Zopiclone is another nonbenzodiazepine that shares all the actions of zolpidem and traditional benzodiazepines. It appears to offer no special advantages or disadvantages.

Partial Agonists at GABA$_A$ Receptors

"Full" GABA agonists such as the benzodiazepines are effective anxiolytics; however their use is limited by rebound anxiety (on discontinuation), physical dependence (with extended use), abuse potential, and side effects that include ataxia, sedation, and memory and cognitive disturbances. Therefore, attempts have been made to identify "partial" agonists of GABA receptors in the hope of providing anxiolytics that may be equally as effective without the side effects that limit use of the benzodiazepines. To date, several have been examined, although none is yet available in the United States.

The best studied of these agents are alpidem, (marketed in Europe), etizolam, imidazenil, abecarnil, and bretazenil. *Alpidem* is a partial agonist at both GABA$_1$ and GABA$_3$ receptors, is more anxiolytic than full GABA agonists, produces little sedation, and appears not to interact with ethanol.[26,27] Unfortunately, reports of drug-induced hepatitis have tempered the enthusiasm for the drug. *Etizolam* is a potent anxiolytic with a profile similar to classical benzodiazepines; it is claimed to have a lower incidence of side effects at comparable efficacy.[28] *Imidazenil* is an effective anxiolytic with minimal disruptive effects on cognition and memory, and it appears to have only minimal side effects.[29] *Abecarnil* has a rapid onset of anxiolytic action and a low incidence of physical dependence.[30] Rickels and co-workers[31] demonstrated the safety and efficacy of abercarnil in the treatment of generalized anxiety disorder, with only minimal discontinuation symptoms. *Bretazenil* has anxiolytic action and presumed lower incidence of side effects and dependence liability.[32] Interestingly, bretazenil also exhibits moderate antipsychotic efficacy.[33] Chapter 17 discusses the role of GABA receptors in schizophrenia in detail. Each of these partial agonists is in various stages of experimentation or trial.

Serotoninergic Drugs as Anxiolytics

Anxiety may, at least in part, result from defects in serotonin neurotransmission, and drugs that augment serotoninergic activity may be useful in the treatment of anxiety disorders. For more than 20 years it has been postulated that

> if it is assumed that disinhibition of behavior under adverse conditions is indicative of anxiolysis, then serotonin is presumed to play a significant role in anxiety and anxiolysis.[34]

Of the 15 or more subtypes of serotonin receptors, most interest has focused on the presynaptic serotonin transporter and on postsynaptic serotonin 5-HT$_{1A}$ and 5-HT$_3$ receptors.

Serotonin 5-HT$_{1A}$ Receptors

Serotonin 5-HT$_{1A}$ receptors are found in high density in the hippocampus, and they are richly distributed in the septum, parts of the amygdala, and the dorsal raphe nucleus,[34] areas all presumed to be involved in fear and anxiety responses. Here, 5-HT$_{1A}$ receptor activity is thought to diminish neuronal activity (these receptors are known to be ligand-gated channels, and activation of such receptors by agonist drugs leads to neuronal inhibition). Mice selectively bred without 5-HT$_{1A}$ receptors display increased fear responses, suggesting that reductions in 5-HT$_{1A}$ receptor activity or density (presumably due to genetic deficits or environmental stressors) result in heightened anxiety.[35]

Serotonin 5-HT$_{1A}$ Agonists

Clinical interest in serotonin anxiolytics began 20 years ago with demonstration of the anxiolytic action of buspirone, a selective serotonin 5-HT$_{1A}$ agonist. In 1986 the drug was approved for clinical use and it is marketed under the trade name BuSpar. Thereafter, other related agents were identified, but they have not yet been marketed. Such drugs include gepirone, ipsapirone, and alnespirone. Collectively, these 5-HT$_{1A}$ agonists are known as second-generation anxiolytics.

Buspirone

Buspirone (BuSpar) is a 5-HT$_{1A}$ agonist with demonstrable anxiolytic properties. It relieves anxiety in a unique fashion:

- Its anxiolysis occurs without significant sedation, drowsiness, or hypnotic action, even in overdosage.
- Amnesia, mental confusion, and psychomotor impairment are minimal or absent.

- It does not potentiate the CNS depressant effects of alcohol, benzodiazepines, or other CNS sedatives (i.e., synergism does not occur).

- It does not substitute for benzodiazepines in treating anxiety or benzodiazepine withdrawal.

- It does not exhibit cross-tolerance or cross-dependence with benzodiazepines.

- It exhibits little potential for addiction or abuse.

- It exhibits an antidepressant effect in addition to its anxiolytic effect, making it potentially useful in depressive disorders with accompanying anxiety.

- Its effect has a gradual onset rather than the immediate onset of the action of the benzodiazepines.

- It is ineffective as a hypnotic to promote the onset of sleep.

Buspirone is a weak agonist at $5\text{-}HT_{1A}$ receptors. As a result, it exerts both an anxiolytic action and an antidepressant action (the antidepressant role of $5\text{-}HT_{1A}$ receptors is discussed in Chapter 16). Buspirone is effective in the treatment of generalized anxiety disorder (addressed later as a special topic). It has also been recommended for patients who suffer from mixed symptoms of anxiety and depression, as well as for elderly individuals with agitated dementia.[36]

Buspirone is most helpful in anxious patients who do not demand immediate gratification or the immediate response they associate with the benzodiazepine response. Slower and more gradual onset of anxiety relief is balanced by the increased safety and lack of dependency-producing aspects of buspirone. To see clinical effects takes several weeks of continuous treatment. Patients who have previously been taking benzodiazepines do poorly on buspirone.

Harvey and Balon[37] summarize the efficacy of buspirone in several psychological disorders, including depression, panic disorder, obsessive-compulsive disorder, schizophrenia, and anxiety. They conclude that the major usefulness of buspirone in treating these disorders may be for the augmentation of the beneficial effects of other psychotropic medications.

Buspirone may reduce irritability, aggression, and temper outbursts in children with developmental disorders and may significantly potentiate the effects of behavioral stimulants in children and adolescents with comorbid attention deficit and oppositional defiant disorders.[38] Similarly, buspirone may enhance the efficacy of cognitive behavioral therapy on individuals with panic or other anxiety disorders.[39]

Chapter 1 (see especially Figure 1.6) presents a likely reason why the effects of buspirone are so subtle: most of the drug is detoxified by first-pass metabolism; only about 5 percent of orally administered drug reaches the bloodstream. Inhibition of metabolism (for example, by concurrent drinking of grapefruit juice) improves its efficacy by increasing its absorption. Apter and Allen[40] review the future directions for the uses of buspirone in various types of anxiety disorders, ADHD, depression, and behavioral disorders.

Gepirone

Gepirone is another 5-HT$_{1A}$ agonist currently in clinical trial. Rickels and co-workers[41] compared diazepam and gepirone in the treatment of generalized anxiety disorder. Gepirone's anxiolytic response was delayed, differing from placebo only after six weeks of treatment (diazepam's response began by the end of the first week). Diazepam was also statistically more effective as an anxiolytic (Figure 6.8). On drug withdrawal, diazepam caused a temporary worsening of anxiety symptoms, while gepirone did not. Gepirone was, in general, not so well tolerated by patients. In mice, gepirone exerts an antiaggression action, also mediated through 5-HT$_{1A}$ receptors.[42]

Alnespirone

Alnespirone exhibits similar anxiolytic and antiaggressive properties, also mediated by 5-HT$_{1A}$ receptor agonism. Protais and colleagues[43] postulate that stimulation of 5-HT$_{1A}$ receptors secondarily modulates the functioning of dopamine receptors. This action appears to be caused by the fact that buspirone, gepirone, and yet another 5-HT$_{1A}$ agonist, ipsapirone, "inhibit the activity of the enzyme tyrosine hydroxylase

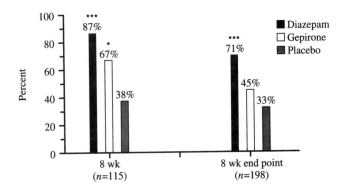

FIGURE 6.8 Percentage of patients experiencing marked or moderate global improvement (in symptoms of generalized anxiety disorder) after eight weeks of drug treatment (diazepam or gepirone) or placebo capsule. Drug/placebo differences: *$p<0.05$; ***$p<0.001$. Statistical difference between diazepam and gepirone responses were not presented. [From Rickels et al.,[41] Figure 3.]

through activation of striatal 5-HT$_{1A}$ heteroreceptors on dopamine nerve terminals."[44] By inhibiting dopaminergic function, these drugs should not be prone to compulsive misuse; a therapeutic advantage over benzodiazepines despite limited efficacy of these second-generation anxiolytics.

As stated, data indicate that some components of anxiety may be related to defects in the serotonin transporter protein.[45,46] Kent and colleagues[47] review the clinical usefulness of selective serotonin reuptake inhibitors (e.g., fluoxetine, Prozac) in treating various anxiety disorders. In comparative trials, these agents are as effective as are the benzodiazepines, with less likelihood of dependence. Use is limited by a slow onset of action. Nevertheless, they are rapidly becoming drugs of choice for treating many of the various anxiety disorders. They are discussed at length in Chapter 15.

Finally, serotonin 5-HT$_3$ receptor antagonists have been studied as anxiolytic agents (these drugs are potent antivomiting agents). Evidence is accumulating that antagonism of 5-HT$_3$ receptors leads to the same clinical outcome (anxiolysis) as 5-HT$_{1A}$ activation. Preliminary data are only modestly optimistic; they indicate anxiolytic effects only slightly greater than the effect of placebo therapy.[48]

STUDY QUESTIONS

1. What are the advantages of benzodiazepines over barbiturates?
2. Describe the mechanism of action of benzodiazepines.
3. Describe evidence for and against a natural anxiolytic in the brain.
4. Describe the structure and function of the benzodiazepine receptor.
5. How might you describe anxiety or panic in terms of receptors or neurochemicals (at this point)?
6. List some of the clinical uses of benzodiazepines.
7. List three processes that might prolong the half-life of a benzodiazepine.
8. Why should the elderly avoid using long-acting benzodiazepines?
9. Describe the most clinically significant drug interaction that involves benzodiazepines.
10. Discuss benzodiazepine withdrawal and its treatment.
11. What is flumazenil and for what purpose can it be used?
12. Compare and contrast the mechanisms of action and clinical uses of benzodiazepines and buspirone.
13. To what benzodiazepine is zolpidem most often compared? Why?
14. Compare and contrast zolpidem and zaleplon.

15. Discuss the future treatment of anxiety disorders with either benzodiazepines or serotonin agonists.

REFERENCES

1. C. F. Reynolds, D. J. Buyse, and D. J. Kupfer, "Treating Insomnia in Older Adults: Taking a Long-term View," *Journal of the American Medical Association* 281 (1999): 1034–1035.
2. C. M. Morin et al., "Behavioral and Pharmacological Therapies for Late-life Insomnia: A Randomized Controlled Trial," *Journal of the American Medical Association* 281 (1999): 991–999.
3. C. Salzman, "An 87-Year-old Woman Taking a Benzodiazepine," *Journal of the American Medical Association* 281 (1999): 1121–1125.
4. A. L. Malizia et al., "Decreased Brain GABA$_A$-Benzodiazepine Receptor Binding in Panic Disorder: Preliminary Results from a Quantitative PET Study," *Archives of General Psychiatry* 55 (1998): 715–720.
5. S. K. Saunders, S. L. Morzorati, and A. Shekhar, "Priming of Experimental Anxiety by Repeated Subthreshold GABA Blockade in the Rat Amygdala," *Brain Research* 699 (1995): 250–259.
6. D. Kerr and J. Ong, "GABA$_B$ Receptors," *Pharmaceutical Therapeutics* 67 (1995): 187–246.
7. G. R. Johnston, "GABA$_C$ Receptors: Relatively Simple Transmitter-gated Ion Channels," *Trends in Pharmaceutical Sciences* 17 (1996): 319–323.
8. W. R. Hobbs, T. W. Rall, and T. A. Verdoorn, "Hypnotics and Sedatives: Ethanol," in J. G. Hardman, L. E. Limbird, P. B. Molinoff, R. W. Ruddon, and A. G. Gilman, eds., *Goodman and Gilman's The Pharmacological Basis of Therapeutics*, 9th ed. (New York: McGraw-Hill, 1996), 365–367.
9. S. Albrecht et al., "The Effects of Age on the Pharmacokinetics and Pharmacodynamics of Midazolam," *Clinical Pharmacology and Therapeutics* 65 (1999): 630–639.
10. J. T. Hanlon et al., "Benzodiazepine Use and Cognitive Function Among Community-dwelling Elderly," *Clinical Pharmacology and Therapeutics* 64 (1998): 684–692.
11. H. P. Rang and M. M. Dale, *Pharmacology*, 2nd ed. (Edinburgh: Churchill Livingstone, 1991), 637.
12. R. B. Pohl, R. M. Wolkow, and C. M. Clary, "Sertraline in the Treatment of Panic Disorder: A Double-blind Multicenter Trial," *American Journal of Psychiatry* 155 (1998): 1189–1195.
13. J. R. T. Davidson, "Use of Benzodiazepines in Panic Disorder," *Journal of Clinical Psychiatry* 58, Suppl. 2 (1997): 26–28.
14. W. E. Bunney et al., "Report of the Institute of Medicine Committee on the Efficacy and Safety of Halcion," *Archives of General Psychiatry* 56 (1999): 349–352.
15. A. J. Rothschild et al., "Comparison of the Frequency of Behavioral Disinhibition on Alprazolam, Clonazepam, or No Benzodiazepine in Hospitalized Psychiatric Patients," *Journal of Clinical Psychopharmacology* 20 (2000): 7–11.
16. F. Barbone et al., "Association of Road-traffic Accidents with Benzodiazepine Use," *The Lancet* 352 (1998): 1331–1336.

17. K. Rickels et al., "Psychomotor Performance of Long-term Benzodiazepine Users Before, During, and After Benzodiazepine Discontinuation," *Journal of Clinical Psychopharmacology* 19 (1999): 107–113.

18. K. Rickels, N. DeMartinis, M. Rynn, and L. Mandos, "Pharmacologic Strategies for Discontinuing Benzodiazepine Treatment," *Journal of Clinical Psychopharmacology* 19, Suppl. 2 (1999): 12S–16S.

19. S. M. Ramin, L. C. Gilstrap, and B. B. Little, "Psychotropics in Pregnancy," in L. C. Gilstrap and B. B. Little, eds., *Drugs and Pregnancy*, 2nd ed. (New York: Chapman & Hall, 1998).

20. G. Kantor, "Flumazenil: A Review for Clinicians," *American Journal of Anesthesiology* 24 (1997): 84–88.

21. D. Ruana et al., "Regional Differences in the Enhancement by GABA of [3H]Zolpidem Binding to Omega-1 Sites in Rat Brain Membranes and Sections," *Brain Research* 600 (1993): 134–140.

22. B. L. Lobo and W. L. Greene, "Zolpidem: Distinct from Triazolam?" *Annals of Pharmacotherapy* 31 (1997): 625–632.

23. N. J. Wesensten et al., "Reversal of Triazolam- and Zolpidem-induced Memory Impairment by Flumazenil," *Psychopharmacology* 121 (1995): 242–249.

24. D. J. Greenblatt et al., "Comparative Kinetics and Dynamics of Zaleplon, Zolpidem, and Placebo," *Clinical Pharmacology and Therapeutics* 64 (1998): 553–561.

25. R. Elie et al., "Sleep Latency Is Shortened During Four Weeks of Treatment with Zaleplon, a Novel Nonbenzodiazepine Hypnotic," *Journal of Clinical Psychiatry* 60 (1999): 536–544.

26. L. Frattola et al., "Comparison of the Efficacy, Safety, and Withdrawal of Alpidem and Alprazolam in Anxious Patients," *British Journal of Psychiatry* 165 (1994): 94–100.

27. M. Hascoet and M. Bourin, "Anticonflict Effect of Alpidem as Compared with the Benzodiazepine Alprazolam in Rats," *Pharmacology, Biochemistry & Behavior* 56 (1997): 317–324.

28. E. Sanna et al., "Molecular and Neurochemical Evaluation of the Effects of Etizolam on GABA$_A$ Receptors Under Normal and Stress Conditions," *Arzneimittel-Forschung* 49 (1999): 88–95.

29. E. Costa and A. Guidotti, "Benzodiazepines on Trial: A Research Strategy for Their Rehabilitation," *Trends in Pharmacological Sciences* 17 (1996): 192–200.

30. B. Aufdembrinke, "Abecarnil, a New Beta-Carboline, in the Treatment of Anxiety Disorders," *British Journal of Psychiatry* 34, suppl. (1998): 55–63.

31. K. Rickels, N. DeMartinis and B. Aufdembrinke, "A Double-Blind, Placebo-Controlled Trial of Abercarnil and Diazepam in the Treatment of Patients with Generalized Anxiety Disorder," *Journal of Clinical Psychopharmacology* 20 (2000): 12–18.

32. J. G. Richards and J. R. Martin, "Binding Profiles and Physical Dependence Liabilities of Selected Benzodiazepine Receptor Ligands," *Brain Research Bulletin* 45 (1998): 381–387.

33. A. Delini-Stula and D. Berdah-Tordjman, "Antipsychotic Effects of Bretazenil, a Partial Benzodiazepine Agonist, in Acute Schizophrenia—A Study Group Report," *Journal of Psychiatric Research* 30 (1996): 239–250.

34. "Sedative-hypnotic and Anxiolytic Drugs," in R. S. Feldman, J. S. Meyer, and L. F. Quenzer, *Principles of Neuropsychopharmacology* (Sunderland, Mass.: Sinauer, 1997), 702–703.

35. S. Rambos et al., "Serotonin Receptor 1A Knockout: An Animal Model of Anxiety-related Disorder," *Proceedings of the National Academy of Sciences* 95 (1998): 14476–14481.

36. D. G. Folks and W. C. Fuller, "Anxiety Disorders and Insomnia in Geriatric Patients," *Psychiatric Clinics of North America* 20 (1997): 137–164.

37. K. V. Harvey and R. Balon, "Augmentation with Buspirone: A Review," *Annals of Clinical Psychiatry* 7 (1995): 143–147.

38. M. D. Gross, "Buspirone in ADHD with ODD," *Journal of the American Academy of Child and Adolescent Psychiatry* 34 (1995): 1260.

39. J. Cottraux et al., "A Controlled Study of Cognitive Behavior with Buspirone or Placebo in Panic Disorder with Agoraphobia," *British Journal of Psychiatry* 167 (1995): 635–641.

40. J. T. Apter and L. A. Allen, "Buspirone: Future Directions," *Journal of Clinical Psychopharmacology* 19 (1999): 86–93.

41. K. Rickels et al., "Gepirone and Diazepam in Generalized Anxiety Disorder: A Placebo-controlled Trial," *Journal of Clinical Psychopharmacology* 17 (1997): 272–277.

42. D. L. Mendoza, H. A. Bravo, and H. H. Swanson, "Antiaggressive and Anxiolytic Effects of Gepirone in Mice and Their Attenuation by WAY 100635," *Pharmacology, Biochemistry and Behavior* 62 (1999): 499–509.

43. P. Protais, M. Lesourd, and E. Comoy, "Similar Pharmacological Properties of 8-OH-DPAT and Alnespirone at Dopamine Receptors: Comparison with Buspirone," *European Journal of Pharmacology* 352 (1998): 179–187.

44. E. A. Johnson, J. L. Fox, and A. J. Azzaro, "The Anxiolytic Serotonin 5-HT$_{1A}$ Receptor Agonists Buspirone, Ipsapirone and Gepirone Are Inhibitors of Tyrosine Hydroxylation in Rat Striatum," *Behavioural Brain Research* 73 (1996): 331–335.

45. J. M. Kent, J. D. Coplan, and J. M. Gorman, "Clinical Utility of the Selective Serotonin Reuptake Inhibitors in the Spectrum of Anxiety," *Biological Psychiatry* 44 (1998): 812–824.

46. S. Katsuragi et al., "Association Between Serotonin Transporter Gene Polymorphism and Anxiety-related Traits," *Biological Psychiatry* 45 (1999): 368–370.

47. J. M. Kent, J. D. Coplan, and J. M. Gorman, "Clinical Utility of the Selective Serotonin Reuptake Inhibitors in the Spectrum of Anxiety," *Biological Psychiatry* 44 (1998): 812–824.

48. W. T. Smith et al., "Pilot Study of Zatosetron (LY277359) Maleate, a 5-Hydroxytryptamine-3 Antagonist, in the Treatment of Anxiety," *Journal of Clinical Psychopharmacology* 19 (1999): 125–131.

PART 3

Drugs That Stimulate Brain Function: Psychostimulants

Classically, a psychostimulant is a drug that tends to increase the behavioral activity of an animal to which such a drug has been administered. In general, a psychostimulant might be thought to elevate mood, increase motor activity, increase alertness, allay sleep, and increase the brain's metabolic and neuronal activity.

As a behavioral description, the term "psychostimulant" does not specify neurotransmitter or receptor processes. Nor does it imply augmentation of excitatory neurotransmission or inhibition of inhibitory neurotransmission (disinhibition). The term says little about therapeutic usefulness, just as it says little about abuse and dependency liabilities. Therefore, each drug in the group known as psychostimulants must be described individually—its pharmacology, its mechanism of action, any therapeutic properties or potential, and its abuse and dependency issues.

The psychostimulants are discussed in the following two chapters. Chapter 7 describes the psychostimulants classically thought to act through potentiation of dopaminergic neurotransmission, thus directly activating the reward system involving the nucleus accumbens and the limbic and frontal cortex. Such drugs include cocaine, the amphetamines, and several nonamphetamine psychostimulants. All of these drugs have uses in medicine and most have significant abuse issues as well. Included is a thorough discussion of the pharmacologic treatment of attention-deficit/hyperactivity disorder.

Chapter 8 details the pharmacology of caffeine and nicotine, the most widely used recreational drugs. Neither drug has much therapeutic value, but both are attractive to users because of their psychostimulant properties. However, their use induces moderate to extreme degrees of habituation or dependence.

Chapter 7

Cocaine, Amphetamines, and Other Behavioral Stimulants

Cocaine and the amphetamines are powerful psychostimulants that markedly affect one's mental functioning and behavior. These drugs act through various mechanisms to augment the synaptic action of several neurotransmitters, most importantly the monoamines dopamine, norepinephrine, and serotonin. Cocaine and the amphetamines exert, in addition to other actions, a direct stimulation on the nucleus accumbens, a structure associated with behavioral reinforcement, compulsive abuse, and drug dependency. They are therefore widely recognized as important drugs of abuse. Paradoxically, certain of these drugs also have therapeutic usefulness in the treatment of such disorders as narcolepsy and attention-deficit/hyperactivity. All psychostimulants have significant side effects, toxicities, and patterns of abuse.

In low doses, cocaine and other psychostimulants evoke an alerting, arousing, or behavior-activating response that is not unlike a normal reaction to an emergency or stress. Physiologically, blood pressure and heart rate increase, pupils dilate, blood flow shifts from skin and internal organs to muscle, and oxygen levels rise, as does the level of glucose in the blood. In the CNS, psychostimulants produce positive and attractive effects that include an elevation of mood, induction of euphoria, increased alertness, reduced fatigue, a sense of increased energy, decreased appetite, improved task performance, and relief from boredom. These effects, however, are offset by many negatives.

Anxiety, insomnia, and irritability are common side effects. As doses increase, irritability and anxiety become more intense, and a pattern of psychotic behavior may appear. Eventually, intense dependence develops, a dependence that so far has resisted widely successful treatment and rehabilitation.

COCAINE

Background

The leaves of *Erythroxylon coca* have been used since ancient times in their native South America for religious, mystical, social, euphoriant, and medicinal purposes—most notably to increase endurance, promote a sense of well-being, reduce fatigue, increase stamina, induce euphoria, and alleviate hunger. Chewing the leaves as an endurant produced a usual total daily dose of cocaine of up to about 200 milligrams, a point that will become more important later in this discussion. Today, the relevant clinical issues related to cocaine's history have to do largely with the changes over time in dosage, route of administration, patterns of use, and technology of production.

The active alkaloid in *E. coca* was isolated in 1855, purified in 1860, and named cocaine. During the same time period, the introduction of the syringe and hypodermic needle led to many attempts to use cocaine to produce local anesthesia for surgery. Perhaps the first medical report of cocaine's local anesthetic action[*] was made by Vassily von Anrep in 1880.[1] Further identification of cocaine's local anesthetic properties were made by several surgeons, and cocaine became widely used for topical anesthesia, spinal anesthesia, and nerve blocks from about 1884 until about 1918, when procaine (Novocaine) was developed as the first synthetic local anesthetic; procaine is devoid of psychological and dependence-producing effects.

In 1884, Sigmund Freud obtained cocaine, studied its psychological effects, used it himself, and prescribed it for his patients. Freud advocated the use of cocaine to treat depression and to alleviate chronic fatigue. He described cocaine as a "magical" and marvelous drug with the ability even to cure opioid (morphine and heroin) addiction.[2] Freud, while using cocaine to relieve his own depression, described cocaine as inducing exhilaration and lasting euphoria, which in no way

---

[*]At that time, no other anesthetics (general or local) had been discovered. Surgical procedures were limited to brief procedures conducted without anesthetic or with the patient under alcohol intoxication.

differs from the normal euphoria of the healthy person. However, he did not immediately perceive its side effects—tolerance, dependence, a state of psychosis, and withdrawal depression. In his later writings, Freud called cocaine the "third scourge" of humanity, after alcohol and heroin. This is perhaps an appropriate description.

In the United States, around 1885, there were no restrictions regarding the sale or consumption of cocaine. Thus, the drug was incorporated (along with caffeine) in numerous patent medicines, including the beverage Coca-Cola, which contained approximately 60 milligrams of cocaine per 8-ounce serving. In the late 1800s, however, concern about cocaine's toxicities increased, with several hundred reports of cocaine intoxication and several reported deaths. About 1910, President Taft proclaimed cocaine as Public Enemy Number 1, and in 1914 the Harrison Narcotic Act banned the incorporation of cocaine in patent medicines and beverages.

With enforcement of the Narcotic Act, cocaine use decreased during the 1930s; this psychostimulant was replaced by the newly available amphetamines. These drugs cost less and produced longer-lasting, yet similar, effects. Cocaine all but disappeared until the late 1960s, when tight federal restrictions on amphetamine distribution raised the cost of amphetamines, once again making cocaine attractive.*

In the late 1970s and early 1980s, a new epidemic of cocaine use began with the widespread availability of inexpensive "crack" cocaine. This cocaine epidemic continues today.[2] It is characterized by concentrated preparations of cocaine, use of which is characterized by high-dose, rapid-onset effects with the rapid development of both toxicity and dependency. One of the most addictive and reinforcing of the abused drugs, cocaine has been used by about 50 million people in the United States alone and more than 6 million Americans use cocaine regularly. Most regular users "snort" (use nasally) the water-soluble salt of cocaine (called cocaine hydrochloride), many smoke crack cocaine, and fewer inject (intravenously) cocaine hydrochloride.[3]

Cocaine-dependent individuals are typically young (12 to 39 years of age), dependent on at least three drugs, and male (75 percent). They tend to have coexisting psychopathology (30 percent have anxiety disorders, 67 percent suffer from clinical depression, and 25 percent exhibit paranoia). About 85 to 90 percent are alcohol dependent. Cocaine use is associated with a range of violent premature deaths, including homicides, suicides, and accidents.

---

*Because their net effects are nearly indistinguishable, cocaine and the amphetamines can be used almost interchangeably as euphoriants. Availability, price, and sociocultural considerations now largely determine the comparative popularity of the two.

Forms of Cocaine

The leaf of *E. coca* contains about 0.5 to 1.0 percent cocaine, or *benzoyl-methylecognine* (Figure 7.1). When the leaves are soaked and mashed, cocaine is extracted in the form of coca paste (60 to 80 percent cocaine).[4] Coca paste is usually treated with hydrochloric acid to form the

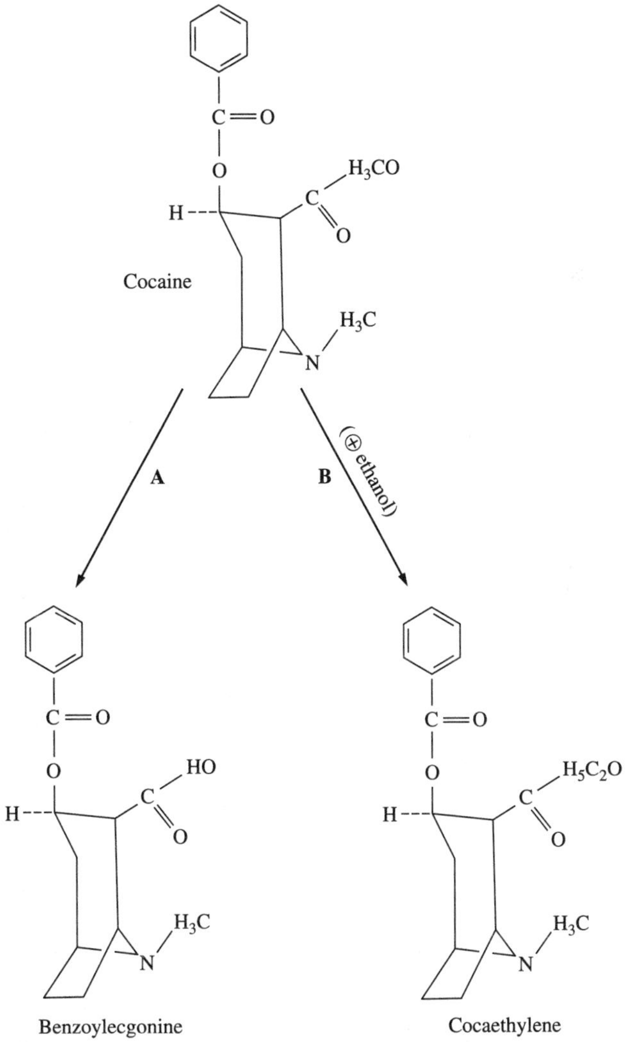

FIGURE 7.1 Structures of cocaine and the products of cocaine metabolism.
A. Normal metabolism to benzoylecognine. **B.** Metabolism to the abnormal, active metabolite cocaethylene, formed from the interaction between cocaine and alcohol. Cocaethylene is the ethyl ester of benzoylecognine.

less potent, water-soluble salt *cocaine hydrochloride* before it is exported. Because cocaine hydrochloride is water soluble, the drug can be injected intravenously or absorbed through the nasal mucosa (snorted). However, in the hydrochloride form, cocaine decomposes when it is heated and is destroyed at the temperature of smoke, making it unsuitable for use by inhalation. In contrast, cocaine base, also known as *freebase* or *crack cocaine,* is insoluble in water but is soluble in alcohol, acetone, or ether. Heating the freebase converts cocaine to a stable vapor that can be inhaled. The name crack is derived from the sound of cocaine crystals popping when smoked. Crack cocaine is readily available and inexpensive; it is therefore the most popular form of cocaine.

Cocaine hydrochloride ("crystal" or "snow"), when snorted as a "line" of drug, provides a dose of about 25 milligrams; a user might sniff about 50 to 100 milligrams of drug at a time. The smoking of crack cocaine yields average doses in the range of 250 milligrams to 1 gram (Table 7.1). The consequences of these higher doses are severe, as will become apparent later in this chapter.

Pharmacokinetics

Absorption

Cocaine is absorbed from all sites of application, including mucous membranes, the stomach, and the lungs. Thus, cocaine can be snorted, smoked, taken orally, or injected intravenously. Table 7.1 presents some pharmacokinetic data for common methods of administration.

Snorted intranasally, cocaine hydrochloride poorly crosses the mucosal membranes since the drug is a potent *vasoconstrictor* (one of its defining pharmacologic actions), constricting blood vessels and limiting its own absorption. As a consequence, only about 20 to 30 percent of the snorted drug is absorbed through the nasal mucosa into blood, with plasma levels not peaking for 30 to 60 minutes. The time course of the pharmacological effects (the subjective "high") parallels the plasma levels, as well as the amount of drug actually in brain tissue. With nasal inhalation, the euphoric effect is prolonged (because the drug is absorbed slowly) and the drug may persist in plasma for up to 6 hours.

When cocaine base is vaporized and smoked, some particles become trapped in the nose while others pass through the nasal pharynx into the trachea and onto lung surfaces, from which absorption is rapid and quite complete. Onset of effects is within seconds, peaks at 5 minutes, and persists for about 30 minutes. Only about 6 to 32 percent of the initial amount vaporized reaches plasma.

Intravenous injection of cocaine hydrochloride bypasses all the barriers to absorption, placing the total dose of drug immediately

TABLE 7.1 Effects of cocaine administration

Administration		Initial onset of action (s)	Duration of "high" (min)	Average acute dose (mg)	Peak plasma levels (ng/mL)	Purity (%)	Bioavailability (% absorbed)
Route	Mode						
Oral	Coca leaf chewing	300–600	45–90	20–50	150	0.5–1	25
Oral	Cocaine HCl	600–1800		100–200	150–200	20–80	20–30
Intranasal	Snorting cocaine HCl	120–180	30–45	5 × 30	150	20–80	20–30
Intravenous	Cocaine HCl	30–45	10–20	25–50	300–400	7–100 × 58	100
				>200	1000–1500		
Smoking	Coca paste	8–10	5–10	60–250	300–800	40–85	6–32
	Free base	8–10	5–10	250–1000	800–900	90–100	6–32
	Crack	8–10	5–10	250–1000	?	50–95	6–32

From Gold,[1] Table 16.5, p. 209.

into the bloodstream. The 30- to 60-second delay in onset of action simply reflects the time it takes the drug to travel from the site of injection through the pulmonary circulation and into the brain. Recall from Chapter 1 that it takes slightly longer for an intravenously administered drug to reach the brain than for a drug that is smoked and absorbed directly into the pulmonary veins.

Although not a common route of administration, cocaine is also absorbed when taken orally. Rush and co-workers[5] studied the physiological and psychological effects of graded doses of cocaine in volunteer, cocaine-experienced individuals. Drug was discernable from placebo within .5 to 1.0 hour, peaked 1 hour after administration, and disappeared gradually. Similar blood levels and comparable behavioral effects are observed with cocaine administered either orally or by intranasal snorting.

Distribution

Cocaine penetrates the brain rapidly; initial brain concentrations far exceed the concentrations in plasma. After it penetrates the brain, cocaine is rapidly redistributed to other tissues. Cocaine freely crosses the placental barrier, achieving levels in the unborn equal to those in the mother.

Metabolism and Excretion

Cocaine has a biological half-life in plasma of only 30 to 90 minutes; it is rapidly and almost completely metabolized by enzymes located both in plasma and in the liver. Although it is rapidly removed from plasma, it is more slowly removed from the brain, in which it can be detected for 8 or more hours after initial use. As a consequence, urine can test positive for cocaine for up to 12 hours. The major metabolite of cocaine is the inactive compound *benzoylecgonine* (Figure 7.1), which can be detected in the urine for about 48 hours and much longer (up to 2 weeks) in chronic users. Urine detection of benzoylecgonine forms the basis of drug testing for cocaine use. The persistence of the metabolite in urine implies that high-dose, long-term users might accumulate drug in their body tissues.

The metabolic interaction between cocaine and ethanol is interesting and important. In individuals who use cocaine and concurrently drink alcohol, a unique ethyl ester of benzoylecgonine is produced by the liver enzymes that metabolize the two drugs.[5,6] This metabolite (called *cocaethylene*) is pharmacologically as active as cocaine in blocking the presynaptic dopamine reuptake transporter, potentiating the euphoric effect of cocaine, increasing the risk of dual dependency, and increasing the severity of withdrawal with chronic patterns of use.[7] The cocaethylene metabolite is actually more toxic than cocaine and exacerbates cocaine's toxicity.[8] The half-life of cocaethylene is about 150 minutes.

Mechanism of Action

Pharmacologically, cocaine has three prominent actions that account for virtually all of its physiological and psychological effects. Indeed, cocaine is the only drug that possesses these three characteristics.

1. It is a potent *local anesthetic*.
2. It is a *vasoconstrictor*, strongly constricting blood vessels.
3. It is a powerful *psychostimulant* with strong reinforcing qualities.

It is the psychostimulant property that leads to compulsive abuse of the drug. Therefore, this section focuses on the actions that lead to its psychostimulation and its behavior-reinforcing properties. Its vasoconstrictive and local anesthetic actions contribute to severe cardiovascular toxicities.

Dopaminergic Actions

For 25 years, cocaine has been known to potentiate the synaptic actions of dopamine, norepinephrine, and serotonin. Such potentiation occurs as a result of cocaine's ability to block the active reuptake of these three transmitters into the presynaptic nerve terminals from which they were released (Figure 7.2). Currently, most focus is on cocaine's blockade of the presynaptic transporter for dopamine as being crucial to its behavior-reinforcing and psychostimulant properties, although blockade of serotonin reuptake is being reexamined. Blockade of the dopamine transporter markedly increases the levels of dopamine within the synaptic cleft, an observation well documented in animal experiments[9] and supported in human studies.[10] Increased dopamine levels in the nucleus accumbens and other components of the dopaminergic reward system seem to be responsible for the euphoric/addictive effects of the drug.[4,11] Both dopamine and cocaine decrease the discharge rate of neurons located in both the ventral tegmental area and the nucleus accumbens, indicating that dopamine exerts inhibitory effects on the postsynaptic receptors (i.e., dopamine is primarily an inhibitory neurotransmitter). Cocaine markedly potentiates this dopamine-induced decrease in discharge rate: such potentiation occurs secondary to blockade of dopamine reuptake, potentiating its inhibitory action on postsynaptic receptors.

In 1991, the presynaptic transporter protein for dopamine, which is blocked by cocaine, was cloned and characterized.[12,13] This transporter protein is a 619-amino-acid protein with 12 putative membrane-spanning regions; both termini of the protein are located in the intracellular cytoplasm of the presynaptic neuron (refer to Figure 2.7). Cocaine competes with dopamine for this receptor, the cocaine blocking the binding of dopamine and prolonging its presence in the synaptic cleft.

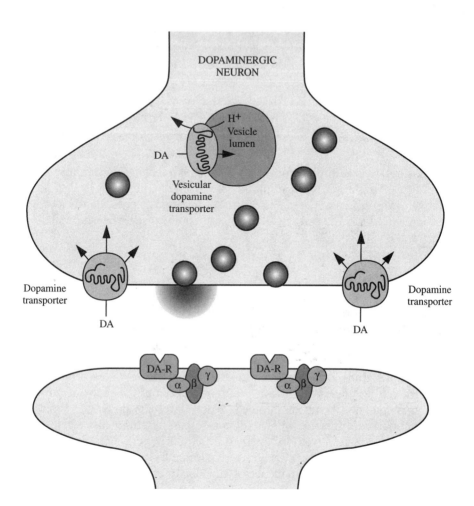

FIGURE 7.2 Transporter proteins involved in the active uptake of dopamine (DA). Two transporters are shown. The first is a vesicular DA transporter located in the cytoplasm of the presynaptic neuron, bound to DA-containing storage vesicles. This transporter carries DA from the cytoplasm into storage. The second type of DA transporter is found on the synaptic membrane of the presynaptic neuron and functions to transport DA from the synaptic cleft into the presynaptic nerve terminal, recycling the transmitter and ending the process of synaptic transmission. It is the second transporter that is blocked by cocaine, prolonging the action of DA in the synaptic cleft. Amphetamines function to induce the release of increased amounts of DA from the storage vesicles into the synaptic cleft. The result is the same: increased amounts of DA at the postsynaptic receptor (DA-R). [From S. G. Amara and M. S. Sonders, "Neurotransmitter Transporters as Molecular Targets for Addictive Drugs," *Drug and Alcohol Dependence* 51 (1998): 87–96.]

Serotoninergic Actions

Augmentation of dopaminergic neurotransmission as a basis for euphoria/reward/dependency has gone nearly unchallenged for many years. In 1998, however, Rocha and co-workers[14,15] studied cocaine effects in mice that genetically lacked either the presynaptic dopamine transporter or the postsynaptic serotonin 5-HT_{1B} receptor. In mice lacking the dopamine transporter, dopamine would not be expected to serve as a positive reinforcer; contrary to expectations, the drug was indeed a reinforcer! Thus, other pathways must be involved, pathways that involve binding of cocaine to the serotonin transporter, supporting the reinforcing effects of cocaine. Rocha and colleagues conclude: "The serotonin system may provide an additional component of reinforcement, which in the case of dopamine-transporter-deficient mice seems to be sufficient to initiate the self-administration behavior."[14] Also, in mice lacking the serotonin 5-HT_{1B} receptor, cocaine's effects were augmented over control and mice were even more motivated to self-administer cocaine. Thus, serotonin 5-HT_{1B} receptors may put the brake on, or antagonize, the reinforcing effects of cocaine.[15]

White[16] editorializes on the significance of the Rocha studies, hinting that perhaps individuals with altered serotonin receptor function may have increased susceptibility to cocaine dependence (Figure 7.3). Little and co-workers[17] test the hypothesis that alterations in brain serotonin transporter exist in chronic users of cocaine and alcohol, lending support to the hypothesis of genetically defective transporter function in drug dependence.

Effects of Short-Term, Low-Dose Use

Low-dose (e.g., 25 to 100 milligrams) nontoxic *physiological responses* to cocaine include increased alertness, motor hyperactivity, tachycardia, vasoconstriction, hypertension, bronchodilation, increased body temperature, pupillary dilation, increased glucose availability, and shifts in blood flow from the internal organs to the muscles. *Psychological effects* of low doses include an immediate euphoria, giddiness, enhanced self-consciousness, and a forceful boastfulness that last only about 30 minutes. This period is followed by one of milder euphoria mixed with anxiety, which can last for 60 to 90 minutes, followed by a more protracted anxious state that spans hours. During acute and subacute intoxication, thoughts typically race, and speech becomes talkative and rapid, often pressured, even garrulous, and sometimes tangential and incoherent. Appetite is markedly suppressed but later rebounds. Sleep is delayed; fatigue is postponed but later rebounds. Conscious awareness and mental acuity are increased but are followed with depression. Motor activity is increased, with agitation, restlessness, and a feeling of constant motion. Perhaps most

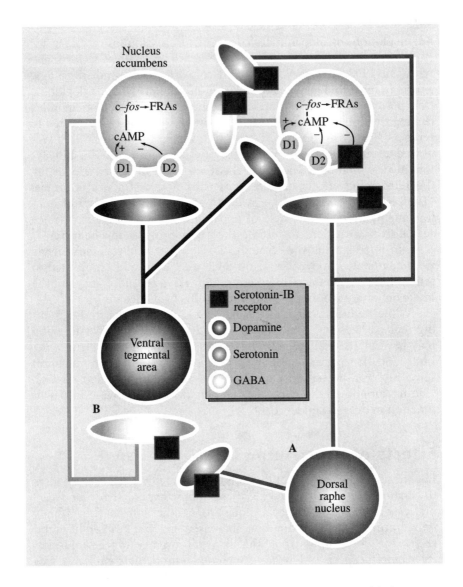

FIGURE 7.3 Possible sites at which function of the dopamine system might be affected by loss of serotonin-1B receptors. **A.** Serotonin-releasing neurons in the dorsal raphe nucleus project to both the ventral tegmental area (VTA) and the nucleus accumbens (NAc). The serotonin-1B receptors act as autoreceptors on serotonin-releasing neurons, regulating this release. If this population of receptors is lost, serotonin transmission is released in both the VTA and the NAc. **B.** Serotonin-1B receptors on the terminals of GABA-releasing neurons in the VTA suppress release of GABA. Loss of this serotonin-1B modulation could lead to activation of DA-releasing neurons, which increase stimulation of dopamine receptors, leading to activation of complicated intracellular transcription factors. Loss of serotonin-1B receptors might increase signaling through dopamine receptors. [From White.[16]]

important, cocaine promotes one's desire to take more cocaine, even instead of such important reinforcers as food.

Low-dose acute effects of cocaine are difficult to maintain because either (1) the perceived effects promote increased use or (2) tolerance develops and higher doses must be taken to perceive continued effects or avoid withdrawal. Thus, a person "graduates" rapidly to the use of higher doses with the onset of increased risks and toxicities.

Cocaine functions as a discriminative stimulus in several species,[18] a fundamental mechanism by which a drug can control behavior. Also, cocaine administration has been reported to be followed by an increase in cocaine craving, "an effect that may, like its positive reinforcing effect, increase the likelihood of additional cocaine consumption."[18] Childress and co-workers[19] studied the effects of viewing cocaine-related videos on limbic system activity in detoxified cocaine users and cocaine-naive controls. Visual cuing induced subjective craving and specific increases in blood flow to limbic regions important in motivation and affect in cocaine-experienced individuals but not in controls.

As the dose or duration of use of cocaine increases, all these effects are intensified, and a rebound depression follows. There is a progressive loss of coordination, followed by tremors and eventually seizures. CNS activation is followed by depression, dysphoria, anxiety, somnolence, and drug craving.

Although sexual interest may be heightened by using cocaine, and high doses (injected or smoked) are sometimes described as orgasmic, cocaine is not an aphrodisiac. Sexual dysfunction is common in heavy users, as they lose interest in interpersonal and sexual interactions. Further, when dysfunction is combined with the isolation that cocaine-dependent individuals experience, normal interpersonal, sensual, and sexual interactions are markedly compromised.

Organ-specific medical and physiological risks and complications of cocaine use are listed in Table 7.2. In the CNS, cocaine may cause local depletions of oxygen (cerebral ischemia), vascular thrombosis, intracranial hemorrhage and hemorrhagic strokes, cerebral atrophy, seizures, and movement disorders.[2] Even drug-abstinent users may show persistent detrimental changes in their brains[20] with associated alterations in memory function.[21] Bartzokis and colleagues[22] demonstrated that, in men who are cocaine dependent, doses of cocaine usually caused a "subclinical" form of brain damage "of the kind usually caused by vascular insufficiency." It is possible that this kind of injury could predispose to early-onset dementia and other neurological syndromes as subtle brain damage accumulates and adds to normal aging.

Cardiac complications include hypertensive crises, cardiac ischemia (lack of oxygen), heart attacks, cardiac arrhythmias, sudden death, heart failure, infected heart tissue or valves, and rupture of the aorta. Complications can occur during prolonged use or with single use.

TABLE 7.2 Organ-specific medical and physiological risks
and complications of cocaine use

Central nervous system
   Ischemic or hemorrhagic strokes
   Seizures
   Movement disorders
   Intracranial hemorrhage

Cardiac complications
   Acute myocardial infarction (heart attack)
   Cardiac arrhythmias
   Sudden cardiac arrest and death
   Heart failure
   Myocarditis (infections of the heart)
   Ruptured aorta

Pulmonary complications
   Nasal septal perforations
   Inhalation injuries
   Immunity-related diseases
   Pulmonary edema, hemorrhage
   Bronchiolitis (inflamation of the bronchial tree)

Gastrointestinal complications
   Ulcers, perforations of the stomach and upper intestine
   Bowel ischemia (lack of oxygen)
   Intestinal infarction

Renal Complications
   Renal failure
   Renal ischemia

Maternal, fetal, and neonatal complications
   Maternal
      Spontaneous abortion, abruptio placentae
      Placenta previa, stillbirth
   Fetal
      Growth retardation, premature delivery
      Congenital anomalies
      Cerebral infarction and/or hemorrhage
   Neonatal
      Drug withdrawal, seizure disorders
      Cardiovascular system complications

Modified from Boghdadi and Henning.[2]

Nasal and pulmonary complications include nasal-septal perforation, pulmonary lesions, hemorrhage, edema, and infections. Gastrointestinal and renal complications (Table 7.2) are reviewed in depth by Boghdadi and Henning.[2]

Toxic and Psychotic Effects of Long-Term, High-Dose Use

Although low doses of cocaine cause CNS stimulation that is pleasurable and euphoric, higher doses produce toxic symptoms, including anxiety, sleep deprivation, hypervigilance, suspiciousness, paranoia, and persecutory fears. A person taking cocaine may become hyperreactive, paranoid, and impulsive and may display a repetitive, compulsive pattern of behavior. The person can have a markedly altered perception of reality and become aggressive or homicidal in response to imagined persecution. These behaviors make up what is called a *toxic paranoid psychosis.*

Other high-dose, long-term effects of cocaine use include interpersonal conflicts (resulting from the sense of isolation and paranoia), depression, dysphoria, and bizarre and violent psychotic disorders that can last days or weeks after a person stops using the drug. In its most extreme form, a cocaine psychosis is characterized by paranoia, impaired reality testing, anxiety, a stereotyped compulsive repetitive pattern of behavior, and vivid visual, auditory, and tactile hallucinations. More subtle changes in behavior may include irritability, hypervigilance, extreme psychomotor activation, paranoid thinking, impaired interpersonal relations, and disturbances of eating and sleeping.

An acutely toxic dose of cocaine has been estimated to be about 1 to 2 milligrams per kilogram of body weight. Thus, 70 to 150 milligrams of cocaine is a toxic one-time dose for a 150-pound (70-kilogram) person. Serious physiological toxicity follows higher doses.

Comorbidity

Chronic cocaine use produces virtually every psychiatric syndrome: affective disorders (mania and depression), schizophrenia-like syndromes, personality disorders, and so on. Rounsaville and colleagues[23] studied 300 cocaine abusers: 56 percent met current criteria and 73 percent met lifetime criteria for the presence of a neuropsychological disorder (major depression, anxiety disorder, bipolar affective disorder, antisocial personality, PTSD, or ADHD). Thus, toxicities or withdrawal complications may indicate either high-dose drug toxicities or the onset of symptoms of a coexisting neuropsychological disorder (or both). Most cocaine-dependent individuals also have problems with other drugs of abuse. According to one report:

Cocaine addicts, like alcoholics and heroin addicts, often show a certain profile on personality tests—they are reckless, rebellious, and have a low tolerance for frustration and a craving for excitement. In fact, most of them have been or will be alcoholics or heroin addicts as well. They use opiates and alcohol either to enhance the effects of cocaine or to medicate themselves for unwanted side effects—calming jitters, dulling perceptions, and reducing paranoia to indifference. Intravenous drug users often take cocaine and heroin together in a mixture known as a speedball. Probably more than half of people treated for cocaine abuse are also alcoholic, and the rate of alcoholism in the families of cocaine addicts is high.[24]

Comorbidity of cocaine dependence with another psychological or drug-dependency disorder is discussed further in the section on treatment of cocaine dependence.

Cocaine and Pregnancy

One of tragedies of the late twentieth century was the birth of hundreds of thousands of infants who were injured intra-utero by cocaine, a drug that produces detrimental effects on the fetus of a drug-using pregnant woman. Figure 7.4 outlines the effects of cocaine on the fetus. Indirect effects result from cocaine's vasoconstrictive action on the mother's blood vessels, decreasing blood flow to the uterus and placenta and reducing oxygen delivery to the fetus. Adverse consequences of blood flow decrease include placental detachment, placental insufficiency, preterm or precipitous labor, fetal death (stillbirth), low birth weight, intrauterine growth retardation, small head size (microcephaly), and possible aberrations in nervous system development. Virtually any body organ of the neonate can be adversely affected if blood flow to that organ is restricted during development. Little and co-workers[26] state:

> Cocaine use during pregnancy should be considered teratogenic and fetotoxic. The exact mechanism of cocaine-induced congenital anomalies is presently uncertain, but it may be related to the placental vasoconstriction and fetal hypoxia produced by the drug, with the resulting intermittent vascular disruptions and ischemia in the embryo and fetus actually causing congenital anomalies.

From Figure 7.4, note that cocaine also exerts adverse direct effects on the fetus. Cocaine easily crosses the placental barrier, and fetal concentrations equal or can actually exceed those in the mother.[2] Direct organ toxicity can involve the heart, the CNS, the urinary system, and the GI tract.

Vasoconstriction in either the mother or the fetus can increase blood pressure in the fetus, leading to intracerebral hemorrhage, thickening

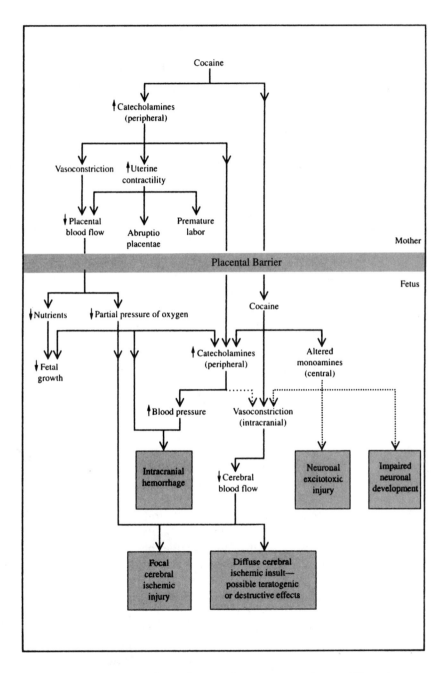

FIGURE 7.4 Deleterious effects of maternal cocaine use on fetuses. Effects that appear plausible on the basis of current information but whose confirmation requires more supporting evidence are indicated by dotted lines. ↑ denotes increase and ↓ denotes decrease. [From Volpe.[25]]

of heart muscle, and various vascular and structural abnormalities.[27] Volpe,[25] reviewing the direct fetotoxic effects of cocaine, notes that, as the brain develops, exposure of the fetus to cocaine may promote serious destructive lesions, leading to a neonatal neurological syndrome typified by abnormal sleep patterns, tremors, poor feeding, irritability, occasional seizures, and an increased risk or incidence of sudden infant death syndrome (SIDS).

Some have tried to define a fetal cocaine syndrome and a cocaine jittery baby syndrome. However, because of the wide spectrum of indirect and direct effects on the fetus, any such syndrome is not as clearly defined as the fetal alcohol syndrome, and cocaine use by the mother is only one of many undesirable influences in the children's lives. Babies born into a drug-using environment, and possibly into poverty, experience little physical or emotional nurturing, so bonding is incomplete or absent.

> Cocaine's effects on the unborn and newborn may also be related to poor nutrition, poor hygiene, and neglect. Cocaine compromises the mother or any caregiver's ability to respond to their new baby through talking, eye contact, and tactile stimulation. Such disconnection and indifference to the infant's behavioral cues, which is necessary for optimal intellectual and emotional infant development, creates additional problems. It has been suggested that drug-dependent mothers are impaired in the ability to respond to their infants; the specific interactional behavior of cocaine-using mothers is still under investigation.[26]

Perhaps 50,000 to 100,000 babies are born each year to mothers who have used at least some cocaine during pregnancy and about 11 percent of pregnant women have used cocaine during pregnancy, with much higher rates among low-income, inner-city women. Birnbach and co-workers[28] noted in a New York City study that 68 percent of pregnant women who were admitted to labor and delivery without previous prenatal care tested positive for cocaine, placing both the pregnant woman and her fetus at risk for life-threatening cardiovascular and CNS complications. While that number may be unique to this population, "between 15 and 25 percent of babies are born with cocaine already in their system."[4]

Cocaine also passes from a nursing mother to a newborn through breast milk. Cocaine can be found in breast milk up to 60 hours after a mother used the drug. The neonatal effects of this are unclear, but certainly the infant is affected.[4]

As cocaine-impaired children enter the school system, they appear to have difficulty developing attachments or dealing effectively with multiple stimuli. They may become either aggressive or withdrawn when they are overstimulated. They have difficulty with unstructured play and a low tolerance for frustration. They also structure input and information poorly, displaying a high incidence of attention-deficit/hyperactivity disorder (ADHD). Certainly, "research is needed to detect the damage to the neurobehavioral and neurophysiologic functioning of these children."[27]

Pharmacological Treatment of Cocaine Dependency

A variety of pharmacological approaches have been suggested for treating cocaine abuse, but as yet there is no consensus regarding any generally accepted successful treatment. Even the expected goals of drug therapy are not agreed on.[29] Several problems complicate attempts at therapy. First is the intensity of both the drug effect and the intense behavior-reinforcing action of cocaine. Second is the pronounced tendency toward relapse, with cocaine-related activities acting as a cue to an increased craving for the drug.[19] Third, most cocaine addicts have a coexisting disorder, involving drug dependencies and/or psychiatric disorders, including major depression, an anxiety disorder, bipolar disorder, borderline personality disorder, and/or antisocial personality disorder.[4] Given these complications, there appear to be three areas of need for pharmacologic intervention:

1. Antiwithdrawal agents intended to restore or enhance the dopaminergic tone of hypoactive limbic system regions. Such agents might be beneficial to ameliorate withdrawal depression.

2. Anticraving agents that block limbic dopaminergic receptors may either reduce cue-induced craving or blunt the euphoric effect of subsequently administered cocaine. For example, Romach and colleagues[30] demonstrated that *ecopipan*, a selective D_1/D_2 blocker, attenuates the euphoric and anxiogenic effects of cocaine as well as the desire to use cocaine.

3. Treatment of comorbid psychological disorders may help reduce the drive that propels a person to self-medicate with cocaine to ameliorate psychological distress.

To date, there are no clearly identified antiwithdrawal agents that work through a process of drug substitution, like methadone in ameliorating withdrawal from heroin or benzodiazepines that help ease the symptoms of alcohol withdrawal. Prolonged cocaine use is associated with a down regulation of dopamine receptors and a reduction in the absolute number of such receptors.[31] Thus, cocaine withdrawal leads to a hypofunctional dopaminergic system, a state that probably persists for weeks or months after drug abstinence. Perhaps an alternate cocaine-like agent with less abuse potential might help maintain receptor activity until new receptors are generated. Methylphenidate (Ritalin) is an example of such a drug.[32] Roache and colleagues[32A] administered methylphenidate to 57 cocaine abusers in treatment. Psychological responses include dysphoria, anxiety, depression, anger, and jitteriness. The authors concluded that "the subjective effects of methylphenidate may not be positive enough for an adequate replacement approach."

More amenable to treatment are disorders that cooccur with cocaine dependency. Thirty to fifty percent of individuals who abuse cocaine have a history of depression and a positive family history for affective illness.[33] Because cocaine blocks the presynaptic dopamine transporter, it resembles mechanistically the pharmacologic actions of the antidepressants such as *bupropion* (Welbutrin; Chapter 16). Margolin and colleagues,[34] however, reported that bupropion was only minimally effective. A few studies have reported favorable effects of tricyclic antidepressants, such as *desipramine* and *imipramine*, in improving mood and prolonging abstinence in patients (with coexisting depression) who have withdrawn from cocaine. Similarly, the serotonin-specific antidepressant *fluoxetine* (Prozac; Chapter 16) has been reported to alleviate comorbid depression and reduce cocaine use, although Mendelson and Mello[35] found fluoxetine to be of little use.

Levin and co-workers[36] note that "35 percent of cocaine abusers seeking treatment have a history of childhood ADHD (attention-deficit/hyperactivity disorder), and approximately 15 percent of cocaine abusers seeking treatment may have adult ADHD." They evaluated the efficacy of long-acting *methylphenidate* (Ritalin SR) on 12 patients with comorbid cocaine dependence abuse and adult ADHD noting that the combined intervention of the drug plus relapse prevention therapy reduced both adult ADHD and cocaine dependency. Other drugs that may, at least theoretically, be useful include *pemoline* and *bromocriptine*, although careful evaluation has not been made. In summary:

> At present, no drug therapy is uniquely effective in treating cocaine abuse and dependence. A number of medications that were initially developed to treat other disorders have been used to treat the behavioral disorders often associated with cocaine abuse and dependence. Unfortunately, none are considered to be highly effective for either cocaine detoxification or the maintenance of abstinence. However, the limitations of the medications currently available should not lead investigators to give up their search, because medication is only one element of humane and comprehensive therapy for persons with drug dependence. There is compelling evidence that many cocaine abusers have had major psychological and psychosocial impairments that contributed to and may have been compounded by subsequent problems

of drug dependence. These impairments include cognitive and learning disorders, interpersonal and social problems, and legal and financial difficulties. [We] stressed the heterogeneity among cocaine abusers
and the need to develop specialized treatment for clinically distinct
subgroups. It is axiomatic that treatment should be selected on the
basis of all biomedical and psychosocial factors associated with the
patient's illness.[35]

Psychosocial Interventions

With the failure of successful pharmacological approaches to the treatment of cocaine dependence, psychosocial interventions offer the most
promise so far. Approaches to treatment are many, from classic 12-step
recovery programs resembling that of Alcoholics Anonymous to interventions utilizing individual and/or group drug counseling, cognitive-
behavioral therapy, supportive-expressive psychodynamic therapy,[37,38]
or behavioral reinforcement approaches.[39] As the recent National
Institute on Drug Abuse Collaborative Study[38] concluded:

> Compared with professional psychotherapy, a manual-guided combi-
> nation of intensive individual drug counseling and group drug coun-
> seling has promise for the treatment of cocaine dependence.

The American Psychiatric Association[40] has published practice guidelines for the treatment of cocaine-related disorders.

AMPHETAMINES AND OTHER BEHAVIORAL STIMULANTS

Amphetamines (Figure 7.5) are a structurally defined group of drugs, all
of which produce a variety of effects on both the CNS and the autonomic
nervous system.* Amphetamines are also called *sympathomimetic agents*

---

*The *autonomic nervous system* (ANS) is frequently called the visceral nervous system because it regulates and maintains the homeostasis of the body's internal organs. It controls the function of the heart, the flow of blood, and the functioning of
the digestive tract, and it regulates other internal functions that are essential for
maintaining the balance necessary for life. The ANS is divided into two subdivi-
sions—the *sympathetic* and the *parasympathetic*. The latter can be viewed as maintaining our "vegetative" functions, while the former functions to handle the body's
response to stress, fright, fear, or other responses that demand an immediate alerting response. Neurotransmitters in the sympathetic division of the ANS include epinephrine (adrenaline), norepinephrine, and dopamine.

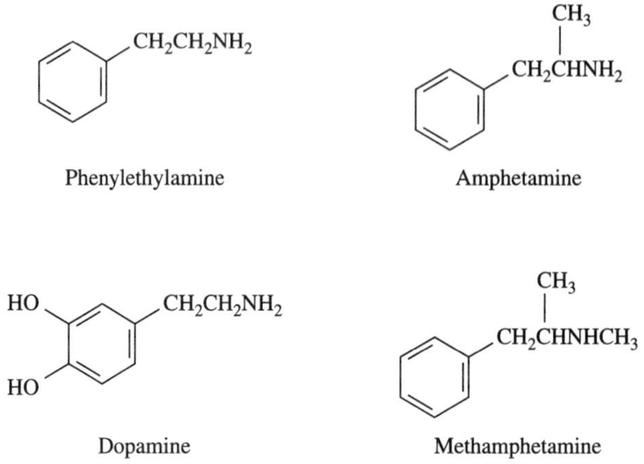

FIGURE 7.5 The basic sympathomimetic amine nucleus (phenylethylamine), the neurotransmitter dopamine (di-hydroxy-phenylethylamine), and the structures of amphetamine and methamphetamine.

because they mimic the actions of adrenaline (epinephrine, one of the transmitters of our "sympathetic" nervous system). Amphetamines produce vasoconstriction, hypertension, tachycardia, and other signs and symptoms of our normal alerting response. These drugs also stimulate the CNS, producing tremor, restlessness, increased motor activity, agitation, insomnia, and loss of appetite (anorexia). These actions result from an indirect action involving the presynaptic release of dopamine and norepinephrine and, to a lesser extent, direct stimulation of post-synaptic catecholamine receptors.

History

For more than 60 years, amphetamines have been used therapeutically to treat a variety of disorders. Between 1935 and 1946, a list of 39 conditions for which amphetamine could be used in treatment was developed. The list included schizophrenia, morphine addiction, tobacco smoking, heart block, head injury, radiation sickness, hypotension, seasickness, severe hiccups, and caffeine dependence. During World War II, amphetamines were used as an aid to fight fatigue and enhance the performance of servicemen.

In some individuals, therapeutic use has led to compulsive abuse. Large-scale abuse (usually oral ingestion of amphetamine tablets) began in the late 1940s, primarily by students and truck drivers in efforts to maintain wakefulness, temporarily increase alertness, and delay sleep. Amphetamines continued to be used (and abused) as appetite suppressants, despite the fact that the anoretic effect persists only over the first two weeks of treatment, after which time it diminishes. In the late 1960s, the abuse pattern of amphetamines changed with the advent of injectable forms of amphetamine. These injectable products (by legitimate manufacturers) have been discontinued.

Today, interest in amphetamine-like compounds involves two areas:

1. Therapeutic use in the treatment of narcolepsy and attention-deficit/hyperactivity disorder

2. Compulsive misuse and dependency, especially with the amphetamine derivative methamphetamine in its various illicit forms and routes of administration (including the smoking of free-base methamphetamine, termed ICE).

Mechanism of Action

The amphetamines exert virtually all of their CNS effects by causing the release of newly synthesized norepinephrine and dopamine from presynaptic storage sites in nerve terminals.[41] The peripheral nervous system effects of the amphetamines probably result from increased norepinephrine levels. The behavioral stimulation and increased psychomotor activity appear to follow from the resulting stimulation of the dopamine receptors in the mesolimbic system (including the nucleus accumbens).[42] The high-dose stereotypical behavior (including constant repetition of meaningless acts) appears to involve dopamine neurons in the caudate nucleus and putamen of the basal ganglia.

The actions leading to an increase in aggressive behavior are complex. Clinically, such behavioral stimulant action is seen primarily in adults suffering from cocaine toxicity and consists of increases in stereotypical, repetitive behaviors. In children, amphetamines are used therapeutically to reduce aggressive behavior and activities characteristic of ADHD; in adults with a history of ADHD, behavioral calming can also occur.

Pharmacological Effects

As stated, amphetamines exert their peripheral and central actions largely by causing the release of newly synthesized norepinephrine and dopamine from presynaptic nerve terminals (Figure 7.2). All the physical and behavioral effects of the amphetamines appear to follow from this action. Note that the release of dopamine increases the amount of dopamine available to the postsynaptic receptor, much as does cocaine. Both drugs have the net effect of increasing the amount of dopamine available (although through two different mechanisms). Indeed, individuals who have used cocaine have difficulty distinguishing between the subjective effects of 8 to 10 milligrams of cocaine and

10 milligrams of dextroamphetamine when both are administered intravenously.

The pharmacological responses to amphetamines vary with the specific drug, the dose, and the route of administration. In general, with amphetamine itself, effects may be categorized as those observed at low to moderate doses (5 to 50 milligrams), usually administered orally, and those observed at high doses (more than approximately 100 milligrams), often administered intravenously. These dose ranges are not the same for all amphetamines. For example, dextroamphetamine is three to four times more potent than amphetamine. Low to moderate doses of dextroamphetamine range from 2.5 to 20 milligrams, while high doses are 50 milligrams or more. Because methamphetamine is even more potent, dose ranges must be lowered even more.

At low doses, all amphetamines increase blood pressure, slow heart rate, relax bronchial muscle, and produce a variety of other responses that follow from the body's alerting response. In the CNS, amphetamine is a potent psychomotor stimulant, producing increased alertness, euphoria, excitement, wakefulness, a reduced sense of fatigue, loss of appetite, mood elevation, increased motor and speech activity, and a feeling of power. Although task performance is improved, dexterity may deteriorate. When short-duration, high-intensity energy output is desired, such as during an athletic competition, a user's performance may be enhanced, despite the fact that his or her dexterity and fine motor skills may be impaired. Amphetamine metabolites are excreted in the urine and are detectable for up to 48 hours.

At moderate doses (20 to 50 milligrams), additional effects of amphetamine include stimulation of respiration, slight tremors, restlessness, a greater increase in motor activity, insomnia, and agitation. In addition, amphetamines prevent fatigue, suppress appetite, promote wakefulness, and cause sleep deprivation.

A person who chronically uses high doses of amphetamine suffers from a different set of drug effects. Stereotypical behaviors include continual, purposeless, repetitive acts, sudden outbursts of aggression and violence, paranoid delusions, and severe anorexia. The harmful effects that are seen in the high-dose user include psychosis and abnormal mental conditions, weight loss, skin sores, infections resulting from neglected health care, and a variety of other consequences that occur both because of the actions of the drug itself and because of poor eating habits, lack of sleep, or the use of unsterile equipment for intravenous injections. Most high-dose users show a progressive deterioration in their social, personal, and occupational affairs. Also seen is amphetamine psychosis with paranoid ideation; many addicts must be hospitalized intermittently for treatment of episodes of psychosis. Today, psychosis is especially seen in people who abuse methamphetamine.

The toxic dose of amphetamine varies widely. Severe reactions can occur from low doses (20 to 30 milligrams). On the other hand, people who have not developed tolerance have survived doses of 400 to 500 milligrams. Even larger doses are tolerated by chronic users. The slogan "Speed kills" refers not only to a direct fatal effect of single doses of amphetamine but also to the deteriorating mental and physical condition that occurs in the addicted user.

The possibility of adverse effects of amphetamines taken either licitly or illicitly during pregnancy have been little studied. There is no clear-cut pattern of congenital anomalies, although there is some consensus that infants born of amphetamine-using mothers have a degree of growth retardation and lower birth weights. An increased rate of intracerebral hemorrhage can be observed, probably brought on by drug-induced increases in blood pressure in both the mother and the fetus. In the long term, there is evidence of psychometric deficits, poor academic performance, behavioral problems, cognitive slowing, and general maladjustment.

Dependence and Tolerance

As a potent psychomotor stimulant and behavior-reinforcing agent, the amphetamines are prone to compulsive abuse. Physical dependence is readily induced in both humans and laboratory animals and follows a classical positive conditioning model (the positive reward leads to further drug use). Once drug use is stopped, the individual experiences a withdrawal syndrome, although it is less dramatic than the withdrawal associated with either narcotics (see Chapter 10) or barbiturates (see Chapter 2). As Bernstein[43] states:

> Withdrawal symptoms associated with the amphetamines include increased appetite, weight gain, decreased energy, and increased need for sleep. Patients may develop a voracious appetite and sleep for several days after amphetamines are discontinued. Paranoid symptoms may persist during drug withdrawal, but generally do not develop as a result of withdrawal. The patient suddenly discontinuing amphetamine use may develop severe depression and become suicidal. Management of amphetamine withdrawal does not require detoxification, but does require appropriate and cautious clinical observation of the patient, recognition of depression, and treatment with an appropriate antidepressant drug if clinically necessary. . . . High-potency antipsychotic drugs, such as haloperidol, may be necessary [to treat paranoid reactions].

Tolerance rapidly develops and can necessitate higher and higher doses, which starts a vicious circle of drug use and withdrawal. At this point, tolerance to the euphoriant effects develops, and periods of prolonged binging begin. This tolerance combined with the memory of drug-induced highs leads to further drug intake, social withdrawal, and a focus on procuring drugs.

ICE: A Free-Base Form of Methamphetamine

Methamphetamine is a more potent drug than dextroamphetamine. Generally considered to be an illicit drug, manufactured in clandestine laboratories, methamphetamine was actually a licit drug, effective in the treatment of ADHD. Today, however, with the negative publicity, it is rarely used legitimately and illicit use dominates. Methamphetamine is easily synthesized from readily obtainable chemicals. In animals, methamphetamine has been implicated as a neurotoxic agent, although toxicity has not been demonstrated in humans. As a drug of abuse, methamphetamine is also known as "speed," "crystal," "crank," "go," and "ICE," with considerable overlap in nomenclature with other amphetamines except for ICE, which refers to the smokable form of methamphetamine.[44]

Like cocaine hydrochloride, methamphetamine (the hydrochloride salt) is broken down at the temperatures that must be achieved for it to be vaporized for smoking. However, when converted to its base, methamphetamine can be effectively vaporized and inhaled in smoke. Methamphetamine hydrochloride is used orally, by intravenous injection, and by snorting; the base form (ICE) is administered by smoking. Absorbed rapidly through the lungs and mucous membranes, the rapidity of ICE's absorption is as rapid or even more rapid than intravenous injection of methamphetamine hydrochloride. Thus, ICE is to methamphetamine as crack is to cocaine: the free-base, concentrated, smokable form of the parent compound. Unlike crack, methamphetamine has an extremely long half-life (about 12 hours), resulting in an intense, persistent drug action. As a form of methamphetamine, ICE is between 90 and 100 percent pure. Chronic use can result in serious and persistent psychiatric, cardiovascular, metabolic, and neuromuscular changes.

Pharmacokinetics

Smoking ICE results in its near-immediate absorption into plasma, with additional absorption continuing over the next 4 hours. The blood level then progressively declines. The biological half-life of methamphetamine is more than 11 hours.[45] After distribution to the brain, about 60 percent of the methamphetamine is slowly metabolized in the liver, and the end products are excreted through the kidneys, along with unmetabolized methamphetamine (about 40 percent is excreted unchanged) and small amounts of the pharmacologically active metabolite amphetamine.

Effects and Toxicity

The effects of methamphetamine closely resemble and are frequently indistinguishable from those of cocaine. Both are potent psychomotor stimulants and positive reinforcers; self-administration is extremely difficult to control and modify, especially in abusers who use the drug either by injection or by smoking. Repeated high doses of methamphetamine are associated with violent behavior and paranoid psychosis. Such doses cause long-lasting decreases in dopamine and serotonin in the brain. These changes appear to be irreversible, because the chemical effects can persist for more than a year after drug administration. This toxic effect is directed at the neurons that manufacture dopamine and serotonin, and the biochemical changes do not appear to be expressed in gross behavioral changes. Permanent neurochemical alterations, however, may be expressed as alterations in sleep or sexual function, depression, movement disorders, or schizophrenia.

Just as prolonged cocaine use can result in psychoses resembling paranoid schizophrenia, smoking ICE produces a pattern of acute delusional and psychotic behavior. However, unlike that of cocaine, ICE-induced psychosis can persist for days or weeks and can occur much earlier. Fatalities have resulted from cardiac toxicity manifested as either pulmonary edema or heart failure.

Nonamphetamine Behavioral Stimulants

An amphetamine is any drug with the basic amphetamine nucleus (Figure 7.5). A nonamphetamine behavioral stimulant does not have this basic nucleus (Figure 7.6), but it shares the same action of potentiating the sympathomimetic actions of the amphetamines. Such drugs include ephedrine (found in nature in Ma-huang; Chapter 20), methylphenidate, pemoline, and sibutramine. The latter three drugs are used in the medical treatment of ADHD, narcolepsy, and obesity, among other medical disorders. *Ephedrine* today has little use in medicine (except perhaps to transiently increase blood pressure); most use is in herbal medicine (discussed in Chapter 20).

Methylphenidate (Ritalin) is a nonamphetamine behavioral stimulant; the regular-release formulation has a half-life of two to four hours (Table 7.1). The sustained-release formulation (Ritalin-SR) has variable absorption, with a half-life varying between three and eight hours. It is erratically absorbed; blood levels are unpredictable, and response can be variable.

Mechanistically, methylphenidate increases the synaptic concentration of dopamine by blocking the presynaptic dopamine transporter

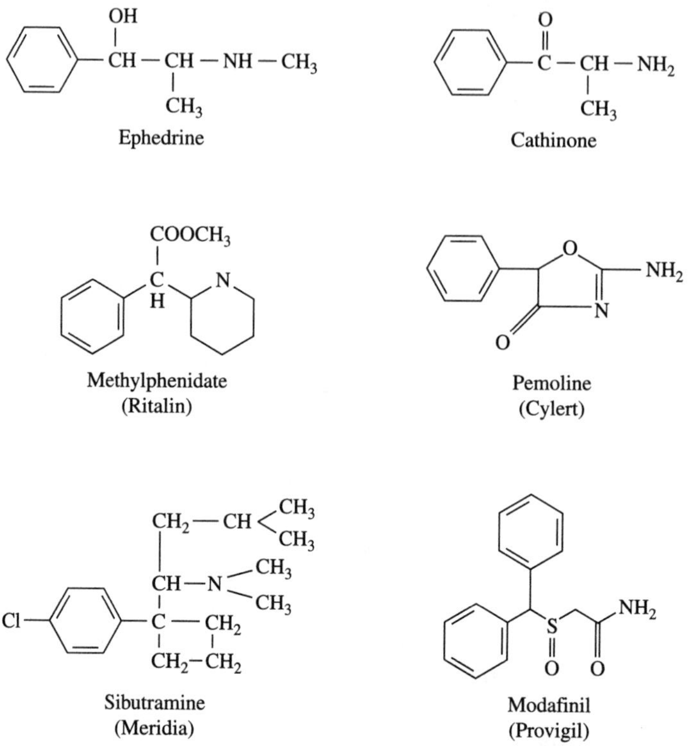

FIGURE 7.6 Structures of two naturally occurring catecholamine psychostimulants— ephedrine (from *Ephedra*, or Ma-huang) and cathinone (from *Catha edulis*, or Khat)]—and four synthetic non-catecholamine psychostimulants used in medicine— methylphenidate (Ritalin), pemoline (Cylert), sibutramine (Meridia), and modafinil (Provigil).

(a cocaine-like action) and also perhaps by slightly increasing the re-lease of dopamine (an amphetamine- or ephedrine-like action). When these drugs are injected intravenously, experienced cocaine users can perceive a cocaine-like or amphetamine-like rush, an action not usu-ally experienced with oral dosage. Volkow and colleagues[46] demon-strated that at clinically relevant doses, methylphenidate blocked more than 50 percent of the dopamine transporters 60 minutes after oral ad-ministration (Figure 7.7). They postulate that the slow uptake of methylphenidate into the brain after oral administration accounts for the low rate of positive reinforcement effects seen with use of the drug.

Behaviorally, methylphenidate is used to calm hyperactivity and improve attention in ADHD. Although this action was thought to be ex-erted through dopaminergic increases, Gainetdinov and co-workers[47] demonstrated in mice that lacked the gene for the dopamine trans-porter that methylphenidate still calmed hyperactivity in a novel

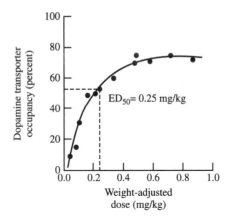

FIGURE 7.7 Levels of dopamine transporter occupancy for weight-adjusted doses of methylphenidate. Also shown is the dose required to occupy 50 percent of the dopamine transporters (ED_{50}). [From Volkow et al.[46]]

environment, presumably by "raising serotonin levels to balance the animal's high brain dopamine level." In these animals, *fluoxetine* (Prozac) exerted a methylphenidate-like action, presumably by also blocking the presynaptic serotonin transporter. Thus, at least in some people, ADHD may represent an imbalance between dopamine and serotonin systems. Dougherty and co-workers[48] demonstrated in six adults with ADHD that dopamine transporter density was increased by 70 percent over levels seen in healthy control adults. Denney and Rapport[49] analyzed the results of methylphenidate therapy in ADHD, noting that academic performance improvements serve as perhaps the best measure of cognitive and behavioral improvements in treated children with ADHD.

Pemoline (Cylert) is a CNS stimulant structurally dissimilar to either methylphenidate or amphetamine (Figure 7.6). Pemoline is presumed to reduce ADHD symptoms by potentiating CNS dopaminergic transmission. Pemoline has a relatively long half-life of 11 to 13 hours. It is thought to have a lower abuse potential than does either methylphenidate or amphetamines. Its use is limited by reports of rare instances of hepatitis, necessitating close monitoring of liver function. Wilens and colleagues[50] studied robust doses of pemoline in 35 adults with ADHD; 50 percent were considered to be positive responders, compared with 17 percent of placebo-treated controls (Figure 7.8). No cases of hepatotoxicity were observed, but this does not rule out the possibility of toxicity in larger populations of drug recipients. Pemoline is no longer recommended for initial therapy of ADHD. If it is used, patients (or their parents) should sign a consent form, and liver function tests are recommended at two-week intervals.

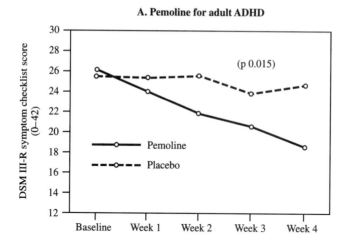

A. Pemoline for adult ADHD

(p 0.015)

○ Pemoline
○ Placebo

DSM III-R symptom checklist score (0–42)

Baseline   Week 1   Week 2   Week 3   Week 4

B. Positive responders
Clinical global impression: Much to very much improved

($p \leq 0.05$)

Percent of sample

Placebo   Pemoline

FIGURE 7.8 A. Reduction in scores on the ADHD symptom checklist (scored 0–42) of subjects on pemoline versus those on placebo. **B.** Subjects on pemoline were significantly improved compared with those on placebo at the end of the active phase. Response rate was determined by clinician's assessment of whether the subject was much or very much improved on the CGI scale. [From Wilens et al.[50]]

Sibutramine (Meridia) is a serotonin, norepinephrine, and (to a lesser extent) dopamine reuptake inhibitor (it blocks their presynaptic transporter proteins) that has recently been marketed as an antiobesity agent. It is structurally related to amphetamine (Figure 7.6), but it is not literally an amphetamine. Sibutramine is rapidly metabolized in the liver to active metabolites that are responsible for the drug's pharmacologic actions. These metabolites reach a peak concentration in plasma in 3 to 4 hours; their half-life is 14 to 16 hours.[51] Modest weight losses for up to one year have been reported, and the drug does not appear to have a potential for compulsive misuse.[52] Significant increases in heart rate and blood pressure have been reported and may limit the use of the drug.

An alternative to sibutramine for weight loss is the drug *orlistat* (Xenical). This drug is not a behavioral stimulant; it is, in fact, not even absorbed into the body. It remains in the intestine where it exerts its pharmacological action. Orlistat is an inhibitor of the pancreatic enzyme *pancreatic lipase* that is secreted from the pancreas into the intestine in response to ingested fat. Pancreatic lipase breaks down fats into absorbable fatty acids. As a result of blockade of enzyme function by orlistat, a portion of ingested fat remains in the intestine. Thus, fat is not broken down or absorbed; the fat is excreted in feces. Orlistat therefore reduces fat absorption, can lower body weight, and can reduce the plasma levels of triglycerides and cholesterol.[53,54] Side effects result from the retention of fats in the intestine: nausea, bloating, and loose stools. Reduction in ingested fats reduces the intensity of these side effects.

Modafinil is a nonamphetamine psychostimulant whose exact mechanism of psychostimulant action remains unclear but is thought to be unique.[55] Modifinil may potentiate excitatory glutamate neurotransmission and inhibit the activity of GABA neurons in the cerebral cortex and the nucleus accumbens, altering the balance between glutamate and GABA transmission.[56] It may not produce dependence and may not lead to compulsive abuse.

Modafinil is used in the treatment of narcolepsy, an inherited disorder of sleep.[57] Potential uses include cognitive improvement in patients with Alzheimer's disease, use in the treatment of ADHD, and potentiation of the action of antidepressant drugs.[58] The drug appears to have only minimal peripheral side effects such as drug-induced hypertension. Modafinil is an important addition to the pharmacologic treatment of narcolepsy as well as an interesting stimulant for evaluation for use in the treatment of other CNS disorders amenable to treatment with a psychostimulant.

Pharmacologic Treatment of ADHD

The medical uses of amphetamines today are limited to two disorders: (1) treatment of narcolepsy, (2) treatment of attention-deficit/hyperactivity disorder. Amphetamine-like drugs have also historically been used in the treatment of obesity, but today this use is considered inappropriate. New drugs for the pharmacologic treatments of obesity (sibutramine and orlistat) and narcolepsy (modafinil) have already been discussed. In this section is recent information on the pharmacologic treatment of ADHD.

Background

Amphetamines have been used since about 1936 for treating attention-deficit/hyperactivity disorder (ADHD) in children and adolescents. Treatment started with the use of amphetamine and dextroamphetamine and has progressed over the years to the extensive use of methylphenidate (Ritalin), pemoline (Cylert), several of the clinical antidepressants, a variety of other compounds, including clonidine, lithium, carbamazepine, and bupropion, and (recently) to a return to amphetamine use (Adderall).[59] Conner and colleagues[60] reviewed the modest efficacy of clonidine and guanfacine in treating ADHD.

ADHD is the most common psychological disorder of childhood, affecting 3 to 5 percent of school-age children.[61] Of these, only 12.5 percent are being treated with stimulant medication:

> Medication treatments are often not used in treating ADHD children identified in the community, suggesting the need for better education of parents, physicians, and mental health professionals about the effectiveness of these treatments. On the basis of these data it cannot be concluded that substantial "overtreatment" with stimulants is occurring across communities in general.[61]

ADHD is characterized by age-inappropriate problems with attention, learning, impulse control, and (usually) hyperactivity. ADHD has been thought to be more prevalent and more severe in boys than in girls. However, recently Biederman and colleagues[62] reported in a study of 140 girls with ADHD that they share with boys the same clustering and intensity of core symptoms of the disorder (Figure 7.9), the same comorbidity profile (Figure 7.10), and the same dysfunction in multiple domains.

ADHD persists beyond childhood and into adulthood in about 40 to 60 percent of affected individuals.[63] In adults, it is associated with a tenfold increase of antisocial personality disorder, up to a fivefold increased risk of drug abuse, a twenty-fivefold increase in risk for institutionalization for delinquency, and up to a ninefold increased risk for incarceration.

A remarkable incidence of comorbid or concomitant disease occurs in individuals affected with ADHD.[61,64] As many as two-thirds of elementary school-age children with ADHD who are referred for clinical evaluation have at least one other diagnosable psychiatric disorder.[65] Concomitant diseases include conduct disorder,[66,67] oppositional defiant disorder,[68] learning disorders, anxiety disorders,[69,70] mood disorders (especially depression[71]), and substance abuse.[72] Pliszka, Carlson, and Swanson[73] discuss the assessment and management of ADHD with comorbid disorders. Disney and co-workers[74] note

A. Symptom profile

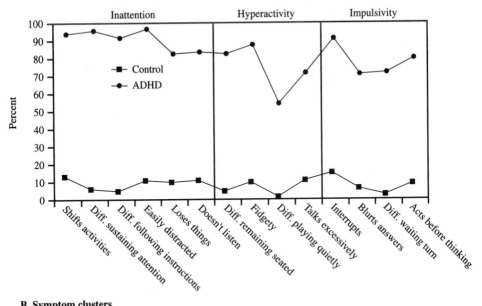

B. Symptom clusters

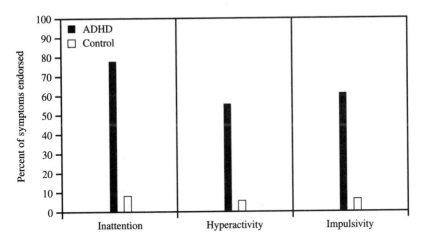

FIGURE 7.9 DSM-III-R symptom profile (**A**) and symptom clusters (**B**) in 140 girls aged 6 to 18 years and 122 non-ADHD controls. Diff. = difficulty. [From Biederman et al.[62]]

that comorbid conduct disorder has been reported in 30 to 50 percent of ADHD cases, and that conduct disorder (rather than ADHD) increases the risk of substance abuse in children and adolescents with ADHD.

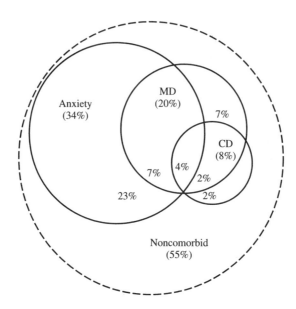

FIGURE 7.10 Psychiatric comorbidity in 140 girls aged 6 to 18 years with ADHD. MD = mood disorder; CD = conduct disorder. Other disorders that aggregated significantly included tics and enuresis. Statistical trends suggested increased risk for panic disorder, obsessive-compulsive disorder, language disorders, alcohol and drug abuse, and cigarette smoking. [From Biederman et al.[62]]

The genetic, neurochemical, and/or functional deficits involved in or responsible for ADHD are still matters for speculation. There does appear to be a genetic link for ADHD; most evidence points to a dopaminergic etiology, specifically to the dopamine D_4 gene.[75] People with altered D_4 gene appear to be "novelty-seeking, impulsive, exploratory, excitable and quick-tempered."[74] Neuroanatomically, Bush and colleagues[76] point to a hypofunctional or dysfunctional anterior cingulate cognitive division playing a central role in attentional processes (Figure 7.11); hypofunction alters stimulus selection as well as response selection. It is currently unknown whether or not ADHD medication will reverse structural dysfunction or how dysfunction interfaces with any dopamine$_4$ receptor abnormality.

Treatment

Stimulant drugs improve behavior and learning ability in 60 to 80 percent of children who are correctly diagnosed. The primary drugs used in treatment include methylphenidate, amphetamines, and pemoline (Table 7.3); other drugs, such as buspirone (BuSpar) and bupropion (Welbutrin), are used in refractory cases. Of these, *methylphenidate*

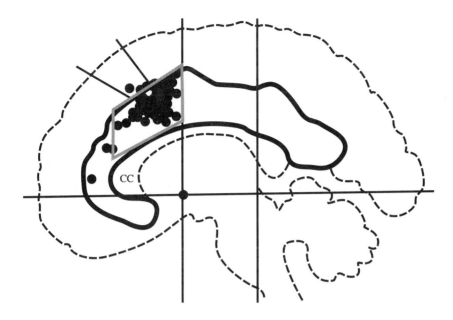

FIGURE 7.11 Localization of the anterior cingulate cognitive division, a functional subdivision of the anterior cingulate cortex (CC) that plays a crucial role in complex cognitive/attentional processing. Adults with ADHD failed to activate this area during an attentional/cognitive interference task. Normal adults strongly activated this area as shown by the dots. [From Bush et al.[76]]

accounts for 90 percent of the prescribed medication. Methylphenidate is of rapid onset and short duration; thus, it must be administered at both breakfast time and lunchtime. It is not administered in the evening to permit the blood level to drop, allowing normal sleep. The short half-life is a problem in some children who experience an end-of-dose rebound in dysfunctional behavior. The sustained-release preparation of methylphenidate has been disappointing. Because orally administered methylphenidate enters the brain slowly, its abuse potential (with oral administration) is low.

Amphetamines still provide a treatment option to methylphenidate; both *dextroamphetamine* (Dexedrine) and an *amphetamine mixture* (Adderall) are promoted for use. Manos, Short, and Findlind[77] compared methylphenidate and Adderall in youths and noted no differences between the two on either teacher or parent ratings of behavior. They concluded:

> Single-dose treatments of Adderall appear to be as effective as two daily doses of methylphenidate and therefore increase the possibility of

TABLE 7.3 Psychostimulants used to treat attention-
deficit/hyperactivity disorder

Feature	Methyl-phenidate	Pemoline	Dextro-amphetamine	Racemic amphetamine (Adderall)
Elimination half-life	2–3[a]	2–12	8	7, 8
Time to peak plasma concentration (T_{max})	1–3	1–5	3–4	3–4
Onset of behavioral effect	1	3–4 weeks	1	1
Duration of behavioral effect	3–4	Not available	6–8	6–8
Daily dose range				
mg/kg/day	0.6–0.7	0.5–3.0	0.3–1.25	0.5–1.25
mg/day	10–60	37.5–112.5	5–40	10–40

Time values are given in hours unless otherwise noted. From P. G. Janicak, J. M. Davis, S. H. Preskorn, and F. J. Ayd, Jr., *Principles and Practice of Psychopharmacotherapy* (Baltimore: Williams & Wilkins, 1993), Table 14.1, p. 493.

managing treatment without involving the school in medication administration. In addition, youths who have previously been unsuccessfully treated with methylphenidate because of adverse side effects or poor response may be successfully treated with Adderall.

This conclusion was reiterated by Pelham and co-workers[78] and by Pliszka and co-workers[78a] who concluded that once-daily Adderall is similar to twice-daily methylphenidate.

Although methylphenidate and amphetamines are the drugs of choice in the treatment of ADHD, about 10 to 30 percent of ADHD individuals do not respond adequately and are considered to be treatment resistant. Therefore, there is need for treatment alternatives. Antidepressants (especially *nortriptyline*, a tricyclic antidepressant; Chapter 15) have been studied; however, rare cases of potentially fatal cardiac toxicities associated with tricyclic antidepressant use in adolescents pose a considerable limitation.[79] Initial reports on other antidepressants indicate some usefulness of *fluoxetine* (Prozac), *bupropion*

(Welbutrin), and buspirone (Buspar).[80] Other drugs reported to have positive effects in the treatment of ADHD include *carbamazepine* (Tegretol) and two CNS-acting antihypertensive (blood pressure–lowering) catecholamine agonists (stimulants)—*clonidine* (Catapres) and *guanfacine* (Tenex). Use of these alternative agents in combination with methylphenidate may result in improved therapy at a lower dose of the stimulant. Indeed, the increasingly recognized comorbidity of ADHD with other psychiatric disorders is leading to increasing utilization of combined pharmacotherapy in individuals who respond less than adequately to a single agent.[81]

Reviews

Recent reviews have discussed the current status of the treatment of ADHD.[82-86] It should be noted that several facets of the treatment of ADHD remain controversial, especially (1) the management of treatment-resistant youths, (2) the combination of drugs in ADHD management, and (3) the management of adults with ADHD and comorbid substance abuse.

In December 1999, the long-awaited results of the "Multimodal Treatment Study of Children with Attention-Deficit/Hyperactivity Disorder" (the MTA study) appeared in print.[87,88] A cohort of 579 children with ADHD were assigned to 14 months of medication management, intensive behavioral treatment, the two combined, or standard community care. Carefully structured medication management resulted in better outcome than intensive behavioral treatment, and combined treatment yielded outcome that was better than behavioral treatment but equivalent to medication management. Thus, for ADHD symptoms,

> carefully crafted medication management was superior to behavioral treatment and to routine community care that included medication. Combined treatment did not yield significantly greater benefits than medication management for core ADHD symptoms, but it may have provided modest advantages for non-ADHD symptoms and positive functioning outcomes.

Since this study covered a period of only 14 months, long-term efficacy is still unknown. Certainly medication benefits are considerable, but they persist only as long as treatment is continued. Since ADHD is now considered a chronic disorder, often persisting into adulthood, ongoing treatment often seems necessary. With the long-term waxing and waning of symptoms, perhaps behavioral treatment can help families actively cope with their child's disorder and make the necessary life accommodations to optimize family functioning, even when behavioral treatment is not so effective as medication in reducing children's ADHD symptoms.[87]

STUDY QUESTIONS

1. Compare and contrast cocaine and amphetamine.

2. What is crack? What is ICE?

3. Describe the three major actions of cocaine.

4. Discuss the effects of cocaine on the fetus.

5. Describe the behavioral states that are observed in high-dose amphetamine users.

6. Describe the effects of amphetamine on neurotransmission, neurotransmitters, and the CNS reward system.

7. Why are amphetamine-like drugs useful in treating children, adolescents, and adults with ADHD?

8. Compare and contrast psychostimulants with clinical antidepressants.

9. What is meant by the phrase "Speed kills"?

10. What is modafinil? How does it differ from amphetamine? What are its potential uses?

11. What are some of the issues and therapeutic approaches to treating cocaine and amphetamine dependence?

12. What are some of the issues and therapeutic approaches to treating ADHD?

REFERENCES

1. S. M. Yentis and K. V. Vlassakov, "Vassily von Anrep, Forgotten Pioneer of Regional Anesthesia," *Anesthesiology* 90 (1999): 890–895.
2. M. S. Boghdadi and R. J. Henning, "Cocaine: Pathophysiology and Clinical Toxicology," *Heart and Lung* 26 (1997): 466–483.
3. D. K. Hatsukami and M. W. Fishman, "Crack Cocaine and Cocaine Hydrochloride: Are the Differences Myth or Reality?" *Journal of the American Medical Association* 276 (1996): 1580–1588.
4. M. S. Gold and N. S. Miller, "Cocaine (and Crack): Neurobiology," in J. H. Lowinson, P. Ruiz, R. B. Millman, and J. G. Langrod, eds., *Substance Abuse: A Comprehensive Textbook*, 3rd ed. (Baltimore: Williams & Wilkins, 1997), 166–181.
5. C. R. Rush, R. W. Baker and K. Wright, "Acute Physiological and Behavioral Effects of Oral Cocaine in Humans: A Dose-response Analysis," *Drug and Alcohol Dependence* 55 (1999): 1–12.
6. P. Jatlow et al., "Alcohol plus Cocaine: The Whole Is More Than the Sum of Its Parts," *Therapeutic Drug Monitoring* 18 (1996): 460–464.
7. E. F. McCance et al., "Cocaethylene: Pharmacology, Physiology, and Behavioral Effects in Humans," *Journal of Pharmacology and Experimental Therapeutics* 274 (1995): 215–223.

8. D. N. Bailey, "Comprehensive Review of Cocaethylene and Cocaine Concentrations in Humans," *American Journal of Clinical Pathology* 106 (1996): 701–704.

9. E. A. Kiyarkin, "Dopamine Mechanisms of Cocaine Addiction," *Addiction* 89 (1994): 1435–1441.

10. T. E. Schlaepfer et al., "PET Study of Competition Between Intravenous Cocaine and [^{11}C]Raclopride at Dopamine Receptors in Human Subjects," *American Journal of Psychiatry* 154 (1997): 1209–1213.

11. R. A. Wise, "Drug Activation of Brain Reward Pathways," *Drug and Alcohol Dependence* 51 (1998): 13–22.

12. S. Shimada et al., "Cloning and Expression of a Cocaine-sensitive Dopamine Transporter Complementary DNA," *Science* 254 (1991): 576–578.

13. J. E. Kilty, D. Lorang, and S. G. Amara, "Cloning and Expression of a Cocaine-sensitive Rat Dopamine Transporter," *Science* 254 (1991): 578–580.

14. B. A. Rocha et al., "Cocaine Self-administration in Dopamine-transporter Knockout Mice," *Nature Neuroscience* 1 (1998): 132–137.

15. B. A. Rocha et al., "Increased Vulnerability to Cocaine in Mice Lacking the Serotonin-1B Receptor," *Nature* 393 (1998): 175–178.

16. F. J. White, "Cocaine and the Serotonin Saga," *Nature* 393 (1998): 118–119.

17. K. Y. Little et al., "Cocaine, Ethanol, and Genotype Effects on Human Midbrain Serotonin Transporter Binding Sites and mRNA Levels," *American Journal of Psychiatry* 155 (1998): 207–213.

18. W. L. Woolverton and K. M. Johnson, "Neurobiology of Cocaine Abuse," *Trends in Pharmacological Sciences* 13 (1992): 193–200.

19. A. R. Childress et al., "Limbic Activation During Cue-induced Cocaine Craving," *American Journal of Psychiatry* 156 (1999): 11–18.

20. L. Chang et al., "Gender Effects on Persistent Cerebral Metabolic Changes in the Frontal Lobes of Abstinent Cocaine Users," *American Journal of Psychiatry* 156 (1999): 716–722.

21. W. G. vanGorp et al., "Declarative and Procedural Memory Functioning in Abstinent Cocaine Abusers," *Archives of General Psychiatry* 56 (1999): 85–89.

22. G. Bartzokis et al., "Magnetic Resonance Imaging Evidence of 'Silent' Cerebrovascular Toxicity in Cocaine Dependence," *Biological Psychiatry* 45 (1999): 1203–1211.

23. B. J. Rounsaville et al., "Psychiatric Diagnoses of Treatment-Seeking Cocaine Abusers," *Archives of General Psychiatry* 48 (1991): 43–51.

24. "Update on Cocaine, Part II," *Harvard Mental Health Letter* 10, no. 3 (September 1993): 2.

25. J. J. Volpe, "Effects of Cocaine Use on the Fetus," *New England Journal of Medicine* 327 (1992): 399–407.

26. B. B. Little, T. T. VanBeveren, and L. C. Gilstrap, "Cocaine Abuse During Pregnancy," in L. C. Gilstrap and B. B. Little, eds., *Drugs and Pregnancy*, 2nd ed. (New York: Chapman & Hall), 1998, 419–444.

27. R. J. Konkol and G. D. Olsen, *Prenatal Cocaine Exposure* (Boca Raton, Fla.: CRC Press, 1996).

28. D. J. Birnbach et al., "Cocaine Screening of Parturients Without Prenatal Care: An Evaluation of a Rapid Screening Assay," *Anesthesia and Analgesia* 84 (1997): 76–79.

29. P. W. Lavori et al., "Plans, Designs, and Analyses for Clinical Trials of Anti-cocaine Medications: Where We Are Today," *Journal of Clinical Psychopharmacology* 19 (1999): 246–256.

30. M. K. Romach et al., "Attenuation of the Euphoric Effects of Cocaine by the Dopamine D1/D5 Antagonist Ecopipan (SCH 39166)," *Archives of General Psychiatry* 56 (1999): 1101–1106.

31. F. J. White and P. W. Kalivas, "Neuroadaptations Involved in Amphetamine and Cocaine Addiction," *Drug and Alcohol Dependence* 51 (1998): 141–153.

32. N. D. Volkow et al., "Association of Methylphenidate-induced Craving with Changes in Right Striato-orbitofrontal Metabolism in Cocaine Abusers: Implications for Addiction," *American Journal of Psychiatry* 156 (1999): 19–26.

32A. J. D. Roache et al., "Laboratory Measures of Methylphenidate Effects in Cocaine-Dependent Patients Receiving Treatment," *Journal of Clinical Psychopharmacology* 20 (2000): 61–68.

33. R. A. Brown et al., "Depression Among Cocaine Abusers in Treatment: Relation to Cocaine and Alcohol Use and Treatment Outcome," *American Journal of Psychiatry* 155 (1998): 220–225.

34. A. Margolin et al., "A Multicenter Trial of Bupropion for Cocaine Dependence in Methadone-maintained Patients," *Drug and Alcohol Dependence* 40 (1995): 125–131.

35. J. H. Mendelson and N. K. Mello, "Management of Cocaine Abuse and Dependence," *New England Journal of Medicine* 334 (1996): 965–972.

36. F. R. Levin et al., "Methylphenidate Treatment for Cocaine Abusers with Adult Attention-Deficit/Hyperactivity Disorder: A Pilot Study," *Journal of Clinical Psychiatry* 59 (1998): 300–305.

37. P. Crits-Christoph et al., "The National Institute on Drug Abuse Collaborative Cocaine Treatment Study: Rationale and Methods," *Archives of General Psychiatry* 54 (1997): 721–726.

38. P. Crits-Christoph et al., "Psychosocial Treatments for Cocaine Dependence: National Institute on Drug Abuse Collaborative Treatment Study," *Archives of General Psychiatry* 56 (1999): 493–502.

39. K. Silverman et al., "Sustained Cocaine Abstinence in Methadone Patients Through Voucher-based Reinforcement Therapy," *Archives of General Psychiatry* 53 (1996): 409–415.

40. Work Group on Substance Use Disorders, "Practice Guidelines for the Treatment of Patients with Substance Use Disorders: Alcohol, Cocaine, Opioids," *Practice Guidelines* (Washington, D.C.: American Psychiatric Association, 1996), 209–319.

41. G. R. King and E. H. Ellinwood, Jr., "Amphetamines and Other Stimulants," in J. H. Lowinson, P. Ruiz, R. B. Millman, and J. G. Langrod, eds., *Substance Abuse: A Comprehensive Textbook*, 3rd ed. (Baltimore: Williams & Wilkins, 1997), 207–223.

42. M. V. Solanto, "Neuropsychopharmacological Mechanisms of Stimulant Drug Action in Attention-deficit Hyperactivity Disorder: A Review and Integration," *Behavioral Brain Research* 94 (1998): 127–152.

43. J. G. Bernstein, *Drug Therapy in Psychiatry*, 3rd ed. (St. Louis: Mosby, 1995), 494–498.

44. D. K. Beebe and E. Walley, "Smokable Methamphetamine ("ICE"): An Old Drug in a Different Form," *American Family Physician* 51 (1995): 449–453.

45. C. E. Cook et al., "Pharmacokinetics of Methamphetamine Self-Administration to Human Subjects by Smoking S-(+)-Methamphetamine Hydrochloride," *Drug Metabolism and Disposition: The Biological Fate of Chemicals* 21 (1993): 717–723.

46. N. D. Volkow et al., "Dopamine Transporter Occupancies in the Human Brain Induced by Therapeutic Doses of Oral Methylphenidate," *American Journal of Psychiatry* 155 (1998): 1325–1331.

47. R. R. Gainetdinov et al., "Role of Serotonin in the Paradoxical Calming Effect of Psychostimulants on Hyperactivity," *Science* 283 (1999): 397–401.

48. J. Marx, "How Stimulant Drugs May Calm Hyperactivity," *Science* 283 (1999): 306.

49. C. B. Denney and M. D. Rapport, "Predicting Methylphenidate Response in Children with ADHD: Theoretical, Empirical, and Conceptual Models," *Journal of the American Academy of Child and Adolescent Psychiatry* 34 (1999): 393–401.

50. T. E. Wilens et al., "Controlled Trial of High Doses of Pemoline for Adults with Attention-Deficit/Hyperactivity Disorder," *Journal of Clinical Psychopharmacology* 19 (1999): 257–264.

51. "Sibutramine for Obesity," *Medical Letter* 40 (March 13, 1998): 32.

52. J. O. Cole et al., "Sibutramine: A New Weight Loss Agent Without Evidence of the Abuse Potential Associated with Amphetamines," *Journal of Clinical Psychopharmacology* 18 (1998): 231–236.

53. M. H. Davidson et al., "Weight Control and Risk Factor Reduction in Obese Subjects Treated for Two Years with Orlistat," *Journal of the American Medical Association* 281 (1999): 235–242.

54. D. F. Williamson, "Pharmacotherapy for Obesity," *Journal of the American Medical Association* 281 (1999): 278–280.

55. D. M. Edgar and W. F. Seidel, "Modafinil Induces Wakefulness Without Intensifying Motor Activity or Subsequent Rebound Hypersomnolence in the Rat," *Journal of Pharmacology & Experimental Therapeutics* 283 (1997): 757–769.

56. L. Ferraro et al., "The Vigilance-promoting Drug Modafinil Increases Extracellular Glutamate Levels in the Medial Preoptic Area and the Posterior Hypothalamus of the Conscious Rat: Prevention by Local $GABA_A$ Receptor Blockade," *Neuropsychopharmacology* 20 (1999): 346–356.

57. U.S. Modafinil in Narcolepsy Multicenter Study Group, "Randomized Trial of Modafinil for the Treatment of Pathological Somnolence in Narcolepsy," *Annals of Neurology* 43 (1998): 88–97.

58. M. A. Menza, K. R. Kaufman and A. Castellanos, "Modafinil Augmentation of Antidepressant Treatment in Depression," *Journal of Clinical Psychiatry* 61 (2000): 378–381.

59. J. M. Swanson et al., "Analog Classroom Assessment of Adderall in Children with ADHD," *Journal of the American Academy of Child and Adolescent Psychiatry* 37 (1998): 519–526.

60. D. F. Conner, K. E. Fletcher, and J. M. Swanson, "A Meta-analysis of Clonidine for Symptoms of Attention-deficit/Hyperactivity Disorder,"

Journal of the American Academy of Child and Adolescent Psychiatry 38 (1999): 1551–1559.

61. P. S. Jensen et al., "Are Stimulants Overprescribed? Treatment of ADHD in Four U.S. Communities," *Journal of the American Academy of Child and Adolescent Psychiatry* 38 (1999): 797–804.

62. J. Biederman et al., "Clinical Correlates of ADHD in Females: Findings from a Large Group of Girls Ascertained from Pediatric and Psychiatric Referral Sources," *Journal of the American Academy of Child and Adolescent Psychiatry* 38 (1999): 966–975.

63. T. Spencer et al., "A Double-blind, Crossover Comparison of Methylphenidate and Placebo in Adults with Childhood-onset Attention-deficit Hyperactivity Disorder," *Archives of General Psychiatry* 52 (1995): 434–443.

64. P. S. Jensen, D. Martin, and D. P. Cantwell, "Comorbidity in ADHD: Implications for Research, Practice and *DSM-V*," *Journal of the American Academy of Child and Adolescent Psychiatry* 36 (1997): 1065–1079.

65. D. P. Cantwell, "Attention Deficit Disorder: A Review of the Past 10 years," *Journal of the American Academy of Child and Adolescent Psychiatry* 35 (1996): 978–987.

66. R. G. Klein et al., "Clinical Efficacy of Methylphenidate in Conduct Disorder With and Without Attention-deficit/Hyperactivity Disorder," *Archives of General Psychiatry* 54 (1997): 1073–1080.

67. P. D. Rigs, S. L. Leon, S. K. Mikulich, and L. C. Pottle, "An Open Trial of Bupropion for ADHD in Adolescents with Substance Abuse Disorders and Conduct Disorder," *Journal of the American Academy of Child and Adolescent Psychiatry* 37 (1998): 1271–1278.

68. R. B. Eiraldi, T. J. Power, and C. M. Nezu, "Patterns of Comorbidity Associated with Subtypes of Attention-deficit/Hyperactivity Disorder Among 6- to 12-Year-Old Children," *Journal of the American Academy of Child and Adolescent Psychiatry* 36 (1997): 503–514.

69. I. R. Diamond, R. Tannock, and R. J. Schachar, "Response to Methylphenidate in Children with ADHD and Comorbid Anxiety," *Journal of the American Academy of Child and Adolescent Psychiatry* 38 (1999): 402–409.

70. A. L. Vance and E. S. Luk, "Attention Deficit Hyperactivity Disorder and Anxiety: Is There an Association with Neurodevelopmental Deficits?" *Australian and New Zealand Journal of Psychiatry* 32 (1998): 650–657.

71. C. Z. Garrison et al., "Incidence of Major Depressive Disorder and Dysthymia in Young Adolescents," *Journal of the American Academy of Child and Adolescent Psychiatry* 36 (1997): 458–465.

72. T. E. Wilens et al., "Attention Deficit Hyperactivity Disorder (ADHD) Is Associated with Early Onset Substance Use Disorders," *Journal of Nervous and Mental Disease* 185 (1997): 475–482.

73. S. R. Pliszka, C. L. Carlson, and J. M. Swanson, eds., *ADHD with Comorbid Disorders* (New York: Guilford, 1999).

74. E. R. Disney, I. J. Elkins, M. McGue, and W. G. Iacono, "Effects of ADHD, Conduct Disorder, and Gender on Substance Use and Abuse in Adolescence," *American Journal of Psychiatry* 156 (1999): 1515–1521.

75. S. V. Faraone et al., "Dopamine D_4 Gene 7-Repeat Allele and Attention Deficit Hyperactivity Disorder," *American Journal of Psychiatry* 156 (1999): 768–770.

76. G. Bush et al., "Anterior Cingulate Cortex Dysfunction in Attention-deficit/Hyperactivity Disorder as Revealed by fMRI and the Counting Stroop," *Biological Psychiatry* 45 (1999): 1542–1552.

77. M. J. Manos, E. J. Short, and R. L. Findling, "Differential Effectiveness of Methylphenidate and Adderall in School-age Youths with Attention-deficit/Hyperactivity Disorder," *Journal of the American Academy of Child and Adolescent Psychiatry* 38 (1999): 813–819.

78. W. E. Pelham et al., "A Comparison of Morning Only and Morning/Late Afternoon Adderall to Morning-only, Twice-daily, and Three-times-daily Methylphenidate in Children with Attention-deficit/Hyperactivity Disorder," *Pediatrics* 104 (1999): 1300–1311.

78A. S. R. Pliszka, R. G. Browne, R. L. Olvera and S. K. Wynne, "A Double-Blind, Placebo-Controlled Study of Adderall and Methylphenidate in the Treatment of Attention-Deficit/Hyperactivity Disorder," *Journal of the American Academy of Child and Adolescent Psychiatry* 39 (2000): 619–626.

79. H. Gutgesell et al., "AHA Scientific Statement: Cardiovascular Monitoring of Children and Adolescents Receiving Psychotropic Drugs," *Journal of the American Academy of Child and Adolescent Psychiatry* 38 (1999): 1047–1050.

80. S. Malhotra and P. J. Santosh, "An Open Trial of Buspirone in Children with Attention-deficit/Hyperactivity Disorder," *Journal of the American Academy of Child and Adolescent Psychiatry* 37 (1998): 364–371.

81. T. E. Wilens et al., "Combined Pharmacotherapy: An Emerging Trend in Pediatric Psychopharmacology," *Journal of the American Academy of Child and Adolescent Psychiatry* 34 (1995): 110–112.

82. L. S. Goldman et al., "Diagnosis and Treatment of Attention-deficit/Hyperactivity Disorder in Children and Adolescents," *Journal of the American Medical Association* 279 (1998): 1100–1107.

83. J. Elia, P. J. Ambrosini, and J. L. Rapoport, "Treatment of Attention-deficit/Hyperactivity Disorder," *New England Journal of Medicine* 340 (1999): 780–788

84. K. Pierce, "Which Stimulant to Choose in ADHD?" *Child & Adolescent Psychopharmacology News* 4 (April, 1999): 1–4.

85. M. Dulcan and the American Academy of Child and Adolescent Psychiatry, "Practice Parameters for the Assessment and Treatment of Children, Adolescents, and Adults with Attention-deficit/Hyperactivity Disorder," *Journal of the American Academy of Child and Adolescent Psychiatry* 36, Suppl. 10 (October, 1997): 85S–121S.

86. "National Institutes of Health Consensus Development Conference Statement: Diagnosis and Treatment of Attention-Deficit/Hyperactivity Disorder (ADHD)" *Journal of the American Academy of Child and Adolescent Psychiatry* 39 (2000): 182–193.

87. MTA Cooperative Group, "A 14-Month Randomized Clinical Trial of Treatment Strategies for Attention-deficit/Hyperactivity Disorder," *Archives of General Psychiatry* 56 (1999): 1073–1086.

88. MTA cooperative Group, "Moderators and Mediators of Treatment Response for Children with Attention-deficit/Hyperactivity Disorder," *Archives of General Psychiatry* 56 (1999): 1088–1096.

Caffeine and Nicotine

CAFFEINE

Caffeine is the most commonly consumed psychoactive drug in the world; in the United States it is consumed daily by up to 80 percent of the adult population.[1] It is found in significant concentrations in coffee, tea, cola drinks, chocolate candy, and cocoa. As shown in Table 8.1, the average cup of coffee contains about 50 to 150 milligrams of caffeine.* A 12-ounce bottle of cola contains about half as much. The caffeine content of chocolate may be as high as 25 milligrams per ounce. Intake of caffeine averages between 80 and 400 milligrams per person per day, correlating with three to five cups of coffee every day. Regulatory agencies impose no restrictions on the sale or use of caffeine, nor is the human consumption of caffeine-containing beverages commonly considered to be drug abuse.[2]

Caffeine has positive effects such as enhanced mental alertness, increased energy, and a sense of well-being. Caffeine also must be reinforcing; data suggest that low doses provide a weak cue that resembles the dopaminergic stimulus discussed in Chapter 7. If caffeine is reinforcing, does the reinforcement mechanism involve the mesolim-

---

*The caffeine content of coffee varies widely. One hundred milligrams is often used as an average. However, among locally popular "gourmet" coffees, one company's coffee averages 200 milligrams per 8 fluid ounces. Thus, a 12-ounce cup of black coffee has 300 milligrams; the 16-ounce "grande" has 400 milligrams. Mixed coffee drinks have less caffeine because of added milk or flavorings. Another company's coffee averages 80 to 90 milligrams; a third's has 100 to 125 milligrams of caffeine per 8 ounces.

TABLE 8.1 Caffeine content in beverages, foods, and medicines

Item	Caffeine content	
	Average (mg)	Range
Coffee (5-ounce cup)	100	50–150
Tea (5-ounce cup)	50	25–90
Cocoa (5-ounce cup)	5	2–20
Chocolate (semisweet, baking) (1 ounce)	25	15–30
Chocolate milk (1 ounce)	5	1–10
Cola drink (12 ounces)	40	35–55
OTC stimulants (No Doz, Vivarin)	100+	
OTC analgesics (Excedrin)	65	
(Anacin, Midol, Vanquish)	33	
OTC cold remedies (Coryban-D, Triaminic)	30	
OTC diuretics (Aqua-ban)	100	

Note: OTC = over the counter.

bic system described for cocaine and the amphetamines, or is its behavioral reinforcement exerted through another mechanism? Also, given the almost universal dependence on caffeinated beverages, what is caffeine's potential for producing toxicities or physical dependency.

Pharmacokinetics

Taken orally, caffeine is rapidly and completely absorbed. Significant blood levels of caffeine are reached in 30 to 45 minutes; complete absorption occurs over the next 90 minutes. Levels in plasma peak at about 2 hours and decrease thereafter.

Caffeine is freely and equally distributed throughout the total body water. Thus, caffeine is found in almost equal concentrations in all parts of the body and the brain. Like all psychoactive drugs, caffeine freely crosses the placenta to the fetus.

Most caffeine is metabolized by the liver before it is excreted by the kidneys. Only about 10 percent of the drug is excreted unchanged. The half-life of caffeine is about 3.5 to 5 hours in most adults, which accounts for nighttime wakefulness in some people. Caffeine's half-life is extended in infants, in pregnant women, and in the elderly. During the latter part of pregnancy, the half-life of caffeine increases from 3 to 10 hours. Postpartum concentrations of caffeine excreted in breast milk equal or even exceed the level that exists in the mother's plasma.

In smokers, caffeine's half-life is shortened; however, when smoking is terminated, caffeine's half-life increases. This reduced metabolism of caffeine when smoking ceases can result in an increase in plasma caffeine levels and may contribute to cigarette withdrawal symptoms in heavy coffee drinkers, particularly since caffeine induces anxiety at high doses.[3]

The metabolism of caffeine is shown in Figure 8.1. The two major metabolites of caffeine, theophylline and paraxanthine, behave similarly to caffeine; a third metabolite, theobromine, does not.[2] Caffeine is metabolized by the CYP1A2 subgroup of hepatic drug-metabolizing enzymes. Interestingly, certain SSRI-type antidepressants such as fluvoxamine (Chapter 17) are potent inhibitors of CYP1A2, and people taking these antidepressants can exhibit unexpected toxicity or intolerance to caffeine as plasma levels of caffeine rise.[4] Antidepressants that do not inhibit CYP1A2 (e.g., venlafaxine)[5] do not alter caffeine's metabolism.

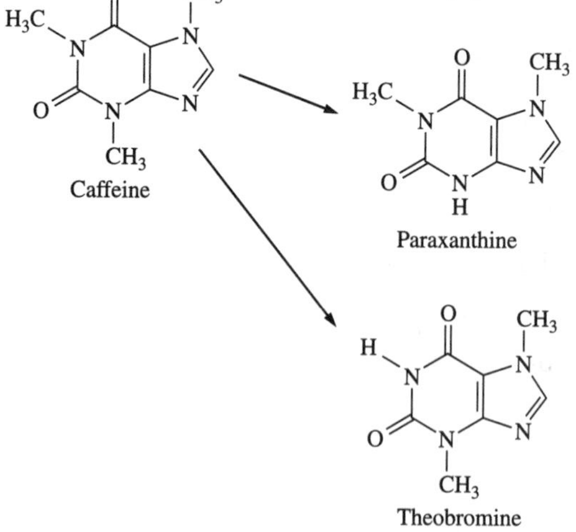

FIGURE 8.1 Metabolism of caffeine to three end products.

Pharmacological Effects

The CNS-stimulant, cardiac, respiratory, and diuretic effects of caffeine have been known for many years. Therapeutically, these effects have been used to treat a variety of disorders including asthma (theophylline is occasionally used for this purpose), narcolepsy (to maintain daytime wakefulness), migraine, and as an adjunct to treat headache and other pain syndromes (used in combination with aspirin or other analgesics).

Caffeine is an effective psychostimulant, ingested to obtain a rewarding effect, usually described as feeling more alert and competent. Behavioral effects seen at the lower doses of caffeine include increased mental alertness, a faster and clearer flow of thought, and wakefulness. Fatigue is reduced and the need for sleep is delayed. This increased mental awareness results in sustained intellectual effort for prolonged periods of time without significant disruption of coordinated intellectual or motor activity. Tasks that involve delicate muscular coordination and accurate timing or arithmetic skills may be adversely affected. These effects occur after oral doses that are as small as 100 or 200 milligrams, that is, one to two cups of coffee. Most individuals adjust, or titrate their intake of caffeine to achieve these beneficial effects while minimizing undesirable effects.

Heavy consumption of coffee (12 or more cups per day, or 1.5 grams of caffeine) can cause agitation, anxiety, tremors, rapid breathing, and insomnia. The lethal dose of caffeine is about 10 grams, which is equivalent to 100 cups of coffee. Thus, death from caffeine is highly unusual, and the drug is usually considered to be relatively nonlethal.

Individuals with anxiety disorders tend to be quite sensitive to the anxiogenic properties of caffeine, especially if they usually avoid caffeinated products and do not develop a tolerance to this effect. In general, individuals with anxiety disorders are wise to totally avoid caffeinated products. Dager and colleagues[6] noted that caffeine-intolerant individuals who developed psychological and physiological distress after caffeine had elevations in brain lactate just as did heavy coffee users who discontinued coffee for two months (and lost tolerance to caffeine) and then resumed the drug. Continuous drinkers did not demonstrate lactate elevations, demonstrating a type of CNS metabolic tolerance that disappears with drug cessation and which does not correlate with anxiogenesis.

Caffeinism is a clinical syndrome, characterized by both CNS and peripheral symptoms, produced by the overuse or overdoses of caffeine. CNS symptoms include increases in anxiety, agitation, insomnia, and mood changes. Peripheral symptoms include tachycardia, hypertension, cardiac arrhythmias, and gastrointestinal disturbances. Caffeinism is usually dose related, with doses higher than about 500 to

1,000 milligrams (1 gram, or 5 to 10 cups of coffee) causing the most unpleasant effects. Cessation of caffeine ingestion resolves these symptoms. Much lower doses of caffeine will produce this syndrome in sensitive individuals, such as those with an underlying anxiety disorder. The usually ingested doses of caffeine do not induce panic attacks in normal individuals. However, in people predisposed to panic disorders, the peripheral and the CNS effects of caffeine are exaggerated.[7]

Outside the CNS, caffeine exerts significant effects, some beneficial and some adverse. Caffeine has a slight stimulant action on the heart. It increases both cardiac contractility (increases the workload of the heart) and cardiac output. While this might predispose a person to hypertension (caffeine does raise blood pressure in adults prone to hypertension[8]), caffeine also dilates the coronary arteries, providing more oxygen to a harder-working heart. Thus, it remains controversial whether or not caffeine increases the incidence of heart disease and deaths due to cardiac disease. Certainly, individuals with hypertension or heart disease might do well to minimize exposure to caffeinated products.

It should be noted that caffeine exerts an opposite effect on cerebral blood vessels; it constricts these vessels, thus decreasing blood flow to the brain by about 30 percent and reducing pressure within the brain. This action can effect striking relief from headaches, especially migraines.[9] Other physical actions of caffeine include bronchial relaxation (an antiasthmatic effect), increased secretion of gastric acid, and increased urine output.

Leitzmann and co-workers[10] demonstrated that males who drink between two and three cups of coffee per day have a greatly reduced incidence of gallstone disease. The mechanism responsible for this advantageous effect is unknown, but the authors speculate on several possible causes.

Mechanism of Action

Caffeine exerts a variety of effects on the CNS at a variety of dose levels. However, at doses routinely consumed by humans, blockade (or *antagonism*) of adenosine receptors represents the major site of action of the drug (Figure 8.2).[2] Four different adenosine receptors (A_1, A_{2A}, A_{2B}, and A_3) exist in humans, and caffeine is most potent at blocking A_1 and A_{2A}, especially the latter. Indeed, in mice in which A_{2A}-adenosine receptors are absent, caffeine has only depressant (not stimulant) effects on behavioral activity.[11]

Since caffeine is an antagonist at these two receptors, one would not expect a pharmacological effect of caffeine unless these receptors were tonically active under stimulation by adenosine.[2] *Adenosine* (Figure 8.3) is a neuromodulator that influences the release of several neurotransmitters in the CNS. There do not appear to be discrete adenosinergic pathways in the CNS; rather, adenosinergic neurons form a diffuse and important

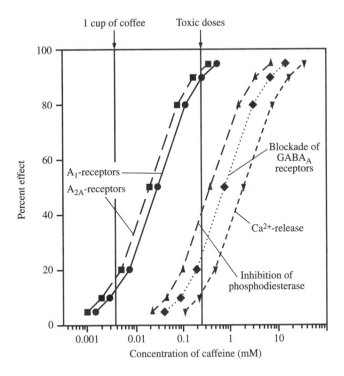

FIGURE 8.2 Adenosine receptors as site of action of caffeine. Concentration-dependent effects of caffeine on adenosine receptors (A_1 and A_{2A}), $GABA_A$ receptors, calcium ion release (Ca^{2+}), and the enzyme phosphodiesterase. At concentrations approximating one cup of coffee, only the adenosine receptors are affected. [From Daly and Fredholm.[2]]

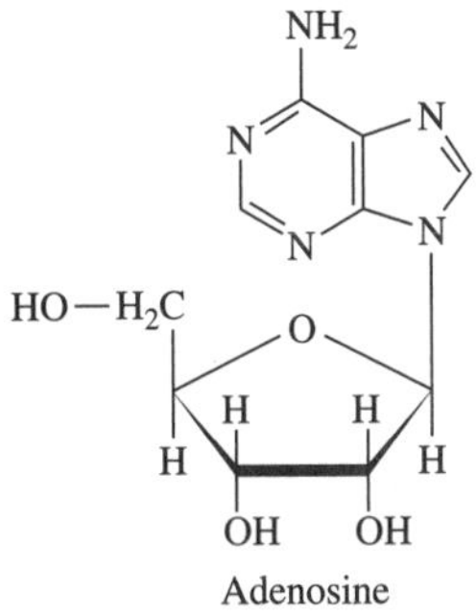

FIGURE 8.3 Structure of adenosine. Note the similarity of adenosine to caffeine (shown in Figure 8.1).

system sometimes labeled a depressant.[7] Adenosine appears to exert sedative, depressant, and anticonvulsant actions; and blockade of adenosine receptors produces actions considered to be stimulating or anxiogenic.

Adenosine receptors decrease the discharge rate of many central neurons, increasing the activity of dopaminergic, cholinergic, glutaminergic, and noradrenergic neurons.[2] Adenosine A_1 receptors inhibit the release of dopamine and glutamate. Blockade of these receptors accounts for the modest reward and the increased vigilance and mental acuity actions of caffeine. A_1 receptor activity also limits the release of acetylcholine; inhibition by caffeine accounts for the behavioral arousal effects of caffeine. A_{2A} receptor activation, through a complex mechanism, tonically inhibits dopaminergic activity; blockade by caffeine increases the potency of endogenous dopamine at D_2 receptors.

> The positive stimulatory effects of caffeine appear in large measure to be due to blockade of A_{2A} receptors that stimulate GABAergic neurons of inhibitory pathways to the dopaminergic reward system of the striatum. However, blockade of striatal A_1 receptors may also play a role.[2]

Furthermore,

> caffeine, as a competitive antagonist at adenosine receptors, may produce its behavioral effects by removing the negative modulatory effects of adenosine from dopamine receptors, thus stimulating dopaminergic activity.[12]

Unlike the actions of cocaine and amphetamine, caffeine does not induce a release of dopamine in the nucleus accumbens; it leads to a release of dopamine in the prefrontal cortex, which is consistent with caffeine reinforcing properties.[13] As Nehlig[13] concludes:

> It appears that although caffeine fulfills some of the criteria for drug dependence and shares with amphetamines and cocaine a certain specificity of action on the cerebral dopaminergic system, it does not act on the dopaminergic structures related to reward, motivation, and addiction.

Reproductive Effects

> Is caffeine safe during pregnancy? Caffeine, the most widely used psychotropic drug, is consumed by at least 75 percent of pregnant women via caffeinated beverages. Despite its widespread use, the safety of this habit during pregnancy is unresolved.[14]

As early as 1980, the U.S. Food and Drug Administration cautioned pregnant women to minimize their intake of caffeine. On the other hand, D'Ambrosio[15] concluded: "It is difficult to implicate caffeine, even at the highest levels of daily consumption, as a genotoxin to humans."

Data in this area are conflicting and controversial. In 1993, the *Journal of the American Medical Association* published two studies on this issue that arrived at contradictory conclusions. The first article reported that caffeine was relatively safe in moderate doses (less than 300 milligrams per day, or less than three medium-size cups of coffee per day).[16] At higher levels, an increased incidence of intrauterine growth retardation was seen. The second study[17] reported that low doses of caffeine (about 160 milligrams per day) in the first trimester of pregnancy increased the risk of intrauterine growth retardation; high consumption (greater than 300 milligrams per day), even in the month before pregnancy, "nearly doubled the risk of spontaneous abortion."[17]

A recent study[18] concluded that the consumption of large amounts of caffeine (perhaps more than 6 to 10 cups of coffee per day), is associated with an increased risk of spontaneous abortion but that moderate consumption does not further increase the risk. It does not appear that caffeine itself is a human teratogen, and caffeine does not appear to affect the course of normal labor and delivery.[19]

Tolerance and Dependence

Chronic use of caffeine is often associated with habituation and tolerance, and discontinuation may produce a withdrawal syndrome.[20] People who drink the most coffee complain of headache, drowsiness, fatigue, and a generally negative mood state upon withdrawal from caffeine. Withdrawal symptoms typically begin slowly, maximize after one or two days and cease within a few days; withdrawal symptoms are rapidly relieved by readministering caffeine. These symptoms certainly indicate the development of a state of mild dependency. Other reported withdrawal signs include impaired intellectual and motor performance, difficulty with concentration, drug (caffeine) craving, and other psychological complaints.[21]

Kendler and Prescott[1] examined the genetics of caffeine in a twin study and found that "genetic differences between individuals contribute substantially in liability to heavy caffeine intake and to caffeine-related sequelae including intoxication, tolerance, and dependence."

In conclusion, Greden and Walters[7] state:

> Caffeine . . . will continue to be the norm in most people. However, caffeinism and caffeine withdrawal also continue to be common and clinically important but unrecognized, underdiagnosed even when recognized, and untreated in many treatment settings. . . . Clinicians

who actively consider the diagnosis of caffeinism in their patients will be surprised at how many afflicted subjects are identified, impressed at how many are helped by removal of the offending agent, and pleased to know that almost all are grateful.

NICOTINE

Together with caffeine and ethyl alcohol, nicotine is one of the three most widely used psychoactive drugs in our society. Despite the fact that nicotine has few or no therapeutic applications in medicine, its potency, its widespread use, and its toxicity give it immense importance. Indeed, nicotine and the other ingredients in tobacco are responsible for a wide variety of health problems, including the deaths of more than 1100 Americans every day.

From the end of World War II to the mid-1960s, cigarette smoking was considered chic. Today, after more than 30 years of U.S. government reports on the adverse health consequences of cigarettes, cigarette smoking is being increasingly shunned as unhealthy and unwise. Nevertheless, each day 6000 American teenagers try their first cigarette and 3000 children become regular smokers,[22] and almost 1000 of them will eventually die from diseases related to smoking. Also, 9 in 10 smokers become addicted before age 21. Today, in the United States, 3 million adolescents are smokers. Advertisements for cigarettes still appeal to children, and in even more subtle ways, the depiction of smoking as okay continues.[23]

On the positive side, half of all persons who have ever smoked cigarettes have quit, and the proportion of American adults who smoke has fallen from 50 percent in 1965 to 25 percent in 1998. About 1 million potential deaths have been averted or postponed by persons who have quit smoking. Millions more deaths will be avoided or postponed in the twenty-first century. Even 30 years ago, the Surgeon General of the United States identified smoking as the major *preventable* cause of death and disability, and this will probably continue to be the case.[24]

In this discussion, it is important to note the following:

- Nicotine is the primary active ingredient in tobacco.
- Nicotine is only 1 of about 4000 compounds released by the burning of cigarette tobacco.
- Nicotine accounts only for the acute pharmacological effects of smoking and for the dependence on cigarettes. The adverse, long-term cardiovascular, pulmonary, and carcinogenic effects of cigarettes are related to other compounds contained in the product.

- While nicotine itself may have some adverse effects, its delivery device (the tobacco cigarette) is responsible for much of its toxicity.

Pharmacokinetics

Nicotine is readily absorbed from every site on or in the body, including the lungs, buccal and nasal mucosa, skin, and gastrointestinal tract. Easy and complete absorption forms the basis for the recreational abuse of smoked or chewed tobacco, as well as the medical use of nicotine (in treating nicotine dependency) in gums, nasal sprays, transdermal skin patches, and smokeless inhalers.

Nicotine is suspended in cigarette smoke in the form of minute particles (tars), and it is quickly absorbed into the bloodstream from the lungs when the smoke is inhaled, although recent research[24] indicates that absorption is much slower than once thought and arterial concentrations of nicotine rise rather slowly. It is likely that, as with pulmonary absorption of anesthetic gases and vapors, blood rapidly saturates with nicotine, and blood leaving the lungs (to the left side of the heart) can carry only a modest amount of drug. Thus, the arterial concentration rises slowly, even though blood carried to the brain at the initiation of smoking is near-saturated with nicotine, accounting for the early "rush" perceived with the first cigarette.

Most cigarettes contain between 0.5 and 2.0 milligrams of nicotine, depending on the brand. Only about 20 percent (between 0.1 and 0.4 milligrams) of the nicotine in a cigarette is actually inhaled and absorbed into the smoker's bloodstream; the remainder is rapidly metabolized by the hepatic enzyme CYP2A6.* Individuals in whom the CYP2A6 enzyme is absent have higher blood levels of nicotine and lower levels of its metabolite.[25]

A smoker can readily avoid acute toxicity, because inhalation as a route of administration offers exceptional controllability of the dose. The user-controlled frequency of breaths, the depth of inhalation, the time the smoke is held in the lungs, and the total number of cigarettes smoked all allow the smoker to regulate the rate of drug intake and thus control the blood level of nicotine. The pharmacokinetic goals of nicotine administration were summarized by Sellers:[26]

> Tobacco smoking is a complex but highly regulated behavior that has as its goal the maintenance of steady-state brain levels of the highly addictive psychoactive agent nicotine. Smokers "self-regulate" the level of nicotine in their system to produce desired effects (e.g., relaxation,

---

*Inhibition of CYP2D6, such as by certain SSRI-type antidepressants, can markedly increase nicotine absorption (by limiting its metabolism).

increased concentration) and to avoid unpleasant adverse effects associated with too-high (e.g., dizziness) or too-low (e.g., desire to smoke or
withdrawal).

When nicotine is administered orally in the form of snuff, chewing tobacco, or gum, blood levels of nicotine are comparable to those
achieved by smoking (Figure 8.4).

Nicotine is quickly and thoroughly distributed throughout the
body, rapidly penetrating the brain, crossing the placental barrier, and
appearing in all bodily fluids, including breast milk. There are no barriers in the body to the distribution of nicotine.

The liver metabolizes approximately 80 to 90 percent of the nicotine administered to a person either orally or by smoking before it is
excreted by the kidneys. The primary metabolite of nicotine is *cotinine*
(Figure 8.5), and this substance serves as a marker of both tobacco use
and exposure to environmental smoke. Recent studies[27,28] have noted

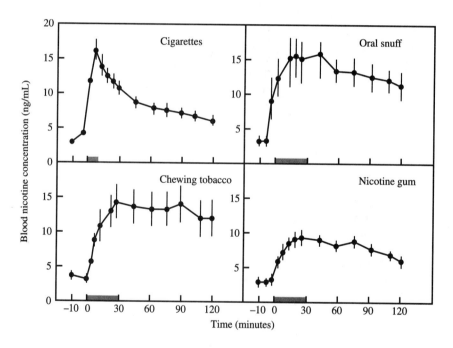

FIGURE 8.4 Blood nicotine concentrations during and after the use of cigarettes,
oral snuff, chewing tobacco, and nicotine gum (two 2-milligram pieces). Data
represent average values for 10 subjects: vertical bars indicate standard errors;
shaded bars above the time axis indicate the period of tobacco or nicotine gum
exposure. [From N. L. Benowitz et al., "Nicotine Absorption and Cardiovascular
Effects with Smokeless Tobacco Use: Comparison with Cigarettes and Nicotine Gum,"
Clinical Pharmacology and Therapeutics 44 (1988), p. 24.]

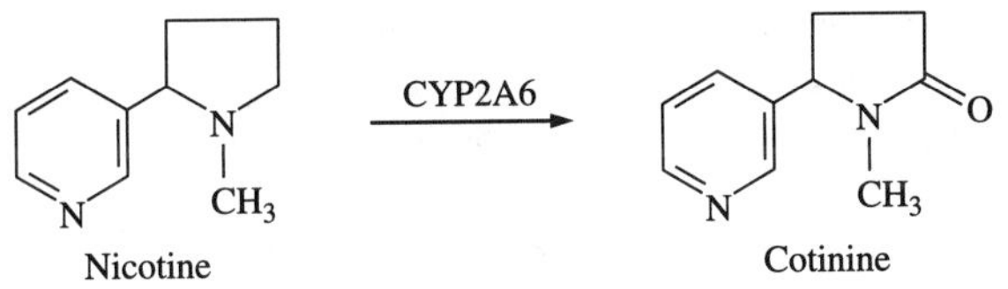

FIGURE 8.5 Structures of nicotine and its metabolite cotinine.

higher cotinine levels in black smokers than in white smokers, "indicating either slower elimination of cotinine or higher intake of nicotine per cigarette in blacks."[27] It may also "explain why blacks find it harder to quit and are more likely to experience higher rates of lung cancer than white smokers."[28] The elimination half-life of nicotine in a chronic smoker is about two hours, necessitating frequent administration of the drug to avoid withdrawal symptoms or drug craving. On awakening in the morning, nicotine levels are so low that a smoker may need to smoke one or two cigarettes rapidly to achieve the desired "therapeutic" level of 20 to 40 nanograms per milliliter of plasma, thus satisfying craving and avoiding withdrawal.

Pharmacological Effects

Nicotine is the only pharmacologically active drug in tobacco smoke apart from carcinogenic tars. It exerts powerful effects on the brain, the spinal cord, the peripheral nervous system, the heart, and various other body structures.

In the early stages of smoking, nicotine causes nausea and vomiting by stimulating both the vomiting center in the brain stem and the sensory receptors in the stomach. Tolerance to this effect develops rapidly. Nicotine stimulates the hypothalamus to release a hormone, antidiuretic hormone (ADH), that causes fluid retention. Nicotine reduces the activity of afferent nerve fibers coming from the muscles, leading to a reduction in muscle tone. This action may be involved (at least partially) in the relaxation that a person may experience as a result of smoking. Nicotine also reduces weight gain, probably by reducing appetite.

Nicotine produces multiple actions in the CNS, resulting in increases in psychomotor activity, cognitive functioning, sensorimotor performance, attention, and memory consolidation. At higher doses, nicotine can induce nervousness and tremors and, in toxic overdosage, seizures. Cigarette smoking is also associated with an increased occurrence of panic attacks and panic disorder.[29]

Nicotine can improve performance in a variety of cognitive tasks, the most consistent being on vigilance and rapid information processing.[30] The beneficial effects of nicotine seems to be greatest for tasks requiring working memory, rather than long-term memory. Smokers often state that they will smoke a cigarette before doing a complex task that requires attention and arousal,[30] perhaps combining the drug's anxiolytic action with its stimulant action. Stein and colleagues[31] delineate the brain regions activated by nicotine; these include areas involved in cognition, working memory, attention, motivation, mood and emotion (frontal lobes and cingulate cortex) and the locus ceruleus (behavioral arousal and vigilance).

Several reports note an antidepressant effect of nicotine as well as the comorbidity of both childhood ADHD and depression with cigarette use[32,33] and of adult depressive disorders with nicotine dependence. Salin-Pascual and co-workers,[34] noting a high frequency of cigarette-smoking among individuals with major depression, found that, in non-smokers, transdermal nicotine patches produced improvement in depression (Figure 8.6). They postulated that the high rate of smoking among depressed individuals may, in part, represent an attempt at self-medication to assist in dealing with some of their depressive symptoms. In agreement with this concept, Fergusson and colleagues,[35] in a study of 16-year-olds, reported:

> There was evidence of clear comorbidity between depressive disorders and nicotine dependence in this cohort of 16-year-olds; subjects

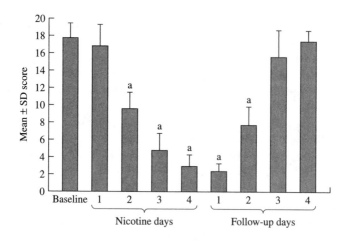

FIGURE 8.6 Hamilton rating scale for depression ratings of 10 depressed patients before, during, and after administration of nicotine patches. A significant reduction was observed on the second day of nicotine patches and continued until the second follow-up day. [From Salin-Pascual et al.[34]]

with depression had odds of nicotine dependence that were more than 4.5 times the odds for those without depression. This relationship was similar for male and female subjects. These results suggest that comorbidities between nicotine dependence and depression are well established by the age of 16 years.

Riggs and co-workers[36] note that "most of the risk for adolescent smoking, as well as the subsequent development of nontobacco substance involvement, is mediated through the presence of conduct disorder." Additional comorbidity, such as ADHD and depression, adds to the already high risk of smoking imparted by conduct disorder. This important study highlights the contribution of comorbidity to smoking initiation, especially conduct disorder, "highlighting the need for coordinated assessment and treatment of smoking cessation along with concurrent treatment of other drug use and psychiatric comorbidity such as ADHD and major depression in such youths."

Anda and co-workers,[37] in a retrospective survey of over 9000 adults, found a strong relationship between smoking behaviors and adverse childhood experiences, including emotional, physical, and sexual abuse, a battered mother, parental separation or divorce, and growing up with a substance-abusing, mentally ill, or incarcerated household member. At least one of these experiences was listed by 63 percent of respondents. As the number of adverse experiences increased, the likelihood of being an early and a current smoker increased, as did the likelihood of being currently depressed. The authors speculated that for these people cigarette smoking may provide a mood-elevating effect and that "unconscious selection of cigarette use could occur in situations of chronic distress," such as depression. How conduct disorder and adult ADHD fit into this pattern was not addressed.

Nicotine exerts a potent behavioral reinforcing action, especially in the early phases of drug use. The reinforcing action of nicotine involves indirect activation of midbrain dopamine neurons. In the veteran smoker, this reinforcing action diminishes, and the user smokes primarily to relieve or avoid withdrawal symptoms. As stated earlier, smokers adjust their nicotine intake to maintain nicotine levels between about 20 to 40 nanograms of nicotine per milliliter of plasma. Because of nicotine's two-hour half-life, there is a very low residual level of nicotine in the blood and brain after a night's sleep. The smoker wakes each morning in a state of drug withdrawal. That first cigarette of the morning has a powerful reinforcing effect because it brings relief of withdrawal discomfort. Thereafter, each cigarette produces a sharp increase in the nicotine concentration within the brain to the desired plasma concentration.

In addition to its effects on the CNS, normal doses of nicotine can increase heart rate, blood pressure, and cardiac contractility. In nonatherosclerotic coronary arteries, nicotine initiates vasodilation, increasing blood flow to meet the increased oxygen demand of the heart muscle. In atherosclerotic coronary arteries (which cannot dilate), however, cardiac ischemia can result when the oxygen supply fails to meet the oxygen demand created by the drug's cardiac stimulation. This occurrence can precipitate angina or myocardial infarction (a heart attack).

Mechanism of Action

Nicotine exerts virtually all of its CNS and peripheral effects by activating certain specific acetylcholine receptors (nicotinic receptors). In the peripheral nervous system, activation of these receptors causes an increase in blood pressure and heart rate, causes release of epinephrine (adrenaline) from the adrenal glands, and increases the tone, secretions, and activity of the gastrointestinal tract.

In the CNS, the nicotine-sensitive acetylcholine receptors are widely distributed and may be located on the presynaptic nerve terminals of dopamine-, acetylcholine-, and glutamine-secreting neurons. Activation of nicotinic receptors by nicotine facilitates the release of these transmitters and increases their actions in the brain.

Nicotine increases dopamine levels in the mesocortico-limbic system involving the ventral tegmentum, nucleus accumbens, and forebrain. This accounts for the behavioral reinforcement, stimulant, antidepressant, and addictive properties of the drug.[30,31,38]

The increased acetylcholine resulting from nicotine administration contributes to the cognitive potentiation and memory facilitation properties of the drug. It may also be responsible for the arousal effects commonly seen with smoking. It is at least theoretically possible that nicotine (if administered other than by cigarette smoking) might have some use to delay the onset of some of the cognitive deficits seen in Alzheimer's disease. Finally, the facilitation of glutaminergic neurotransmission would likely contribute to the improvement in memory functioning seen with nicotine.

Tolerance and Dependence

Nicotine does not appear to induce any pronounced degree of biological tolerance. On the other hand, nicotine clearly induces both physiological and psychological dependence in a majority of smokers. Only a minority appear capable of abrupt cessation of smoking without abstinence symptoms, and even these individuals are prone to craving and relapse. As early as 1988, the Surgeon General of the United States made the following conclusions:

- Cigarettes and other forms of tobacco are addicting.
- Nicotine is the drug in tobacco that causes addiction.
- The pharmacologic and behavioral processes that determine tobacco addiction are similar to those that determine addiction to drugs such as heroin and cocaine.
- More than 300,000 cigarette-addicted Americans die yearly as a consequence of their addiction. (Today this number approaches 450,000 per year.)

Despite all the verbal exchanges between public, regulatory, medical, political, and industry sources, today the scientific case that nicotine is addictive is overwhelming:

> Patterns of use by smokers and the remarkable intractability of the smoking habit point to compulsive use as the norm. Studies in both animal and human subjects have shown that nicotine can function as a reinforcer, albeit under a more limited range of conditions than with some other drugs of abuse. In drug discrimination paradigms, there is some cross-generalization between nicotine on the one hand, and amphetamine and cocaine on the other. A well-defined withdrawal syndrome has been delineated which is alleviated by nicotine replacement. Nicotine replacement also enhances outcomes in smoking cessation, roughly doubling success rates. In total, the evidence clearly identifies nicotine as a powerful drug of addiction, comparable to heroin, cocaine, and alcohol.[39]

Withdrawal from cigarettes is characterized by an abstinence syndrome that is usually not life-threatening. Abstinence symptoms include a severe craving for nicotine, irritability, anxiety, anger, difficulty in concentrating, restlessness, impatience, increased appetite, weight gain, and insomnia. The period of withdrawal may be intense and persistent, often lasting for many months. The difficulty in handling cigarette dependence is illustrated by the fact that cigarette smokers who seek treatment for other drug and alcohol problems often find it harder to quit cigarette smoking than to give up the other drugs. Even Sigmund Freud continued his cigar habit (20 per day) until death, in spite of an endless series of operations for mouth and jaw cancer (the jaw was eventually totally removed), persistent heart problems that were exacerbated by smoking, and numerous attempts at quitting.[40]

It is of note that abstinent smokers displaying signs of withdrawal often tend to increase their caffeine (coffee) consumption; blood caffeine levels increase and remain elevated for as long as six months. "A review of 86 studies of nicotine withdrawal, caffeine withdrawal, and caffeine toxicity suggests that the symptoms are similar enough to be confused, and that reported nicotine withdrawal symptoms may be a mixture of nicotine withdrawal and caffeine toxicity."[41]

Toxicity

As discussed, both the acute pharmacologic effects and the withdrawal signs seen on cessation of smoking result from the nicotine in tobacco. The *tar* in tobacco is mainly responsible for the diseases associated with long-term tobacco use. Of the 450,000 persons in the United States who die annually from tobacco use, 82,000 deaths are caused by noncancerous lung diseases, 115,000 are caused by lung cancer, 30,000 are caused by cancers of other body organs, and more than 200,000 result from heart and vascular diseases. A person's life is shortened 14 minutes for every cigarette smoked. In other words, a person who smokes two packs of cigarettes a day for 20 years loses an estimated 8 years of his or her life. More than 50 million people (one out of every five Americans) alive today will die prematurely from the effects of smoking cigarettes. Cigarette smoking, the nation's greatest public health hazard, is, ironically, the nation's most preventable cause of premature death, illness, and disability.

Cardiovascular Disease

The carbon monoxide in smoke decreases the amount of oxygen delivered to the heart muscle, while nicotine increases the amount of work the heart must do (by increasing the heart rate and blood pressure). Both carbon monoxide and nicotine increase the incidence of atherosclerosis* (narrowing) and thrombosis (clotting) in the coronary arteries. These three actions (and others as well) seem to underlie the dramatic increase in the risk of death from coronary heart disease in smokers as compared to nonsmokers. Howard and colleagues[44] document this cigarette-induced increase in atherosclerosis, noting that current cigarette smoking was associated with a 50 percent increase in the progression of atherosclerosis when compared with people who had never smoked. As shown in Figure 8.7, past smoking was associated with a 25 percent

---

*Atherosclerosis first appears as fatty deposits inside large arteries and progresses to occlusion of the arteries throughout the body; the result is clinically manifested as strokes or peripheral vascular ischemic disease. Atherosclerosis is not a disease of the elderly; it begins in youth and is readily apparent during the 15- to 34-year age span.[42] In a large study of arteries collected from young men who had died of violent causes, a history of cigarette smoking was associated with a threefold to fourfold increase in atherosclerosis of the coronary arteries and abdominal aorta.[43] This report emphasizes that in males, cigarette-induced atherosclerosis begins at a young age, and it reinforces the fact that smoking must be controlled for the long-range prevention of adult vascular disease.

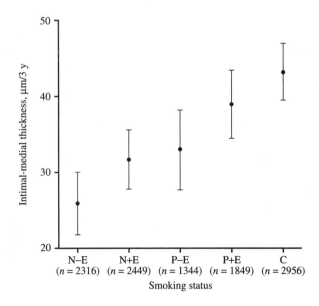

FIGURE 8.7 Mean and 95 percent confidence intervals of three-year progression in the wall thickness of the carotid artery, shown by smoking status category, after adjustment for demographic characteristics, cardiovascular risk factors, and lifestyle variables. N = nonsmoker. P = past smoker. C = current smoker. +E = with exposure to environmental tobacco smoke. –E = without exposure to environmental tobacco smoke. [From Howard et al.[44]]

increase (or a 50 percent improvement over current smokers), and exposure to environmental tobacco smoke was associated with a 20 percent increase. If a smoker has preexisting hypertension or diabetes, the risk is magnified.[44]

Finally, besides occurring in the coronary arteries, atherosclerosis occurs in other arteries as well, most notably the aorta (in the abdomen), the carotid arteries (in the neck), and the femoral and other arteries of the legs. Cigarette-induced occlusion of these vessels blocks the blood flow to important body organs and results in ischemic damage, strokes, and other disorders, causing great discomfort and disability and necessitating continuing and often futile surgical interventions.

Pulmonary Disease

In the lungs, chronic smoking results in a smoker's syndrome, characterized by difficulty in breathing, wheezing, chest pain, lung congestion, and increased susceptibility to infections of the respiratory tract.[45] Cigarette smoking impairs ventilation and greatly increases the risk of emphysema (a form of irreversible lung damage). Smoke exposure also reduces the efficacy of the immune defense mechanisms in the lungs. About 9 million Americans suffer from cigarette-induced chronic bronchitis and emphysema. Indeed, 70 percent of pulmonary diseases and deaths are tobacco related; 57,000 deaths per year result from emphysema.

Cancer

Although nicotine itself is not carcinogenic, the relationship between smoking and cancer is now beyond question. Cigarette smoking is the major cause of lung cancer in both men and women, causing approximately 112,000 deaths in the United States every year. Denissenko and co-workers[46] implicated cigarette smoke as a causative agent in cigarette-induced lung cancers:

> Benzo[a]pyrene, which occurs in amounts of 20–40 nanograms per cigarette, is . . . one of the most potent mutagens and carcinogens known. The compound requires metabolic activation to become the ultimate carcinogenic metabolite, BPDE (benzo[a]pyrene diol epoxide).

BPDE damages a cancer suppressor gene, resulting in the cancer-causing transformation of human lung tissue. This fact "provides a direct link between a defined cigarette smoke carcinogen and human cancer mutations."[46]

Smoking is also a major cause of cancers of the mouth, voice box, and throat. Concomitant alcohol ingestion greatly increases the incidence of these problems. In addition, cigarette smoking is a primary cause of more than 50 percent of the nearly 10,000 deaths every year that result from bladder cancer; it is a primary cause of pancreatic cancer, and it increases the risk of cancer of the uterine cervix twofold. Of all cancer deaths in the United States, 30 percent (154,000 annually) would be prevented if no one smoked.[47]

Ayanian and Cleary[48] and Iribarren and colleagues[49] recently reviewed two important smoking topics. The first paper documents misperceptions about the risks of smoking, noting that most smokers do not view themselves at increased risk of heart disease and cancer. The second report delineated the adverse health risks of cigar smoking in men.

Effects of Passive Smoke

In addition to the direct effects of cigarettes on smokers, the environmental pollution caused by smokers can have adverse consequences for nonsmokers.[47] About 4000 Americans die annually from lung cancer caused by other persons' smoking (so-called passive smoke), and an additional 37,000 deaths every year follow from heart disease contracted as a result of inhaling passive smoke. Nonsmokers exposed to passive smoking have a coronary death rate 20 to 70 percent higher than nonsmokers not exposed to passive smoking.

Effects During Pregnancy

Cigarette smoking adversely affects the developing fetus, leading to increases in the rates of spontaneous abortion, stillbirth, early postpartum death, and preterm deliveries.[50] The risk of intrauterine growth retardation is increased 40 percent, and low birth weights are common, although smoker's offspring with low birth weight usually rises to normal at about 18 months of age.[51] Lower birth-weight children are even seen in women exposed to passive smoke inhalation. More than 2,000 infant deaths per year are attributed to maternal smoking.

Cigarette smoking reduces oxygen delivery to the developing fetus, causing a variable degree of fetal hypoxia, which can result in long-term, irreversible intellectual and physical deficiencies. Milberger and co-workers[52] presented evidence that school-age children born of mothers who smoked during pregnancy have lower intelligence quotients (IQs) and an increased prevalence of ADHD when compared with children born of nonsmoking mothers. Thus, a paramount question is whether maternal smoking causes neurobehavioral deficits later in life.[51]

There is now increasing evidence that maternal smoking results in offspring at increased risk of developing later childhood externalizing problems, including ADHD, oppositional defiant behavior, or conduct disorder. Fergusson and co-workers[53] extended these data and confirmed validity in adolescents to age 18 years. Weissman and colleagues[54] conducted a 10-year longitudinal study of offspring of women who smoked during pregnancy (with appropriate controls of offspring of women who did not smoke during pregnancy). They noted through young adulthood a fourfold increase in conduct disorder in males and a fivefold increase in risk of substance abuse in young women who were offspring of smoking mothers. Finally, Brennan and co-workers[55] report an adverse dose-response relationship between amounts of maternal prenatal smoking and arrests of male offspring (to age 34 years) for both nonviolent and violent crimes.

A developing consensus is that nicotine input to the developing dopaminergic motivational and reward system in the fetal brain could predispose the brain, during a critical period of its development, to subsequent addictive influences and that because of its potential effect on the dopamine system, in utero exposure to nicotine might be related to an increased risk of substance abuse as the offspring matures.[54] The same analogy applies to ADHD, conduct disorder, and other externalizing behaviors.

Therapy for Nicotine Dependence

The late 1990s saw dramatic advances both in the recognition of nicotine dependence as a biological reality and in its treatment. Perhaps the most important advance was the development and clinical application of nicotine replacement therapies, specifically nicotine-containing gum, transdermal nicotine-containing patches, and nicotine-containing nasal spray and inhalers. Besides nicotine replacement therapies, additional efforts have been made to identify agents that reduce cigarette cravings, relieve the distress of comorbid psychiatric illnesses, or relieve withdrawal symptoms.

Efforts began in 1996 with the publication of practice guidelines for the treatment of nicotine-dependent individuals. The first guideline was compiled by the U.S. Agency for Health Care Policy and Research (AHCPR) and was titled "Smoking Cessation Clinical Practice Guideline."[56] The second guideline, published by the American Psychiatric Association, was titled "Practice Guidelines for the Treatment of Patients with Nicotine Dependence."[57]

The AHCPR panel of experts identified nicotine replacement therapy (nicotine patches and nicotine gum at that time) as the only pharmacotherapy then shown to be effective as an aid to smoking cessation. They recommended that, unless there is a clear medical contraindication, all patients planning a quit attempt should be offered nicotine replacement therapy. While both the nicotine patch and nicotine gum were found to be efficacious, the panel felt that the patch is preferable for routine clinical use because of greater compliance and ease of use.[56]

Cromwell and co-workers[58] estimated the cost effectiveness of implementing the smoking cessation guidelines, calculating that "society could expect to gain 1.7 million new quitters (of smoking) at an average cost of $3,779 per quitter, $2,587 per life-year saved, and $1,915 for every quality-adjusted life year saved." Discouragingly, Thorndike and co-workers[59] noted that American physician practices fall far short of national health objectives: they are not meeting the published practice guidelines, either in offering counseling or in prescribing or monitoring nicotine replacement programs. Ferry and co-workers[60] surveyed 122 medical schools and determined that a majority of medical school graduates are not adequately trained to treat nicotine dependence. Although 70 percent of smokers visit a physician each year, most are not advised or assisted in an attempt to quit.

Since publication of the guidelines in 1996, several events have occurred that have substantially changed pharmacotherapy for smoking cessation: nicotine gum and two brands of nicotine-containing skin patches are available over the counter (without a physician's prescription), and nicotine nasal spray, nicotine inhalers, and bupropion hydrochloride (Zyban) are approved as prescription medications by the U.S. Food and Drug Administration.[61] A major question today involves the comparable efficacy of different nicotine-containing products and nonnicotine therapy, either alone or in combination with other therapy.

All methods of nicotine replacement appear to be equally efficacious, approximately doubling the quit rate of smokers attempting to quit without assistance. The gum and patch provide a low, constant blood level of nicotine (about 10 to 20 nanograms per milliliter of plasma). The nasal spray delivers nicotine more rapidly than gum, patch, or inhaler, but less rapidly than a cigarette. The inhaler is a plastic rod with a nicotine plug that provides a nicotine vapor when pulled on. The device does not deliver much nicotine to the lungs (as one might expect it might); the device deposits nicotine on the buccal mucosa from which it is absorbed. Each inhaler contains about 300 doses of nicotine (each dose containing 0.016 mg of drug). The pharmacokinetics of the inhaler resemble the gum more than the spray. The major difference of the inhaler versus other nicotine replacement therapies is that the inhaler substitutes for some of the behavioral features of smoking—although this apparently does not vastly improve quit rates. Blondal and co-workers[62] found that using a patch for five months followed by nasal spray for one year improved quit rates over those achieved with a patch alone.

A number of studies have noted that smokers are more likely to have a history of depression than nonsmokers; perhaps smokers use nicotine to self-medicate for relief of depression.[63] This has led to examination of the efficacy of antidepressants in treating nicotine dependence. Hall and co-workers[64] reported the efficacy of nortriptyline (an antidepressant; Chapter 15), noting the supra-additive effect of the drug plus cognitive-behavioral therapy. Hurt and coworkers[65] reported the efficacy of bupropion (again, doubling the quit rate); Jorenby and co-workers[66] extended this therapy to a combination of bupropion plus a nicotine patch, with the patch only slightly improving results over use of bupropion alone (Figure 8.8). Interestingly, bupropion is equally effective whether the smoker is or is not clinically depressed, suggesting that bupropion's efficacy is not solely due to its antidepressant effect.[67]

Krishman-Sarin and co-workers[68] noted that nicotine-dependent persons (compared to nonsmokers) experienced nicotine craving following intravenous naloxone (a narcotic antagonist; Chapter 9), suggesting that nicotine dependence may involve alterations in the activity of the endogenous opioid system. Finally, Tyndale and co-workers[69] reported that administration of a blocker of nicotine metabolism (recall that nicotine is metabolized to cotinine by CYP2A6) allows for effective oral absorption of nicotine; this might provide "a new approach to treatment of tobacco dependence by making an oral nicotine replacement therapy feasible." More on this novel idea should be forthcoming.

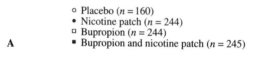

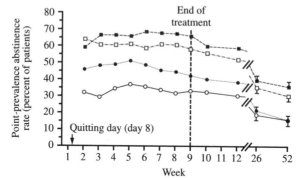

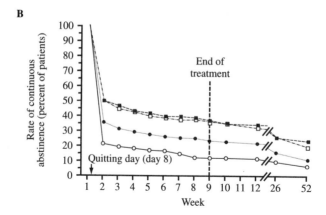

FIGURE 8.8 Point-prevalence rates of abstinence (**A**) and rates of continuous abstinence (**B**) during treatment (weeks 1–9) and follow-up (weeks 10–52). All treatment groups were superior to placebo; the two bupropion groups were superior to the nicotine patch-only group. There was no statistical difference between bupropion alone and bupropion in combination with the nicotine patch. [From Jorenby et al.[66]]

STUDY QUESTIONS

1. Differentiate the CNS stimulant actions of caffeine from those of amphetamine and cocaine.

2. Describe the mechanism of action of caffeine. How does this mechanism explain the clinical effects of the drug?

3. What is the relationship between panic attacks and caffeine?

4. Discuss the effects of caffeine in the cardiovascular system.

5. What evidence is there for and against the use of caffeine by women who are pregnant or breast feeding?

6. Discuss the political, health, and economic issues related to tobacco. Should the FDA regulate nicotine as a drug?

7. List some of the statistics that are relevant to the health effects of cigarettes.

8. Discuss the antidepressant property of nicotine. Might this contribute to cigarette dependence? Why?

9. Are cigarettes addicting or are they merely habit forming? Defend your position.

10. Discuss the clinical uses and limitations of nicotine replacement devices. How might their efficacy be boosted?

11. If nicotine exerts an antidepressant action, what drugs or therapies might assist in withdrawal and relapse prevention?

REFERENCES

1. K. S. Kendler and C. A. Prescott, "Caffeine Intake, Tolerance, and Withdrawal in Women: A Population-based Twin Study," *American Journal of Psychiatry* 156 (1999): 223–228.
2. J. W. Daly and B. B. Fredholm, "Caffeine—An Atypical Drug of Dependence," *Drug and Alcohol Dependence* 51 (1998): 199–206.
3. R. S. Feldman, J. S. Meyer, and L. F. Quenzer, *Principles of Neuropsychopharmacology* (Sunderland, Mass.: Sinauer, 1997), 612.
4. B. B. Rasmussen, T. L. Nielsen, and K. Brosen, "Fluvoxamine Is a Potent Inhibitor of the Metabolism of Caffeine in Vitro," *Pharmacology and Toxicology* 83 (1998): 240–245.
5. J. Amchin et al., "Effect of Venlafaxine on CYP1A2-Dependent Pharmacokinetics and Metabolism of Caffeine," *Journal of Clinical Pharmacology* 39 (1999): 252–259.
6. R. R. Dager et al., "Human Brain Metabolic Response to Caffeine and the Effects of Tolerance," *American Journal of Psychiatry* 156 (1999): 229–237.
7. J. F. Greden and A. Walters, "Caffeine," in J. H. Lowinson, P. Ruiz, R. B. Millman, and J. G. Langrod, eds., *Substance Abuse: A Comprehensive Textbook,* 3rd ed. (Baltimore: Williams & Wilkins, 1997), 294–307.
8. C. Rachima-Maoz, E. Peleg, and T. Rosenthal, "The Effect of Caffeine on Ambulatory Blood Pressure in Hypertensive Patients," *American Journal of Hypertension* 11 (1998): 1426–1432.
9. R. B. Lipton et al., "Efficacy and Safety of Acetaminophen, Aspirin, and Caffeine in Alleviating Migraine Headache Pain: Three Double-blind,

Randomized, Placebo-controlled Trials," *Archives of Neurology* 55 (1998): 210–217.

10. M. F. Leitzmann et al., "A Prospective Study of Coffee Consumption and the Risk of Symptomatic Gallstone Disease in Men," *Journal of the American Medical Association* 281 (1999): 2106–2112.

11. C. Ledent et al., "Aggressiveness, Hypoalgesia, and High Blood Pressure in Mice Lacking the Adenosine A_{2A} Receptor," *Nature* 388 (1997): 674–678.

12. B. E. Garrett and R. R. Griffiths, "The Role of Dopamine in the Behavioral Effects of Caffeine in Animals and Humans," *Pharmacology, Biochemistry and Behavior* 57 (1997): 533–541.

13. A. Nehlig, "Are We Dependent Upon Coffee and Caffeine? A Review on Human and Animal Data," *Neuroscience and Biobehavioral Reviews* 23 (1999): 563–576.

14. B. Eskenazi, "Caffeine During Pregnancy: Grounds for Concern," *Journal of the American Medical Association* 270 (1993): 2973–2974.

15. S. M. D'Ambrosio, "Evaluation of the Genotoxicity Data on Caffeine," *Regulatory Toxicology & Pharmacology* 19 (1994): 243–281.

16. J. L. Mills et al., "Moderate Caffeine Use and the Risk of Spontaneous Abortion and Intrauterine Growth Retardation," *Journal of the American Medical Association* 269 (1993): 593–597.

17. C. Infante-Rivard et al., "Fetal Loss Associated with Caffeine Intake Before and During Pregnancy," *Journal of the American Medical Association* 270 (1993): 2940–2943.

18. M. A. Klebanoff et al., "Maternal Serum Paraxanthine, a Caffeine Metabolite, and the Risk of Spontaneous Abortion," *New England Journal of Medicine* 341 (1999): 1639–1644.

19. T. S. Hints et al., "The Effect of Caffeine on Pregnancy Outcome Variables," *Nutrition Reviews* 54 (1996): 203–207.

20. S. M. Evans and R. R. Griffiths, "Caffeine Withdrawal: A Parametric Analysis of Caffeine Dosing Conditions," *Journal of Pharmacology & Experimental Therapeutics* 289 (1999): 285–294.

21. B. B. Fredholm et al., "Actions of Caffeine in the Brain with Special Reference to Factors that Contribute to Its Widespread Use," *Pharmacological Reviews* 51 (1999): 83–133.

22. C. E. Coop, "Adverse Anesthesia Events in Children Exposed to Environmental Tobacco Smoke," *Anesthesiology* 88 (1998): 1141–1142.

23. A. O. Goldstein, R. A. Sobel, and G. R. Newman, "Tobacco and Alcohol Use in G-rated Children's Animated Films," *Journal of the American Medical Association* 281 (1999): 1131–1136.

24. J. E. Rose, F. M. Behm, E. C. Westman, and R. E. Coleman, "Arterial Nicotine Kinetics During Cigarette Smoking and Intravenous Nicotine Administration: Implications for Addiction," *Drug and Alcohol Dependence* 56 (1999): 99–107.

25. M. Nakajima et al., "Deficient Cotinine Formation from Nicotine Is Attributed to the Whole Deletion of the CYP2A6 Gene in Humans," *Clinical Pharmacology and Therapeutics* 67 (2000): 57–69.

26. E. M. Sellers, "Pharmacogenetics and Ethnoracial Differences in Smoking," *Journal of the American Medical Association* 280 (1998): 179–180.

27. E. J. Perez-Stable et al., "Nicotine Metabolism and Intake in Black and White Smokers," *Journal of the American Medical Association* 280 (1998): 152–156.

28. R. S. Caraballo et al., "Racial and Ethnic Differences in Serum Cotinine Levels of Cigarette Smokers," *Journal of the American Medical Association* 280 (1998): 135–139.

29. N. Breslau and D. F. Klein, "Smoking and Panic Attacks," *Archives of General Psychiatry* 56 (1999): 1141–1147.

30. M. R. Picciotto, "Common Aspects of the Action of Nicotine and Other Drugs of Abuse," *Drug and Alcohol Dependence* 51 (1998): 165–172.

31. E. A. Stein et al., "Nicotine-induced Limbic Cortical Activation in the Human Brain: A Functional MRI Study," *American Journal of Psychiatry* 155 (1998): 1009–1015.

32. S. Milberger et al., "ADHD Is Associated with Early Initiation of Cigarette Smoking in Children and Adolescents," *Journal of the American Academy of Child and Adolescent Psychiatry* 36 (1997): 37–44.

33. R. A. Brown et al., "Cigarette Smoking, Major Depression, and Other Psychiatric Disorders Among Adolescents," *Journal of the American Academy of Child and Adolescent Psychiatry* 35 (1996): 1602–1610.

34. R. J. Salin-Pascual et al., "Antidepressant Effect of Transdermal Nicotine Patches in Nonsmoking Patients with Major Depression," *Journal of Clinical Psychiatry* 57 (1996): 387–389.

35. D. M. Fergusson, M. T. Lynskey, and L. J. Horwood, "Comorbidity Between Depressive Disorders and Nicotine Dependence in a Cohort of 16-Year-Olds," *Archives of General Psychiatry* 53 (1996): 1043–1047.

36. P. D. Riggs, S. K. Mikulich, E. A. Whitmore, and T. J. Crowley, "Relationship of ADHD, Depression, and Non-tobacco Substance Use Disorders to Nicotine Dependence in Substance-dependent Delinquents," *Drug and Alcohol Dependence* 54 (1999): 195–205.

37. R. F. Anda et al., "Adverse Childhood Experiences and Smoking During Adolescence and Adulthood," *Journal of the American Medical Association* 282 (1999): 1652–1658.

38. E. M. Pich et al., "Common Neural Substrates for the Addictive Properties of Nicotine and Cocaine," *Science* 275 (1997): 83–86.

39. I. P. Stolerman and M. J. Jarvis, "The Scientific Case That Nicotine Is Addictive," *Psychopharmacology* 117 (1995): 2–10.

40. P. K. Gessner, "Substance Abuse Treatment," in C. M. Smith and A. M. Reynard, eds., *Textbook of Pharmacology* (Philadelphia: W. B. Saunders, 1992), 1160.

41. J. A. Swanson, J. W. Lee, and J. W. Hopp, "Caffeine and Nicotine: A Review of Their Joint Use and Possible Interactive Effects in Tobacco Withdrawal," *Addictive Behaviors* 19 (1994): 229–256.

42. J. P. Strong et al., "Prevalence and Extent of Atherosclerosis in Adolescents and Young Adults: Implications for Prevention from the Pathological Determinants of Atherosclerosis in Youth Study," *Journal of the American Medical Association* 281 (1999): 727–735.

43. Pathobiological Determinants of Atherosclerosis in Youth (PDAY) Research Group, "Relationship of Atherosclerosis in Young Men to Serum Lipoprotein Cholesterol Concentrations and Smoking," *Journal of the American Medical Association* 264 (1990): 3018–3024.

44. G. Howard et al., "Cigarette Smoking and Progression of Atherosclerosis: The Atherosclerosis Risk in Communities (ARIC) Study," *Journal of the American Medical Association* 279 (1998): 119–124.

45. J. P. Nuorti et al., "Cigarette Smoking and Invasive Pneumococcal Disease," *New England Journal of Medicine* 342 (2000): 681–689.

46. M. F. Denissenko, A. Pao, M. Tang, and G. P. Pfeifer, "Preferential Formation of Benzo[a]pyrene Adducts at Lung Cancer Mutational Hotspots in P53," *Science* 274 (October 18, 1996): 430–432.

47. H. Witschi, J. P. Joad, and K. E. Pinkerton, "The Toxicology of Environmental Tobacco Smoke," *Annual Review of Pharmacology and Toxicology* 37 (1997): 29–52.

48. J. Z. Ayanian and P. D. Cleary, "Perceived Risks of Heart Disease and Cancer Among Cigarette Smokers," *Journal of the American Medical Association* 281 (1999): 1019–1021.

49. C. Iribarren et al., "Effect of Cigar Smoking on the Risk of Cardiovascular Disease, Chronic Obstructive Pulmonary Disease, and Cancer in Men," *New England Journal of Medicine* 340 (1999): 1773–1780.

50. S. Cnattingius, F. Granath, G. Petersson, and B. L. Harlow, "The Influence of Gestational Age and Smoking Habits on the Risk of Subsequent Preterm Deliveries," *New England Journal of Medicine* 341 (1999): 943–948.

51. B. B. Little and L. C. Gilstrap, "Tobacco Use in Pregnancy," in L. C. Gilstrap and B. B. Little, eds., *Drugs and Pregnancy*, 2nd ed. (New York: Chapman & Hall), 1998, 463–472.

52. S. Milberger et al., "Is Maternal Smoking During Pregnancy a Risk Factor for Attention Deficit Hyperactivity Disorder in Children?" *American Journal of Psychiatry* 153 (1996): 1138–1142.

53. D. M. Fergusson, L. J. Woodward, and J. Horwood, "Maternal Smoking During Pregnancy and Psychiatric Adjustment in Late Adolescence," *Archives of General Psychiatry* 55 (1998): 721–727.

54. M. M. Weissman et al., "Maternal Smoking During Pregnancy and Psychopathology in Offspring Followed to Adulthood," *Journal of the American Academy of Child and Adolescent Psychiatry* 38 (1999): 892–899.

55. P. A. Brennan, S. A. Grekin, and S. Mednick, "Maternal Smoking During Pregnancy and Adult Male Criminal Outcomes," *Archives of General Psychiatry* 56 (1999): 215–219.

56. M. C. Fiore et al., "Smoking Cessation Clinical Practice Guideline" (Rockville, Md.: Agency for Health Care Policy and Research, Public Health Service, U.S. Department of Health and Human Services, 1996).

57. American Psychiatric Association, "Practice Guidelines for the Treatment of Patients with Nicotine Dependence," *American Journal of Psychiatry* 153, suppl. (October 1996), 1–31.

58. J. Cromwell et al., "Cost-effectiveness of the Clinical Practice Recommendations in the AHCPR Guideline for Smoking Cessation," *Journal of the American Medical Association* 278 (1997): 1759–1766.

59. A. N. Thorndike et al., "National Patterns in the Treatment of Smokers by Physicians," *Journal of the American Medical Association* 279 (1998): 604–608.

60. L. H. Ferry, L. M. Grissino, and P. S. Runfola, "Tobacco Dependence Curricula in U.S. Undergraduate Medical Education," *Journal of the American Medical Association* 282 (1999): 825–829.

61. J. R. Hughes et al., "Recent Advances in the Pharmacotherapy of Smoking," *Journal of the American Medical Association* 281 (1999): 72–76.
62. T. Blondal et al., "Nicotine Nasal Spray with Nicotine Patch for Smoking Cessation: Randomized Trial with Six-year Follow-up," *British Medical Journal* 318 (1999): 285–289.
63. N. Breslau et al., "Major Depression and Stages of Smoking," *Archives of General Psychiatry* 55 (1998): 161–166.
64. S. H. Hall et al., "Nortriptyline and Cognitive-Behavioral Therapy in the Treatment of Cigarette Smoking," *Archives of General Psychiatry* 55 (1998): 683–690.
65. R. D. Hurt et al., "A Comparison of Sustained-release Bupropion and Placebo for Smoking Cessation," *New England Journal of Medicine* 337 (1997): 1195–1202.
66. D. E. Jorenby et al., "A Controlled Trial of Sustained-release Bupropion, a Nicotine Patch, or Both for Smoking Cessation," *New England Journal of Medicine* 340 (1999): 685–691.
67. K. E. Hayford et al., "Effectiveness of Bupropion for Smoking Cessation in Smokers with a Former History of Major Depression or Alcoholism," *British Journal of Psychiatry* 174 (1999): 173–178.
68. S. Krishnan-Sarin, M. I. Rosen, and S. S. O'Malley, "Naloxone Challenge in Smokers: Preliminary Evidence of an Opioid Component in Nicotine Dependence," *Archives of General Psychiatry* 56 (1999): 663–668.
69. R. F. Tyndale et al., "Inhibition of Nicotine's Metabolism: A Potential New Treatment for Tobacco Dependence," *Clinical Pharmacology and Therapeutics* 65 (1999): 145.

PART 4

Drugs That Relieve Pain: Opioid and Nonopioid Analgesics

There are three types of drugs available for use as analgesics: (1) opioid ("narcotic") analgesics, (2) nonopioid ("nonnarcotic") analgesics, and (3) other drugs not usually thought of as analgesics, which act as adjuvants when given with opioid or nonopioid analgesics or have analgesic activity of their own in some types of pain. Drugs in the third category include certain antidepressants (discussed in Chapter 15) and certain antimanic drugs (discussed in Chapter 16).

Both opioid and nonopioid analgesics have been used for millennia. Naturally occurring opioid analgesics are obtained from the opium poppy; morphine and codeine are the primary analgesic compounds found therein. Salicylates are also found in nature, but they are not widely used for pain relief. In fact, the synthetic derivatives that have been developed are the most commonly used pain relievers.

Chapter 9 explores the pharmacology of the opioid analgesics, drugs that act in the CNS to produce analgesic and euphoriant effects. Opioids (both naturally occurring and synthetically produced) are irreplaceable in medicine as the most important drugs for the relief of severe pain. Unfortunately, these drugs have a marked propensity for producing abuse and dependence. Chapter 9 also addresses the pharmacologic effects and side effects of opioids, their abuse complications, and the treatment of opioid abuse and dependence.

Chapter 10 covers the use of the nonnarcotic analgesic drugs and their use in treatment of mild to moderate pain and the pain that accompanies such diseases as rheumatoid arthritis or osteoarthritis. This chapter presents the pharmacology of aspirin, acetaminophen, and a newer class of drugs called COX-2 inhibitors intended both for the relief of pain and for the reduction of inflammation associated with arthritis and other inflammatory diseases.

Chapter 9

Opioid Analgesics

Pain can be defined as an unpleasant sensory or emotional process often associated with actual or potential tissue damage. When body tissues are damaged, tissue injury is accompanied by the activation of small-diameter sensory (afferent) fibers of peripheral nerves. These pain-sensing (*nociceptive*) sensory neurons are located in our skin, muscles, joints, and abdominal viscera. They are activated by various mechanical, thermal, and chemical injuries that cause us pain when these tissues are injured.[1] Because these neurons are activated by noxious (painful) stimuli, their receptors are called *nociceptors* (Figure 9.1). The action potentials (electrical discharge) in these neurons are conducted to their synaptic terminals, which are located in the dorsal horn of the spinal cord and where (in its simplest concept) they induce the release of a variety of chemical neurotransmitters, including the neuropeptide substance P, nerve growth factor, neurotropic factors, and the amino acid neurotransmitter glutamate.[2]

The release of pain-signaling neurotransmitters is regulated intrinsically by endogenous endorphins and/or by any drug that we refer to as an opioid agonist, since it mimics the analgesic action of our endogenous endorphins, acting upon the same set of receptors. Endorphins and opioids exert much of their analgesic action by acting presynaptically on the different sensory neurons to inhibit substance P release. In other words, opioids and endorphins exert presynaptic inhibition on the terminals of afferent sensory neurons to inhibit the release of pain-signaling neurotransmitters.

When any of these pain-induced transmitters are released, they activate receptors located on small spinal cord neurons, which in turn

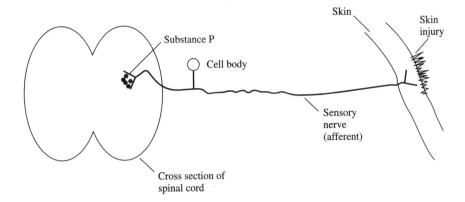

FIGURE 9.1 Activation of peripheral nociceptive (pain) fibers results in the release of substance P and other pain-signaling neurotransmitters from nerve terminals in the dorsal horn of the spinal cord. The cell body for the nerve is located in the dorsal root ganglion.

rapidly transmit information about noxious stimuli from the spinal cord to the brain, where the information is processed and integrated and the person becomes consciously aware of injury and discomfort (Figure 9.2). Thus, pain is perceived by activation of nociceptive receptors and is carried to the spinal cord by afferent nerve fibers. This perception is relayed to the brain stem and the thalamus and, eventually, to higher centers in the brain (such as the limbic system and the somatosensory cortex) for interpretation. In addition to all this, certain brain structures (such as the thalamus, brain stem, and limbic system) are rich in opioid receptors, which serve as additional sites of action of opioids and endorphins.[3]

As Figure 9.3 illustrates, two pathways, which originate in the lower brain stem, can modulate the transmission of pain impulses by activating descending pain-inhibitory systems. Activation of these two pathways, which consist of descending (brain stem to spinal cord) norepinephrine- and serotonin-releasing neurons, activates endorphin neurons in the dorsal horn of the spinal cord, which, in turn, exerts an analgesic action by inhibiting release of transmitters from the primary afferent nociceptive neurons.[4,5] It is these descending pathways on which certain antidepressants act to exert their own analgesic actions, separate and distinct from their antidepressant action.

Besides the physical component of pain, there is an affective component that determines emotional response to real or perceived distress. The affective component may be the underlying factor in the mechanism of chronic pain for which no objective cause can be identified. States of

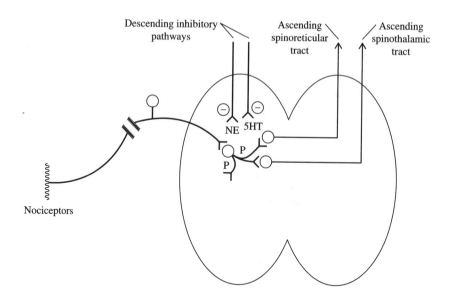

FIGURE 9.2 Release of substance P in the dorsal horn of the spinal cord with transmission of secondary relay pathways to higher centers. Descending inhibitory pathways (–) are also shown (expanded in Figure 10.3). NE = norepinephrine; 5HT = serotonin.

chronic pain may arise from deficits in the central processing of nociceptive afferent actions; input that might be innocuous in most people debilitates others, and treatment with opioids is not very effective (and sometimes even harmful because dependence can develop). For people with chronic pain, treatment focuses on behavior modification, cognitive-behavioral therapy, or self-management approaches that include biopsychosocial models of therapy. Drug therapy for these individuals relies on treatment algorithms[6] and judicious use of opioid analgesics.[7] Finally, the efficacy of the *placebo response* cannot be overlooked, especially since placebo analgesia may well be mediated by release of our own endogenous endorphins.[8]

History

Opium is extracted from poppy seeds (*Paper somniforum*) and has been used for thousands of years to produce euphoria, analgesia, sleep, and relief from diarrhea and cough. In pre-Christian centuries, opium was used primarily for its constipating effect and later for its sleep-inducing properties (noted by writers such as Homer, Hippocrates, Discorides, Virgil, and Ovid). Even in those times, recreational abuse and addiction were common.

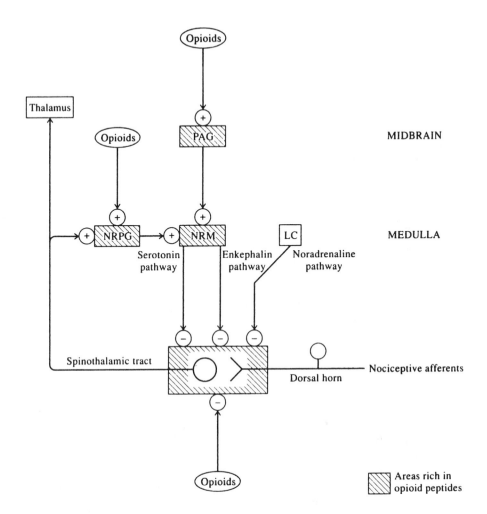

FIGURE 9.3 Sites of action of opioids on pain transmission. Opioids excite neurons in the periaqueductal gray matter (PAG) and in the midbrain and medulla. From there, serotoninergic and enkephalinergic neurons run to the dorsal horn and exert an inhibitory influence on transmission. Opioids also act directly on the dorsal horn. The locus coeruleus (LC) sends noradrenergic neurons to the dorsal horn, which also inhibits transmission. The pathways shown in this diagram represent a considerable oversimplification, but they depict the general organization of the supraspinal control mechanisms.

From the early Greek and Roman days through the sixteenth and seventeenth centuries, the medicinal and recreational uses of opium were well established. Combined with alcohol, the mixture was called *laudanum* (named by Paracelsus in 1520), meaning "something to be praised," and it was referred to as the "stone of immortality."[9] Thereafter, opium and laudanum were used for practically every known disease. It was not until the early 1800s that morphine was isolated from opium as its active ingredient. Since then, morphine has been used throughout the world as the premier agent for treating severe pain. Recognition of the addictive properties of opium, morphine, and other opioids has led to restrictions on their use to the treatment of conditions for which they are known to be effective.

After the Civil War (when opioid addiction was referred to as "soldier's disease") and the invention of the hypodermic needle in 1856, a new type of drug user appeared in the United States—one who self-administered opioids by injection.[9] By about 1910, concern began to mount about the dangers of opioids and the dependence they could induce. In 1914 the Harrison Narcotic Act was passed, and the use of most opioid products was strictly controlled. Nonmedical uses of opioids were banned, although today nonmedical use continues, despite intense efforts to eradicate it. The use of opioids is deeply entrenched in society; it is widespread and impossible to stop. Opioids exert pleasurable effects, produce tolerance and physiological dependence, and have a potential for compulsive misuse, all liabilities that are likely to resist any efforts at legal control. Also, the opioids will continue to be used in medicine because they are irreplaceable as pain-relieving agents. Goldstein[10] writes of the opioids: "They dramatically relieve emotional as well as physical pain. This property contributes to making them extremely seductive for self-administration."

Terminology

Before proceeding, some terms should be defined. *Opium* is a Greek word that means "juice"; more specifically, it refers to the juice or exudate from the poppy *Papaver somniferum*. An *opiate* is a drug extracted from the exudate of the poppy; the term is restricted to two drugs that are naturally found in the exudate, morphine and codeine. An *opioid* is any exogenous drug (natural or synthetic) that binds to an opiate receptor and produces agonist, or morphine-like, effects. Conversely, an *opioid antagonist* is any drug that binds to an opiate receptor and antagonizes the effects of morphine, displacing the morphine from the receptor. In opioid-dependent persons, an opioid antagonist precipitates withdrawal signs and symptoms. Finally, several opioids are classified as *mixed agonist-antagonist opioids*, since they have a weak analgesic action at opiate receptors but (because they are "weaker" than morphine) precipitate withdrawal in opioid-dependent persons.

Endorphin is a generic, all-inclusive term that applies to any endogenous substance (i.e., one naturally formed in the body) that exhibits pharmacological properties of morphine. There are three families of endogenous opioid peptides—*enkephalins, dynorphins,* and *beta-endorphins.* The topic of endogenous opioids is large and complex. The interested reader is referred to the review by Akil and co-workers.[11]

The term *narcotic* is derived from the Greek word *narke*, meaning "numbness," "sleep," or "stupor." Originally referring to any drug that induced sleep, the term later became associated with opioids, such as morphine and heroin. Today, it is an imprecise and pejorative term, sometimes used in a legal context to refer to a wide variety of abused substances that includes nonopioids, such as cocaine and marijuana. The term is not useful in a pharmacological context, and its use in referring to opioids is discouraged. It is not used in this chapter.

Opioids are agonists at highly specific receptor sites, and the analgesic potency of the agonist correlates with the affinity of the agonist for the opioid receptor. There is general agreement on the existence of at least three types of opioid receptors: *mu*, *kappa*, and *delta*. The genes encoding these three families, as well as the receptors themselves, have been cloned, sequenced, and well studied.[12]

Opioids occur in nature in two places: in the juice of the opium poppy (morphine and codeine) and within our own bodies as any of the endorphins. All other opioids are prepared either from morphine (*semisynthetic opioids*, such as heroin) or are synthesized from other precursor compounds (*synthetic opioids*, such as fentanyl).

Opioid Receptors

Receptors upon which endorphins and exogenous opioids act are widely distributed throughout the CNS, and each type of opioid receptor is differentially distributed. Some regions (e.g., the spinal cord) have all three types of receptors; other regions have predominantly one type (e.g., the thalamus has primarily mu receptors). The clinical significance of this distribution is still unclear. However, overall, it seems that mu-receptor agonists display the best and strongest analgesic actions but also the highest abuse liability.[12] Mu receptors are of two types: mu-1 and mu-2. Mu-1 receptors are located outside the spinal cord (are supraspinal) and are responsible for the central interpretation of pain. Mu-2 receptors are located throughout the CNS and are responsible for respiratory depression, spinal analgesia, bradycardia, physical dependence and euphoria. Morphine is an example of a mu agonist; it activates both mu-1 and mu-1 receptors. Thus, it exerts powerful effects on the brain (especially in the thalamus and striatum), the brain stem (where it slows respiration), and the spinal cord (where it exerts a strong analgesic action). In contrast, the delta-receptor agonists exhibit little addictive potential, but are also poor analgesics. Delta receptors are thought to modulate the activity of mu receptors. Kappa agonists exert modest analgesic effects, little or no respiratory depression, miosis (pinpoint pupils), and little or no dependence effects. In fact, activation of kappa receptors may serve to antagonize mu-receptor-mediated actions in the brain.[13] The use of kappa agonists is limited because strong dysphoric responses can accompany their use.[12]

Despite this knowledge about receptor subtypes, it was not until the 1990s that the opioid receptors were isolated, purified, cloned, and sequenced and their three-dimensional structures modeled.[14] Studies have revealed that all opioid receptors belong to a superfamily of G-protein-coupled receptors, all of which possess seven membrane-spanning regions (Figure 9.4), similar to the receptors we have seen earlier. Each receptor type (mu, kappa, delta) arises from its own gene and is expressed through a specific messenger RNA (mRNA). Each receptor is a chain of approximately 400 amino acids, with the amino acid sequences being about 60 percent identical to one another and 40 percent different (Figure 9.4). The diversity is responsible for the specific fit of an endogenous endorphin or an exogenous opioid to a specific receptor.[14] A fit for a fentanyl derivative for a mu receptor is illustrated in Figure 9.5. In this figure, note that the flat, two-dimensional drawing

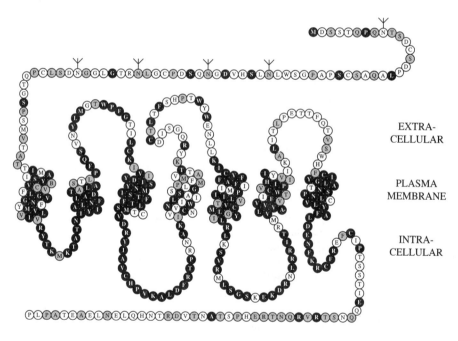

FIGURE 9.4 Two-dimensional model of the rat mu-opioid receptor. The receptor is a chain of about 390 amino acids (the letter in each circle is the first letter of the individual amino acid), with seven transmembrane coils and a terminal chain both intracellular (linked to a G-protein, not illustrated) and extracellular (binds the transmitter). Amino acids conserved in mu, delta, and kappa receptors are shown in black; amino acids conserved in mu and *either* delta or kappa receptors are shown in gray; amino acids preset only in this mu receptor (not in delta or kappa) are shown in white. [From M. Satoh and M. Minami, "Molecular Pharmacology of the Opioid Receptors," *Pharmacology and Therapeutics* 68 (1995): 343–364.]

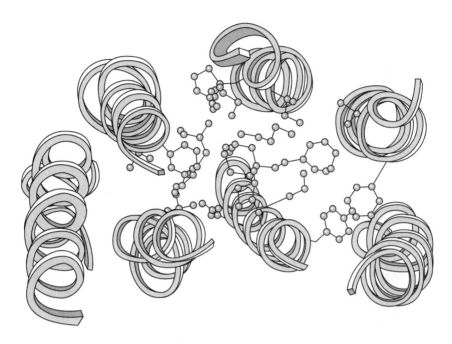

FIGURE 9.5 Speculative three-dimensional depiction of interaction of the mu-opioid receptor with the potent pure mu-agonist lofentanyl. Transmembrane helices are depicted by coils. The cell membrane within which the coils reside is not illustrated. Lofentanyl structure is shown by the connected small circles, which represent carbon molecules of the drug. Specific side chains of amino acids on the receptor helices bind with specific portions of the lofentanyl molecule. [Modified from Uhl, Childers, and Pasternak.[15] Original details by H. Moereels, L. M. Kaymans, J. Leysen, and P. Janssen (Janssen Research Foundation, Beerse, Belgium).]

of the receptor shown in Figure 9.4 is now depicted more realistically as a three-dimensional receptor with seven helical coils embedded in the membrane and three amino acid loops and a terminal chain (located in the extracellular, synaptic space) forming a fit with the opioid.[15]

What is the consequence of the binding of an opioid agonist to a mu receptor? In recent years it has become clear that the primary effect of opioid receptor activation (by either an endorphin or an opioid) is reduction in or inhibition of neurotransmission, which occurs largely through opioid-induced presynaptic inhibition of neurotransmitter release (Figure 9.6). Some of this depressant action involves alterations in transmembrane ion conductance such as drug-induced increase in potassium conductance (leading to hyperpolarization) and calcium channel inactivation, which produces reductions in neurotransmitter release. These actions, however, do not explain many of the excitatory effects of opioids (e.g., tolerance,

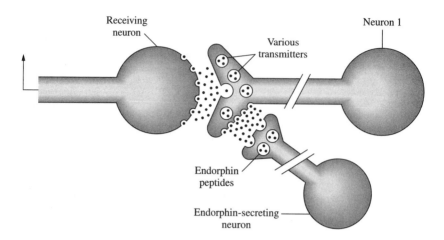

Receiving neuron

Neuron 1

Various transmitters

Endorphin peptides

Endorphin-secreting neuron

FIGURE 9.6 Simplified illustration demonstrating the presynaptic inhibition (exerted by an endorphin-secreting neuron) on neuron 1, inhibiting its release of transmitter. In the spinal cord, neuron 1 would be a primary afferent (sensory pain neuron), with enkephalin-inhibiting substance P release. In the ventral tegmentum, neuron 1 might be a GABA-secreting neuron, with an endorphin-inhibiting GABA release, disinhibiting a dopaminergic neuron, a mechanism of opioid-induced reward.

dependence/addiction, muscle rigidity). To explain this, Gutstein and co-workers[16] demonstrated that opioids strongly activate important intracellular cascades, which induce changes in cellular function to the level of nuclear proteins. Changes were different for each receptor type and may explain the differences in receptor function (e.g., mu-receptor action induces euphoria and is a positive reinforcer, while kappa-receptor activation causes dysphoria and is a negative reinforcer).

Mu Receptors

Mu opioid receptors (and the messenger RNA that expresses the receptor protein) are present in all structures in the brain and spinal cord involved in morphine-induced analgesia. The structures include the periaquaductal gray, spinal trigeminal nucleus, caudate and geniculate nuclei, thalamus, and spinal cord (dorsal horn). Mu receptors are also present in brain-stem nuclei involved in control of respiration and in morphine's depression of respiration, in brain-stem structures involved in initiation of nausea and vomiting, and in the nucleus accumbens, an area involved in the compulsive abuse of opioids, behavioral stimulants, and other drugs subject to compulsive abuse. Few or no mu receptors (or its mRNA) are found in the cerebral cortex or cerebellum.

Kappa Receptors

Kappa receptors (and the mRNA that expresses the receptor protein) are found in high concentrations in the basal ganglia, nucleus accumbens, ventral tegmentum, deep layers of cerebral cortex, hypothalamus, periaquaductal gray, dorsal horn of spinal cord, and other areas.

As stated, kappa receptors may actually antagonize mu-receptor activity.[13] Kappa receptors produce modest amounts of analgesia, dysphoria (as opposed to mu-receptor-induced euphoria, possibly because of the blockade of dopamine release), psychotomimetic effects (disorientation, depersonalization feelings), and mild respiratory depression. The mixed agonist-antagonist drugs, such as pentazocine (Talwin), are agonists at the kappa receptors. Dynorphin is the endorphin with the greatest affinity for the kappa receptor.

Delta Receptors

The enkephalins are the endogenous endorphins for the delta receptors. These receptors are involved in analgesia at both the spinal and brain levels, but further pharmacologic characterization is open to investigation. Delta receptors are also found in the nucleus accumbens and limbic system, possibly playing a role in the emotional responses to opioids.

Classification of Opioid Analgesics

Classification of opioids can be confusing. Clinically, opioids can be classified according to their receptor interactions (agonist, partial agonist, mixed agonist-antagonist, or pure antagonist), the pain intensity (moderate or severe) for which they are conventionally used, their half-lives (short or long), or the specific opioid receptors with which a specific drug interacts. Table 9.1 shows the putative effects mediated by

TABLE 9.1 Responses mediated by opioid receptors

Receptor	Response on activation
μ (mu)	Analgesia, respiratory depression, miosis, euphoria, reduced gastrointestinal motility
κ (kappa)	Analgesia, dysphoria, psychotomimetic effects, miosis, and respiratory depression

From Cherny,[17] p. 715.

an agonist opioid acting on mu and kappa receptors. The strong opioids, such as morphine, primarily act on mu receptors, and their pharmacological effects, including analgesia, respiratory depression, miosis, euphoria, reward, and constipation, all follow from this action. With this knowledge of opioid receptors, the opioid analgesics can be classified. First, the activity of each drug at each type of receptor can be tabulated and indication made whether it activates (agonistic action) or inhibits (antagonistic action) the function of any of the three specific opioid receptors. We can thus categorize each drug as a pure agonist (at a given receptor), a pure antagonist, a partial agonist, or a mixed agonist-antagonist (Table 9.2).

Pure Agonists

As discussed in Chapter 1, an agonist is a drug that has an affinity for (binds to) cell receptors to induce changes in the cell characteristic of the natural ligand (here, for example, an endorphin) for that receptor. Morphine, the prototype opioid analgesic (Table 9.1), methadone, an orally active, long-acting opioid used to treat heroin dependency, and fentanyl, a short-acting opioid with clinical use in anesthesia, bind specifically to mu receptors (Table 9.3). As stated, mu agonism invariably results in both analgesia and euphoria and has a propensity to cause dependence. So far, all attempts to separate analgesia from euphoria and dependence have been unsuccessful and are likely remain so for the forseeable future.

Pure Antagonists

Pure antagonists have affinity for a receptor (here, the mu receptor, because most clinically useful opioids are mu agonists), but after attaching they elicit no change in cellular functioning. They do, however, block access of both endogenous ligands (here, endorphins) or an exogenous drug (e.g., morphine) either present in the body (precipitating withdrawal) or administered with or after the antagonist (resulting in no effect of the agonist). An example of the latter is the clinical use of an opioid antagonist (e.g., *naltrexone*) in treatment programs for heroin addicts, where heroin taken after the antagonist elicits no analgesic or euphoric effects.

Mixed Agonist-Antagonists

A mixed agonist-antagonist drug produces an agonist effect at one receptor and an antagonistic effect at another. Clinically useful mixed drugs are kappa agonists and weak mu antagonists (they bind to both kappa and mu receptors, but only the kappa receptor is activated). In contrast to a pure agonist, a mixed agonist-antagonist usually displays a ceiling effect for analgesia;[17] in other words, it has decreased efficacy compared to a pure agonist and usually is not so effective in treating severe pain. Also, when a mixed agonist-antagonist is administered to an opioid-dependent

TABLE 9.2 Classification of opioid analgesics by analgesic properties

Pure agonists	Mixed agonist/antagonists	Pure antagonists	Partial agonists
Morphine	Nalbuphine (Nubain)	Naloxone (Narcan)	Buprenorphine (Buprene)
Codeine	Butorphanol (Stadol)	Naltrexone (Trexan,	Tramadol (Ultram)[a]
Heroin	Pentazocine (Talwin)	ReVia)	
Meperidine (Demerol)	Dezocine (Dalgan)	Nalmefene (Revex)	
Methadone (Dolophine)			
Oymorphone (Numorphan)			
Hydromorphone (Dilaudid)			
Fentanyl (Sublimaze)			

[a] Tramadol also blocks reuptake of norepinephrine and serotonin.

TABLE 9.3 Classification of opioid analgesics by actions at opioid receptors

Compound	Receptor types[a]		
	Mu	**Kappa**	**Delta**
Morphine	+++	+	+
Naloxone	−	−	−
Pentazocine	+/0	+	NA
Butorphanol	+/0	+	NA
Nalbuphine	−	+	NA
Buprenorphine	++	+	+
Fentanyl	+++	+	+
Dezocine	+	+	+

[a] The mu receptor is thought to mediate supraspinal analgesia, respiratory depression, euphoria, and physical dependence; the kappa receptor, spinal analgesia, miosis, and sedation. Categorizations are based on best inferences about actions in humans. See text for further explanation. Agonists are indicated by one or more plus signs, antagonists by a minus sign, and agents that have no significant action at the receptor by zero. NA = data not available.

person, the antagonist effect at a mu receptor precipitates an acute withdrawal syndrome. *Pentazocine* (Talwin) is the prototype agonist-antagonist (it and several related drugs are discussed later).

Partial Agonists

A partial agonist binds to opioid receptors but has a low intrinsic activity (low efficacy). It therefore exerts an analgesic effect, but the effect has a ceiling at less than the maximal effect produced by a pure agonist. *Buprenorphine* (Buprenex) is the prototype partial agonist opioid. When administered to a naive individual, analgesia is observed; when administered to an opioid-dependent individual, however, blockade of the pure agonist can occur and withdrawal can be precipitated. Compared to a mixed agonist-antagonist, the partial agonist buprenorphine binds to all three types of opioid receptors, although with lower efficacy. Its potential for producing respiratory depression is also reduced, compared with that produced by morphine.

Morphine: A Pure Agonist Opioid

Two analgesics (morphine and codeine) are found in the opium poppy. Morphine (Figure 9.7) is the more potent and represents about 10 percent of the crude exudate. Codeine is much less potent and constitutes

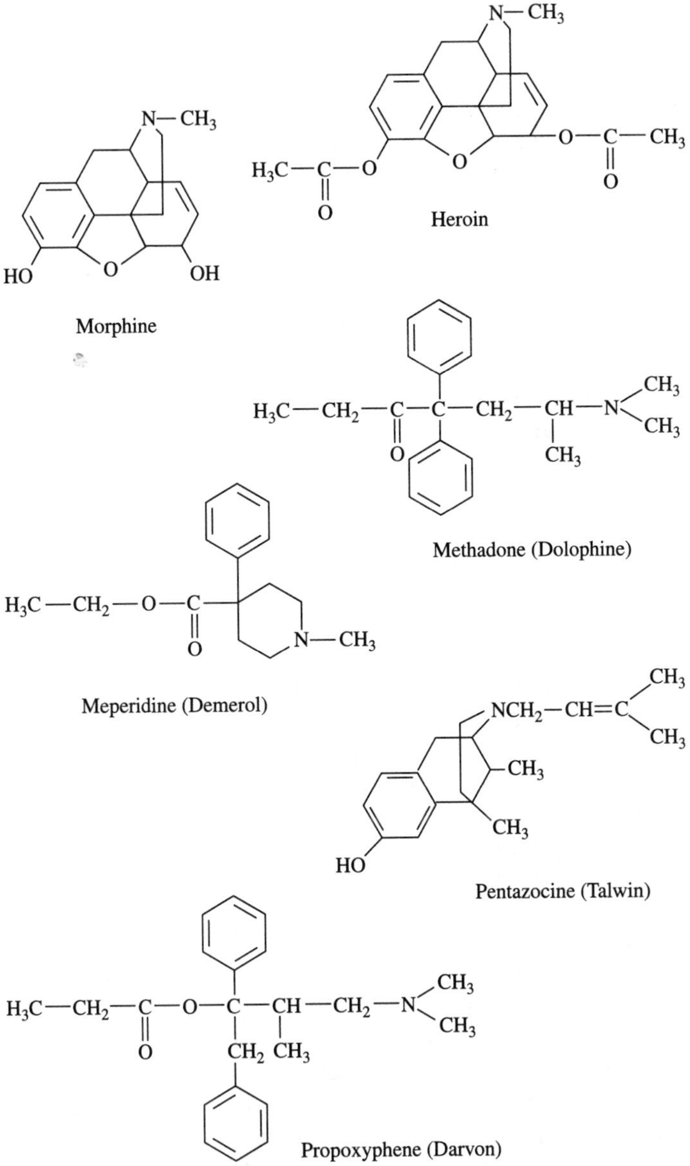

FIGURE 9.7 Structures of morphine, heroin, and four synthetic analgesics.

only 0.5 percent of the crude exudate. Despite decades of research, no other drug has been found that exceeds morphine's effectiveness as an analgesic, and no other drug is clinically superior for treating severe pain.

Pharmacokinetics

Morphine is administered orally, rectally, or by injection. In general, absorption of morphine from the gastrointestinal tract is slow and incomplete compared to absorption following injection. Absorption through the rectum is adequate, and several opioids (morphine, hydromorphone, and oxymorphone) are available in suppository form. Such preparations might be indicated in patients suffering from muscle-wasting diseases who cannot tolerate other routes of administration.

Earlier discussion of opioid action in the dorsal horn of the spinal cord leads us to discussion of a novel use of morphine: administering it directly into the spinal canal (through small catheters). This places the drug right at its site of action, avoiding its effects both on higher CNS centers (maintaining wakefulness and avoiding respiratory depression) and in the periphery (avoiding drug-induced constipation). In medicine, this technique is used to control the pain of obstetric labor and delivery, to treat postoperative pain, and (for long-term use) to relieve otherwise intractable pain associated with terminal cancer and chronic pain problems. This technology is revolutionizing the treatment of patients who suffer from chronic, severe pain.[18]

More commonly, however, morphine is administered by intravascular injection, but injections must be given with great care to avoid potentially fatal respiratory depression. As is known from the history of opium smoking in Asian cultures, the opioids may also be administered by inhalation, most commonly by inhaling the smoke from burning crude opium. The rapidity of onset of drug action rivals that following intravenous injection. Morphine itself is rarely abused in this manner.

Morphine only fairly slowly crosses the blood-brain barrier, as it is more water soluble than lipid soluble. Other opioids (such as heroin and fentanyl) cross it much more rapidly. Only about 20 percent of administered morphine reaches the CNS. This may explain why the "flash" or "rush" following intravenous injection of heroin is so much more intense than that perceived after injecting morphine.

Opioids reach all body tissues, including the fetus; infants born of addicted mothers are physically dependent on opioids and exhibit withdrawal symptoms that require intensive therapy. The habitual use of morphine or other opioids during pregnancy does not seem to increase the risk of congenital anomalies; thus these drugs are not considered to be teratogenic. However, there may be an increase in birth-related problems and fetal growth retardation Other delays and impairments observed in the development of opioid-exposed children may relate more to environmental and social-developmental problems.

Morphine is metabolized by the liver, and one of its metabolites (morphine-6-glucuronide) is actually ten- to twentyfold more potent as an analgesic than is morphine. Indeed, much of the analgesic action of morphine is mediated by this active metabolite. The half-lives of morphine and morphine-6-glucuronide are both 3 to 5 hours. Patients with impaired kidney function tend to accumulate the metabolite and thus may be more sensitive to morphine administration. Metabolite accumulation would also tend to prolong the analgesic actions of drug and metabolite.

Urine-screening tests can be used to detect codeine and morphine as well as their metabolites. Because heroin is metabolized to morphine, and because street heroin also contains acetylcodeine (which is metabolized to codeine), heroin use is suspected when both morphine and codeine are present in a patient's urine. However, such tests cannot accurately determine which specific drug (heroin, codeine, or morphine) has been used. Furthermore, codeine is widely available in cough syrups and analgesic preparations, and even poppy seeds contain small amounts of morphine. Thus, depending on the drug that was taken, morphine and codeine metabolites may be detected in a patient's urine for 2 to 4 days.

Pharmacological Effects

Morphine produces a syndrome characterized by analgesia, relaxed euphoria, sedation, a sense of tranquility, reduced apprehension and concern, respiratory depression, suppression of the cough reflex, and pupillary constriction (Table 9.1).

Analgesia. Morphine produces intense analgesia and indifference to pain, reducing the intensity of pain and thus reducing the associated distress by altering the central processing of pain. Morphine analgesia occurs without loss of consciousness and without affecting other sensory modalities. Indeed, the pain may persist as a sensation, but patients "feel more comfortable"[10] and are not bothered by the fact that they hurt. In other words, the perception of the pain is significantly altered. An injection of naloxone (Narcan) displaces morphine from the mu receptors and blocks the analgesic effect.

Euphoria. Morphine produces a pleasant euphoric state, which includes a strong feeling of contentment, well-being, and lack of concern. Indeed, this is part of the affective, or reinforcing, response to the drug.

Opioids, like cocaine, are used for their positive effects. Use of exogenous opioids gives the addict access to the reinforcement system . . . in the locus coeruleus and elsewhere. This positive reward system, normally reserved to reward the performance of species-specific survival behaviors, once reached by exogenous self-administration of drugs of abuse, provides the user with an experience that the brain equates with profoundly important events like eating, drinking, and sex. Opioid use becomes an acquired drive state that permeates all aspects of human life. Withdrawal from opioid use is mediated by separate neural pathways that cause withdrawal events to be perceived as life-threatening, and the subsequent physiologic reactions often lead to renewed opioid consumption.[19]

Regular users of morphine describe the effects of intravenous injection in ecstatic and often sexual terms, but the euphoric effect becomes progressively less intense after repeated use. At this point, users inject the drug for one or more of several possible reasons: to try to re-experience the extreme euphoria experienced after the first few injections, to maintain a state of pleasure and well-being, to prevent mental discomfort that may be associated with reality, or to prevent withdrawal symptoms.

Because morphine exerts powerful effects on pain and emotion, we might ask what role the endorphins play as natural analgesics or euphoriants. The answer is unknown, since intravenous naloxone does not precipitate feelings of pain, dysphoria, or any other major response. In marathon runners, however, it has been reported that endorphin levels in plasma increase fourfold;[20] these natural analgesics reduce depression and provide an overall feeling of well-being (a "runner's high"). Endorphins may therefore be part of a natural euphoric reward system and a determinant of our mood.

The mechanism of morphine's positive reinforcing and euphoria-producing action probably involves more than mu receptors, especially the dopaminergic.[21,22] Opioids activate mu receptors within the mesolimbic dopamine reward system by means of the ventral tegmental–nucleus accumbens pathway that is involved in the rewarding effects of cocaine, the benzodiazepines, and alcohol. This receptor action is illustrated in Figure 9.8. Simonato[20] summarizes the complexity of this action:

> In the ventral tegmental area, morphine inhibits GABA neurons via mu opioid receptors, thus disinhibiting dopaminergic neurons and increasing dopamine input in the nucleus accumbens and in other areas; this phenomenon may be involved in the mechanism of reward, i.e., the positive reinforcer to opioid addiction.

Sedation and Anxiolysis.   Morphine produces anxiolysis, sedation, and drowsiness, but the level of sedation is not so deep as that produced by the CNS depressants. Although persons who are taking morphine will

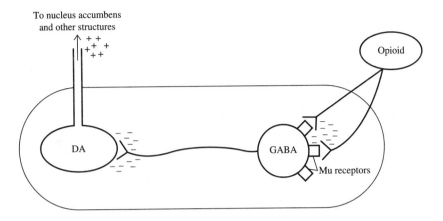

To nucleus accumbens
and other structures

FIGURE 9.8 Schematic illustration of how dopamine-secreting neurons in the ventral tegmental area are excited by opioids. Dopamine-containing neurons are hyperpolarized by GABA acting at $GABA_A$ receptors. GABA-containing neurons are hyperpolarized by opioids acting at mu receptors. Thus, opioids reduce the inhibition exerted by GABA on dopamine neurons. DA = dopamine.

doze, they can usually be awakened readily. During this state, "mental clouding" is prominent, which is accompanied by a lack of concentration, apathy, complacency, lethargy, reduced mentation, and a sense of tranquility. Obviously, in such a state, cognitive impairment results.

Depression of Respiration.   Morphine causes a profound depression of respiration by decreasing the respiratory center's sensitivity to higher levels of carbon dioxide in the blood. Respiratory rate is reduced even at therapeutic doses; at higher doses, the rate slows even further, respiratory volume decreases, breathing patterns become shallow and irregular, and, at sufficiently high levels, breathing ceases. Respiratory depression is the single most important acute side effect of morphine and is the cause of death from acute opioid overdosage. The combination of morphine (or other opioid) with alcohol or other sedatives is especially dangerous.

Suppression of Cough.   Opioids suppress the "cough center," which is also located in the brain stem. Thus, opioid narcotics have historically been used as cough suppressants, codeine being particularly popular for this purpose. Today, however, less addicting drugs are used as cough suppressants; opioids are inappropriate choices for treating persistent cough.

Pupillary Constriction.   Morphine (as well as other mu and kappa agonists) causes pupillary constriction (miosis). Indeed, pupillary constriction in the presence of analgesia is characteristic of opioid ingestion.

Nausea and Vomiting. Morphine stimulates receptors in an area of the medulla that is called the chemoreceptor trigger zone. Stimulation of this area produces nausea and vomiting, which are the most characteristic and unpleasant side effects of morphine and other opioids, but they are not life threatening.

Gastrointestinal Symptoms. Morphine and the other opioids relieve diarrhea as a result of their direct actions on the intestine, the most important action of morphine outside the CNS. Opioids cause intestinal tone to increase, motility to decrease, feces to dehydrate, and intestinal spasm (and cramping) to occur. This combination of decreased propulsion, increased intestinal tone, decreased rate of movement of food, and dehydration harden the stool and further retard the advance of fecal material. All these effects contribute to the constipating effect of opioids. Nothing more effective than the opioids has yet been developed for treating severe diarrhea. In recent years two opioids have been developed that only very minimally cross the blood-brain barrier into the CNS. The first is *diphenoxylate* (the primary active ingredient in Lomotil), and the second is *loperamide* (Imodium). These two drugs are exceedingly effective opioid antidiarrheals but are not analgesics, nor are they prone to compulsive abuse, because they do not reach the CNS.

Other Effects. Morphine can release histamine from its storage sites in mast cells in the blood. This can result in localized itching or more severe allergic reactions, including bronchoconstriction (an asthma-like constriction of the bronchi of the lungs). Opioids also affect white blood cell function, perhaps producing complex alterations in the immune system.[23] It is wise, perhaps, to avoid the use of morphine in patients with compromised immune function.

Tolerance and Dependence

The development of tolerance and dependence with repeated use is a characteristic feature of all opioid drugs, including morphine. Use of opioids is severely limited because of the development of *tolerance*, the presence of uncomfortable side effects, and their potential for compulsive abuse.

The molecular basis of tolerance is now thought to involve glutaminergic mechanisms. In 1997, Gies and colleagues[24] stated that activation of glutamate NMDA receptors correlates with resistance to opioids and the development of tolerance. Mu-receptor mRNA levels are regulated by activation of these receptors. Recently, Celerier and colleagues[25] demonstrated that following the dissipation of opioid-induced analgesia, a prolonged period of sustained decrease in the pain threshold (a hypergesic state) occurs. The NMDA receptor blocker *ketamine* (Chapter 12) prevented the development of this late-onset and long-lasting enhancement in pain sensitivity after the initial analgesic effect dissipated.

Thus, glutaminergic NMDA receptors may regulate mu-receptor mRNA, accounting for the development of tolerance to the continuous presence of opioid. Akil and co-workers[11] review the intracellular alterations induced by morphine and its relation to the development of tolerance after prolonged exposure to such drugs. Several other research articles and reviews enhance current understanding of the complex interaction among glutamate, NMDA receptor blockade, analgesia, and the development of tolerance and dependence.[26–30]

The rate at which tolerance develops varies widely. When morphine or other opioids are used only intermittently, little, if any, tolerance develops. Thus, when a person's sprees of drug use are separated by prolonged periods without using drugs, the opioids retain their initial efficacy. When administration is repeated, tolerance may become so marked that massive doses have to be administered to either maintain a degree of euphoria or prevent withdrawal discomfort (avoidance of discomfort is more common). The degree of tolerance is illustrated by the fact that the dose of morphine can be increased from clinical doses (i.e., 50 to 60 milligrams per day) to 500 milligrams per day over as short a period as 10 days.[31]

Tolerance to one opioid leads to cross-tolerance to all other natural and synthetic opioids, even if they are chemically dissimilar. Cross-tolerance, however, does not develop between the opioids and the sedative hypnotics. In other words, a person who has developed a tolerance for morphine will also have a tolerance for heroin but not for alcohol or barbiturates.

Physical dependence was described in Chapter 1 as an altered state of biology induced by a drug whereby withdrawal of a drug is followed by a complex set of biological events typical for that class of drugs. Acute withdrawal from opioids has been well studied, since it can be easily precipitated in drug-dependent individuals by injecting the opioid antagonist naloxone (Narcan). Withdrawal results in a profound reduction in the release of dopamine in the nucleus accumbens,[21] and a threefold increase in the release of norepinephrine in various structures, including the hippocampus, nucleus accumbens, and locus coeruleus.[32] As stated by Simonato:[21]

> The firing rate of the locus coeruleus is actively inhibited by morphine, returns to baseline levels with tolerance, and rises dramatically during withdrawal; these phenomena may be involved in the mechanism of dependence, i.e., the negative reinforcer to opioid addiction.

Symptoms of withdrawal are, in general, the opposite of pharmacological effects (Table 9.4) and include restlessness, dysphoria, drug craving, sweating, extreme anxiety, depression, irritability, fever, chills, retching and vomiting, increased respiratory rate (panting), cramping,

TABLE 9.4 Acute effects of opioids and rebound withdrawal symptoms

Acute action	Withdrawal sign
Analgesia	Pain and irritability
Respiratory depression	Hyperventilation
Euphoria	Dysphoria and depression
Relaxation and sleep	Restlessness and insomnia
Tranquilization	Fearfulness and hostility
Decreased blood pressure	Increased blood pressure
Constipation	Diarrhea
Pupillary constriction	Pupillary dilation
Hypothermia	Hyperthermia
Drying of secretions	Lacrimation, runny nose
Reduced sex drive	Spontaneous ejaculation
Peripheral vasodilation; flushed and warm skin	Chilliness and "gooseflesh"

From R. S. Feldman, J. S. Meyer, and L. F. Quenzer, *Principles of Neuropsycholpharmacology* (Sunderland, Mass.: Sinauer, 1997), Table 12.8, p. 533.

insomnia, explosive diarrhea, and intense aches and pains. The magnitude of these acute withdrawal symptoms depends on the dose of opioid, the frequency of previous drug administration, and the duration of drug dependence. Acute opioid withdrawal is not considered to be life-threatening, although it can seem unbearable to the person experiencing it.

To help alleviate the symptoms of acute withdrawal, several approaches have been tried. One newer method is termed *rapid opioid detoxification* or, perhaps more appropriately, *rapid anesthesia-aided detoxification* (RAAD).[33] A pure opioid antagonist, such as naloxone or naltrexone, and the sympathetic blocker clonidine are administered intravenously to the opioid-dependent person while he or she is asleep under general anesthesia. The procedure goes on for several hours, during which time the withdrawal signs are blunted.[34] The objective is to enable the patient to tolerate high doses of an opioid antagonist and thus undergo complete detoxification in a matter of hours while unconscious, rather than over several days or weeks while awake and suffering from severe withdrawal symptoms.[35] After awakening, the patient is maintained on orally administered naltrexone, to reduce opioid craving, and undergoes supportive psychotherapy and group therapies for relapse prevention and to address the underlying causes of addiction. The RAAD technique is controversial, in part because it is expensive, it involves the risks of anesthesia, and it is rather elaborate.

No matter the method of opioid withdrawal, following acute withdrawal, focus is directed toward the so-called *protracted abstinence syndrome*,[31] beginning when the acute phase of opioid withdrawal ends and persisting for up to six months. Symptoms of this syndrome include depression, abnormal responses to stressful situations, drug hunger, decreased self-esteem, anxiety, and other psychological disturbances. Complicating the diagnosis of prolonged abstinence syndrome is the high prevalence of other psychiatric disorders (e.g., affective and personality disorders) in opioid-dependent individuals.[6] Brooner and co-workers[36] documented psychiatric comorbidity in 47 percent of 716 treatment-seeking opioid abusers; antisocial personality disorder (25 percent) and major depression (15 percent) are the most common diagnoses. Nunes and co-workers[37] reported a "robust antidepressant effect of *imipramine*" (an antidepressant; Chapter 15) in 57 percent of 84 depressed opioid-dependent people. Oliveto and co-workers[38] reported that another antidepressant, *desipramine*, increased opioid (and cocaine) abstinence in opioid-dependent cocaine abusers.

Several behavioral theories have been posited to account for continued opioid use:[21]

- Continued use avoids the distress and dysphoria associated with withdrawal (a negative reinforcing effect).
- The euphoria produced by the opioids leads to their continued use (a positive reinforcing effect).
- Preexisting dysphoric or painful affective states are alleviated. This presumes that the opioids were initially used as a type of self-medication to treat these symptoms, and dependence gradually developed.
- The euphoric response is an atypical response to opioids that occurs in individuals with preexistent psychopathology.
- Preexisting psychopathology may be the basis for initial experimentation and euphoria, but repeated use is prompted by the desire to avoid withdrawal.
- Some individuals have deficient endorphin systems that are corrected by the use of opioids.
- Repeated use of opioids leads to permanent dysfunction in the endorphin system to the point that normal function requires the continued use of exogenous opioids.
- Drug effects and drug withdrawal can become linked through environmental cues and internal mood states. Emotions and external cues recall the distress of withdrawal or the memory of opioid euphoria or opioid reduction of dysphoria or painful affective states.

To varying degrees, all these theories are probably involved in a given individual's use of opioids. Opioid tolerance and dependence lie not merely in a few predisposed individuals; they can develop in anyone who uses the drugs repeatedly, not necessarily people who are abusing them. A patient in the chronic pain of terminal illness should not be denied opioids, despite the inevitable development of tolerance and dependence, a condition that can be controlled with even small amounts of drug.[7]

Other Pure Agonist Opioids

Codeine occurs naturally in opium and is one of the most commonly prescribed opioid drugs. For medical use, it is usually combined with aspirin or acetaminophen for the relief of mild to moderate pain. These products are frequently sought drugs of abuse. About 40 percent of people who use them meet the criteria for codeine dependence,[39] and the use of codeine-containing products is strongly associated with endogenous depression—again a dual-diagnosis problem.[40] The plasma half-life and duration of action is about 3 to 4 hours.

Pharmacokinetically, codeine is metabolized by hepatic cytochrome CYP2D6 enzymes to morphine, and many of the clinical effects attributed to codeine (e.g., pain relief and euphoria) may, in fact, result from the actions of morphine. Interestingly, serotonin-specific antidepressants can block the pain relief of codeine, as they block the conversion of codeine to morphine. Here, in such patients, an analgesic drug other than codeine may have to be selected.

Heroin (diacetylmorphine) is three times more potent than morphine and is produced from morphine by a slight modification of chemical structure (Figure 9.7). The increased lipid solubility of heroin leads to faster penetration of the blood-brain barrier, producing an intense rush when it is either smoked or injected intravenously. Heroin is metabolized to monoacetylmorphine and morphine, the latter being eventually metabolized and excreted. Heroin is legally available in Great Britain and Canada,[17] where it can be used clinically. The drug is not legal in the United States, but it is widely used illicitly. When heroin is smoked together with crack cocaine, euphoria is intensified, the anxiety and paranoia associated with cocaine are tempered, and the depression that follows after the effects of cocaine wear off is reduced. Unfortunately, this combination creates a multidrug addiction that is extremely difficult to treat.

Hydromorphone (Dilaudid) and *oxymorphone* (Numorphan) are both structurally related to morphine. Both of these drugs are as effective as morphine; they are 6 to 10 times more potent than morphine. Somewhat less sedation but equal respiratory depression is observed.

Meperidine (Demerol) is a synthetic opioid whose structure differs from that of morphine (Figure 9.7). Because of this structural difference, meperidine was originally thought to be free of many of the undesirable properties of the opioids. However, meperidine is addictive; it can be substituted for morphine or heroin in addicts and is widely prescribed medically. It is one-tenth as potent as morphine, produces a similar type of euphoria, and is equally likely to cause dependence. Meperidine's side effects differ from morphine's and include more excitatory effects, such as tremors, delirium, hyperreflexia, and convulsions. These effects are produced by a metabolite of meperidine (normeperidine) that appears to be responsible for the CNS excitation. Meperidine and normeperidine can accumulate in individuals who have kidney dysfunction or who use only meperidine for their opioid addiction. Withdrawal symptoms will develop more rapidly than with morphine because of the shorter duration of action of meperidine.

Methadone (Dolophine) is a synthetic mu-agonist opioid, the pharmacological activity of which is very similar to that of morphine. Methadone was first shown to cover for and block the effects of heroin withdrawal in 1948. In 1965 it was introduced as substitution treatment for opioid dependency and since then has become the principal pharmacologic agent for prevention of abstinence symptoms and signs. The outstanding properties of methadone are its effective analgesic activity, its efficacy by the oral route, its extended duration of action in suppressing withdrawal symptoms in physically dependent individuals, and its tendency to show persistent effects with repeated administration.

> The main objectives of opioid treatment programs are rehabilitation of the dependent individual and reduction in needle-associated diseases, illicit drug use, and crime. Randomized controlled trials of methadone maintenance programs have shown that they generally fulfill these aims. . . . Although there are a number of predictors of the success of a program, the most important is the magnitude of the daily methadone dose. Programs that prescribe average daily doses exceeding 50 mg have higher retention rates and lower illicit drug use rates than those in which the average dose is less than 50 mg.[41]

Even where liberal doses are used, about one-third of the clients regularly experience withdrawal (they are called *nonholders*) and two-thirds (called *holders*) do not during a once-daily dosing schedule. Thus, to maintain compliance, prescribers must be free to regulate doses to meet individual requirements. (The generally accepted half-life of methadone is 24 hours.) Dyer and co-workers[41] determined that this variability was a pharmacokinetic (not a receptor or pharmacodynamic) consequence, as some clients appear to metabolize methadone more quickly; small changes in plasma concentration can lead to relatively large changes in clinical effect (e.g., can precipitate withdrawal).

Strain et al.[42] and Preston et al.[42A] reported improved compliance and reduced heroin use with higher doses (80 to 100 mg/day) compared with doses of 40 to 50 mg/day. Dyer and colleagues[41] concluded that (1) once-daily dosage is not suitable for at least one-third of clients; (2) dividing the daily dose may be more appropriate for nonholders; (3) use of a longer-acting opioid might be considered. Here, levo-alpha acetylmethadol (LAAM) and slow-release morphine are promising candidates. The Dyer team also makes a case for the development of a slow-release formulation of methadone.˙

LAAM (levo-alpha acetylmethadol) is related to methadone and is an oral opioid analgesic that was approved in mid-1993 for the clinical management of opioid dependence in heroin addicts. LAAM is well absorbed from the gastrointestinal tract. It has a slow onset and a long duration of action (about 72 hours). It is metabolized to compounds that are also active as opioid agonists. Its primary advantage over methadone is its long duration of action; in maintenance therapy it is administered by mouth three times a week. With LAAM, a major controversy, like that over methadone, relates to dose-related efficacy. Eissenberg and co-workers[43] studied opioid-dependent volunteers who were given thrice-weekly doses of LAAM (25/25/35 mg, 50/50/70 mg, and 100/100/140 mg, Monday, Wednesday, and Friday). They noted that heroin use decreased as the LAAM dose was increased (presumably with fewer people experiencing withdrawal symptoms as the dose increased). Interestingly, self-reported cocaine use also decreased, although the magnitude of the decrease did not correlate with the LAAM dosage. Jones and co-workers[44] verified these data; however, they noted that the high-dose group had more dropouts because of "agonist adverse effects." At higher doses, opioid use, opioid craving, and withdrawal symptoms were all reduced.

Propoxyphene (Darvon) is an analgesic compound that is structurally similar to methadone (Figure 9.7). As an analgesic for treating mild to moderate pain, it is less potent than codeine but more potent than aspirin. When propoxyphene is taken in large doses, opioid-like effects are seen; when it is used intravenously, it is recognized by addicts as an opioid. Taken orally, propoxyphene does not have much potential for abuse. Some cases of drug dependence have been reported, but to date they have not been of major concern. Because commercial intravenous preparations of propoxyphene are not available, intravenous abuse is encountered only when someone attempts to inject solutions of the powder that is contained in capsules, which are intended for oral use.

Fentanyl (Sublimaze) and three related compounds, *sufentanil* (Sufenta), *alfentanil* (Alfenta), and *remifentanyl* (Ultiva) are short-acting, intravenously administered, agonist opioids that are structurally related to meperidine. These four compounds are intended to be used during and after surgery to relieve surgical pain. Fentanyl is now also available both in a transdermal skin patch and as an oral lozenge on a stick (a "lollipop").[45] The transdermal route of drug delivery offers prolonged, rather steady levels of drug in blood; the lollipop is used for the short-term treatment of surgical pain in children.

Fentanyl and its three derivatives are 80 to 500 times as potent as morphine as analgesics and profoundly depress respiration. Death from these agents is invariably caused by respiratory failure. In illicit use, fentanyl is known as "China white." Numerous derivatives (such as methylfentanyl) can be manufactured illegally; they emerge periodically and have been responsible for many fatalities. Peng and Sandler[46] review the pharmacology and analgesic properties of fentanyl.

Remifentanyl has the shortest half-life of any known opioid: only 10 to 20 minutes because the drug is rapidly metabolized by specific enzymes (esterases) present in blood. Little drug remains to be metabolized in the liver. Remifentanyl is intended to be used to control brief, intense pain during surgery. Because of its short half-life, remifentanyl is administered by continuous intravenous infusion.[47]

Partial Agonist Opioids

Buprenorphine (Buprenex) is a newer, semisynthetic, partial agonist opioid whose action is characterized by a limited stimulation of mu receptors, which is responsible for its analgesic properties. As a partial agonist, however, there is a ceiling to its analgesic effectiveness as well as to its potential for inducing euphoria and respiratory depression. Buprenorphine has a very long duration of action (about 24 hours), because it binds very strongly to mu receptors, limiting its reversibility by naloxone when reversal is considered necessary. Perry and coworkers,[48] in a study of the use of buprenorphine in treating opioid dependence, found that, because of its ceiling effect, doses four times the daily maintenance dose could be given twice weekly without either agonist effects or withdrawal symptoms occurring. This certainly offers additional variety for special situations where variable dosage becomes a clinical necessity.

Buprenorphine can be administered by oral, parenteral, or sublingual routes. Currently being developed is a sublingual tablet.[49] At low doses, buprenorphine can substitute for morphine (in morphine-dependent individuals) and it is analgesic (in nontolerant individuals).

Buprenorphine has been evaluated as an alternative or a subsequent step to methadone for opioid detoxification and maintenance programs. Schottenfeld and co-workers[50] compared buprenorphine and methadone maintenance for treatment of concurrent opioid dependence and cocaine abuse. Despite theoretical advantages over methadone, superiority over methadone in reducing illicit opioid (heroin) use was not demonstrated; although high daily doses (12 mg sublingual) were about as effective as high daily doses (65 mg) of methadone. Buprenorphine exerted no beneficial effect on illicit cocaine use. Johnson and co-workers[51] reported that at comparable doses, methadone, LAAM, and buprenorphine "are efficacious treatments for opioid dependence." Umbricht and co-workers[52] used buprenorphine as a "tapering" medication for rapid opioid detoxification, following buprenorphine with successful opioid antagonist therapy (naltrexone). The combination "is an acceptable and safe treatment for shortened opioid detoxification and induction of naltrexone maintenance." The availability of buprenorphine should offer clinicians yet another pharmacologic option for the treatment of opioid dependence.

Tramadol (Ultram), available in Europe for many years, became available for use as an analgesic in the United States in 1995. The drug exhibits a unique dual analgesic action: (1) it is a partial agonist at mu receptors, and (2) it blocks the presynaptic reuptake of norepinephrine[53] and serotonin,[54,55] producing both an antidepressant and an analgesic action. (Chapter 15 discusses the analgesic actions of antidepressants.) In the United States, tramadol is available only for oral use. Well absorbed orally, the drug undergoes a two-step metabolism, and the first metabolite (mono-demethyl tramadol) is as active or more active than the parent compound.[56] As a partial agonist, the drug exhibits a ceiling effect on analgesia (but not so analgesic as morphine), which limits respiratory depression and abuse potential. Side effects are considerable and include drowsiness and vertigo, nausea, vomiting, constipation, and headache. Additive sedation with CNS depressants is observed. The analgesic efficacy of tramadol is now well documented.[57] Reports of its use in treating opioid dependency are not available.

Finally, there has been concern about the combination of tramadol and serotonin-type antidepressant drugs: the combination may increase the toxicity of the antidepressants (causing a serotonin syndrome; Chapter 15). This drug combination should probably be avoided, if possible.

Mixed Agonist-Antagonist Opioids

There are four commercially available drugs classified pharmacologically as mixed agonist-antagonist opioids: pentazocine, butorphanol, nalbuphine, and dezocine (Figure 9.9). Each of these drugs binds with varying affinity to the mu and kappa receptors. The drugs are weak mu agonists; most of their analgesic effectiveness (which is quite limited) results from their stimulation of kappa receptors (Table 9.3). Low doses cause moderate analgesia; higher doses produce little additional

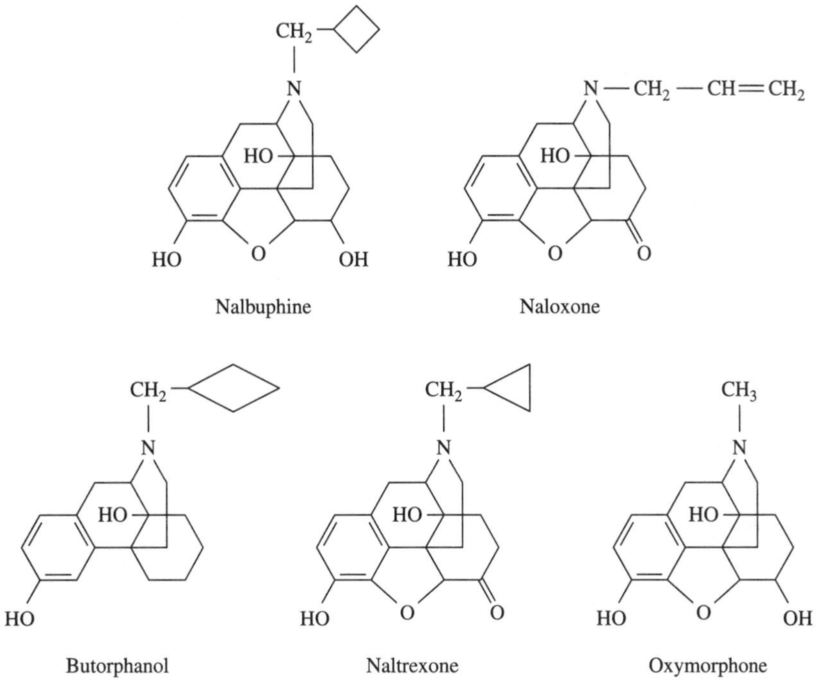

FIGURE 9.9 Structural formulas of oxymorphone and four analogues. Oxymorphone is a pure mu agonist. Nalbuphine and butorphanol have mixed agonistic/antagonistic properties, while naloxone and naltrexone are pure antagonists.

analgesia. In opioid-dependent individuals, these drugs precipitate withdrawal. A high incidence of adverse psychotomimetic side effects (dysphoria, anxiety reactions, hallucinations, and so on) are associated with the use of these agents, limiting their therapeutic use but increasing their attraction for illicit use.

Pentazocine (Talwin) and *butorphanol* (Stadol) are prototypical mixed agonist-antagonists. Neither has much potential for producing respiratory depression or physical dependence. In 1993 butorphanol, previously available for use by injection, became available as a nasal spray, the first analgesic so formulated. After spraying into the nostrils, peak plasma levels (and maximal effect) are achieved in one hour, with a duration of 4 to 5 hours. Use of the nasal spray can be euphoric and abuse of this preparation appears to be increasing.

The abuse of pentazocine has also been increasing, particularly in combination with tripelennamine, an antihistamine. This combination of drugs, called "Ts and blues," has caused serious medical complications, including seizures, psychotic episodes, skin ulcerations, abscesses, and muscle wasting. (The latter three effects are caused by the repeated injections rather than by the drugs themselves.)

Nalbuphine (Nubain) is primarily a kappa agonist of limited analgesic effectiveness. Because it is also a mu antagonist, it is not likely to produce either respiratory depression or patterns of abuse.

Dezocine (Dalgan) was introduced in 1990 as the newest of the agonist-antagonist drugs. As a moderate mu agonist and a weak delta and kappa agonist, dezocine can substitute for morphine. Its clinical efficacy and potential for abuse appear limited.

Antagonist Opioids

Three clinically available drugs, naloxone, naltrexone, and nalmefene, are structural derivatives of oxymorphone, a pure opioid agonist (Figure 9.9). All three have an affinity for opioid receptors (especially mu receptors), but after binding they exert no agonist effects of their own. Therefore, they antagonize the effects of agonist opioids and are termed *pure opioid antagonists.*

Naloxone (Narcan) is the prototype antagonist. It has little or no effect when injected into nonopioid-dependent persons, but it rapidly precipitates withdrawal when injected into opioid-dependent persons. Naloxone is neither analgesic nor subject to abuse. Because naloxone is not absorbed from the gastrointestinal tract, it must be given by injection. Furthermore, its duration of action is very brief, in the range of 15 to 30 minutes. Thus, for continued opioid antagonism, it must be reinjected at short intervals to avoid "renarcotization." Naloxone is used to reverse the respiratory depression that follows acute opioid intoxication (overdoses) and to reverse opioid-induced respiratory depression in newborns born of opioid-dependent mothers. The limitations of naloxone include its short duration of action and its parenteral route of administration.

Naltrexone (Trexan, ReVia) became clinically available in 1985 as the first orally absorbed, pure opioid antagonist. Its actions resemble those of naloxone, but naltrexone is well absorbed orally and has a long duration of action, necessitating only a single daily dose of about 40 to 80 milligrams. Naltrexone is used clinically in treatment programs when it is desirable to maintain a person on chronic therapy with an opioid antagonist rather than an agonist such as methadone. In people who take naltrexone daily, any injection of a pure opioid agonist is ineffective. The clinical use of naltrexone is somewhat limited by nausea (which can be quite severe in some persons) and dose-dependent liver toxicity, which can be a problem in patients with pre-existing liver disease.

As discussed in Chapter 4, naltrexone is also used in the treatment of alcoholism to reduce the craving for alcohol during the maintenance period of treatment.[58] It is likely that such action follows from the antagonism of endorphin action rather than from an as yet unidentified action outside the opioid system. Anton and co-workers[59] studied the effects of cognitive behavioral therapy (CBT) combined with either naltrexone or placebo medication for the treatment of outpatient alcoholics. CBT-treated patients medicated with naltrexone drank less, took longer to relapse, and had more time to relapse than did CBT-treated placebo-medicated patients. They also exhibited more resistance to and control over alcohol-related thoughts and urges. Overall, 62 percent of the naloxone group did not relapse into heavy drinking, in comparison with 40 percent of the placebo group. The authors concluded that "the therapeutic effects of CBT and naltrexone may be synergistic."

Naltrexone has also been reported to have some efficacy in the treatment of autism,[60,61] self-injurious behaviors,[62,63] and borderline personality disorder,[64] three disorders where some evidence points to a role of the endogenous opioid system. While naltrexone does not treat any core etiology of autism, it can reduce characteristic hyperactivity, irritability, and self-injurious behaviors. Self-injurious behavior can be used to maintain a high level of endogenous opioids, either to prevent decreases in endorphins or to experience the euphoric effect of opioid stimulation following injury. In the study by Roth and co-workers,[62] the self-injurious behavior of six out of seven female patients ceased entirely during naltrexone therapy, with resumption of injurious behavior when the drug was withdrawn.

Nalmefene (Revex), introduced in 1996, is an injectable pure opioid antagonist with a half-life of about 8 to 10 hours, in contrast to the short half-life of naloxone. The drug is useful by injection for the treatment of acute opioid-induced respiratory depression caused by overdosage. With its long half-life, the incidence of "renarcotization" is greatly reduced. If administered to an addict, however, the precipitation of withdrawal can be prolonged and require additional medical treatment. Mason and co-workers[65] studied the effects of orally administered nalmefene* as an alternative to naltrexone in alcoholic patients (see Figure 4.9). Treatment for 12 weeks was effective in preventing relapse. The oral preparation is not yet available commercially.

Pharmacotherapy of Opioid Dependence

Opiate dependence is a brain-related medical disorder (characterized by predictable signs and symptoms) that can be effectively treated with

---

*Nalmefene is currently available only in injectable form. For this study, tablets of nalmefene were supplied by the manufacturer as an experimental preparation.

significant benefits for the patient and society, and society must make a commitment to offer effective treatment for opiate dependence to all who need it. All persons dependent on opiates should have access to methadone hydrochloride maintenance therapy under legal supervision, and the U.S. Office of National Drug Control Policy and the U.S. Department of Justice should take the necessary steps to implement this recommendation. . . . The unnecessary regulations of methadone maintenance therapy and other long-acting agonist treatment programs should be reduced and coverage for these programs should be a required benefit in public and private insurance programs.[66]

In any treatment of opioid dependence, pharmacotherapy is the foundation, involving more than use of methadone:

1. LAAM and/or buprenorphine for treatment-resistant individuals, or nonholders
2. Opioid antagonist therapy for individuals for whom it is more appropriate than agonist therapy
3. Treatment of comorbid disorders, especially affective disorders such as depression: "Comorbid psychiatric disorders require treatment."[66]

In addition to appropriate pharmacotherapy, "nonpharmacologic supportive services are pivotal to successful methadone maintenance therapy."[66] Both are needed for success, but how much nonpharmacologic supportive service is optimal? Can there be too little? Can there be too much? Kraft and co-workers[67] determined that large amounts of support to methadone-maintained clients was not cost-effective, but moderate amounts of support are better than minimal amounts. They concluded that there is a floor below which supplementary support should not fall. Similarly, Avants and co-workers[68] reported that intensive day-treatment programs for unemployed, inner-city methadone patients cost twice as much and were no more effective than a program of enhanced methadone maintenance services, which consisted of standard methadone maintenance plus a weekly skills training group and referral to on-site and off-site services.

What about the duration of methadone maintenance? Should a goal be eventual withdrawal from methadone? While data are poor, it is felt that total abstinence from all opioids need not be an objective for all addicts. Goals, however, must include prevention of relapse to the use of illicitly obtained, injectable opioids (such as heroin). Continuing, medically managed, supportive opioid therapy may be necessary for many addicts, an approach that follows models of medical illness. Sees and co-workers[69] reported that continued methadone maintenance more effectively reduced heroin use and HIV risk behaviors than did detoxification supplemented with intensive psychosocial therapies.

Until very recently, the objective has been medically managed withdrawal to an opioid-free state. This can be successful in patients who are highly motivated to remain opioid-free. Examples include addicted medical personnel whose continued licensure to practice their profession is contingent on complete abstention from opioids. The supervised ingestion of naltrexone implies that an agonist opioid will be ineffective. In many addicts, however, naltrexone therapy is unacceptable, and continued opioid therapy is needed. For these, the benefits of maintenance therapy, including significant reductions in illicit opioid use, increases in treatment retention, and improved psychosocial functioning, have been clearly demonstrated within the methadone maintenance model. Under newly proposed regulations, U.S. physicians practicing outside traditional methadone clinics could prescribe methadone to patients with opioid dependence (they cannot do this now). Weinrich and Stuart[70] describe the Scottish experience with such a program.

Goldstein[10] reviewed more than 20 years of administering methadone maintenance therapy to 1000 heroin addicts in New Mexico. More than half of the patients were traced and analyzed. Of these, more than one-third are now dead; causes include violence, overdosage, and alcoholism. About one-quarter are still enmeshed in the criminal justice system. Another one-quarter go on and off methadone maintenance, indicating that opioid dependence, whether on heroin or on methadone, is a lifelong condition for a considerable fraction of the addict population. With half of the treated population of 1000 addicts unaccounted for, the data are obviously incomplete. It is likely that many of these unaccounted-for former addicts are either drug-free or are stabilized on an opioid and are functional in their communities. The successful graduates of therapy are the most difficult to track, usually preferring to remain anonymous in their communities.

Regardless, treatment of opioid dependence leads to a productive lifestyle in only a minority of cases. The most interesting data now support lifelong opioid maintenance (e.g., methadone) as a treatment possibility, with LAAM or buprenorphine maintenance or naltrexone treatment as options when necessary. When opioid-withdrawn individuals relapse, they must be readmitted to methadone (or LAAM) maintenance immediately and receive both adequate doses and the necessary supportive therapies. Unfortunately, many people still see physical dependence on an opioid as "bad" in and of itself. These attitudes must be changed before widespread attempts at long-term opioid maintenance can be fully evaluated.

STUDY QUESTIONS

1. Describe the location of opioid receptors in the brain and in the spinal cord.

2. How are pain impulses modulated as they enter the spinal cord?

3. What is substance P and how is it influenced by narcotic analgesics?

4. What might be the effects of the endorphins?

5. What is an opioid agonist? What is an opioid antagonist? What is a mixed agonist-antagonist? A partial agonist? Give an example of each.

6. What might lead a person to misuse or abuse opioids? What are the signs of opioid misuse/abuse?

7. Differentiate between naloxone and naltrexone. How might each be used?

8. Describe the various ways that opioid dependence might be handled or treated.

9. Why are tricyclic antidepressants analgesic?

10. Differentiate between the opioid modulation of afferent pain impulses and the affective component of pain.

11. Give your thoughts for and against the existence of endogenous opioid peptides (endorphins) that serve as natural opioids.

12. If a patient suffers from chronic pain, what two classes of drugs should be optimized before starting opioid therapy? If opioid therapy is started, how should the opioids be administered?

13. Differentiate the use of opioids in individuals with chronic, nonmalignant pain and in those with pain due to a terminal malignancy.

14. What is buprenorphine? What are its potential uses?

15. Discuss the various options in the pharmacological management of opioid withdrawal and in the prevention of relapse.

REFERENCES

1. L. S. Sorkin, "Basic Pharmacology and Physiology of Acute Pain Processing," *Anesthesiology Clinics of North America* 15 (1997): 235–249.
2. M. O. Urban and G. F. Gebhart, "Central Mechanisms in Pain," *Medical Clinics of North America* 83 (1999): 585–596.
3. T. L. Yaksh, "Spinal Systems and Pain Processing: Development of Novel Analgesic Drugs with Mechanistically Defined Models," *Trends in Pharmacological Sciences* 20 (1999): 329–337.

4. C. Zhang, M. F. Davies, T.-Z. Guo, and M. Maze, "The Analgesic Action of Nitrous Oxide Is Dependent on the Release of Norepinephrine in the Dorsal Horn of the Spinal Cord," *Anesthesiology* 91 (1999): 1401–1407.

5. H. Baba et al., "Norepinephrine Facilitates Inhibitory Transmission in Substantia Gelatinosa of Adult Rat Spinal Cord," *Anesthesiology* 92 (2000): 473–492.

6. D. A. Fishbain, "Approaches to Treatment Decisions for Psychiatric Comorbidity in the Management of the Chronic Pain Patient," *Medical Clinics of North America* 83 (1999): 737–757.

7. S. R. Savage, "Opioid Use in the Management of Chronic Pain," *Medical Clinics of North America* 83 (1999): 761–785.

8. G. ter Riet et al., "Is Placebo Analgesia Mediated by Endogenous Opioids? A Systematic Review," *Pain* 76 (1998): 273–275.

9. F. J. Spielman, "God's Own Medicine," *American Journal of Anesthesiology* 25 (1998): 43–44.

10. A. Goldstein, *Addiction: From Biology to Drug Policy* (New York: W. H. Freeman and Company, 1994).

11. H. Akil et al., "Endogenous Opioids: Overview and Current Issues," *Drug and Alcohol Dependence* 51 (1998): 127–140.

12. B. L. Kieffer, "Opioids: First Lessons from Knockout Mice," *Trends in Pharmacological Sciences* 20 (1999): 19–26.

13. Z. Z. Pan, "Mu-opposing Actions of the Kappa-opioid Receptor," *Trends in Pharmacological Sciences* 19 (1998): 94–98.

14. R. J. Knapp et al., "Molecular Biology and Pharmacology of Cloned Opioid Receptors," *Federation of the American Society for Experimental Biology (FASEB) Journal* 9 (1995): 516–525.

15. G. R. Uhl, S. Childers, and G. Pasternak, "An Opiate-receptor Gene Family Reunion," *Trends in Neurological Sciences* 17 (1994): 89–93.

16. H. B. Gutstein et al., "Opioid Effects on Mitogen-activated Protein Kinase Signaling Cascades," *Anesthesiology* 87 (1997): 1118–1126.

17. N. I. Cherny, "Opioid Analgesics: Comparative Features and Prescribing Guidelines," *Drugs* 51 (1996): 713–737.

18. P. M. Dougherty and P. S. Staats, "Intrathecal Drug Therapy for Chronic Pain: From Basic Science to Clinical Practice," *Anesthesiology* 91 (1999): 1891–1918.

19. M. S. Gold, "Opiate Addiction and the Locus Coeruleus: The Clinical Utility of Clonidine, Naltrexone, Methadone, and Buprenorphine," *Psychiatric Clinics of North America* 16 (1993): 65.

20. D. A. Mahler et al., "Beta-endorphin Activity and Hypercapnic Ventilatory Responsiveness After Marathon Running," *Journal of Applied Physiology* 66 (1989): 2431–2436.

21. M. Simonato, "The Neurochemistry of Morphine Addiction in the Neocortex," *Trends in Pharmacological Sciences* 17 (1996): 410–415.

22. T. S. Shippenberg, R. Bals-Kubik, and A. Herz, "Examination of the Neurochemical Substrates Mediating the Motivational Effects of Opioids: Role of the Mesolimbic Dopamine System and D-1 Versus D-2 Dopamine Receptors," *Journal of Pharmacology and Experimental Therapeutics* 265 (1993): 53–59.

23. C. J. Nelson, L. A. Dykstra, and D. T. Lysle, "Comparison of the Time Course of Morphine's Analgesic and Immunologic Effects," *Anesthesia and Analgesia* 85 (1997): 620–626.

24. E. K. Gies et al., "Regulation of Mu Opioid Receptor mRNA Levels by Activation of Protein Kinase C in Human SH-SY5Y Neuroblastoma Cells," *Anesthesiology* 87 (1997): 1127–1138.

25. E. Celerier et al., "Long-lasting Hyperalgesia Induced by Fentanyl in Rats: Preventive Effect of Ketamine," *Anesthesiology* 92 (2000): 465–472.

26. H. Zhu, R. W. Rockhold, and I. K. Ho, "The Role of Glutamate in Physical Dependence on Opioids," *Japanese Journal of Pharmacology* 76 (1998): 1–14.

27. C. N. Sang et al., "AMPA/Kainate Antagonist LY293558 Reduces Capsaicin-evoked Hyperalgesia but Not Pain in Normal Skin in Humans," *Anesthesiology* 89 (1998): 1060–1067.

28. Z. Wiesenfeld-Hallin, "Combined Opioid-NMDA Antagonist Therapies: What Advantages Do They Offer for the Control of Pain Syndromes?" *Drugs* 55 (1998): 1–4.

29. D. Christensen, G. Guilbaud, and V. Kayser, "Complete Prevention but Stimulus-dependent Reversion of Morphine Tolerance by the Glycine/NMDA Receptor Antagonist (+) -HA966 in Neuropathic Rats," *Anesthesiology* 92 (2000): 786–794.

30. T. Nishiyama, T. L. Yakish, and E. Weber, "Effects of Intrathecal NMDA and Non-NMDA Antagonists on Acute Thermal Nociception and Their Interaction with Morphine," *Anesthesiology* 89 (1998): 715–722.

31. J. H. Jaffe, C. M. Knapp, and D. A. Ciraulo, "Opiates: Clinical Aspects," in J. H. Lowinson, P. Ruiz, R. B. Millman, and J. G. Langrod, eds., *Substance Abuse: A Comprehensive Textbook*, 3rd ed. (Baltimore: Williams & Wilkins, 1997), 158–166.

32. M. J. Christie, J. T. Williams, P. B. Osborne, and C. E. Bellchambers, "Where's the Locus in Opioid Withdrawal?" *Trends in Pharmacological Sciences* 18 (1997): 134–140.

33. C. G. Gold et al., "Rapid Opioid Detoxification During General Anesthesia: A Review of 20 Patients," *Anesthesiology* 91 (1999): 1639–1647

34. P. Keinbaum et al., "Profound Increase in Epinephrine Plasma Concentration and Cardiovascular Stimulation Following Mu-opioid Receptor Blockade in Opioid-addicted Patients During Barbiturate Anesthesia for Acute Detoxification," *Anesthesiology* 88 (1998): 1154–1161.

35. R. E. Solomon and S. F. Markowitz, "Does Anesthesia Permanently Alter Brain Chemistry?" *Anesthesiology* 90 (1999): 329–330.

36. R. K. Brooner et al., "Psychiatric and Substance Abuse Comorbidity Among Treatment-seeking Opioid Abusers," *Archives of General Psychiatry* 54 (1997): 71–80.

37. E. V. Nunes et al., "Imipramine Treatment of Opiate-dependent Patients with Depressive Disorders," *Archives of General Psychiatry* 55 (1998): 153–160.

38. A. H. Oliveto et al., "Desipramine in Opioid-dependent Cocaine Abusers Maintained on Buprenorphine vs. Methadone," *Archives of General Psychiatry* 56 (1999): 812–820.

39. B. A. Sproule et al., "Characteristics of Dependent and Nondependent Regular Users of Codeine," *Journal of Clinical Psychopharmacology* 19 (1999): 367–372.

40. M. K. Romach et al., "Long-term Codeine Use Is Associated with Depressive Symptoms," *Journal of Clinical Psychopharmacology* 19 (1999): 373–376.

41. K. R. Dyer et al., "Steady-state Pharmacokinetics and Pharmacodynamics in Methadone Maintenance Patients: Comparison of Those Who Do and Do Not Experience Withdrawal and Concentration-effect Relationships," *Clinical Pharmacology and Therapeutics* 65 (1999): 685–694.

42. E. C. Strain, G. E. Bigelow, I. A. Liebson, and M. L. Stitzer, "Moderate- vs. High-dose Methadone in the Treatment of Opioid Dependence: A Randomized Trial," *Journal of the American Medical Association* 281 (1999): 1000–1005.

42A. K. L. Preston, A. Umbricht and D. H. Epstein, "Methadone Dose Increase and Abstinence Reinforcement for Treatment of Continued Heroin Use During Methadone Maintenance," *Archives of General Psychiatry* 57 (2000): 395–404.

43. T. Eissenberg et al., "Dose-related Efficacy of Levomethadyl Acetate for Treatment of Opioid Dependency," *Journal of the American Medical Association* 277 (1997): 1945–1951.

44. H. E. Jones et al., "Induction with Levomethadyl Acetate: Safety and Efficacy," *Archives of General Psychiatry* 55 (1998): 729–736.

45. L. E. Basskin, "Oral Transmucosal Fentanyl Citrate: A New Dosage Form for Breakthrough Malignant Pain," *American Journal of Pain Management* 9 (1999): 129–138.

46. P. W. H. Peng and A. N. Sandler, "A Review of the Use of Fentanyl Analgesia in the Management of Acute Pain in Adults," *Anesthesiology* 90 (1999): 576–599.

47. M. Black, J. L. Hill, and J. P. Zacny, "Behavioral and Physiological Effects of Remifentanil and Alfentanil in Healthy Volunteers," *Anesthesiology* 90 (1999): 718–726.

48. N. M. Petry, W. K. Bickel, and G. J. Badger, "A Comparison of Four Buprenorphine Dosing Regimens in the Treatment of Opioid Dependence," *Clinical Pharmacology and Therapeutics* 66 (1999): 306–314.

49. K. J. Schuh and C.-E. Johanson, "Pharmacokinetic Comparison of the Buprenorphine Sublingual Liquid and Tablet," *Drug and Alcohol Dependence* 56 (1999): 55–60.

50. R. S. Schottenfeld et al., "Buprenorphine vs. Methadone Maintenance Treatment for Concurrent Opioid Dependence and Cocaine Abuse," *Archives of General Psychiatry* 54 (1997): 713–720.

51. R. E. Johnson et al., "First Randomized Controlled Trial of Methadone, Levomethadyl Acetate (LAAM), and Buprenorphine in Opioid Dependence Treatment," *Clinical Pharmacology and Therapeutics* 65 (1999): 145.

52. A. Umbricht et al., "Naltrexone-shortened Opioid Detoxification with Buprenorphine," *Drug and Alcohol Dependence* 56 (1999): 181–190.

53. D. Franceschini, M. Lipartiti, and P. Giusti, "Effect of Acute and Chronic Tramadol on [^{3}H]-norepinephrine Uptake in Rat Cortical Synaptosomes," *Progress in Neuro-Psychopharmacology and Biological Psychiatry* 23 (1999): 485–496.

54. M. Gobbi and T. Mennini, "Release Studies with Rat Brain Cortical Synaptosomes Indicate that Tramadol is a 5-Hydroxytryptamine Uptake Blocker and Not a 5-Hydroxytryptamine Releaser," *European Journal of Pharmacology* 370 (1999): 23–26.

55. J. S. Markowitz and K. S. Patrick, "Venlafaxine-tramadol Similarities," *Medical Hypotheses* 51 (1998): 167–168.
56. L. L. Norton and M. J. Ferrill, "Tramadol: Establishing a Place in Therapy," *American Journal of Pain Management* 6 (1996): 42–50
57. M. Naguib et al., "Perioperative Antinociceptive Effects of Tranadol. A Prospective, Randomized, Double-blind Comparison with Morphine," *Canadian Journal of Anaesthesia* 45 (1998): 1168–1175.
58. R. M. Weinreib and C. P. O Brien, "Naltrexone in the Treatment of Alcoholism," *Annual Review of Medicine* 48 (1997): 477–487.
59. R. F. Anton et al., "Naltrexone and Cognitive Behavioral Therapy for the Treatment of Outpatient Alcoholics: Results of a Placebo-controlled Trial," *American Journal of Psychiatry* 156 (1999): 1758–1764.
60. M. Campbell, "Resolved: Autistic Children Should Have a Trial of Naltrexone," *Journal of the American Academy of Child and Adolescent Psychiatry* 35 (1996): 246–250.
61. S. H. Willemsen-Swinkels, J. K. Buitelaar, F. G. Weijnen, and H. Van Engeland, "Placebo-controlled Acute Dosage Naltrexone Study in Young Autistic Children," *Psychiatry Research* 58 (1995): 203–215.
62. A. S. Roth, R. B. Ostroff, and R. E. Hoffman, "Naltrexone as a Treatment for Repetitive Self-injurious Behavior: An Open-label Trial," *Journal of Clinical Psychiatry* 57 (1996): 233–237.
63. J. A. Casner, B. Weinheimer, and C. T. Gualtieri, "Naltrexone and Self-injurious Behavior: A Retrospective Population Study," *Journal of Clinical Psychopharmacology* 16 (1996): 389–394.
64. M. J. Bohus et al., "Naltrexone in the Treatment of Dissociative Symptoms in Patients with Borderline Personality Disorder: An Open-label Trial," *Journal of Clinical Psychiatry* 60 (1999): 598–603.
65. B. J. Mason et al., "A Double-blind, Placebo-controlled Study of Oral Nalmefene for Alcohol Dependence," *Archives of General Psychiatry* 56 (1999): 719–724.
66. National Consensus Development Panel on Effective Management of Opiate Addiction, "Effective Medical Treatment of Opiate Addiction," *Journal of the American Medical Association* 280 (1998): 1936–1943.
67. M. K. Kraft et al., "Are Supplementary Services Provided During Methadone Maintenance Really Cost-effective?" *American Journal of Psychiatry* 154 (1997): 1214–1219.
68. S. K. Avants et al., "Day Treatment Versus Enhanced Standard Methadone Services for Opioid-dependent Patients: A Comparison of Clinical Efficacy and Cost," *American Journal of Psychiatry* 156 (1999): 27–33.
69. K. L. Sees et al., "Methadone Maintenance vs 180-Day Psychosocially Enriched Detoxification for Treatment of Opioid Dependence: A Randomized Controlled Trial," *Journal of the American Medical Association* 283 (2000): 1303–1310.
70. M. Weinrich and M. Stuart, "Provision of Methadone Treatment in Primary Care Medical Practices: Review of the Scottish Experience and Implications for U.S. Policy," *Journal of the American Medical Association* 283 (2000): 1343–1348.

Nonnarcotic, Anti-inflammatory Analgesics

There are two classes of analgesic (pain-relieving) drugs. The first consists of the centrally acting opioid analgesics, such as morphine (Chapter 9). The second consists of peripherally acting analgesics, such as aspirin, ibuprofen (Advil, Motrin), acetaminophen (Tylenol), celecoxib (Celebrex), rofecoxib (Vioxx), and many others. All are considered in the general classification *nonsteroidal analgesic, anti-inflammatory agents* or NSAIDs. These drugs act at the local (peripheral) site of tissue injury to reduce pain and inflammation by interfering with the synthesis of prostaglandin hormones. The nonopioid NSAID-type analgesics are a group of chemically unrelated drugs (Figure 10.1) that produce both analgesic and anti-inflammatory effects.[1] They block the generation of peripheral pain impulses by inhibiting the synthesis and release of chemical mediators called *prostaglandins*. NSAIDs do not bind to opioid receptors.

Prostaglandins are body hormones that perform a variety of functions including the production of local inflammatory responses. NSAIDs inhibit the enzyme cyclooxygenase. *Cyclooxygenase* (also called *prostaglandin synthetase*) functions to convert a precursor substance (arachidonic acid) to prostaglandins.* There are two isomeric forms

---

*Studies suggest that the inhibition of prostaglandin synthesis is only part of aspirin's action;[3] the local anti-inflammatory action also results from aspirin's ability to disrupt white blood cell responsiveness to tissue injury, thus preventing the cellular release of tissue-disruptive enzymes.

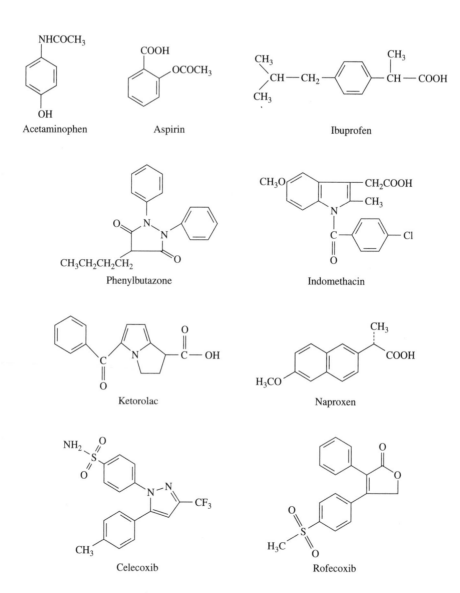

FIGURE 10.1 Structural formulas of representative anti-inflammatory analgesics.

of cyclooxygenase, COX-1 and COX-2. COX-1 primarily functions to mediate the production of prostaglandins that protect and regulate cell function in the gastrointestinal (GI) tract and in blood platelets, during normal physiologic conditions. Among other things, this allows normal platelet function as initiators of blood clotting. COX-2 has fewer roles under normal conditions; however, in response to stressors such as inflammation, COX-2 is markedly induced by chemical mediators associated with inflammation.[2] Such induction by immune or inflammatory stimuli leads to the production of prostaglandins that mediate inflammation and pain. Immune instigators include such autoimmune diseases as osteoarthritis and rheumatoid arthritis, for which antiinflammatory drugs are so effective therapeutically.

Most NSAIDs nonselectively inhibit the cyclooxygenase enzyme (both COX-1 and COX-2). Therefore, they would be expected to affect the GI tract and platelet function, as well as reducing the inflammatory response. Three newer drugs, celecoxib (Celebrex), rofecoxib (Vioxx), and meloxicam, are selective inhibitors of the COX-2 enzyme at therapeutic concentrations. They do not inhibit the COX-1 enzyme, so they would be expected to have less effect on the GI tract and on platelet function.

The effects of anti-inflammatory analgesic drugs include the following:

- Reduction of inflammation (an anti-inflammatory effect)
- Reduction in body temperature when the patient has a fever (an antipyretic effect)
- Reduction of pain without sedation (an analgesic effect)
- Inhibition of platelet aggregation (an anticoagulant effect)

The prototype NSAID is *aspirin*; hence all similar drugs can be referred to as aspirin-like drugs. The term "NSAID" does not describe their full spectrum of effects (at least until one understands what that spectrum encompasses). These drugs are widely used (and are quite irreplaceable) to reduce both the inflammation and the pain associated with the various forms of arthritis. Gastric irritation tends to limit their long-term usefulness.

The prototype selective COX-2 inhibitor is *celecoxib* (Celebrex). COX-2 inhibitors have become wildly popular for the treatment of various forms of arthritis, largely because of their heavy promotion both to physicians and directly to patients through the mass media. Other, more rarely used NSAIDs available in the United States include *mefenamic acid* (Ponstel), *meclofenamate sodium* (Meclomen), *tolmetin* (Tolectin), *diclofenac* (Voltaren, Cataflam), *piroxicam* (Feldene), and *nabumetone* (Relafen). These drugs are primarily used in the treatment of arthritis.

Nonselective Cyclooxygenase Inhibitors

Aspirin

In the United States, between 10,000 and 20,000 tons of aspirin are consumed each year.[1] Aspirin is the most popular and most effective analgesic, antipyretic, and anti-inflammatory drug. Because it is a nonselective COX-inhibitor, aspirin is an inhibitor of both COX-1 and COX-2. It therefore exerts effects on inflammation, on blood platelets, and on the GI tract.

As an analgesic, aspirin is most effective for low-intensity pain, as increased doses rapidly reach a ceiling beyond which additional drug provides no more analgesia than do lower doses (all NSAIDs demonstrate this ceiling effect against pain). The ceiling is reached with doses of between about 650 mg and 1300 mg.

Aspirin's antipyretic (fever-lowering) effect follows the inhibition of prostaglandin synthesis in the hypothalamus, a structure in the brain that modulates body temperature. However, one caution is necessary regarding the use of aspirin to reduce fever in children. An association exists between the use of aspirin for the fever that accompanies varicella (chicken pox) or influenza and the subsequent development of Reye's syndrome, including severe liver and brain damage and even death.[3] Therefore, in children, aspirin use is precluded for the treatment of virus-induced febrile illness.[1]

Aspirin exerts important effects on blood coagulation. For blood to coagulate, platelets* must first be able to aggregate, an action requiring the presence of prostaglandins. Aspirin binds to blood platelets, irreversibly inhibiting their function for the 8- to 10-day lifetime of the platelet. This results in inhibition of hemostasis, reducing the tendency for blood to clot.[4] In daily low doses (1/2 tablet), aspirin is used to prevent blood from clotting in diseased coronary arteries, reducing the risks of a stroke or a heart attack.

Aspirin increases oxygen consumption by the body, which increases the production of carbon dioxide, an effect that stimulates respiration. Therefore, an overdose of aspirin is often characterized by a marked increase in respiratory rate, which causes the overdosed person to appear to pant. This occurrence results in other severe metabolic consequences that are beyond this discussion.

Side effects of aspirin are common. First, gastric upset occurs frequently and can range from mild upset and heartburn to severe, destructive ulcerations and bleeding of the stomach or upper intestine. Second, poisoning due to aspirin overdosage is not infrequent and can be fatal. Third, mild intoxication can produce ringing in the ears, auditory and visual difficulties, mental confusion, thirst, and hyperventilation. Fourth, in aspirin-sensitive individuals, a single dose of aspirin can precipitate an asthma attack.

---

*Platelets are small components of the blood that adhere to vascular membranes after injury to a vessel. They form an initial plug, over which a blood clot eventually forms to limit bleeding from a lacerated blood vessel.

Acetaminophen

Acetaminophen (Tylenol) is an effective alternative to aspirin both as an analgesic and as an antipyretic agent:

> Acetaminophen is as effective as aspirin, similar in potency and, in single analgesic doses, has the same time-effect curve, but does not have the adverse effects characteristic of aspirin.[4]

Unlike that of aspirin, acetaminophen's anti-inflammatory effect is minor, and the drug is not clinically useful in treating either acute inflammation or chronic arthritis.[1] Also, because acetaminophen does not inhibit platelet aggregation, it is not useful for preventing vascular clotting or for prophylaxis against heart attacks or stroke. No reports have associated acetaminophen with Reye's syndrome; therefore, it has an improved margin of safety in children.

It should be noted that an acute overdose (either accidental or intentional) may produce severe or even fatal liver damage. Alcoholics appear to be especially susceptible to the hepatotoxic effects of even moderate doses of acetaminophen. Indeed, alcoholics should avoid acetaminophen while they persist in heavy consumption of alcohol.

Acetaminophen generally produces less gastric distress and less ringing in the ears. It has been proven to be a reasonable substitute for aspirin when analgesic or antipyretic effectiveness is desired, especially in children and in patients who cannot tolerate aspirin.

Ibuprofen and Related Drugs

Ibuprofen, ketoprofen (Orudis), and phenoprofen (Nalfon) exert aspirin-like analgesic, antipyretic, and anti-inflammatory effects (Table 10.1). These agents are often better tolerated than aspirin. Their effectiveness is comparable to or greater than that of acetaminophen, aspirin, codeine, aspirin with codeine, and propoxyphene.[2] Like other NSAIDs, their actions result from drug-induced inhibition of prostaglandin synthesis. The incidence and severity of side effects produced by these agents are somewhat lower than those of aspirin, but gastric distress and the formation of peptic ulcers have occasionally been reported. Like aspirin (but unlike acetaminophen), these compounds inhibit platelet aggregation and therefore interfere with the clotting process. These drugs should be used with caution in patients who suffer from peptic ulcer disease or bleeding abnormalities. Ibuprofen and related drugs are not recommended for use by pregnant women. They are not secreted in breast milk.

FDA-approved indications for ibuprofen and related drugs include use as analgesics and use in the symptomatic treatment of various forms of arthritis, tendinitis, bursitis, and for dysmenorrhea (painful menstrual cramps). The anti-inflammatory effect is comparable to that

TABLE I0.1 Ibuprofen and related drugs: Available formulations and recommendations for anti-inflammatory therapy

Nonproprietary name	Trade name	Formulation	Usual anti-inflammatory dose
Ibuprofen	Motrin, Advil, Nuprin, Medipren	Tablets	400 mg, three to four times a day
Naproxen	Naprosyn, Aleve, Anaprox	Tablets, suspension	250–500 mg, twice a day
Fenoprofen	Nalfon	Tablets, capsules	300–600 mg, three to four times a day
Ketoprofen	Orudis, Oravail	Capsules	150–300 mg, two to four times a day
Flurbiprofen	Ansaid, others	Tablets	50–75 mg, two to four times a day
Oxaprozin	Daypro	Tablets	600–1200 mg, once a day
Mefenamic acid	Ponstel	Tablets	250 mg, three to four times a day
Celecoxib	Celebrex	Capsules	100 mg, twice a day
Rofecoxib	Vioxx	Tablets, suspension	12.5–25 mg, once a day

of aspirin. The generally lower level of gastrointestinal side effects must be measured against the generally greater expense of these drugs.

Phenylbutazone

Phenylbutazone (Butazolidin) is an older effective anti-inflammatory agent (available since 1949) that was once widely used to relieve the inflammation associated with rheumatoid arthritis. However, significant serious side effects limit its long-term usefulness. Most patients who take phenylbutazone experience gastric distress and skin rashes. More severe problems include ulcer formation, allergies, liver and renal dysfunction, and a variety of severe abnormalities in various types of blood cells.

Unlike most of the other NSAIDs, the half-life of phenylbutazone is quite long (about 2 days). At present, phenylbutazone is considered to be a distant choice for clinical use.

Indomethacin, Sulindac, and Etodolac

Indomethacin (Indocin), available since 1963, is an effective anti-inflammatory drug that is used primarily for treating rheumatoid arthritis and similar disorders. Like phenylbutazone, its use is limited because of its toxicity. Indomethacin is an analgesic, antipyretic, and anti-inflammatory agent. Its clinical effects closely resemble those of aspirin. Side effects occur in about 50 percent of the patients who take indomethacin; gastric dysfunction is the most prominent. Paradoxically, drug-induced headache limits its use in about 50 percent of patients. Other side effects are rare but potentially serious.

Sulindac (Clinoril) and *etodolac* (Lodine) are two newer NSAIDs that are structurally and pharmacologically related to indomethacin. Sulindac is itself inactive, but its metabolite (sulindac sulfide) is very active. Its efficacy is comparable to that of indomethacin but perhaps with a lower level of gastrointestinal toxicities (less than indomethacin, but greater than many other NSAIDs). Etodolac is an effective analgesic and anti-inflammatory drug. Its side effects, which include skin rashes, headache, and gastrointestinal irritation and ulceration, appear to be fewer than those caused by many other NSAIDs.

Ketorolac

Ketorolac (Toradol) is a newer analgesic and anti-inflammatory agent; it is the first NSAID available in injectable form for use in the treatment of postsurgical pain. Administered either intramuscularly or intravenously, it is effective in the short-term treatment of moderate to severe pain.[5,6] Because it does not produce the accompanying "rush" or pleasure associated with intravenous opioid use, ketorolac is not a drug of abuse. Like the other NSAIDs, ketorolac indirectly inhibits prostaglandin synthesis. Its analgesic potency is comparable to that of low doses of morphine, and it offers an anti-inflammatory action not offered by morphine. Its concomitant use with morphine offers synergistic action, reducing the required analgesic dose of morphine by about 50 percent. The half-life of ketorolac is about 4 to 6 hours in most persons, but it is longer in the elderly. Ketorolac is not recommended for use in obstetrics, because it and all other inhibitors of prostaglandin synthesis can adversely affect uterine contraction and fetal circulation.

Side effects of ketorolac include excessive bleeding (due to platelet inhibition) and renal failure; the latter is minimized by limiting the use of the drug to 24 to 48 hours after surgery. Available also in tablet form for oral use, analgesic efficacy differs little from other orally administered NSAIDs.

Bromfenac

Bromfenac (Duract) was introduced into the United States in 1997 as an orally administered NSAID intended for the short-term treatment of pain. It was not indicated for the long-term treatment of pain and inflammation associated with rheumatoid or osteoarthritis. Hepatotoxicity was noted to develop with courses of therapy longer than about 10 days. Like all NSAIDs, there was a risk of GI effects, including bleeding and ulceration or perforation of the stomach or intestine. Because of a high incidence of idiosyncratic liver toxicity (some cases of which required liver transplantation[7]), it was withdrawn from sale in 1999 pending investigation of these adverse events.[8]

Selective COX-2 Inhibitors

Only since the mid- to late-1990s have the roles of cyclooxygenase enzymes in health and disease begun to be understood, in particular, the role of inducible COX-2 in inflammation.[9,10] In addition, a possible role in the prevention of cancers of the colon is being identified.[11] To date, two selective COX-2 inhibitors have been marketed for use as anti-inflammatory and analgesic compounds, and others, including meloxicam,[12] are under study. They have not been approved for the treatment or prevention of cancer.

Celecoxib (Celebrex) was released in 1998 as the first COX-2 inhibitor. In industry-sponsored clinical trials, it has been shown to be as effective as aspirin in reducing the pain and inflammation of rheumatoid arthritis and osteoarthritis, without the gastrointestinal toxicity and platelet blockade produced by aspirin.[13,14] Therefore, it may have equal efficacy but lower acute toxicity than does aspirin. Conversely, it has no use in the prevention of clotting afforded by aspirin in patients with coronary artery disease. Interestingly, preliminary studies have demonstrated efficacy against both skin cancer[15] and colon cancers.[16] This antitumor action is exerted in the colon and probably involves "a mechanism involving the inhibition of cyclooxygenase-2 which is overexpressed in malignant adenomatous polyps and colon cancer."[16] In skin cancers, ultraviolet light induces COX-2, which may be involved in carcinogenesis; NSAIDs decrease this tumorigenic effect of ultraviolet light.[15]

Celecoxib is well absorbed orally, reaches peak blood level in three hours, and has a half-life of about 11 hours. It inhibits the activity of CYP2D6, and some drug interactions can be predicted, even with psychotropics such as antidepressants and antipsychotic agents. Abdominal pain, diarrhea, and gastric upset have been reported; however, the incidence of drug-induced gastric ulcerations approaches placebo levels, much lower than that seen with naproxen. Celcoxib does not prolong bleeding time and therefore does not appear to interact with blood platelets. Time will be required to determine the place of this drug in therapy.[18] The drug is not recommended in pregnancy and should be avoided in the third trimester of pregnancy.

Rofecoxib (Vioxx) is the second and newest COX-2 inhibitor introduced into medicine.[2] It is approved for the treatment of osteoarthritis, acute pain, and menstrual pain.[19] It is fairly rapidly absorbed orally, reaches peak plasma levels in about 3 hours, is metabolized before excretion, and has a half-life of about 17 hours. Clinical trials comparing this drug to celecoxib are as yet unavailable. It appears to be as effective as the traditional nonselective COX inhibitors.[19] In addition to its analgesic and anti-inflammatory effects, COX-2 inhibition appears to underlie the antipyretic effect of NSAIDs. To demonstrate this, Schwartz and colleagues[20] showed that rofecoxib reduces fever as well as diclofenac (a nonselective COX inhibitor). Thus, it is the COX-2 isoform of the COX enzyme that "is primarily involved in the genesis of fever in humans."

The usual side effects and toxicities of NSAIDs are reported: nausea, diarrhea, abdominal pain, and dyspepsia. Some GI toxicities are reported, but the incidence is less than that with aspirin and other NSAIDs[21] but more than with placebo. Wolfe and colleagues[22] reviewed the GI toxicities of all the NSAIDs, both those that are aspirin-like and those that are selective COX-2 inhibitors. Reviewing rofecoxib, the *Medical Letter*[19] concludes:

> How rofecoxib compares with celecoxib and whether either of these drugs with long-term use will cause less serious gastrointestinal bleeding than older NSAIDs remains to be established.

Like celecoxib, the drug should probably be avoided during pregnancy. A symposium on clinically available and experimental COX-2 inhibors was published in 1999.[23]

Advances beyond COX-2 inhibition are being explored. An interesting example is a class of *nitroaspirins* that release both aspirin and nitric oxide, are safe to the intestine, and yet retain aspirin's analgesic, antipyretic, and antiplatelet effects.[24] The released nitric oxide is protective to the gastrointestinal mucosa and offsets the adverse effects of COX-1 inhibition.[24]

STUDY QUESTIONS

1. What is an *NSAID*? What does this term mean?

2. List the various actions of aspirin. How might each be used therapeutically? Which might present clinical problems?

3. What is meant by the term *COX inhibitor*?

4. Differentiate between COX-1 and COX-2.

5. How is the anticoagulant action of aspirin "good"? How is it "bad"?

6. Describe the theoretical advantages of COX-2 inhibitors over NSAIDs (nonselective COX-inhibitors).

7. What is the correlation between COX enzyme and tumorigenesis? How might COX inhibitors be of benefit?

REFERENCES

1. P. A. Insel, "Analgesic-antipyretic and Anti-inflammatory Agents and Drugs Employed in the Treatment of Gout," in J. G. Hardman, L. E. Limbird, P. B. Molinoff, R. W. Ruddon, and A. G. Gilman, eds., *Goodman and Gilman's The Pharmacological Basis of Therapeutics*, 9th ed. (New York: McGraw-Hill, 1996), 617–657.

2. E. W. Ehrich et al., "Characterization of Rofecoxib as a Cyclooxygenase-2 Isoform Inhibitor and Demonstration of Analgesia in the Dental Pain Model," *Clinical Pharmacology and Therapeutics* 65 (1999): 336–347.

3. P. Pinsky, E. S. Hurwitz, L. B. Schonberger, and W. J. Gunn, "Reye's Syndrome and Aspirin: Evidence for a Dose-response Effect," *Journal of the American Medical Association* 260 (1988): 657–661.

4. "Drugs for Pain," *Medical Letter on Drugs and Therapeutics* 40 (August 14, 1998): 79–84.

5. M.-T. Buckley and R. N. Brogden, "Ketorolac: Review of Its Pharmacodynamic and Pharmacokinetic Properties, and Therapeutic Potential," *Drugs* 39 (1990): 86–109.

6. J. C. Gillis and R. N. Brogden, "Ketorolac: A Reappraisal of Its Pharmacodynamic and Pharmacokinetic Properties and Therapeutic Use in Pain Management," *Drugs* 53 (1997): 139–188.

7. E. B. Hunter et al., "Bromfenac (Duract)-associated Hepatic Failure Requiring Liver Transplantation," *American Journal of Gastroenterology* 94 (1999): 2299–2301.

8. N. M. Skjodt and N. M. Davies, "Clinical Pharmacokinetics and Pharmacodynamics of Bromfenac," *Clinical Pharmacokinetics* 36 (1999): 399–408.

9. M. K. O'Banion, "Cyclooxygenase-2: Molecular Biology, Pharmacology, and Neurobiology," *Critical Reviews in Neurobiology* 13 (1999): 45–82.

10. L. J. Marnett and A. S. Kalgutkar, "Cyclooxygenase-2 Inhibitors: Discovery, Selectivity, and the Future," *Trends in Pharmacological Sciences* 20 (1999): 465–469.

11. M. M. Taketo, "Cyclooxygenase-2 Inhibitors in Tumorigenesis," *Journal of the National Cancer Institute* 90 (1998): 1529–1536.

12. D. E. Baker, "Melaxicam: A New COX-2 Seletive Agent," *American Journal of Pain Management* 10 (2000): 14–24.

13. G. S. Geis, "Update on Clinical Developments with Celecoxib, a New, Specific COX-2 Inhibitor: What Can We Expect?" *Journal of Rheumatology* 56, Suppl. 26 (1999): 31–36.

14. J. Fort, "Celecoxib, a COX-2-specific Inhibitor: The Clinical Data," *American Journal of Orthopedics* 28, Suppl. 3 (1999): 13–18.

15. S. M. Fischer et al., "Chemoprotective Activity of Celecoxib, a Specific Cycooxygenase-2 Inhibitor, and Indomethacin Against Ultraviolet Light-induced Skin Carcinogenesis," *Molecular Carcinogenesis* 25 (1999): 231–240.

16. T. Kawamori, C. V. Rao, K. Seibert, and B. S. Reddy, "Chemoprotective Activity of Celecoxib, a Specific Cycooxygenase-2 Inhibitor, Against Colon Carcinogenesis," *Cancer Research* 58 (1998): 409–412.

17. L. S. Simon et al., "Anti-inflammatory and Upper Gastrointestinal Effects of Celecoxib in Rheumatoid Arthritis: A Ranomized Controlled Trial," *Journal of the American Medical Association* 282 (1999): 1921–1928.

18. W. L. Peterson and B. Cryer, "COX-1-sparing NSAIDs: Is the Enthusiasm Justified?" *Journal of the American Medical Association* 282 (1999): 1961–1963.

19. "Rofecoxib for Osteoarthritis and Pain," *Medical Letter on Drugs and Therapeutics* 41 (July 2, 1999): 59–61.

20. J. I. Schwartz et al., "Cycooxygenase-2 Inhibition by Rofecoxib Reverses Naturally Occurring Fever in Humans," *Clinical Pharmacology and Therapeutics* 65 (1999): 653–660.

21. M. J. Langman et al., "Adverse Upper Gastrointestinal Effects of Rofecoxib Compared with NSAIDs," *Journal of the American Medical Association* 282 (1999): 1929–1933.

22. M. M. Wolfe, D. R. Lichtenstein, and G. Singh, "Gastrointestinal Toxicity of Nonsteroidal Antiinflammatory Drugs," *New England Journal of Medicine* 340 (1999): 1888–1899.

23. R. H. Hunt, "Rationalizing Cyclooxygenase Inhibition for Optimization of Efficacy and Safety Profiles: Proceedings of a Symposium," *American Journal of Medicine* 107, Suppl. 6A (December 13, 1999): 1S–60S.

24. P. del Soldato, R. Sorrentino, and A. Pinto, "No-aspirins: A Class of New Antiinflammatory and Antithrombotic Agents," *Trends in Pharmacological Sciences* 20 (1999): 319–323.

Drugs That Possess Hallucinogenic or Psychedelic Properties

Chapters 11 and 12 focus on drugs whose actions are characterized primarily by alterations in cortical functions, including cognition, perception, and mood. These alterations occur as the drugs' primary psychobiological actions in the presence of an otherwise clear sensoria.

In the 1990s, much was learned about the mechanisms of action of these drugs. This knowledge allows not only description of the physical and mental effects of these drugs but interpretation of their effects in terms of receptor mechanisms. For example, until recently tetrahydrocannabinol (THC; Chapter 11) was classified as a somewhat unusual sedative-hypnotic drug. Now, with understanding of its actions on specific receptors in the CNS, THC can be classified as an anandamide partial agonist. Isolation of these receptors has allowed for development of numerous synthetic agonists and even of an antagonist. Such drugs contribute mightily to our understanding of THC's actions as well as offering the potential for improved therapeutic utility of drugs that act on anandamide receptors.

The pharmacology of the psychedelic drugs is presented in Chapter 12. Several naturally occurring psychedelics are discussed (for example, mescaline and psilocybin) as well as a variety of "designer" psychedelics including NMDA ("ecstacy"). Also discussed is the pharmacology of phencyclidine and ketamine: two dissociative psychedelics that also serve as model drugs for investigations into the psychobiology of schizophrenia. (The pathophysiology of schizophrenia in discussed in Chapter 17).

Chapter 11

Tetrahydrocannabinol

The hemp plant *Cannabis sativa*, commonly called marijuana, grows throughout the world and flourishes in most temperate and tropical regions. The major psychoactive ingredient of the marijuana plant is *delta-9-tetrahydrocannabinol* (THC), with *cannaninol* and *cannabidiol* present in lesser amounts. These three ingredients, as well as newly developed synthetic *cannabinoids*, produce the characteristic motor, cognitive, psychedelic, and analgesic effects that are described in this chapter. Names for *Cannabis* products include marijuana, hashish, charas, bhang, ganja, and sinsemilla. *Hashish* and *charas*, which consist of the dried resinous exudate of the female flowers, are the most potent preparations, with a THC content averaging between 10 and 20 percent. *Ganja* and *sinsemilla* refer to the dried material found in the tops of the female plants, where the THC content averages about 5 to 8 percent. *Bhang* and *marijuana* are lower-grade preparations taken from the dried remainder of the plant, and their THC content varies between 2 to 5 percent.

Until about 1990, marijuana was classified according to its behavioral effects, usually as a mild sedative-hypnotic agent, with effects similar to low doses of alcohol and the benzodiazepines. Unlike sedatives, however, higher doses of THC do not depress respiration and are not lethal. Also, little cross-tolerance occurs between THC and the sedative-hypnotics. THC also produces a unique spectrum of pharmacologic effects, including disruption in attention mechanisms, impairment of short-term memory, altered sensory awareness, analgesia, altered control of motor movements and postural control, and a possible immunosuppressive action.[1,2] This spectrum of action has led to possible uses in the treatment of various symptoms associated with disorders ranging from multiple sclerosis to AIDS to terminal cancer.

The chemical structure of THC is unique, resembling that of neither the sedatives nor the psychedelics (Figure 11.1). There is now conclusive evidence that THC binds to specific *cannabinoid receptors* and mimics the actions of endogenous cannabinoids, which exert important biological effects of their own. In addition, cannabinoid receptors exist in the brain at levels higher than most other G-protein-coupled receptors, approaching or exceeding levels observed for the amino acid receptors glutamate and GABA.[1,3]

History

The use of *Cannabis sativa* dates from several thousand years B.C. (Figure 11.2), when it was used as a mild intoxicant, somewhat milder than alcohol. It is much less useful for religious and psychedelic experiences than naturally occurring psychedelic drugs because it produces much less sensory distortion. Over the years, products from *Cannabis sativa* have been claimed to have a wide variety of medical uses, although few persist in native cultures.

Cannabis sativa is rather new to Western culture; it probably was introduced in the 1850s. During the early 1920s, marijuana was portrayed as being evil, part of underground activities, and a menace. Claiming that an association existed between marijuana and crime, laws were passed to outlaw its use. By the mid-1930s, marijuana was looked on as a "narcotic" and as a drug responsible for crimes of violence. By 1940 the public was convinced that marijuana was a "killer drug" that (1) induced people to commit crimes of violence, (2) led to heroin addiction, and (3) was a great social menace. The emotional campaign against marijuana continued, and to some degree it persists today. Disquieting is the fact that, like alcohol, marijuana is widely used by youth and is part of the culture of many individuals under the age of 21 years. In 1997, approximately 35 percent of U.S. high school

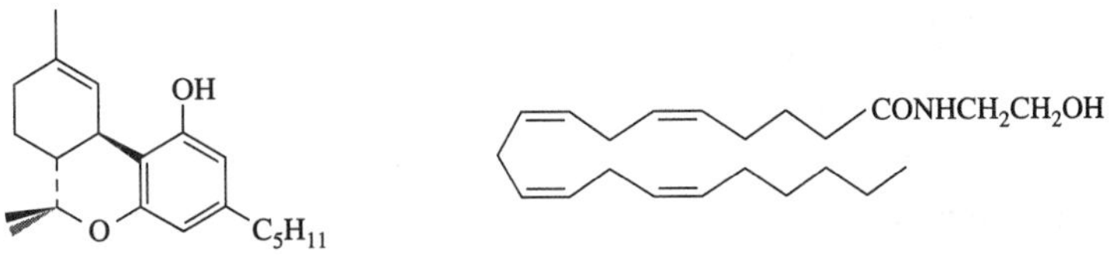

FIGURE 11.1 Structures of delta-9-tetrahydrocannabinol (THC) and anandamide, the endogenous ligand (neurotransmitter) of the cannabinoid receptor.

A. The ancient world to the present

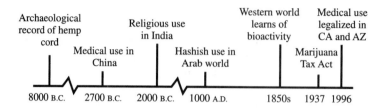

B. *Cannabis* research developments

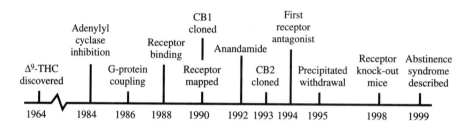

FIGURE 11.2 Two timelines of marijuana history. **A.** Brief history of cannabis use throughout the world. **B.** Advances in research into actions of cannabis. [Modified from Childers and Breivogel.[1]]

seniors reported having used marijuana at least once in the preceding 12 months; daily use was estimated at 4.6 percent of these students.

Since 1996, voters in several states have approved ballot initiatives to permit the legal use of marijuana for purported medical purposes (Figure 11.2). Approval of these initiatives signaled the first time since the repeal of Prohibition some 70 years ago that the public has approved a pullback in the "war on drugs." But medical efficacy of marijuana is controversial; no double-blind studies have compared the relative efficacy of marijuana to any drug of proven efficacy. Passage of these initiatives thus raises several issues:

- Should marijuana (or the active drug THC) be made available for *medical use* throughout the United States, and for what medical uses is THC (or crude marijuana) efficacious?

- Should marijuana (or the active drug THC) be made available for *recreational use by adults* in the United States?

- How should society deal with the use of marijuana (or the active drug THC) as well as ethyl alcohol by those under the age of 21 years?

Mechanism of Action: The Cannabinoid Receptor

THC was isolated from marijuana as its pharmacologically active ingredient (Figure 11.2) in 1964. Evidence gathered from then until the mid-1980s led to the hypothesis that THC and other cannabinoids act via a pharmacologically distinct set of receptors. In 1986 Howlett and co-workers[4] demonstrated that THC inhibits the intracellular enzyme *adenylate cyclase*, and that the inhibition requires the presence of a G-protein complex, similar to the opioid receptors discussed in Chapter 9. In about 1990, it was shown that THC does not directly inhibit adenylate cyclase;[5] rather, it acts on a specific receptor in such a way that the enzyme is ultimately inhibited.

In 1990 Matsuda and co-workers[6] isolated the receptor and cloned it. They found that it was a specific G-protein–coupled receptor that both inhibited adenylate cyclase and bound cannabinoids. Today, we know that cannabinoid receptors are primarily found on presynaptic nerve terminals and act to inhibit calcium ion flux and facilitate potassium channels.[1,2,7] As a result, stimulation of cannabinoid receptors inhibits the release of other neurotransmitters from presynaptic nerve terminals. It is thought that this presynaptic inhibition at nerve terminals accounts for the psychoactive effects of cannabinoids.

The cannabinoid receptor is a chain of 473 amino acids with seven hydrophobic domains that extend through the cell membrane (Figure 11.3); each region is composed of one hydrophobic domain.[8,9] As shown by Childers and Breivogel,[1] when THC binds to its receptors, it activates G-proteins that act on various effectors including the second-messenger enzyme adenylate cyclase and both potassium and calcium ion channels (Figure 11.4).

Thus, the cannabinoid receptor was isolated and cloned, its transmembrane and three-dimensional structures proposed, and its cellular transduction mechanisms delineated. The identification of a naturally occurring ligand that binds to the cannabinoid receptor and thus might function as a natural THC remained to be demonstrated. In the search for this ligand, Devane and co-workers[10] in 1992 isolated an arachidonic acid derivative named *anandamide* (Figure 11.1), which not only bound to the cannabinoid receptor but produced cannabinoid-like pharmacological effects. Many additional reports since then demonstrated that anandamide produces behavioral, hypothermic, and analgesic effects that parallel those caused by psychotropic cannabinoids. Anandamide exhibits the essential criteria required to be classified as the endogenous ligand at cannabinoid receptors.[1,2,7] In 1999, Ameri, Wilhelm, and Simmet[11] verified that anandamide acting on hippocampal cannabinoid receptors controls neuronal excitability by reducing excitatory neurotransmission at a presynaptic site. Shen and

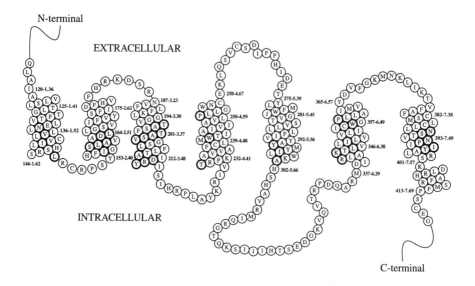

FIGURE 11.3 Two-dimensional representation of the anandamide receptor, a protein consisting of a chain of more than 450 amino acids (the first letter of each amino acid is shown). Like the opioid receptors, the anandamide receptor is a G-protein-linked, seven membrane-spanning structure with three extracellular loops. [Model from Bramblett et al.[9]]

Thayer[12] demonstrated that THC acts as a partial agonist at hippocampal glutamate-releasing neurons to "reduce, but not totally block, excitatory transmission." From their findings comes the knowledge that both THC and anandamide function as partial agonists that are unable to fully activate G-proteins at maximally effective concentrations.[13] There are huge numbers of cannabinoid receptors in the brain, perhaps 10 to 20 times as many as there are opioid receptors, perhaps more than any other type of receptor.[13] Anandamide, as a partial agonist, activates perhaps only 50 percent of available receptors; THC activates only about 20 percent. In fact, THC is probably effective not because of any inherent efficacy but because of the tremendous number of receptors for it in the brain. Even in the spinal cord, cannabinoid receptors are expressed in sensory nociceptive cells located in the dorsal root ganglion from whence the receptors are carried by axoplasmic flow both to peripheral sensory nerve endings and to nerve terminals in the dorsal horn of the spinal cord.[14,15]

As can be seen from Figure 11.1, anandamide is structurally dissimilar to THC. Thomas and co-workers[16] constructed three-dimensional pharmacologic models of THC and anandamide and demonstrated that in this conformation the molecules are in actuality quite similar (Figure

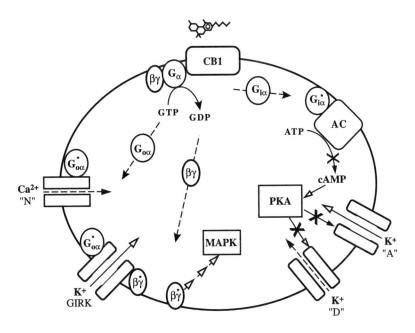

FIGURE 11.4 Several proposed signal transduction mechanisms of cannabinoid receptors. After THC (or anandamide) binds (*top*), the CB1 receptor activates G-proteins, which in turn act on various effectors including adenylate cyclase (AC), calcium (Ca^2), and mitogen-activated protein kinase (MAPC). Inhibition of adenylate cyclase and subsequent decreases in cAMP decreases activation of cAMP-dependent protein kinase (PKA), which leads to decreased potassium (K^+) channel fluxes. Stimulatory effects are shown by open arrows and inhibitory effects by filled arrows. The open or closed states of the channels and X's over some arrows reflect the final effects of cannabinoid agonists. [From Childers and Breivogel.[1]]

11.5) and would be predicted to interact with the same receptor. As the 1990s progressed, the first cannabinoid antagonist was synthesized, and mice lacking the cannabinoid receptor were bred and demonstrated a lack of response to canninoid drugs.[17] Anandamide antagonists have also been used to study dependence on THC.[18] In 1999, Haney and co-workers[19] described more clearly a marijuana abstinence syndrome (discussed on page 320).

Cadas and co-workers[20] studied the biosynthesis of anandamide and determined that it is synthesized within neurons by a condensation reaction between arachidonic acid and ethanolamine, under the regulation of calcium ions and cyclic adenosine monophosphate enzyme. It is broken down by a process of hydrolysis after carrier-mediated neuronal and astrocyte reuptake by an amidase for rapid hydrolysis.[21] Shen and co-workers[12] also studied rat hippocampus and demonstrated that anandamide, THC, and other anandamide-receptor

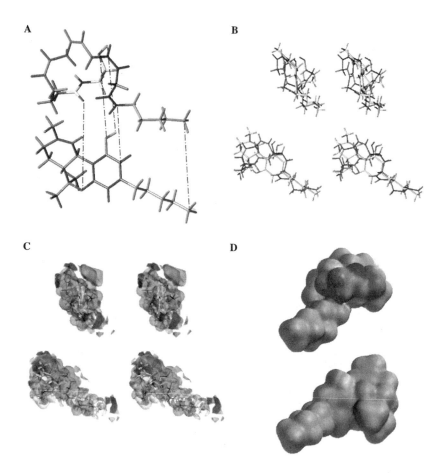

FIGURE 11.5 Several structural comparisons of anandamide and THC. **A.** Stick model showing alignment of the two molecules with dashed lines signifying the five atoms used for superpositioning. **B.** Views of the overlaid structures that predict three-dimensional similarity and thus affinity for the same receptor. **C.** Stereoviews of overlaid structures show nonoverlapping molecular volumes. **D.** Another view of the steric shape and bulk of anandamide (*top*) and THC (*bottom*). [From Thomas et al.[16]]

agonists inhibit the presynaptic release of the excitatory neurotransmitter glutamate via an inhibitory G-protein, as illustrated in Figure 11.4. These data are all consistent with marijuana-induced detrimental effects on cognitive functioning and on neuronal excitability secondary to reduction in excitatory glutamate neurotransmission. Thus, the hippocampus, cerebral cortex, cerebellum, and basal ganglia appear to be major loci of action of THC because these structures are involved in cognition, learning, memory, mood, and other higher intellectual functions, as well as motor functions, all of which are affected by THC.

Herkenham and co-workers[22,23] delineated the unique pattern of localization of cannabinoid receptors in the brain (Figures 11.6 and 11.7). First, large numbers of receptors found in the basal ganglia and cerebellum are involved in many forms of movement and postural control that are affected by smoking marijuana. Second, the cerebral cortex, especially the frontal cortex, is rich in cannabinoid receptors. Binding of THC here likely mediates at least some of the psychoactive effects of the drug, including the distortions of the sense of time, sound, color, and taste; alterations in the ability to concentrate; and production of a dreamlike state. Cannabinoid receptors are also dense in the hippocampus; this fact may account for THC-induced disruption of memory, memory storage, and coding of sensory input. Because brain-stem structures do not bind cannabinoids, THC does not affect basal body functions, including respiration. The lack of cannabinoid-anandamide receptors in the brain stem explains the relative nonlethality of THC. Perhaps in the near future the cannabinoid receptor may be redefined as the anandamide receptor, named for the endogenous neurotransmitter for the receptor in the same way that other transmitter-activated receptors are named.

In 1994 Lynn and Herkenham[24] studied the peripheral effects of cannabinoids and reported cannabinoid receptors outside the brain of a slightly different type than those found in the brain (the brain receptors, as well as certain cannabinoid receptors in the peripheral nervous system, are termed *cannabinoid$_1$ receptors*). *Cannabinoid$_2$* receptors are found in specific components of the lymphoid system, indicating that the

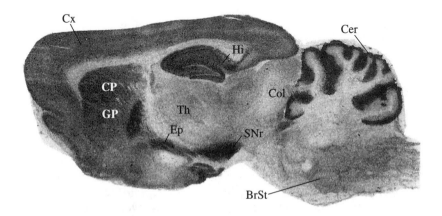

FIGURE 11.6 Autoradiographic binding of potent cannabinoid-to-cannabinoid receptors in the rat brain. BrSt = brain stem; Cer = cerebellum; Col = colliculi; CP = caudate putamen; Cx = cerebral cortex; Ep = entopeduncular nucleus; GP = globus pallidus; Hi = hippocampus; SNr = substantia nigra; Th = thalamus.

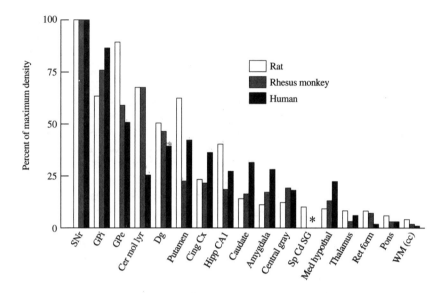

FIGURE 11.7 Relative densities of cannabinoid receptors across brain structures in rat, rhesus monkey, and human. Cer mol lyr = cerebellum, molecular layer; Cing Cx = cingulate cortex; Dg = dentate gyrus; GPe = external globus pallidus; GPi = internal globus pallidus; Hipp CA1 = hippocampal field CA1; Med hypothal = medial hypothalamus; Ret form = reticular formation; Sp Cd SG = substantia gelatinosa of spinal cord (*only rat measured); WM (cc) = white matter of corpus callosum.

immunosuppressive activity of THC is cannabinoid receptor mediated. Cannabinoid receptors are also found in the retina of the eye, where they probably play a role in retinal physiology and perhaps in vision in general.[25] Nonspecific binding of cannabinoids was found in several areas, including the heart, lungs, endocrine system, and reproductive organs.

Pharmacokinetics

Most marijuana available in the United States has a THC content that does not exceed 8 percent and usually averages 4 to 6 percent. THC is usually administered in the form of a hand-rolled marijuana cigarette (the average marijuana cigarette contains between 0.5 and 1 gram of plant material). Thus, if a marijuana cigarette contains 1 gram of plant material with a THC content of about 5 percent, the cigarette contains approximately 50 milligrams of THC. In general, about one-fourth to one-half of the THC present in a marijuana cigarette is actually available in the smoke. Thus, if a cigarette contains 50 milligrams of THC, about 12 to 25 milligrams are available in the smoke. In practice, the amount of THC *absorbed* into the bloodstream as a result of the social smoking of one marijuana cigarette is probably in the range of 0.4 to 10 milligrams. The absorption of THC from the smoking of marijuana is rapid and complete.

The behavioral effects of THC in smoked marijuana occur almost immediately after smoking begins and correspond with the rapid attainment of peak concentrations in plasma (Figure 11.8). Unless more is smoked, the effects seldom last longer than 3 to 4 hours (Figure 11.9). Peak blood levels of THC of 80 and 150 nanograms of drug per milliliter of plasma (ng/mL) occur about 10 minutes after initiation of smoking cigarettes containing 1.75 percent and 3.55 percent THC, respectively. Within 2 hours, levels fall below 5 ng/mL but remain detectable for up to 12 hours after smoking a single cigarette. Heart rate and blood pressure both increase, while skin temperature decreases. The subjective "high" is of rapid onset and persists for more than 12 hours, indicating either persistence of drug in the CNS or a threshold of about 5 ng/mL, above which the "high" is perceived.

THC is also absorbed when it is administered orally, but the absorption is slow and incomplete. The onset of action usually takes 30 to 60 minutes, with peak effects occurring 2 to 3 hours after ingestion. THC is approximately three times more effective when it is smoked than when it is taken orally, indicating possible first-pass metabolism with oral administration.

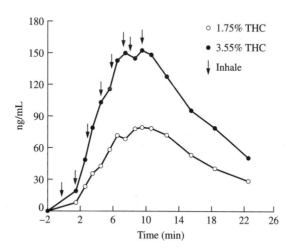

FIGURE 11.8 Mean plasma concentrations of total THC for smoked marijuana and infused THC on days 1 and 22. One marijuana cigarette was smoked from 0 to 15 minutes and was followed by intravenous infusion from 15 to 65 minutes, as indicated by arrows. Results from day 22 were obtained after daily smoking of marijuana and suggest that tolerance failed to develop. [From M. Perez-Reyes et al., "The Pharmacological Effects of Daily Marijuana Smoking in Humans," *Pharmacology, Biochemistry, and Behavior* 40 (1991): 691–694.]

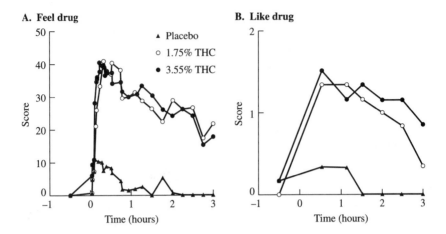

FIGURE 11.9 Mean ratings of "high" from the combination of smoked marijuana and infused THC on days 1 and 22. As in Figure 11.8, the lack of development of tolerance is apparent. [From M. Perez-Reyes et al., "The Pharmacological Effects of Daily Marijuana Smoking in Humans," *Pharmacology, Biochemistry, and Behavior* 40 (1991): 691–694.

Once THC is absorbed, it is *distributed* to the various organs of the body, especially those that have significant concentrations of fatty material. Thus, THC readily penetrates the brain; the blood-brain barrier does not appear to hinder its passage. Similarly, THC readily crosses the placental barrier and reaches the fetus.

THC is almost completely *metabolized* by hepatic cytochrome P450 enzymes to an active metabolite (11-hydroxy-delta-9-THC) that is subsequently converted to an inactive metabolite (11-nor-9-carboxy-delta-9-tetrahydrocannabinol, or THC-COOH) that is then excreted.[26] The metabolism of THC itself is quite slow; an elimination half-life of about 30 hours is generally accepted, although some researchers report longer half-life. Therefore, THC can persist in the body for several days to about 2 weeks. Such a delay tends to prolong and intensify the activity of subsequently smoked marijuana, forming a type of "reverse tolerance" to the drug, where the persistent low levels are potentiated by subsequently smoked THC cigarettes.

Like most psychoactive drugs, only minute quantities of THC are *excreted* in the urine of persons who use the drug. Therefore, urine testing for THC focuses primarily on identification of its metabolites. THC-COOH is only slowly excreted and the half-lives of THC-COOH in urine vary from about 30 hours to 60 hours,[27] even longer in obese individuals. Chronic smokers, even if they smoke only two to three times weekly, have persistently positive urine tests for THC metabolites. A heavy smoker who stops smoking may show positive urine tests for about a month after cessation. Thus, a positive urinalysis can indicate either recent use or use that occurred several weeks earlier. In addition, a positive urine test does not necessarily mean that a person was under the influence of marijuana at the time the urine specimen was collected; there may be little or no correlation between the presence of THC-COOH metabolite in urine and the presence of a pharmacologically significant amount of THC in the blood.

Pharmacological Effects of THC and Anandamide in Animals

In some animals, THC and other cannabinoids produce a unique syndrome of behavioral effects, including cognitive alterations and euphoria. Anandamide exerts similar effects, accompanied by "reductions in nigrostriatal dopaminergic neuronal activity."[28] Mice lacking the cannabinoid receptor have increased mortality rates, are less active, and have lower pain thresholds.[29]

One of the major effects of marijuana in humans is disruption of memory, which follows from reduction in hippocampal activity. THC disrupts both the encoding and the retrieval processes.[30,31] Memory impairments can be attenuated by cannabinoid antagonists,[32] implying that THC- and anandamide-induced memory disruption is mediated by cannabinoid receptors and not by any indirect sedative mechanism. THC and anandamide are both analgesic (at both spinal and brain stem levels).[33,34] "Cannabinoids produced analgesia by modulating the rostral ventromedial medulla neuronal activity in a manner similar to, but pharmacologically dissociable from, that of morphine."[35] THC in rodents potentiates the analgesic action of morphine, increasing morphine's potency; this action is blocked by cannabinoid antagonists.[36] As discussed, cannabinoid receptors are present in both the peripheral and central terminals of afferent nociceptive neurons.[14,15] Thus THC can exert analgesic effects by modulating both sensory input from peripheral sites of tissue injury as well as reducing the release of nociceptive neurotransmitters, such as substance P and glutamic acid, in the dorsal horn of the spinal cord. THC therefore exerts important analgesic actions in the brain, the spinal cord, and the periphery at the site of tissue injury.[37]

THC also exerts a variety of other effects in animals. THC decreases body temperature, calms aggressive behavior, potentiates the effects of barbiturates and other sedatives, blocks convulsions, and depresses reflexes. In primates, specifically, THC decreases aggression, decreases the ability to perform complex behavioral tasks, seems to induce hallucinations, and appears to cause temporal distortions. THC causes monkeys to increase the frequency of their social interactions. High doses can depress ovarian function, lower the concentration of female sex hormones, decrease ovulation, and possibly decrease sperm production. Finally, THC can disrupt appetite regulation, inducing overeating in rats exposed to anandamide, which provides "evidence for the involvement of a central cannabinoid system in the normal control of eating."[38]

Pharmacological Effects in Humans

Central Nervous System

The CNS effects of THC in humans vary with dose, route of administration, experience of the user, vulnerability to psychoactive effects, and setting of use. In general, the senses may be enhanced and the perception of time is usually altered. Users report an increased sense of well-being, mild euphoria, relaxation, and relief from anxiety. The subjective effects include dissociation of ideas. Illusions and hallucinations occur infrequently.

During intoxication, THC impairs cognitive functions, perception, reaction time, learning, and memory. Impairment persists for several hours beyond the perception of the high. Impairments have obvious implications for psychomotor functioning, for example, in the operation of a motor vehicle.[39] As a cognitive inhibitor, drug use is inappropriate and impairs performance in the workplace and at school.

At higher doses of THC, the user experiences an intensification of emotional responses and alterations in sensation that resemble mild sensory distortions and even mild hallucinations. Few people who smoke marijuana socially are seeking these effects.

At very high doses, acute depressive reactions, acute panic reactions, or mild paranoia have been observed, probably brought on by drug-induced alterations in perception; some panic responses may follow the feeling of a loss of mental control. Several surveys indicate that 50 to 60 percent of marijuana users have reported at least one anxiety experience. Only at psychotoxic doses of THC do delusions, paranoia, hallucinations, confusion and disorientation, depersonalization, altered sensory perception, and loss of insight occur, and these reactions are unusual and generally short lasting. Common predisposing factors include preexisting personality disturbances or schizophrenia.

The effects of marijuana on cognition, learning, memory, and attention certainly may be the major adverse effects resulting from the use of THC. Acute use certainly impairs the ability to perform complex functions requiring attention and mental coordination. In chronic use, the situation may be different, either because of the persistence of drug in the body or because of chronic down regulation of cannabinoid receptors. Ehrenreich and co-workers[40] studied a cohort of chronic marijuana users who started smoking before the age of 16 years (compared with users who started later). They concluded that "beginning cannabis use during early adolescence may lead to enduring effects on specific attentional functions in adulthood." Solowij and co-workers[41] had stated earlier:

> Chronic users have difficulty in setting up an accurate focus of attention and in filtering out irrelevant information. The data suggest a dysfunction in the allocation of attentional resources and stimulus evaluation strategies. These results imply that long-term cannabis use may impair the ability to efficiently process information.

Such impairments were discussed in the driving study by Kurzthaler and co-workers:[39]

> Immediately after smoking cannabis, subjects were not able to profit from their own test experience from the day before. . . . a driver under acute cannabis influence would not be able to use acquired knowledge from earlier experiences adequately to ensure road safety. Consequently, an impairment of driving ability immediately after drug consumption must be assumed.

Lundqvist[42] and Solowij[43] describe a marijuana-induced impaired ability to focus attention and filter out irrelevant information. Users demonstrate weakness in attention and synthetic skills, difficulty making subtle distinctions in relevance and memory, decreased psychospatial skills, poor mental representations of the environment, and poor routines of daily life. These impairments are associated with feelings of alienation and that life is not under their control and lacks meaning. During therapy users will "begin to show improvement in cognitive functioning within 14 days of abstinence combined with therapy, and function normally at the end of 6 weeks of therapy."[42]

Fletcher and co-workers[44] studied two cohorts of long-term cannabis users and nonusers in Costa Rican men over a 20-year period. The cohorts were compared with younger, shorter-term users and nonusers. Older users demonstrated greater impairment in complex learning tasks of memory and recall, selective attention, and divided attention. To place these detrimental effects of marijuana in perspective, the Fletcher study concluded:

> The deficiencies observed . . . are subtle. The older long-term users are largely functional and employable, and they do not demonstrate the types of dementia and amnesic syndromes associated with alcohol use of comparable magnitude. The health of the subjects continues to be adequate over time, and no evidence exists for the severity of health risks associated with the use of other drugs, such as alcohol. Nevertheless, the

risks of long-term use of even smaller amounts of cannabis are likely magnified in a more technological society. . . . Certain occupations may carry particular risk because of safety issues and effects on productivity and learning. . . . The findings suggest a need to focus efforts on the prevention of cannabis use through balanced educational programs for children and their parents. It is clear that the younger cohort and, to a lesser extent, the older cohort began to move toward polydrug use, a pattern consistent with studies of North American subjects. This pattern underscores the need for preventive efforts to reduce the risk of consumption of drugs by young people.

Kouri and co-workers[45] studied cohorts of heavy versus occasional marijuana smokers in a college population. By objective measurement of psychiatric functioning (diagnosed DSM disorders), the two groups were indistinguishable. They differed, however, in the level of use of other drugs, with one-third of heavy marijuana users displaying a history of some form of substance abuse or dependence (Tables 11.1 and 11.2).

TABLE 11.1 Lifetime substance use among heavy versus occasional marijuana smokers

	Heavy smokers ($n = 45$)	Occasional smokers ($n = 44$)
	n(%)	n(%)
SUBJECTS WHO HAD EVER USED		
Hallucinogens	44 (98)	23 (42)[c]
Hallucinogens > 10 times	36 (80)	5 (11)[c]
Cocaine	32 (71)	8 (18)[c]
Cocaine > 10 times	20 (44)	0[c]
Inhalants	11 (24)	3 (7)[a]
Stimulants	14 (31)	7 (16)
Sedative-hypnotics	27 (60)	7 (16)[c]
Opioids	12 (27)	1 (2)[b]
Any of the above	45 (100)	26 (59)[c]
SUBJECTS CURRENTLY USING		
Cigarettes ≥ 1 pack/day	17 (38)	5 (11)[b]
Alcohol > 10 drinks/week	17 (38)	9 (20)

Significance of differences between groups: [a]$p < .05$; [b]$p < .01$; [c]$p < .001$.
From Kouri et al.[45]

TABLE 11.2 Lifetime diagnoses of substance abuse and dependence in heavy versus occasional marijuana smokers

	Heavy smokers (n = 45)	Occasional smokers (n = 44)
	n(%)	n(%)
SUBSTANCE		
Cannabis	45 (100)	0
Alcohol	11 (24)	5 (11)
Cocaine	6 (13)	0
Hallucinogens	3 (7)	0
Sedative-hypnotics	1 (2)	0
Polysubstance	2 (4)	0
ANY SUBSTANCE OTHER THAN CANNABIS[a]	15 (33)	5 (11)

[a]Total for heavy users is less than the sum of the individual diagnoses because some subjects reported more than one form of substance abuse or dependence.
Significance of differences: cannabis, $p < .001$; cocaine, $p = .03$; any substance other than cannabis, $p = .01$.
From Kouri et al.[45]

To understand the behavioral attractiveness of marijuana, Gardner and Lowinson[46] reviewed marijuana's interactions with brain reward systems, particularly in the dopamine-mediated, medial forebrain bundle projection. They stated:

> Acute enhancement of brain reward mechanisms appears to be the single essential commonality of abuse prone drugs, and the hypothesis that recreational and abused drugs act on these brain mechanisms to produce the subjective reward that constitutes the "high" or "rush" or "hit" sought by drug users is, at present, the most compelling hypothesis available on the neurobiology of recreational drug use and abuse.

Also involved are synaptic interconnections of opioid and many other neurotransmitters. Gardner and Lowinson argue that THC acts on this system as do other abused drugs, inducing the release of dopamine in reward loci including the basal ganglia, the nucleus accumbens, and the prefrontal cortex.[46]

Tanda and colleagues[47] reported that THC increased dopaminergic activity in the nucleus accumbens, probably "through a common mu-opioid receptor mechanism located in the ventral tegmentum." This action may account for both the pleasurable and the analgesic actions of THC. Manzanares and colleagues[48] expanded on this concept and concluded that there is a functional link between opioids and cannabinoid pathways, especially regarding the antinociceptive (analgesic) actions of cannabinoids. They suggest that cannabinoids induce the synthesis or release (or both) of opioid peptides; a potential mechanism to explain the augmentation of morphine-induced analgesia by THC as well as the ability of THC to ameliorate the symptoms of opioid withdrawal (both potential therapeutic uses of natural and synthetic cannabinoids). On the other hand, the Manzanares team states that "the hypothesis that marijuana consumption might enhance the reinforcing potential of opioids (by increasing opioid receptor expression) needs to be more extensively studied."[48]

An amotivational syndrome has long been associated with chronic marijuana use: it compels users to "drop out" because of a loss of interest in goal-oriented endeavors. The etiology of this syndrome is unclear, although Musty and Kaback[49] report that between 40 and 50 percent of adolescents admitted to a treatment program were found to have depressive symptoms at admission (indicating comorbidity of substance abuse with depression). They summarized:

> Both light and heavy users with symptoms of depression had significantly lower scores than those without depressive symptoms, on the overall Orientation to Life questionnaire and on each subscale measuring Meaningfulness, Manageability and Comprehensibility. These data suggest that amotivational symptoms observed in heavy marijuana users in treatment are due to depression.

Cardiovascular System

An increase in heart rate and blood pressure are two commonly observed physiological effects of THC. Blood vessels of the cornea can dilate, which results in bloodshot eyes that can be observed in persons who have just smoked marijuana. THC users frequently report increased appetite, dry mouth, occasional dizziness, and slight nausea. Respiratory depression is not observed.

Although the increased heart rate could be a problem for people with cardiovascular disease, dangerous physical reactions to marijuana are almost unknown. No human being is known to have died of overdosage. By extrapolation from animal experiments, the ratio of lethal to effective (intoxicating) dose is estimated to be on the order of thousands to one.

Interestingly, peripheral cannabinoid$_2$ receptors in the heart function in an intrinsic defense of the heart against potentially fatal ischemic attacks.[50] This protective effect of cannabinoids may eventually be an important therapeutic intervention in the prevention of heart attacks.

Pulmonary System

The gaseous and particulate components of both marijuana and tobacco smoke provide some insights into the potential for marijuana to cause pulmonary damage. In a 25-year-old classic study, Hoffman and co-workers[51] performed such an analysis (Table 11.3) and noted that,

TABLE 11.3 Gases and particulates in marijuana and tobacco smoke

	Marijuana cigarette	Tobacco cigarette
GAS PHASE ANALYSIS		
Carbon monoxide (vol %)	3.99	4.58
(mg)	17.6	20.2
Carbon dioxide (vol %)	8.27	9.38
(mg)	57.3	65.0
Ammonia (µg)	228	178
HCN (µg)	532	498
Isoprene (µg)	83	310
Acetaldehyde (µg)	1200	980
Acetone (µg)	443	578
Acrolein (µg)	92	85
Acetonitrile (µg)	132	123
Benzene (µg)	76	67
Toluene (µg)	112	108
Dimethylnitrosamine (ng)	75	84
Methylethylnitrosamine (ng)	27	30
PARTICULATE MATTER ANALYSIS		
Phenol (µg)	76.8	138.5
o-cresol (µg)	76.8	24
m-, p-cresol (µg)	54.4	65
2,4- and 2,5-dimethylphenol (µg)	6.8	14.4
Cannabidiol (µg)	190	——
Delta-9-tetracannabinol	820	——
Nicotine	——	2850
Naphthalene (ng)	3000	1200
1-methylnaphthalene (ng)	6100	3650
2-methylnaphthalene (ng)	3600	1400
Benzo(a)anthracene (ng)	75	43
Benzo(a)pyrene (ng)	31	22.1

From Hoffman, Brunemann, Gori, and Wynder.[51]

with the exception of the presence of THC in marijuana and nicotine in tobacco, both inhalants are remarkably similar, with marijuana smoke containing more tars and many of the same carcinogenic compounds identified in tobacco smoke.

Reports of altered lung function due to smoking marijuana show evidence of bronchial irritation and inflammation. Tashkin and co-workers initially noted changes in heavy marijuana smokers consistent with tobacco-induced lung injury, although a 1997 study by the same researchers[52] noted that tobacco smoking but not marijuana smoking is associated with a decline in lung function:

> These findings do not support an association between regular marijuana smoking and chronic COPD [chronic obstructive pulmonary disease] but do not exclude the possibility of other adverse respiratory effects.

Aside from its irritant effects, the obvious question is whether marijuana smoke causes lung cancer. No direct evidence shows that chronic marijuana smoking causes lung cancer, but cannabis-induced lung cancer may be in a prodromal phase. Certainly no scientist would state with absolute certainty that chronic smoking of marijuana is safe to pulmonary tissue; it seems extremely unlikely that the pulmonary toxicities seen with cigarettes will not be seen to some degree in heavy marijuana smokers.

Immune System

As noted earlier, cannabinoid$_2$ receptors are found primarily in the immune system. Long-term marijuana use is associated with a degree of immunosuppression, which might be thought to potentially render the smoker susceptible to infections or disease. Although data in this area are controversial and implications have not been proven, marijuana smoking, in some circumstances, may partially suppress immunity. The clinical significance of this occurrence is not known, but it should be noted that other depressant drugs, such as alcohol, barbiturates, benzodiazepines, and anticonvulsants, share this immunosuppressive action.

Because both the spleen and the lymphocytes (white blood cells) are important to the body's immune response, they have been investigated to determine how they are affected by cannabinoids. Cabral and co-workers[53] reported that both THC and anandamide inhibit the function of specialized tumor-killing cells. The implications of such actions and the physiological role of anandamide in immunomodulation are unknown. To put the immunosuppressive action of marijuana in perspective, in humans marijuana-induced immune suppression is subtle and in many cases insignificant. There is, at this time, little evidence for cannabinoid-induced immunosuppression as a causative agent in disease.

Reproductive System

Evidence of THC-induced suppression of sexual function and reproduction is being gathered. The chronic use of marijuana by males can reduce levels of the hormone testosterone and sperm formation. Reductions in male fertility and sexual potency, however, have not been reported. In females, the levels of the hormones FSH (follicle-stimulating hormone) and LH (luteinizing hormone) are reduced by the use of marijuana. Menstrual cycles can be affected and anovulatory cycles have been reported. All these actions reverse when drug use is discontinued.

Marijuana freely crosses the placenta, and so its use probably should be avoided during pregnancy. However, estimated prevalence rates of cannabis use during pregnancy range from 3 percent to more than 20 percent of pregnant women.[54] To date, the only medical risk reasonably ascribed to marijuana use during pregnancy appears to be mild fetal growth retardation and maternal lung damage (both similar to that seen with tobacco smoking).[54]

One of the greatest risks appears to be the high probability that a pregnant female who smokes marijuana during pregnancy may also use other, more fetotoxic drugs. Infants born of marijuana-smoking mothers display mild withdrawal signs, including tremulousness and abnormal responses to stimuli. These signs appear to be transient in nature.

An important consideration is the long-term effects of prenatal marijuana exposure on child development. Fried[55] evaluated the effects of maternal marijuana use on offspring and notes a relative lack of effect in children aged 1 to 3 years. At 4 years, however, children displayed "increased behavioral problems and decreased performance on visual perceptual tasks, language comprehension, sustained attention and memory." Prenatal marijuana exposure may affect "executive functioning—goal-directed behavior that include[s] planning, organized search, and impulse control." Fried concludes:

> Such an interpretation would be consistent with the literature . . . suggesting that chronic marijuana use may impact prefrontal lobe functioning.

In any case, "to evaluate the long-term effects of interuterine marijuana exposure on child intellectual, language and behavioral development, more research is needed."[54]

Side Effects

The major acute side effects associated with marijuana use are dose-related extensions of its recreational uses: sedation, altered motor coordination, impaired cognition, and reduced short-term memory. Marijuana impairs a person's ability to drive an automobile safely, much as alcohol does. With marijuana intoxication, however, impairment can persist well beyond the time of actually feeling impaired. Such unperceived impairment can persist for several hours. Brookoff and co-workers[56] studied reckless drivers who tested negative for alcohol use: 13 percent tested positive for cocaine, 33 percent tested positive for marijuana, and 12 percent tested positive for both cocaine and marijuana. Ninety-four of the 150 drivers were considered intoxicated (to trained observers) and 80 of those (85 percent) tested positive for cocaine or marijuana. Intoxicated drivers testing positive for alcohol were not tested for the coexistence of marijuana, although one would predict that the number of positives would be significant.

Tolerance and Dependence

Tolerance to *Cannabis sativa* does occur, and it appears to result from two separate mechanisms. The first involves a cannabinoid-induced down regulation and desensitization of brain cannabinoid receptors.[57] The second is more complicated and involves a rapid receptor internalization following agonist binding and receptor activation.[58] Potent synthetic cannabinoid agonists cause rapid internalization; THC causes little, if any. Thus, with the weak agonist THC, down regulation is the primary mechanism of tolerance and withdrawal of THC results in rapid normalization of receptor responsiveness.

Until recently, it was generally thought that physical dependence on THC probably did not develop, and if it did, any symptoms were mild and transient:

> Cannabinoids are not generally self-administered by animals, indicating that they are not reinforcing. However, recent studies have indicated that cannabinoids increase dopamine levels in the mesolimbic dopamine system of rats, a pathway associated with reinforcement.[1]

Recently, Haney and co-workers[19] defined a marijuana withdrawal syndrome in more detail. Withdrawal symptoms consist of restlessness, irritability, agitation, anxiety, depression, reduced food intake, insomnia, sleep disturbances, nausea, and cramping. The withdrawal syndrome begins within 48 hours after cessation of drug administration and lasts at least 2 days and perhaps 4 to 6 days. Duffy and Milin[59] describe three cases in adolescents indicating that the withdrawal syndrome may be more serious than is generally appreciated and that drug craving contributes to the persistent use of cannabis in adolescents despite motivation to stop. They conclude:

The importance of gaining an appreciation for cannabis withdrawal in adolescent users is underscored by the high prevalence of cannabis use among adolescents, the association of cannabis use with the subsequent use of hard drugs, and the serious psychosocial sequelae associated with chronic cannabis use. Systematic study is warranted to understand better the magnitude of the problem of cannabis dependence in adolescents. We need to ask about withdrawal symptoms in adolescent cannabis users to identify significant symptoms and intervene as required, perhaps necessitating brief admission, extended care, and/or pharmacotherapy.

Brook, Balka, and Whiteman[60] conducted a five-year study of 1182 youths of African American and Puerto Rican ancestry in East Harlem, New York, focusing on marijuana use (used at least monthly) as the only independent variable. An increase in marijuana use was associated with a reduced likelihood of graduating from high school, with delinquency, with a tripling of the risk of self-deviancy, and with an increase in the risk of multiple other problem behaviors. While marijuana smoking in early adolescence is correlated or associated with later educational, job, and psychosocial problems, no causal inferences can be drawn. Marijuana use may indeed predispose one to future problems, or it may merely be one of many factors incorporated into the life of adolescents who chose one pathway versus another. The cognitive effects of THC, however, would, at a minimum, interfere with academic success. In any case, no one of reasonable mind advocates the availability of marijuana to minors. However society moves toward or away from marijuana availability for medical or recreational use, availability to youth must be restricted.

As with other psychoactive drugs, marijuana dependence is defined by three critical elements:

1. Preoccupation with the acquisition of the drug

2. Compulsive use of the drug

3. Relapse to or recurrent use of the drug

To date, these elements have not been major problems with marijuana used alone, although the reports by Duffy and Milin[59] and by Brook, Balka, and Whiteman[60] are disconcerting. The criteria are far more commonly met in multidrug dependence. Therefore, few treatment programs are oriented solely toward marijuana abuse, as both multidrug dependence and comorbid disease are invariably present. Treatments such as psychotherapy can be appropriate for frequent users of marijuana, but this is not therapy for marijuana abuse: it is therapy for an underlying psychopathology (such as depression), one symptom of which is the abuse of cannabis. Grinspoon and Bakalar[61] write:

> Being attached to cannabis is not so much a function of any inherent psychopharmacologic property of the drug as it is emotionally driven by the underlying psychopathology. Success in curtailing cannabis use requires dealing with that pathology.

Childers and Brievogel[1] conclude:

> Thus, while cannabinoids appear to be conforming to some of the neurobiological effects of other drugs abused by humans, the underlying mechanisms of these actions and their significance in determining the reinforcement and dependence liability of cannabinoids are still undetermined.

Therapeutic Uses

Currently, there is one approved and several possible therapeutic uses for THC and its various derivatives. *Dronabinol* (Marinol), which is synthetic THC formulated in sesame oil, has been available for more than 10 years for use as an appetite stimulant in patients with AIDS and for use in the treatment of nausea and vomiting associated with chemotherapy in cancer patients. Schwartz, Voth, and Sheridan[62] reviewed the use of smoked marijuana and oral dronabinol in this population of patients and compared these THC-containing products with physician-prescribed antiemetic compounds. The latter had superior efficacy in treating chemotherapy-induced nausea and vomiting. Other potential uses of dronabinol are to reduce the muscle spasms and pain of multiple sclerosis and reduce the intraocular pressure of glaucoma. Antidepressant and analgesic effects are also claimed, with analgesic actions best described in animal studies. Finally, both marijuana[63] and non-psychoactive synthetic cannabinoids[64] effectively protect the brain from permanent injury following head trauma, stroke, or ischemic insults. Further work into the cardioprotective and neuroprotective effects of cannabinoids is essential.

The passage of initiatives legalizing the medical use of marijuana has reopened the issue of therapeutics. Does marijuana have therapeutic efficacy equal to or greater than those of existing agents? The answer is muddied both by smoking as a route of administration and by the use of a crude product containing THC, which is only a weak agonist at cannabinoid receptors. The synthesis of pure anandamide agonists, specific antagonists, and now psychotropic agonists may aid the development of compounds that lack the undesirable side effects of marijuana plant material.

A 1999 report from the Institute of Medicine[65] concluded that cannabinoids have potential applicability for some human symptoms. However, it also suggests that those components should be delivered by a mechanism other than inhaling smoke, for example, inhaling non-smoked molecules of either natural THC from marijuana or a totally synthetic compound. The institute made six major recommendations:

1. Research should continue into the physiological effects of synthetic and plant-derived cannabinoids and the natural function of cannabinoids found in the body. Because different cannabinoids appear to have different effects, cannabinoid research should include but not be restricted to effects attributable to THC alone.

2. Clinical trials of cannabinoid drugs for symptom management should be conducted with the goal of developing rapid-onset, reliable, and safe delivery systems.

3. Psychological effects of cannabinoids such as anxiety reduction and sedation, which could influence perceived medical benefits, should be evaluated in clinical trials.

4. Studies to define the individual health risks of smoking marijuana should be conducted, particularly among populations in which marijuana use is prevalent.

5. Clinical trials of marijuana use for medical purposes should be conducted in the following limited circumstances: trials should involve only short-term marijuana use (less than six months); be conducted in patients with conditions for which there is reasonable expectation of efficacy; be approved by institutional review boards; and collect data with efficacy.

6. Short-term use of smoked marijuana (less than six months) for patients with debilitating symptoms (such as intractable pain or vomiting) must meet the following conditions:

   • Failure of all approved medications to provide relief has been documented.

   • The symptoms can reasonably be expected to be relieved by rapid-onset cannabinoid drugs.

   • Treatment is administered under medical supervision in a manner that allows for assessment of treatment effectiveness.

   • Treatment involves an oversight strategy comparable to an institutional review board process that could provide guidance within 24 hours of a submission by a physician to provide marijuana to a patient for a specified use.

It is hoped that the federal government will move forward with support for research along these guidelines. In addition, it is hoped that states in which voters have approved "medical marijuana" legislation will control use along the same guidelines. At a minimum, it is hoped that the institute's report will encourage the federal government to become involved in well-designed experimentation of cannabinoid pharmacology and therapeutics. Hollister[66] addresses the medical marijuana controversy and the swamp of conflict between voters' desires in favor of medical marijuana and federal legislation opposed to it. He lists potential indications for medical marijuana:

- Nausea and vomiting associated with cancer chemotherapy or other causes
- Weight loss associated with debilitating illnesses
- Spasticity secondary to neurological diseases
- Chronic pain syndromes

Further, Hollister outlines a rational approach to the problem, including additional clinical research, availability of smoked marijuana to qualified patients, and exclusion from criminal penalty for prescribing, supplying, or using marijuana for medical purposes. None of this would require new legislation or funding; "Executive orders would provide a start to settling the issue of medical use of marijuana."[66]

As early as 1997, in an editorial in the *New England Journal of Medicine*, Kassirer[67] stated:

> I believe that a federal policy that prohibits physicians from alleviating suffering by prescribing marijuana for seriously ill patients is misguided, heavy-handed, and inhumane. Federal authorities should rescind their prohibition of the medical use of marijuana for seriously ill patients and allow physicians to decide which patients to treat. The government should change marijuana's status from that of a Schedule 1 drug [considered to be potentially addictive and with no current medical use] to that of a Schedule 2 drug [potentially addictive but with some accepted medical use] and regulate it accordingly.

Most certainly, the debate over marijuana and cannabinoid use and availability will continue for many years.

STUDY QUESTIONS

1. How are the effects of THC similar to those of the nonselective depressants? How are they dissimilar?
2. How are the effects of THC similar to those of the psychedelic drugs? How are they dissimilar?

3. How does the half-life of THC reflect a person's ability to become intoxicated more easily and with a smaller amount of drug after its repeated use?

4. Discuss some of the concerns and side effects that are associated with varying degrees of THC use by young people.

5. What does THC do to cognition?

6. Are there any long-term effects of marijuana on the brain? The body? Society?

7. Are there any potential long-term effects that might be associated with chronic use of marijuana?

8. Does dependence on marijuana develop? Discuss both views.

9. Discuss the cannabinoid receptor, its location, and its endogenous neurotransmitter.

10. How might a treatment program be organized for persons who become dependent on marijuana.

11. What do you think society's response should be to the continued illicit use of marijuana? Should marijuana be legalized for either medical or recreational use? If so, how should it be regulated or restricted?

12. Discuss evidence for or against medical uses of marijuana. If it has medical uses, how might efficacy and societal acceptance be improved?

13. How do you see the future of marijuana and cannabinoid research?

REFERENCES

1. S. R. Childers and C. S. Breivogel, "Cannabis and Endogenous Cannabinoid Systems," *Drug and Alcohol Dependence* 51 (1998): 173–187.
2. C. C. Felder and M. Glass, "Cannabinoid Receptors and Their Endogenous Agonists," *Annual Review of Pharmacology and Toxicology* 38 (1998): 179–200.
3. S. A. Deadwyler, R. E. Hampson, and S. R. Childers, "Functional Significance of Cannabinoid Receptors in Brain," in R. G. Pertwee, ed., *Cannabinoid Receptors* (London: Academic Press, 1995), 205–231.
4. A. C. Howlett, J. M. Qualy, and L. L. Khachatrian, "Involvement of G_i in the Inhibition of Adenylate Cyclase by Cannabimimetic Drugs," *Molecular Pharmacology* 29 (1986): 307–313.
5. C. A. Audette, S. H. Burstein, S. A. Doyle, and S. A. Hunter, "G-Protein Mediation of Cannabinoid-induced Phospholipase Activation," *Pharmacology, Biochemistry, and Behavior* 40 (1991): 559–563.
6. L. A. Matsuda et al., "Structure of a Cannabinoid Receptor and Functional Expression of the Cloned cDNA," *Nature* 346 (1990): 561–564.

7. R. G. Pertwee, "Pharmacological, Physiological and Clinical Implications of the Discovery of Cannabinoid Receptors: An Overview," in R. G. Pertwee, ed., *Cannabinoid Receptors* (London: Academic Press, 1995), 1–34.

8. A. C. Howlett, T. M. Champion-Dorow, L. L. McMahon, and T. M. Westlake, "The Cannabinoid Receptor: Biochemical and Cellular Properties in Neuroblastoma Cells," *Pharmacology, Biochemistry, and Behavior* 40 (1991): 565–569.

9. R. D. Bramblett, A. M. Panu, J. A. Ballesteros, and P. H. Reggio, "Construction of a 3D Model of the Cannabinoid CB1 Receptor: Determination of Helix Ends and Helix Orientation," *Life Sciences* 56 (1995): 1971–1982.

10. W. A. Devane et al., "Isolation and Structure of a Brain Constituent That Binds to the Cannabinoid Receptor," *Science* 258 (1992): 1946–1949.

11. A. Ameri, A. Wilhelm, and T. Simmet, "Effects of the Endogenous Cannabinoid, Anandamide, on Neuronal Activity in Rat Hippocampal Slices," *British Journal of Pharmacology* 126 (1999): 1831–1839.

12. M. Shen and S. A. Thayer, "Delta9-tetrahydrocannabinol Acts as a Partial Agonist to Modulate Glutamatergic Synaptic Transmission Between Rat Hippocampal Neurons in Culture," *Molecular Pharmacology* 55 (1999): 8–13.

13. S. R. Childers, "G-protein-coupled Mechanisms of Cannabinoid Receptors in Brain," *Proceeding of the Western Pharmacology Society* (2000): in press.

14. A. G. Hohmann and M. Herkenham, "Localization of Central Cannabinoid CB1 Receptor Messenger RNA in Neuronal Subpopulations of Rat Dorsal Root Ganglia: A Double-label In Situ Hybridization Study," *Neuroscience* 90 (1999): 923–931.

15. A. G. Hohmann and M. Herkenham, "Cannabinoid Receptors Undergo Axonal Flow in Sensory Nerves," *Neuroscience* 92 (1999): 1171–1175.

16. B. F. Thomas et al., "Structure-activity Analysis of Anandamide Analogs: Relationship to a Cannabinoid Pharmacophore," *Journal of Medicinal Chemistry* 39 (1996): 471–479.

17. C. Ledent et al., "Unresponsiveness to Cannabinoids and Reduced Addictive Effects of Opiates in CB_1 Receptor Knockout Mice," *Science* 283 (1999): 401–403.

18. S. A. Cook, J. A. Lowe, and B. R. Martin, "CB1 Receptor Antagonist Precipitates Withdrawal in Mice Exposed to Delta9-Tetrahydrocannabinol," *Journal of Pharmacology and Experimental Therapeutics* 285 (1998): 1150–1156.

19. M. Haney et al., "Abstinence Symptoms Following Smoked Marijuana in Humans," *Psychopharmacology* 141 (1999): 395–404.

20. H. Cadas et al., "Biosynthesis of an Endogenous Cannabinoid Precursor in Neurons and Its Control by Calcium and cAMP," *Journal of Neuroscience* 16 (1996): 3934–3942.

21. D. Piomelli et al., "Structural Determinants for Recognition and Translocation by the Anandamide Transporter," *Proceedings of the National Academy of Sciences of the United States of America* 96 (1999): 5802–5807.

22. M. Herkenham, "Cannabinoid Receptor Localization in Brain: Relationship to Motor and Reward Systems," *Annals of the New York Academy of Sciences* 654 (1992): 19–32.

23. W. Y. Ong and K. Mackie, "A Light and Electron Microscopic Study of the CB1 Cannabinoid Receptor in Primate Brain," *Neuroscience* 92 (1999): 1177–1191.
24. A. B. Lynn and M. Herkenham, "Localization of Cannabinoid Receptors and Nonsaturable High-density Cannabinoid Binding Sites in Peripheral Tissues of the Rat: Implications for Receptor-mediated Immune Modulation by Cannabinoids," *Journal of Pharmacology and Experimental Therapeutics* 268 (1994): 1612–1623.
25. A. Straiker et al., "Cannabinoid CB1 Receptors and Ligands in Vertebrate Retina: Localization and Function of an Endogenous Signaling System," *Proceedings of the National Academy of Sciences of the United States of America* 96 (1999): 14565–14570.
26. T. Matsunaga et al., "Metabolism of Delta^9-Tetrahydrocannabinol by Cytochrome P450 Isozymes Purified from Hepatic Microsomes of Monkeys," *Life Sciences* 56 (1995): 2089–2095.
27. M. A. Huestis and E. J. Cone, "Urinary Excretion Half-life of 11-Nor-9-carboxy-delta9-tetrahydrocannabinol in Humans," *Therapeutic Drug Monitoring* 20 (1998): 570–576.
28. J. Romero et al., "The Endogenous Cannabinoid Receptor Ligand, Anandamide, Inhibits the Motor Behavior: Role of Nigrostriatal Dopaminergic Neurons," *Life Sciences* 56 (1995): 2033–2040.
29. A. Zimmer et al., "Increased Mortality, Hypoactivity, and Hypoalgesia in Cannabinoid CB1 receptor Knockout Mice," *Proceedings of the National Academy of Sciences of the United States of America* 96 (1999): 5780–5785.
30. R. E. Hampson and S. A. Deadwyler, "Cannabinoids, Hippocampal Function and Memory," *Life Sciences* 65 (1999): 715–723.
31. R. E. Hampson and S. A. Deadwyler, "Role of Cannabinoid Receptors in Memory Storage," *Neurobiology of Disease* 5 (6, Part B, 1998): 474–482.
32. P. E. Mallet and R. J. Beninger, "The Cannabinoid CB1 Receptor Antagonist SR141716A Attenuates the Memory Impairment Produced by Delta9-Tetrahydrocannabinol or Anandamide," *Psychopharmacology* 140 (1998): 11–19.
33. W. J. Martin et al., "An Examination of the Central Sites of Action of Cannabinoid-induced Antinociception in the Rat," *Life Sciences* 56 (1995): 2103–2109.
34. A. G. Hohmann, W. J. Martin, K. Tsou, and J. M. Walker, "Inhibition of Noxious Stimulus-evoked Activity of Spinal Cord Dorsal Horn Neurons by the Cannabinoid WIN-55,212-2," *Life Sciences* 56 (1995): 2111–2118.
35. I. D. Meng et al., "An Analgesic Circuit Activated by Cannabinoids" *Nature* 395 (1998): 381–383.
36. F. L. Smith, D. Cichewicz, Z. L. Martin, and S. P. Welch, "The Enhancement of Morphine Antinociception in Mice by Delta9-Tetrahydrocannabinol," *Pharmacology, Biochemistry, and Behavior* 60 (1998): 559–566.
37. M. C. Ko and J. H. Woods, "Local Administration of Delta9-tetrahydro-cannabinol Attenuates Capsaicin-induced Thermal Nociception in Rhesus Monkeys: A Peripheral Cannabinoid Action," *Psychopharmacology* 143 (1999): 322–326.
38. C. M. Williams and T. C. Kirkham, "Anandamide-induced Overeating: Mediation by Central Cannabinoid (CB!) Receptors," *Psychopharmacology* 143 (1999): 315–317.

39. I. Kurzthaler et al., "Effect of Cannabis Use on Cognitive Functions and Driving Ability," *Journal of Clinical Psychiatry* 60 (1999): 395–399.
40. H. Ehrenreich et al., "Specific Attentional Dysfunction in Adults Following Early Start of Cannabis Use," *Psychopharmacology* 142 (1999): 295–301.
41. N. Solowij, P. T. Michie, and A. M. Fox, "Effects of Long-term Cannabis Use on Selective Attention: An Event-related Potential Study," *Pharmacology, Biochemistry, and Behavior* 40 (1991): 683.
42. T. Lundqvist, "Specific Thought Patterns in Chronic Cannabis Smokers Observed During Treatment," *Life Sciences* 56 (1995): 2141–2144.
43. N. Solowij, "Do Cognitive Impairments Recover Following Cessation of Cannabis Use?" *Life Sciences* 56 (1995): 2119–2126.
44. J. M. Fletcher et al., "Cognitive Correlates of Long-term Cannabis Use in Costa Rican Men," *Archives of General Psychiatry* 53 (1996): 1051–1057.
45. E. Kouri, H. G. Pope, D. Yurgelun-Todd, and S. Gruber, "Attributes of Heavy Versus Occasional Marijuana Smokers in a College Population," *Biological Psychiatry* 38 (1995): 475–481.
46. E. L. Gardner and J. H. Lowinson, "Marijuana's Interaction with Brain Reward Systems: Update 1991," *Pharmacology, Biochemistry, and Behavior* 40 (1991): 571.
47. G. Tanda, F. E. Pontieri and G. DiChiara, "Cannabinoid and Heroin Activation of Mesolimbic Dopamine Transmission by a Common Mu-opioid Receptor Mechanism," *Science* 276 (1997): 2048–2054.
48. J. Manzanares et al., "Pharmacological and Biochemical Interactions Between Opioids and Cannabinoids," *Trends in Pharmacological Sciences* 20 (1999): 287–294.
49. R. E. Musty and L. Kaback, "Relationships Between Motivation and Depression in Chronic Marijuana Users," *Life Sciences* 56 (1995): 2151–2158.
50. J.-F. Bouchard and D. Lamontagne, "Cardioprotection Induced by Endogenous Cannabinoids," *Proceedings of the Western Pharmacology Society* (2000): in press.
51. D. I. Hoffman, K. D. Brunemann, G. B. Gori, and E. L. Wynder, "On the Carcinogenicity of Marijuana Smoke," *Recent Advances in Phytochemistry* 9 (1975): 63–81.
52. D. P. Tashkin, M. S. Simmons, D. L. Sherrill, and A. H. Coulson, "Heavy Habitual Marijuana Smoking Does Not Cause an Accelerated Decline in FEV_1 with Age," *American Journal of Respiratory and Critical Care Medicine* 155 (1997): 141–148.
53. G. A. Cabral et al., "Anandamide Inhibits Macrophage-mediated Killing of Tumor Necrosis Factor-sensitive Cells," *Life Sciences* 56 (1995): 2065–2072.
54. B. B. Little, T. T. VanBeveren, and L. C. Gilstrap, "Cannabinoid Use During Pregnancy," in L. C. Gilstrap and B. B. Little, eds., *Drugs and Pregnancy*, 2nd ed. (New York: Chapman & Hall), 1998: 413–417.
55. P. A. Fried, "The Ottawa Prenatal Prospective Study (OPPS): Methodological Issues and Findings—It's Easy to Throw the Baby Out with the Bath Water," *Life Sciences* 56 (1995): 2159–2168.
56. D. Brookoff, C. S. Cook, C. Williams, and C. S. Mann, "Testing Reckless Drivers for Cocaine and Marijuana," *New England Journal of Medicine* 331 (1994): 518–522.

57. C. S. Breivogel et al., "Chronic Delta-9-tetrahydrocannabinol Treatment Produces a Time-dependent Loss of Cannabinoid Receptors and Cannabinoid Receptor-activated G-proteins in Rat Brain," *Journal of Neurochemistry* 73 (1999): 2447–2459.

58. C. Hsieh, S. Brown, C. Derleth, and K. Mackie, "Internalization and Recycling of the CB1 Cannabinoid Receptor," *Journal of Neurochemistry* 73 (1999): 493–501.

59. A. Duffy and R. Milin, "Case Study: Withdrawal Syndrome in Adolescent Chronic Cannabis Users," *Journal of the American Academy of Child and Adolescent Psychiatry* 35 (1996): 1618–1621.

60. J. Brook, E. B. Balka, and M. Whiteman, "The Risks for Late Adolescence of Early Adolescence Marijuana Use," *American Journal of Public Health* 89 (1999): 1549–1554.

61. L. Grinspoon and J. B. Bakalar, "Marijuana," in J. H. Lowinson, P. Ruiz, R. B. Millman, and J. G. Langrod, eds., *Substance Abuse: A Comprehensive Textbook*, 3rd ed. (Baltimore: Williams & Wilkins, 1997), 199–206.

62. R. H. Schwartz, E. A. Voth, and M. J. Sheridan, "Marijuana to Prevent Nausea and Vomiting in Cancer Patients: A Survey of Clinical Oncologists," *Southern Medical Journal* 90 (1997): 167–172.

63. T. Nagayama et al., "Cannabinoids and Neuroprotection in Global and Focal Cerebral Ischemia and in Neuronal Cultures," *Journal of Neuroscience* 19 (1999): 2987–2995.

64. A. Biegon and A. B. Joseph, "Development of HU-211 (Dexanabinol) as a Neuroprotectant for Ischemic Brain Damage," *Neurological Research* 17 (1995): 275–280.

65. Institute of Medicine, "Marijuana and Medicine: Assessing the Science Base," (Washington, D.C.: National Academy Press, 1999). [Available on line at www.nap.edu]

66. L. E. Hollister, "An Approach to the Medical Marijuana Controversy," *Drug and Alcohol Dependence* 58 (2000): 3–7.

67. J. P. Kassirer, "Federal Foolishness and Marijuana," *New England Journal of Medicine* 336 (1997): 366–367.

Chapter 12

Psychedelic Drugs: Mescaline, LSD, and Other Hallucinogens

This chapter introduces a group of heterogeneous compounds that alter cortical functions, including cognition, perception, and mood.[1,2] Characteristically, these drugs can induce hallucinations, separating people who use them from reality. Because of the wide range of psychological effects they produce, the single term that might best be used to classify these agents has long been debated. The term *hallucinogen* is used because these agents can, in high enough doses, induce hallucinations. However, that term is somewhat inappropriate because illusory phenomena and perceptual distortions are more common than are true hallucinations. The term *psychotomimetic* has also been used because of the alleged ability of these drugs to mimic psychoses or induce psychotic states. However, most of these drugs do not produce the same behavioral patterns that are observed in people who experience psychotic episodes. Others have used a descriptive term, such as *phantasticum* (proposed by Lewin in 1924) or *psychedelic* (proposed by Osmond in 1957), to imply that these agents all have the ability to alter sensory perception. In this book the term *psychedelic* is used because it allows for more flexibility in grouping together a disparate array of effects into a quantifiable and recognizable syndrome.[3]

Abraham, Aldridge, and Gogia[4] define a psychedelic drug as "any agent that causes alterations in perception, cognition, and mood as its primary psychobiological actions in the presence of an otherwise clear sensorium." This definition separates the pure psychedelic drugs from other substances that can cause altered states of thinking and perception, such as *poisons* that affect the mind (not discussed in this book) and *deliriants* that produce clouding of consciousness and amnesia. This chapter covers both the true psychedelics and certain deliriants that are commonly abused (scopolamine and two anesthetic psychedelics, phencyclidine and ketamine).

Many psychedelic agents occur in nature; others are synthetically produced. Naturally occurring psychedelic drugs have been inhaled, ingested, worshipped, and reviled since prehistory.[4] Some may even be viewed as having magical or mystical properties. Prior to the 1960s, most nonnative people were barely aware of their existence. During the late 1960s and 1970s, however, some people advocated their use to enhance perception, expand reality, promote personal awareness, and stimulate or induce comprehension of the spiritual or supernatural. These drugs heighten awareness of sensory input, often accompanied by both an enhanced sense of clarity and diminished control over what is experienced. Frequently, there is a feeling that one part of the self seems to be a passive observer, while another part of the self participates and receives the vivid and unusual sensory experiences. In this state, the slightest sensation may take on profound meaning. Today, many of these drugs are used not only for sensory expansion but for an intoxicating effect.

Most psychedelic drugs structurally resemble one of four neurotransmitters: acetylcholine, two catecholamines (norepinephrine and dopamine), and serotonin. These structural similarities lead to three classes for categorizing psychedelic drugs (see Table 12.1): *anticholinergic, catecholamine-like,* and *serotonin-like.* Table 12.1 includes a fourth class of psychedelic drugs, the *psychedelic anesthetics,* which exert their psychedelic actions by affecting a specific subclass of glutamate receptors, the NMDA receptors. Intoxicants—for example, alcohol (Chapter 4), GHB (Chapter 5), kava (Chapter 20), and the inhalants of abuse (Chapter 4)—do not produce hallucinations or profound sensory distortion in doses below intoxicating doses; therefore they are not included as psychedelic drugs.

Anticholinergic Psychedelics: Scopolamine

Scopolamine, an acetylcholine receptor antagonist, is the classic example of an anticholinergic psychedelic drug (Figure 12.1). Having receptor affinity but devoid of intrinsic activity, scopolamine blocks the access of acetylcholine to its receptors—hence the term anticholinergic.

Historical Background

The history of scopolamine is long and colorful.[5] The drug is distributed widely in nature, found in especially high concentrations in the plants *Atropa belladonna* (belladonna, or deadly nightshade), *Datura*

TABLE 12.1 Classification of psychedelic drugs

ANTICHOLINERGIC PSYCHEDELIC DRUG
Scopolamine

CATECHOLAMINE-LIKE PSYCHEDELIC DRUGS
Mescaline
DOM, MDA, DMA, MDMA, TMA, MDE
Myristin, elemicin

SEROTONIN-LIKE PSYCHEDELIC DRUGS
Lysergic acid diethylamide (LSD)
Dimethyltryptamine (DMT)
Psilocybin, psilocin, bufotenine
Ololiuqui (morning glory seeds)
Harmine

PSYCHEDELIC ANESTHETIC DRUGS
Phencyclidine (Sernyl)
Ketamine (Ketalar)

---

stramonium (Jamestown weed, jimsonweed, stinkweed, thorn apple, or devil's apple), and *Mandragora officinarum* (mandrake). Both professional and amateur poisoners of the Middle Ages frequently used deadly nightshade as a source of poison. In fact, the plant's name, *Atropa belladonna*, is derived from Atropos, the Greek goddess who supposedly cuts the thread of life. Belladonna means "beautiful woman," which refers to the drug's ability to dilate the pupils when it is applied topically to the eyes (eyes with widely dilated pupils were presumably a mark of beauty). Accidental ingestion of berries from *Datura* has even been associated with the incapacitation of whole armies, for example, the defeat of Marc Antony's army in 36 B.C. and the defeat of British soldiers by settlers in the rebellion known as Bacon's Revolution near Jamestown, Virginia, in 1676 (hence the name Jamestown weed).

Plants that contain *atropine* (another drug found in scopolamine-containing plants) and scopolamine have been used and misused for centuries. For example, the delirium caused by these substances may have persuaded certain people that they could fly—and that they were witches (associated with the Halloween customs involving flying witches). Marijuana and opium preparations from the Far East were once fortified with material from *Datura stramonium*. Today, cigarettes

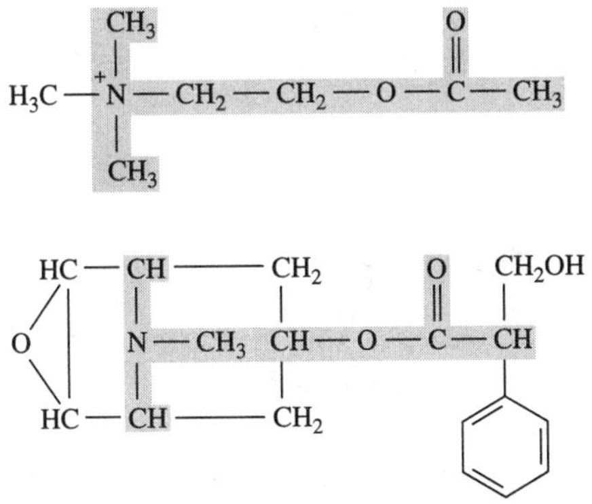

FIGURE 12.1 Structural formulas of acetylcholine (a chemical transmitter) and the anticholinergic psychedelic scopolamine, which acts by blocking acetylcholine receptors. The shaded portion of each molecule illustrates structural similarities, which presumably contribute to receptor fit.

made from the leaves of *Datura stramonium* and *Atropa belladonna* are smoked occasionally to induce intoxication. Throughout the world, leaves of plants that contain atropine or scopolamine are still used to prepare intoxicating beverages.

Pharmacological Effects

Scopolamine acts on the peripheral nervous system to produce an anticholinergic syndrome consisting of dry mouth, reduced sweating, dry skin, increased body temperature, dilated pupils, blurred vision, tachycardia, and hypertension. Scopolamine in the CNS functions as a deliriant and intoxicant. Low doses produce drowsiness, mild euphoria, profound amnesia, fatigue, delirium, mental confusion, dreamless sleep, and loss of attention. Rather than expanding consciousness, awareness, and insight, scopolamine clouds consciousness and produces amnesia; it does not expand sensory perception. As doses progress, psychiatric symptoms include restlessness, excitement, hallucinations, euphoria, and disorientation.

In higher and much more toxic doses, a behavioral state that resembles a toxic psychosis occurs. Delirium, mental confusion, stupor, coma, and respiratory depression dominate. While scopolamine intoxication can convey a sense of excitement and loss of control to the user, the clouding of consciousness and the reduction in memory of the episode render scopolamine rather unattractive as a psychedelic drug. Indeed, it is more appropriate to refer to it as a somewhat dangerous intoxicant, amnestic, and deliriant. Scopolamine is classically stated to make one "hot as a hare, blind as a bat, dry as a bone, red as a beet, and mad as a hen."

Catecholamine-like (Phenethylamine) Psychedelics

Norepinephrine and dopamine receptors are important sites of action for a large group of psychedelic drugs that are structurally similar to both catecholamine neurotransmitters and the amphetamines (Figure 12.2). Structurally, the catecholamine psychedelics resemble norepinephrine, dopamine, and the amphetamines in that they contain the basic phenyl ring, a ethyl side chain with an attached nitrogen or amine ring; hence the classification as a phenethylamine psychedelic.[1] They differ structurally from the normal neurotransmitters by the addition of one or more methoxy (OCH_3) groups to the phenyl ring structure; these methoxy groups, varied as they are (Figure 12.2), seem to confer psychedelic properties on top of their amphetamine-like psychostimulant properties. Methoxylated amphetamine derivatives include mescaline, DOM (also called STP), MDA, MDE, MDMA (ecstasy), MMDA, DMA, and certain drugs that are obtained from nutmeg (myristin and elemicin).

As would be predicted from their structures, phenethylamine psychedelics exert amphetamine-like psychostimulant actions, presumably on dopaminergic neurons (Chapter 7). However, their psychedelic actions are probably ultimately exerted by augmentation of serotonin neurotransmission; they are probably full agonists at postsynaptic serotonin 5-HT_{2A} receptors. This action would account for their LSD-like effects.[1] The combination of catecholamine and serotonin actions points to a complex interaction between dopamine and serotonin and explains their "intermediate position between stimulants and (LSD-like) hallucinogens."[6]

As early as the late 1960s, most psychedelics were known to produce a remarkably similar set of effects, including enhanced emotional responses; sensory-perceptual distortion; altered perceptions of colors, sounds, and shapes; complex hallucinations; dreamlike feelings; depersonalization; and somatic effects (tingling skin, weakness, tremor, and so on). During the 1980s, it was noted that psychedelic drugs produce marked alterations in brain serotonin. As serotonin receptors were characterized in the early 1990s, it became clear that LSD was a serotonin receptor agonist and that the catecholamine-like psychedelics functioned ultimately as indirectly acting serotonin agonists. Today, the focus of attention has been on activation of a subgroup of the 5-HT_2 receptors, specifically the 5-HT_{2A} receptor.[1] These psychedelics can therefore be safely classified as mixed dopamine and serotonin agonists, with 5-HT_2 receptors certainly involved.

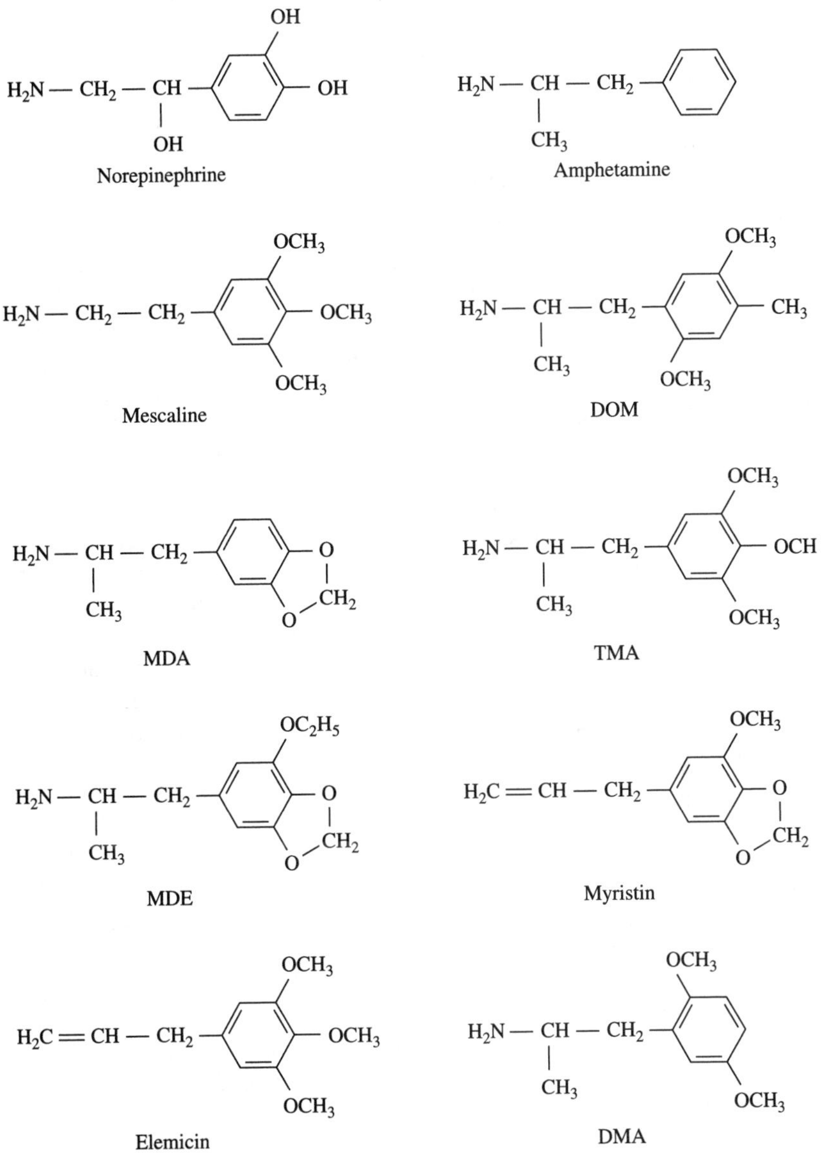

FIGURE 12.2 Structural formulas of norepinephrine (a chemical transmitter), amphetamine, and eight catecholamine-like psychedelic drugs. These eight drugs are structurally related to norepinephrine and are thought to exert their psychedelic actions by altering the transmission of nerve impulses at norepinephrine and serotonin synapses in the brain.

Mescaline

Peyote (*Lophophora williamsii*) is a common plant in the southwestern United States and in Mexico. It is a spineless cactus that has a small crown, or "button," and a long root. When the plant is used for psychedelic purposes, the crown is cut from the cactus and dried into a hard brown disk. This disk, which is frequently referred to as a "mescal button," is later softened in the mouth and swallowed. The psychedelic chemical in the button is mescaline.

Historical Background. The use of peyote extends back to pre-Columbian times, when the cactus was used in the religious rites of the Aztecs and other Mexican Indians. Currently, peyote is legally available for use in the religious practice of the Native American Church of North America, whose members regard peyote as sacramental. The use of peyote for religious purposes is not considered to be abuse, and peyote is seldom abused by members of the Native American Church. Today, the federal government and 23 states permit its sacramental use.

Pharmacological Effects. Early research on the peyote cactus led in 1896 to the identification of mescaline as its pharmacologically active ingredient. After the chemical structure of mescaline was elucidated in 1918, the compound was produced synthetically. Because of its structural resemblance to norepinephrine, a wide variety of synthetic mescaline derivatives has now been synthesized, and all have methoxy (OCH_3) groups or similar additions on their benzene rings (Figure 12.2). Methoxylation of the benzene ring apparently adds psychedelic properties to the drug, presumably due to increased affinity and full agonist activity at the 5-HT_{2A} receptor subtype.[7]

When taken orally, mescaline is rapidly and completely absorbed, and significant concentrations are usually achieved in the brain within 1 to 2 hours. Between 3.5 and 4 hours after drug intake, mescaline produces an acute psychotomimetic state, with prominent effects on the visual system. The effects of a single dose of mescaline persist for approximately 10 hours. The drug does not appear to be metabolized before it is excreted. In functional brain imaging using SPECT, mescaline produced in healthy volunteers "a 'hyperfrontal' pattern with an emphasis on the right hemisphere, which was correlated with mescaline-induced psychotomimetic psychopathology. This questions the validity of the concept of hypofrontality as an explanation for acute psychotic symptomatology."[8]

Interest in mescaline focuses on the fact that it produces unusual psychic effects and visual hallucinations. The usual oral dose (5 mg/kg) in the average normal subject causes anxiety, sympathomimetic effects, hyperreflexia of the limbs, tremors, and visual hallucinations that consist of brightly colored lights, geometric designs, animals, and occasionally people; color and space perception is often concomitantly impaired, but otherwise the sensorium is normal and insight is retained.

The psychotic effects were mainly concerned with the dissolution of ego boundaries, visual hallucinations, and dimensions of "oceanic boundlessness," often mixed with anxious passivity experiences.[9]

Synthetic Amphetamine Derivatives

DOM, MDA, DMA, MDE, TMA, and MDMA are structurally related to mescaline and methamphetamine and, as might be expected, produce similar effects. They have moderate behavioral-stimulant effects at low doses, but like LSD, psychedelic effects dominate as doses increase. These derivatives are considerably more potent and more toxic than mescaline.

DOM (dimethoxy-methamphetamine) has effects that are similar to those of mescaline; doses of 1 to 6 milligrams produce euphoria, which is followed by a 6- to 8-hour period of hallucinations. DOM is 100 times more potent than mescaline but much less potent than LSD. The use of DOM is associated with a high incidence of overdose (because it is potent and street doses are poorly controlled). Acute toxic reactions are common; they consist of tremors that may eventually lead to convulsive movements, prostration, and even death. Because toxic reactions are common, the use of DOM is not widespread.

MDA (methylene-dioxy-amphetamine), *DMA* (dimethoxy-methylamphetamine), *MDE* (methylene-dioxy-ethylamphetamine, or Eve), *TMA* (trimethoxy-amphetamine), and other structural variations of amphetamine are encountered as "designer psychedelics." MDA is also a metabolite of MDMA,[10] and much of MDMA's effect may be due to the presence of MDA. In general, the pharmacological effects of these drugs resemble those of mescaline and LSD; they reflect the mix of catecholamine and serotonin interactions. Side effects and toxicities (including fatalities) are similar to those of MDMA.

Gouzoulis-Mayfrank and colleagues,[6] in their SPECT-scan study of MDE, noted that MDE induced hypermetabolism in the cerebellum and right anterior cingulate with hypometabolism in the cortex. They referred to MDE as an *entactogen*,[*] constituting "an intermediate position between stimulants and hallucinogens."

MDMA. MDMA (methylene-dioxy-methamphetamine, also called ecstasy, XTC, and Adam) resembles MDA in structure but may be less hallucinogenic, inducing a less extreme sense of disembodiment and visual distortion. MDMA is also a potent and selective neurotoxin in animals.[11] PET scan studies on human users suggest memory impairment and

---

[*]Gouzoulis-Mayfrank and colleagues[6] use the term *entactogen* to distinguish mechanisms of drug-induced enhancement of emotional responses (entactogenic effects) from mechanisms responsible for hallucinogenic effects and stimulant effects (such as increased drive and energy).

reduced serotonin transporter binding, both consistent with neurotoxicity. It is now generally agreed that MDMA in animals is a potent and selective serotonin neurotoxin. Mechanistically, such neurotoxicity involves damage to the presynaptic serotonin transporter:

> Prolonged activation of protein kinase C within the 5-HT nerve terminal may contribute to lasting changes in the homeostatic function of 5-HT neurons, leading to the degeneration of specific cellular elements after repeated MDMA exposure.[12]

In human studies, MDMA users (compared with matched controls) performed several attentional and short-term memory tasks less accurately and more slowly than controls, with selective lowering of the spinal fluid serotonin metabolite 5-HIAA, reflecting reduced serotonin turnover.[13] In a SPECT-scan study of MDMA users, Semple and co-workers[14] reported significant reductions in serotonin transporter binding in the sensorimotor cortex with associated subtle cognitive deficits. Morgan[15] administered a test battery to MDMA users (who also used other illicit substances), non-MDMA-using drug abusers, and drug nonuser controls. MDMA users were "more psychologically disturbed and impulsive than non-drug controls." Compared with non-MDMA-using drug abusers, MDMA users were more impulsive, an observation "consistent with previous evidence that elevated levels of impulsivity in humans are associated with reduced levels of serotoninergic function."

In a controversial set of studies, Vollenweider and colleagues[16,17,18] examined the effects of a single dose of MDMA in 13 MDMA-naive healthy volunteers. At a dose of 1.7 mg/kg body weight,

> MDMA produced an affective state of enhanced mood, well-being, and increased emotional sensitiveness, little anxiety, but no hallucinations or panic reactions. Mild depersonalization and derealization phenomena occurred together with moderate thought disorder, first signs of loss of body control, and alterations in the meaning of percepts. Subjects also displayed changes in the sense of space and time, heightened sensory awareness, and increased psychomotor drive.

Despite these generally positive emotional effects, "somatic" effects were significant. One subject experienced a dramatic hypertensive effect (reaching 240/145 mmHg), while the blood pressure of other subjects peaked at 160/100 mmHg).* Other somatic effects included jaw clenching, suppressed appetite, restlessness, insomnia, impaired gait, and rest-

---

*The hypertensive effect should not be underestimated, particularly in persons with latent cardiovascular problems.[17]

less legs. Adverse sequelae after 24 hours included lack of energy and appetite, fatigue, restlessness, difficulty concentrating, and brooding.

Concern about MDMA is increasing as use of the drug increases around the world, especially at dance clubs and "raves." Surveys indicate that between 1.5 and 3.5 percent of 15- to 30-year olds have used ecstasy within the last year. In a recent study in Australia, Topp and colleagues[19] noted that early studies of ecstasy users found generally self-limiting patterns of use, low levels of intravenous use, and few adverse health effects. In their study, the situation was radically different. Extensive polydrug use was the norm (Table 12.2), high rates of intravenous use were reported, and many physical, psychological, financial, relationship, and occupational problems occurred as a result of ecstasy use (Tables 12.3 and 12.4). Twenty percent of users had received

TABLE 12.2 Patterns of drug use of 329 ecstasy users

Drug class	Ever used (%)	Used in last 6 months (%)	No. days used in last 6 months (median)[a]
Ecstasy	100	100	10
Alcohol	99.1	93.6	24
Cannabis	98.8	92.1	48
Amphetamine	94.2	81.8	10
LSD	93.3	68.1	4
Tobacco	85.4	74.8	180
Amyl nitrate	75.4	46.5	3
Cocaine	61.4	40.7	2
Nitrous oxide	61.1	35.3	4
Benzodiazepines	56.8	43.2	5.5
MDA	50.5	31.3	3
Other opiates	32.0	20.7	3
Heroin	30.1	17.3	12
Antidepressants	23.1	13.4	6
Ketamine	18.2	10.0	4
Ethyl chloride	10.0	5.8	2
Methadone	7.3	2.7	20
Anabolic steroids	4.3	1.5	20
GHB	2.7	1.8	1.5
Other drugs[b]	—	5.2	2

[a]Among those who had used.
[b]Other drugs included hallucinogenic mushrooms, DMT, and 2CB.
From Topp et al.[19]

TABLE 12.3 Physical side effects of ectasy ($n = 329$)

Symptom	Last 6 months (%)	While using ecstasy[a]	While coming down[a]	At other times[b]	Median length of worst case[b]	Only related to ecstasy(%)[b]
Loss of energy	64.9	7.7	61.2	19.4	2 days	46.0
Muscular aches	59.9	10.7	57.6	11.6	2 days	34.7
Hot/cold flushes	48.0	39.2	25.5	4.9	1 h	52.5
Blurred vision	47.1	45.9	12.5	4.0	1 h	69.0
Numbness/tingling	45.6	42.2	14.9	6.4	1 h	59.3
Profuse sweating	42.6	38.9	18.0	4.9	3 h	40.6
Weight loss	42.6				21 days	26.1
Dizziness	41.9	31.0	21.3	9.7	20 min	46.4
Tremors/shakes	41.9	30.1	25.2	8.8	2 h	46.4
Heart palpitations	40.7	37.1	16.1	7.6	30 min	38.8
Headaches	40.4	11.2	35.3	7.9	4 h	35.3
Stomach pains	37.7	25.5	22.8	6.4	2 h	48.0
Joint pains/stiffness	35.0	7.9	33.4	7.6	2 days	31.3
Inability to urinate	34.7	34.3	5.8	1.5	3 h	77.9
Vomiting	33.9	30.0	7.6	5.5	5 min	64.9
Teeth problems	33.1	15.2	23.2	12.2	2 days	44.0
Shortness of breath	26.4	22.8	6.7	2.1	30 min	34.5
Blackout/memory lapse	24.9	14.3	12.8	3.2	3 h	31.3
Chest pains	15.8	8.8	9.4	4.9	1 h	25.0
Fainting/passing out	6.4	4.9	1.8	1.5	3.5 min	47.6
Fits/seizures[c]	(3)	(2)	(2)	(0)	30 s	(1)

[a]Proportion of total sample [b]Among those reporting the symptom [c]Figures in parentheses refer to ns. From Topp et al.[19]

TABLE 12.4 Psychological side effects of ectasy (n = 329)

Symptom	Last 6 months (%)	While using ecstasy[a]	While coming down[a]	At other times[b]	Median length of worst case[b]	Only related to ecstasy (%)[b]
Irritability	61.9	3.4	59.8	20.4	2 days	46.8
Trouble sleeping	55.9	23.1	52.0	16.1	12 h	43.2
Depression	55.6	4.6	49.8	24.3	3 days	49.7
Confusion	47.4	30.4	45.6	10.6	12 days	53.2
Anxiety	45.0	26.7	32.5	14.0	4 h	45.9
Paranoia	40.4	22.2	30.7	10.9	3 h	39.8
Visual hallucinations	28.0	27.1	8.2	5.5	1.5 h	52.2
Sound hallucinations	20.7	18.5	7.3	3.3	45 min	54.4
Flashbacks	14.6	0	4.9	12.2	5 min	52.1
Panic attacks	12.8	10.0	4.6	4.0	1 h	42.9
Loss of sex urge	12.2	8.2	7.6	5.2	24 h	52.5
Suicidal thoughts[c]	10.3	(2)	8.2	6.7	24 h	26.5
Violent behavior[c]	(9)	(2)	(5)	(5)	60 min	(2)
Suicide attempts[c]	(3)	0	(1)	(2)	—	0

[a]Proportion of total sample [b]Among those reporting the symptom [c]Figures in parentheses refer to ns. From Topp et al.[19]

treatment for an ecstasy-related problem, and 15 percent wanted formal treatment. Jansen[20] reports on three cases of physical dependence on ecstasy.

It is possible that MDMA is potentially too dangerous for human use: abuse of MDMA may lead to severe toxicities, including fatalities. During periods of intense activity, such as skiing[21] and dancing at "rave" parties,[10,22,23] symptoms include hyperthermia, tachycardia, disorientation, dilated pupils, convulsions, rigidity, and breakdown of skeletal muscle, and kidney failure. Despite these consequences, the "intense euphoric high" promotes continued use.[22]

As a side note, "herbal ecstasy" is an alternative drug of abuse, usually containing both ephedrine and caffeine. Zahn and co-workers[24] report a case of severe cardiovascular toxicity after four capsules of herbal ecstacy; toxicity consisted of severe hypertension and cardiac arrhythmias. Aggressive emergency room treatment led to resolution of symptoms in about 9 hours. (Further discussion of herbal combinations of ephedrine and caffeine appears in Chapter 20.)

The combined use of MDMA with LSD, called "candyflipping," produces a synergistic effect demonstrable in rodents.[25] Use of this combination appears to be increasing.

Myristin and Elemicin. Nutmeg and mace are common household spices sometimes abused for their hallucinogenic properties.[26] Myristin and elemicin, the pharmacologically active ingredients in nutmeg and mace, are responsible for this psychedelic action. Ingestion of large amounts (1 to 2 teaspoons—5 to 15 grams—usually brewed in tea) may, after a delay of 2 to 5 hours, induce feelings of unreality, confusion, disorientation, euphoria, visual hallucinations, acute psychotic reactions, and feelings of impending doom, depersonalization, and unreality. Considering the close structural resemblance of myristin and elemicin to mescaline (Figure 12.2), these psychedelic actions are not unexpected. Ingestion of nutmeg, however, produces many unpleasant side effects, including vomiting, nausea, and tremors. After nutmeg or mace has been taken to produce its psychedelic action, the side effects usually dissuade users from trying these agents a second time.[27]

Serotonin-like (Indoleamine) Psychedelic Drugs

The serotonin-like psychedelic drugs include lysergic acid diethylamide (LSD), psilocybin and psilocin (both from the mushroom *Psilocybe mexicana*), dimethyltryptamine (DMT), and bufotenine (Figure 12.3). Because of their structural resemblance to each other and to serotonin, it has long been presumed that these agents somehow exerted

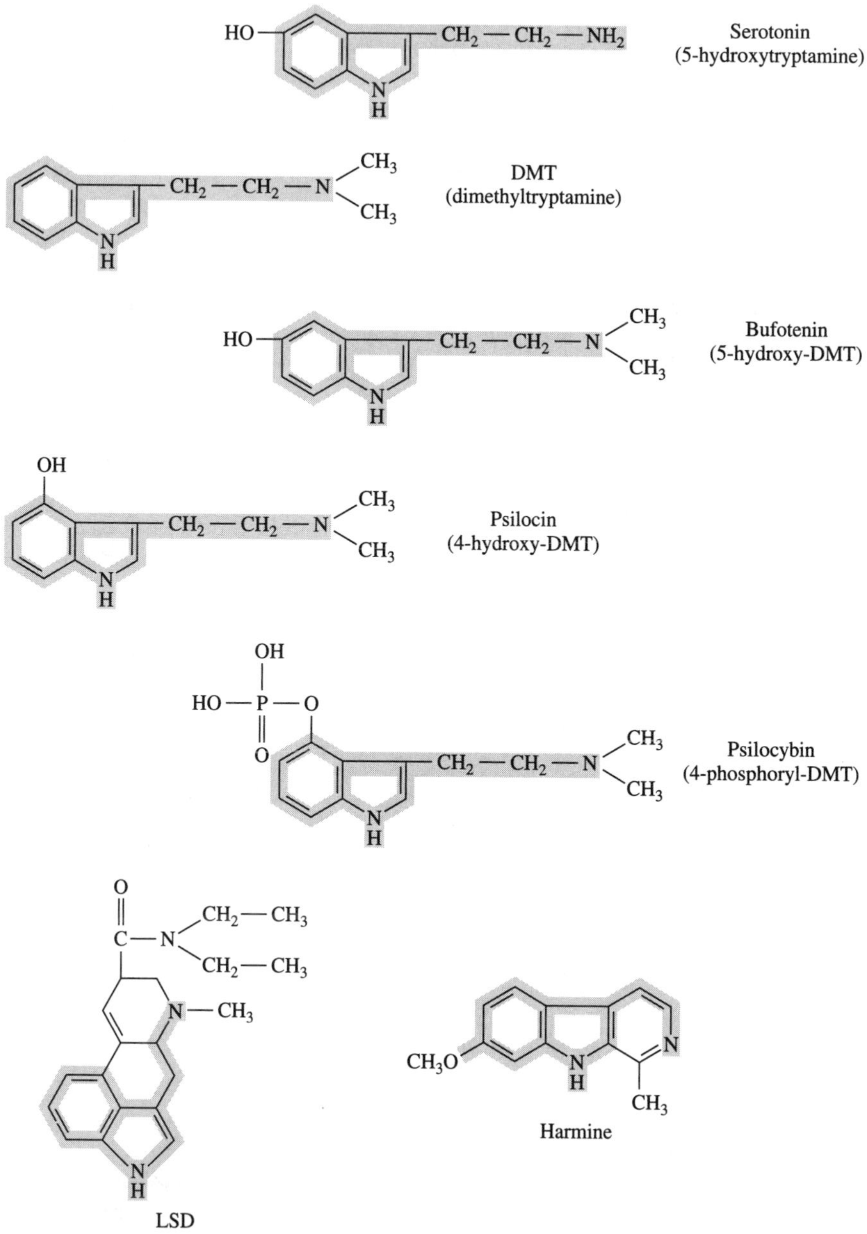

FIGURE 12.3 Structural formulas of serotonin (a chemical transmitter) and six serotonin-like psychedelic drugs. These six drugs are structurally related to serotonin (as indicated by the shading) and are thought to exert their psychedelic actions through alterations of serotonin synapses in the brain. Although LSD is structurally much more complex than serotonin, the basic similarity of the two molecules is apparent.

their effects through interactions at serotonin synapses. Identification of such interactions has, however, been difficult.

Almaula and co-workers[28] mapped the binding site for LSD on the $5-HT_{2A}$ receptor and correlated the binding with receptor activation. Penington and Fox[29] claim that LSD exerts a spectrum of agonist-antagonist effects on a variety of 5-HT receptor subtypes, but they think that the best candidate appears to be agonist actions on $5-HT_{1C}$ receptors. Egan and co-workers[30] and Krebs-Thompson and colleagues[31] argue for an agonist action at both $5-HT_{2A}$ and $5-HT_{2C}$ receptors. Grailhe and co-workers[32] suggest the $5-HT_{5A}$ receptor as a site of action of LSD. Giacomelli and colleagues[33] argue for a complex interaction between the serotoninergic system and the dopaminergic system (LSD acting as a partial agonist at dopaminergic D_2 receptors). Finally, Marek and Aghajanian[1,2] argue for an agonist action at $5-HT_{2A}$ receptors.

With all this focus of agonist action on serotonin receptors, a major question remains unanswered: Why does serotonin not induce psychotomimetic effects? In particular, psychotomimetic effects are not seen after administration of SSRI-type antidepressants or any other treatment that increases serotonin availability at its postsynaptic receptors. Even in the serotonin syndrome (Chapter 15), psychotomimetic effects are rarely seen. Marek and Aghajanian[1] address this problem but are unable to provide an answer.

Regardless of receptor mechanisms, these drugs do produce a characteristic psychedelic syndrome. One speculation about the process by which hallucinogens manifest their impressive alterations of mood, perception, and thought is that the pontine (dorsal) raphe, a major center of serotonin activity, serves as a filtering station for incoming sensory stimuli. It screens the flood of sensations and perceptions, eliminating those that are unimportant, irrelevant, or commonplace. A drug like LSD may disrupt the sorting process, allowing a surge of sensory data and an overload of brain circuits. Dehabituation, in which the familiar becomes novel, is noted under LSD. It may also be caused by indirectly lowering the sensory gates by inhibition of the raphe activity.[34]

Lysergic Acid Diethylamide (LSD)

During the 1960s and early 1970s, lysergic acid diethylamide (LSD) became one of the most remarkable and controversial drugs known. In doses that are so small that they might even be considered infinitesimal, LSD induces remarkable psychological change in a person, enhancing self-awareness and altering internal reality, while causing relatively few alterations in the general physiology of the body.

Historical Background. LSD was first synthesized in 1938 by Albert Hofmann, a Swiss chemist, as part of an organized research program to investigate possible therapeutic uses of compounds obtained from ergot, a natural product derived from a fungus (*Claviceps purpurea*). Early pharmacological studies of LSD in animals failed to reveal anything unusual; the psychedelic action was neither sought nor expected. Thus, LSD remained unnoticed until 1943, when Doctor Hofmann had an unusual experience:

> In the afternoon of 16 April, 1943, . . . I was seized by a peculiar sensation of vertigo and restlessness. Objects, as well as the shape of my associates in the laboratory, appeared to undergo optical changes. I was unable to concentrate on my work. In a dreamlike state I left for home, where an irresistible urge to lie down overcame me. I drew the curtains and immediately fell into a peculiar state similar to drunkenness, characterized by an exaggerated imagination. With my eyes closed, fantastic pictures of extraordinary plasticity and intensive color seemed to surge toward me. After two hours, this state gradually wore off.[35]

Hofmann correctly hypothesized that his experience resulted from the accidental ingestion of LSD. To further characterize the experience, Hofmann self-administered what seemed to be a minuscule oral dose (only 0.25 milligram).[36] We now know, however, that this dose is about 10 times the dose required to induce psychedelic effects in most people. As a result of this miscalculation, his response was quite spectacular:

> After 40 minutes, I noted the following symptoms in my laboratory journal: slight giddiness, restlessness, difficulty in concentration, visual disturbances, laughing. . . . Later, I lost all count of time. I noticed with dismay that my environment was undergoing progressive changes. My visual field wavered and everything appeared deformed as in a faulty mirror. Space and time became more and more disorganized and I was overcome by a fear that I was going out of my mind. The worst part of it being that I was clearly aware of my condition. My power of observation was unimpaired. . . . Occasionally, I felt as if I were out of my body. I thought I had died. My ego seemed suspended somewhere in space, from where I saw my dead body lying on the sofa. . . . It was particularly striking how acoustic perceptions, such as the noise of water gushing from a tap or the spoken word, were transformed into optical illusions. I then fell asleep and awakened the next morning somewhat tired but otherwise feeling perfectly well.[35]

In 1949 the first North American study of LSD in humans was conducted, and during the 1950s large quantities of LSD were distributed to scientists for research purposes. A significant impetus to research was the notion that the effects of LSD might constitute a model for psychosis, which would provide some insight into the biochemical and physiological processes of mental illness and its treatment. Some therapists tried LSD as an adjunct to psychotherapy to help patients verbalize their problems and gain some insight into the underlying causes, but this has not proven to be an effective treatment.

Pharmacokinetics.   LSD is usually taken orally, and it is rapidly absorbed by that route. Usual doses range from about 25 micrograms to more than 300 micrograms. Because such amounts are so small, LSD is often added to other substances, such as squares of paper, the backs of stamps, or sugar cubes, which can be handled more easily. LSD is absorbed within about 60 minutes, reaching peak blood levels in about 3 hours. It is distributed rapidly and efficiently throughout the body; it diffuses easily into the brain and readily crosses the placenta. The largest amounts of LSD in the body are found in the liver, where the drug is metabolized before it is excreted. The usual duration of action is 6 to 8 hours.

Because of its extreme potency, only minuscule amounts can be detected in urine. Thus, conventional urine-screening tests are inadequate to detect LSD. When the use of LSD is suspected, urine is collected (up to 30 hours after ingestion) and an ultrasensitive radioimmunoassay is performed to verify the presence of the drug. Simpson and colleagues[37] discuss problems associated with screening for LSD and other drugs of abuse.

Physiological Effects.   Although the LSD experience is characterized by its psychological effects, subtle physiological changes also occur. A person who takes LSD may experience a slight increase in body temperature, dilation of the pupils, slightly increased heart rate and blood pressure, increased levels of glucose in the blood, and dizziness, drowsiness, nausea, and other effects that, although noticeable, seldom interfere with the psychedelic experience.

LSD is known to possess a low level of toxicity; the effective dose is about 50 micrograms while the lethal dose is about 14,000 micrograms. These figures provide a therapeutic ratio of 280, making the drug a remarkably nonlethal compound. This calculation does not include any fatal accidents or suicides that occur when a person is intoxicated by LSD. Indeed, most deaths attributed to LSD result from accidents, homicides, or suicide. The use of LSD during pregnancy is certainly unwise, although a distinct fetal LSD syndrome has not been described.

Psychological Effects.   The psychological effects of LSD are quite intense. At doses of 25 to 50 micrograms, pupillary dilation and a glassy-eyed appearance may be noticed. These effects are accompanied by alterations in perception, thinking, emotion, arousal, and self-image. Time is slowed or distorted; sensory input intensifies. Cognitive alterations include enhanced power to visualize previously seen or imagined objects and decreased vigilance and logical thought. Visual alterations are the most characteristic phenomenon; they typically include colored lights, distorted images, and vivid and fascinating images and shapes. Colors can be heard and sounds may be seen. The loss of boundaries and the fear of fragmentation create a need for a structuring or supporting environment and experienced companions. During the "trip," thoughts and memories can emerge under self-guidance, sometimes to the user's distress. Mood may be labile, shifting from depression to gaiety, from elation to fear. Tension and anxiety may mount and reach panic proportions.

The LSD-induced psychedelic experience typically occurs in three phases:

1. The *somatic phase* occurs after absorption of the drug and consists of CNS stimulation and autonomic changes that are predominantly sympathomimetic in nature.
2. The *sensory* (or perceptual) *phase* is characterized by sensory distortions and pseudohallucinations, which are the effects desired by the drug user.
3. The *psychic phase* signals a maximum drug effect, with changes in mood, disruption of thought processes, altered perception of time, depersonalization, true hallucinations, and psychotic episodes. Experiencing this phase is considered a "bad trip."

Tolerance and Dependence. Tolerance of both the psychological and physiological alterations that are induced by LSD readily and rapidly develops, and cross-tolerance occurs between LSD and other psychedelics. Tolerance is lost within several days after the user stops taking the drug.

Physical dependence on LSD does not develop, even when the drug is used repeatedly for a prolonged period of time. In fact, most heavy users of the drug say that they ceased using LSD because they tired of it, had no further need for it, or had enough. Even when the drug is discontinued because of concern about bad trips or about physical or mental harm, few withdrawal signs are exhibited. Laboratory animals do not self-administer LSD.

Adverse Reactions and Toxicity. The adverse reactions attributed to LSD generally fall into five categories:

- Chronic or intermittent psychotic states
- Persistent or recurrent major affective disorder (i.e., depression)
- Exacerbation of preexisting psychiatric illness
- Disruption of personality or chronic brain syndrome, known as "burnout"

- Post-hallucinogenic perceptual disorder (i.e., flashbacks characterized by the periodic hallucinogenic imagery months or even years
after the immediate effect of LSD has worn off)

Dimijian[38] wrote:

> Unpleasant experiences with LSD are relatively frequent and may in-
> volve an uncontrollable drift into confusion, dissociative reactions,
> acute panic reactions, a reliving of earlier traumatic experiences, or
> an acute psychotic hospitalization. Prolonged nonpsychotic reactions
> have included dissociative reactions, time and space distortion, body
> image changes, and a residue of fear or depression stemming from
> morbid or terrifying experiences under the drug. . . . With the failure
> of usual defense mechanisms, the onslaught of repressed material
> overwhelms the integrative capacity of the ego, and a psychotic reac-
> tion results. It appears that [LSD-induced] disruption of long-
> established patterns of adapting may be a lasting or semipermanent
> effect of the drug.

LSD reduces a person's normal ability to control emotional reactions, and drug-induced alterations in perception can become so intense that they overwhelm one's ability to cope. There is also the
possible problem of persistent flashbacks, which may occur weeks or
even months after the last use of the drug.[39] Today, the term flashback
has been supplanted by the diagnostic entity *hallucinogen persisting
perception disorder*. Treatment success has been only partial.[3] Halpern
and Pope[40] review evidence for and against drug-induced residual neurotoxicity that would account for a hallucinogen persisting perceptual
disorder. They conclude:

> There are few, if any, long-term neuropsychological deficits attribut-
> able to hallucinogen use. . . . however, to better resolve this issue, it
> will be important to study larger samples of chronic, frequent hallu-
> cinogen users who have not often used other types of drugs.

This controversy over long-term consequences of use of LSD and other
hallucinogens will undoubtedly persist for as long as hallucinogens are
used.

Other Serotonin-like Hallucinogens

DMT. DMT (dimethyl-tryptamine) is a short-acting, naturally occurring psychedelic compound that can be synthesized easily and that
structurally is related to serotonin. DMT produces LSD-like effects in
the user, and, like LSD, it has been shown to bind to serotonin 5-HT$_2$

receptors. Widely used throughout much of the world, DMT is an active ingredient of various types of South American plants, such as *Virola calophylla* and *Mimosa hostilis*; it is snorted or smoked, often on a marijuana cigarette. (DMT is destroyed by stomach acid before it is absorbed; therefore it is not taken orally.) DMT appears to be largely metabolized by the enzyme monoamine oxidase (MAO).

In 1994, Strassman and colleagues[41,42] conducted controlled investigations of DMT in "highly motivated," experienced hallucinogen users. Administered intravenously (0.04 mg/kg to 0.4 mg/kg body weight), onset of action occurred within 2 minutes and was negligible at 30 minutes. DMT elevated blood pressure, heart rate, and temperature, dilated pupils, and increased body endorphin and hormone levels. The psychedelic threshold dose was 0.2 mg/kg body weight; lower doses were primarily "affective and somaesthetic."[42] Hallucinogenic effects included

> a rapidly moving, brightly colored visual display of images. Auditory effects were less common. "Loss of control," associated with a brief, but overwhelming "rush," led to a dissociated state, where euphoria alternated or coexisted with anxiety. These effects completely replaced subjects' previously ongoing mental experience and were more vivid and compelling than dreams or waking awareness.[42]

Thus, DMT produces intense visual hallucinations, intoxication, and often a loss of awareness of the user's surroundings. After the 30-minute period of effect, the user returns to normal feelings and perceptions; thus the nicknames "lunch-hour drug," "businessman's lunch," and "businessman's LSD."

Bufotenine.   Bufotenine (5-hydroxy DMT), like LSD and DMT, is a potent serotonin agonist hallucinogen with an affinity for several types of serotonin receptors. The name bufotenine comes from the name for a toad of the genus *bufo*, whose skin secretions supposedly produce hallucinogenic effects when ingested. Fuller and co-workers[43] studied the pharmacokinetics of bufotenine administered to rats. After subcutaneous injection, the half-life is about 2 hours with MAO responsible for metabolism (as it is for DMT).

In humans, research in the 1960s attempted to correlate the presence of bufotenine in urine (in humans bufotenine is formed from an unusual metabolic pathway for the metabolism of serotonin) with various psychiatric disorders. Lately, there has been increasing interest in this correlation. Takeda[44] reviews the breakdown of serotonin (Figure 12.4), noting that the pathway to bufotenine is an abnormal metabolic pathway, "an unusual route that is associated with the production of venoms or hallucinogens and is not associated with normal

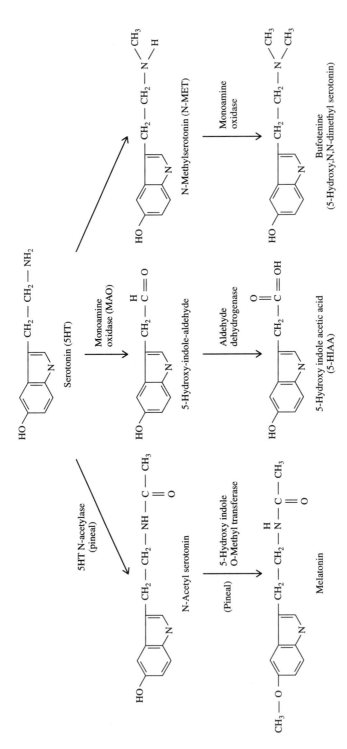

FIGURE 12.4 Metabolic pathways for serotonin (5-HT). The major pathway, shown in the center, leads to production of 5-HIAA, which is excreted by the kidneys. The pathway shown at the left occurs in the pineal gland and leads to the production of the neurohormone melatonin. The pathway at the right is an abnormal metabolic pathway leading to methylation of the terminal nitrogen group, and ultimately to the formation of bufotenine, a putative psychogenic substance. See text for discussion.

homeostasis in animals." Takeda and co-workers[45] studied urine specimens obtained from controls and from inpatients on a psychiatry ward. All patients were Japanese. Only 2 of 200 control urine specimens were positive for bufotenine; in 18 autistic patients with mental retardation and epilepsy, urine was positive in all; in autistic patients with mental retardation (no epilepsy), 32 of 47 were positive; in 18 patients with depression, urine was positive in 15; 13 of 15 schizophrenic patients tested positive for bufotenine. They concluded that the presence of bufotenine in urine may serve as a marker for some psychiatric disorders.

Karkkainen and co-workers[46] studied the urinary excretion of bufotenine in 112 Finnish male violent offenders. Suspiciousness was positively correlated, and socialization was negatively correlated with urinary bufotenine excretion. This and other results indicated that violent offenders with paranoid personality traits have higher urinary levels of bufotenine than other violent offenders.

These intriguing reports raise important questions about the role of altered metabolic pathways of serotonin (producing methylated derivatives) in the etiology of human psychiatric disorders such as autism and paranoia.

Psilocybin and Psilocin.   Psilocybin (4-phosphoryl-DMT) and psilocin (4-hydroxy-DMT) are two psychedelic agents that are found in many species of mushrooms that belong to the genera *Psilocybe, Panaeolus, Copelandia,* and *Conocybe.* These mushrooms grow throughout much of the world, including the northwestern United States. Psilocin and psilocybin are approximately 1/200 as potent as LSD, peak in about 2 hours, and their effects last about 6 to 10 hours.[47] Unlike DMT, psilocin and psilocybin are absorbed effectively when taken orally; the mushrooms are eaten raw to induce psychedelic effects.

There is great variation in the concentration of psilocybin and psilocin among the different species of mushrooms, as well as significant differences among mushrooms of the same species. For example, the usual oral dose of *Psilocybe semilanceata* (liberty caps) may consist of 10 to 40 mushrooms, while the dose for *Psilocybe cyanescens* may be only 2 to 5 mushrooms. Also, some extremely toxic species of mushrooms are not psychoactive, but they bear a superficial resemblance to the mushrooms that contain psilocybin and psilocin. Because the effects of psilocybin so closely resemble those produced by LSD, the "psilocybin" sold illicitly may be LSD, and ordinary mushrooms laced with LSD may be sold as "magic mushrooms."

As Figure 12.3 shows, the only difference between psilocybin and psilocin is that psilocybin contains a molecule of phosphoric acid. After the mushroom has been ingested, phosphoric acid is enzymatically removed from psilocybin, thus producing psilocin, the active psychedelic agent.

Although the psychedelic effects of *Psilocybe mexicana* have long been part of Indian folklore, *Psilocybe* intoxication was not described until 1955, when Gordon Wasson, a New York banker, traveled through Mexico. He mingled with native tribes and was allowed to participate in a *Psilocybe* ceremony, in which he consumed the magic mushroom. Wasson said:

> It permits you to travel backward and forward in time, to enter other planes of existence, even to know God. . . . Your body lies in the darkness, heavy as lead, but your spirit seems to soar and leave the hut, and with the speed of thought to travel where it listeth, in time and space, accompanied by the shaman's singing. . . . At least you know what the ineffable is, and what ecstasy means. Ecstasy! The mind harks back to the origin of that word. For the Greeks, ekstasis meant the flight of the soul from the body. Can you find a better word to describe this state?[48]

As might be predicted, the hallucinations and sensory distortions that are caused by psilocybin resemble those produced by LSD. Weil[49] narrates his experiences with psilocybin mushrooms.

Vollenweider and colleagues[50,51] view psilocybin intoxication as inducing a schizophrenia-like psychosis, via a serotonin 5-HT$_{2A}$ agonist action with a hyperfrontal metabolic pattern in the cerebral cortex, consistent with the observations of Gouzoulis-Mayfrank and co-workers.[5] The Gouzoulis-Mayfrank team[52] also describes psilocybin-induced alterations in "prepulse inhibition" of the startle reflex in humans, further indication of a drug-induced schizophrenia-like effect and of psilocybin producing a "model psychosis."

Ololiuqui.   Ololiuqui is a naturally occurring hallucinogen in morning glory seeds that is used by Central and South American natives both as an intoxicant and as a hallucinogen. The drug is used ritually for spiritual communication, as are extracts of most plants that contain psychedelic drugs. The use of ololiuqui seeds in Central and South America was first described by the Spaniard Hernandez, who stated, "When the priests wanted to commune with their Gods, [they ate ololiuqui seeds and] a thousand visions and satanic hallucinations appeared to them."[53]

The seeds were analyzed in Europe by Albert Hofmann, the discoverer of LSD, who identified several ingredients, one of which was lysergic acid amide (not lysergic acid diethylamide, LSD). The lysergic acid amide that Hofmann identified is approximately one-tenth as active as LSD as a psychoactive agent. However, considering the extreme potency of LSD, lysergic acid amide is still quite potent.

Side effects of ololiuqui include nausea, vomiting, headache, increased blood pressure, dilated pupils, and sleepiness. These side effects are usually quite intense and serve to limit the recreational use of ololiuqui. Ingestion of 100 or more seeds produces sleepiness, distorted perception, hallucinations, and confusion. Flashbacks have been reported, but they are infrequent.

Harmine. Harmine is a psychedelic agent that is obtained from the seeds of *Peganum harmala,* a plant native to the Middle East, and from *Banisteriopsis caapi* of the South American tropics. Intoxication by harmine is usually accompanied by nausea and vomiting, sedation, and finally sleep. The psychic excitement that users experience consists of visual distortions that are similar to those induced by LSD. (A psychedelic agent structurally similar to harmine, *ibogaine,* is discussed as an anticraving drug in Chapter 14.)

Grob and co-workers[54] and Dobkin de Rios[55] describe a hallucinogenic concoction of potent psychoactive plants indigenous to the Brazilian and Peruvian Amazon. The active hallucinogen, termed *hoasca* or *ayahuasca,* contains harmine and two closely related compounds, harmaline and tetrahydroharmine. Less potent and longer-acting than DMT, hoasca is incorporated into native religious ceremonies as a psychoactive sacrament, similar to the way peyote is used in the United States.

Phencyclidine and Ketamine: Psychedelic Anesthetics, Amnestics, and Deliriants

Phencyclidine (PCP, angel dust) and ketamine (Figure 12.5) are referred to as psychedelic anesthetics because they were first developed as amnestic and analgesic drugs for use in anesthesia; later it was found that they also produced a psychedelic or dissociative state of being. These two drugs are structurally unrelated to the other psychedelic agents, and their psychedelic effects are unique; the do not involve actions on serotonin, acetylcholine, or dopamine neurons.

Phencyclidine was developed in 1956 and was briefly used as an anesthetic in humans before being abandoned because of a high incidence of

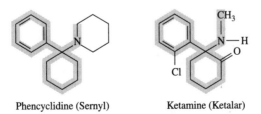

Phencyclidine (Sernyl)   Ketamine (Ketalar)

FIGURE 12.5 Structural formulas of the psychedelic anesthetic drugs phencyclidine and ketamine.

bizarre and serious psychiatric reactions, including agitation, excitement, delirium, disorientation, and hallucinatory phenomena (considered undesirable in the surgical patient!). The altered perception, disorganized thought, suspiciousness, confusion, and lack of cooperation that were exhibited resembled a schizophrenic state that consisted of both positive and negative symptoms.[56-58] Phencyclidine is still used as a veterinary anesthetic, primarily as an immobilizing agent.

Ketamine (Ketalar) was developed shortly after the prominent psychedelic properties of phencyclidine were identified. Introduced in 1960, ketamine induces a phencyclidine-like anesthetic state in low doses with only a moderate number of bothersome psychiatric side effects. Ketamine is occasionally used as anesthesia in patients who cannot tolerate the cardiovascular depressant effects of other anesthetics.

> Ketamine, a PCP analog still used in human anesthesia, has been reported to cause reactions similar to but not as severe as those caused by PCP, including brief, reversible "positive" and "negative" schizophrenia-like symptoms. Both PCP and ketamine can exacerbate psychosis in schizophrenia.[59]

Abuse of phencyclidine and ketamine began in the mid-1960s. Today, abuse of phencyclidine and ketamine still persists, with periodic resurgences in popularity. Phencyclidine is the more commonly abused of the two, and has appeared in the form of powders, tablets, leaf mixtures, and "rock" crystals. It is commonly sold as crystal, angel dust, hog, PCP, THC, cannabinol, or mescaline. When phencyclidine is sold as crystal or angel dust (terms also used for methamphetamine), the drug is usually in concentrations that vary between 50 and 90 percent. When it is purchased under other names or in concoctions, the amount of phencyclidine falls to between 10 and 30 percent, with the typical street dose being about 5 milligrams.[60] Phencyclidine can be eaten, snorted, or injected, but it is most often smoked, sprinkled on tobacco, parsley, or marijuana.

Pharmacokinetics

PCP is well absorbed whether taken orally or smoked. When it is smoked, peak effects occur in about 15 minutes, when about 40 percent of the dose appears in the user's bloodstream. Oral absorption is slower; maximum blood levels are reached about 2 hours after the drug has been taken. The elimination half-life is about 18 hours but ranges from about 11 to 51 hours. A positive urine assay for PCP is assumed to indicate that PCP was used within the previous week. Because false-positive test results are common, a positive assay requires secondary confirmation.

Mechanism of Action

Phencyclidine and ketamine both exert their psychotomimetic, analgesic, amnestic actions and schizophrenic actions as a result of binding as noncompetitive antagonists of the N-methyl-D-aspartate (NMDA)/ glutamate receptors (Chapter 3).* Several lines of evidence now implicate involvement of NMDA receptor dysfunction in the pathophysiology of schizophrenia (discussed in Chapter 17). Since ketamine (and phencyclidine) are NMDA antagonists and induce a schizophrenic-like state, Adler and co-workers[62] conducted a neuropsychological comparison of normal volunteers to whom ketamine was administered and patients with schizophrenia. The results are illustrated in Figure 12.6. As can be seen, the ketamine-induced thought disorder is not dissimilar to that seen in patients with schizophrenia, providing support for the involvement of NMDA receptor dysfunction in the disease.

Jentsch and Roth[58] attempted to integrate this single action on NMDA receptors, especially as it affects dopaminergic neurons, traditionally implicated in the etiology of schizophrenia (Chapter 17). Although acute doses of PCP and ketamine can induce a toxic psychosis, repeated doses induce a more persistent schizophrenic symptomatology, including psychosis, hallucinations, flattened affect, delusions, formal thought disorder, cognitive dysfunction, and social withdrawal.

> Glutamate receptors play a fundamental role in the function and dysfunction of the brain. These receptors are classified in two major classes according to their physiological and pharmacological properties: the NMDA and the non-NMDA receptors. NMDA receptors are highly permeable to calcium and are considered crucial for induction of synaptic plasticity and neurotoxicity. NMDA receptors, in contrast to non-NMDA receptors, are targets of potent psychotropic agents such as the dissociative anesthetic phencyclidine, and the anticonvulsant and anxiolytic dizolcipine, collectively known as noncompetitive NMDA antagonists. PCP is an open channel blocker of the NMDA receptor, transiently occluding the pore. It . . . has . . . a promising strategy to prevent glutamate-mediated neuronal cell death and associated disorders such as stroke, epilepsy, and Huntington's disease.[63]

---

*Ikin and co-workers[61] isolated and analyzed the NMDA/PCP receptor complex. The receptor has a molecular weight of 203,000 and is composed of four membrane-spanning polypeptides (molecular weights of 67,000, 57,000, 46,000, and 33,000), which cluster together to form an ion channel that resembles the benzodiazepine-GABA receptor. Here, however, the drug-binding site (the PCP receptor) is located within the lumen of the ion channel. Attachment of PCP to the receptor occludes the channel and inhibits calcium ion influx when the transmitter (glutamate) attaches to its receptor on the outer surface.

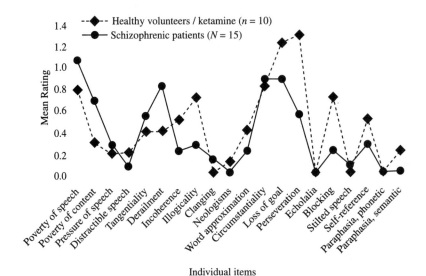

Individual items

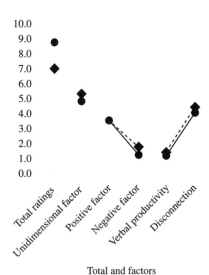

Total and factors

FIGURE 12.6 Comparison of total, factor, and individual item scores for the assessment of thought, language, and communication of 10 healthy volunteers with ketamine-induced thought disorder and 15 patients with schizophrenia (schizophrenic patients were ketamine-free). [From Adler et al.[62]]

NMDA receptors are also involved in synaptic plasticity and in long-term enhancement of synaptic efficacy (i.e., long-term potentiation), thought to be the basis of processes involved in learning and memory. NMDA blockers such as phencyclidine are among the best amnestic drugs known. NMDA antagonists have also been proposed as potentially advantageous as neuroprotective agents, potentially useful for the treatment of CNS ischemia and head trauma. Experimental NMDA antagonists being evaluated for use as neuroprotectants following head injury or stroke include *selfotel* and *aptiganel* (Cerestat).[64,65]

Orser, Pennefather, and MacDonald[66] investigated the mechanism of action of ketamine and concluded that it inhibits NMDA receptors by two mechanisms: (1) blockade of the open channel by occupying a site within the channel in the receptor protein (as discussed earlier for phencyclidine), and (2) reduction in the frequency of NMDA channel opening by drug binding to a second attachment site on the outside of the receptor protein. Phencyclidine probably shares this duality of action.

Psychological Effects

Phencyclidine dissociates individuals from themselves and their environment. It induces an unresponsive state with intense analgesia and amnesia, although the patient's eyes remain open (with a blank stare), and he or she may even appear to be awake. When not used under controlled conditions, phencyclidine in low doses produces mild agitation, euphoria, disinhibition, or excitement in a person who appears to be grossly drunk and exhibits a blank stare. The subject may be rigid and unable to speak. In many cases, however, the patient is communicative, although he or she does not respond to pain.

> PCP acutely induces a psychotic state in which subjects become withdrawn, autistic, negativistic, and unable to maintain a cognitive set, and manifest concrete, impoverished, idiosyncratic, and bizarre responses to proverbs and projective testing. Some subjects show catatonic posturing. These schizophrenic-like alterations in brain functioning went beyond the symptom level. . . . Any person under the influence of even a small amount of PCP . . . will have profound alterations of higher emotional functions affecting judgment and cognition.[60]

High doses of phencyclidine induce a state of coma or stupor. However, abusers tend to titrate their dose to maximize the intoxicant effect while attempting to avoid unconsciousness. Blood pressure usually becomes elevated, but respiration does not become depressed. The patient may recover from this state within 2 to 4 hours, although a state of confusion may last for 8 to 72 hours. The disruption of sensory input by PCP causes unpredictable exaggerated, distorted, or violent reactions to environmental stimuli. Such reactions are augmented by PCP-induced analgesia and amnesia.

Massive oral overdoses, involving up to 1 gram of street-purchased phencyclidine, result in prolonged periods of stupor or coma. This state may last for several days and may be marked by intense seizure activity, increased blood pressure, and a depression of respiration that is potentially lethal. Following this stupor, a prolonged recovery phase, marked by confusion and delusions, may last as long as 2 weeks. In some people, this state of confusion may be followed by a psychosis that lasts from several weeks to a few months.

Side Effects and Toxicity

The course of recovery from a PCP-induced schizophrenic-like psychotic state is variable for reasons that are poorly understood. The intoxicated state may lead to severe anxiety, aggression, panic, paranoia, and rage. A user can also display violent reactions to sensory input, leading to such problems as falls, drowning, burns, driving accidents, and aggressive behavior. Self-inflicted injuries and injuries sustained while physical restraints are applied are frequent, and the potent analgesic action certainly contributes to the lack of response to pain. Respiratory depression, generalized seizure activity, and pulmonary edema have all been reported.

Tolerance, Dependence, and Abuse

PCP is the only psychedelic drug self-administered by monkeys. In humans, this pattern of compulsive abuse is also seen. By inference, therefore, phencyclidine seems to stimulate brain reward areas and therefore places the user at risk of compulsive abuse despite negative health consequences. This probably is true, because there is an interaction between dopaminergic and glutaminergic neurons;[58] phencyclidine indirectly increases extracellular concentrations of dopamine.[67,68] In addition, ketamine binds with opioid receptors, functioning as a mu and kappa antagonist.[69] This implies that the dependence-producing liability of ketamine may be limited and also that its analgesic actions are the result of a nonopioid mechanism, probably the result of NMDA/glutamate antagonism in the spinal cord.[70]

Therapy for PCP intoxication is aimed at reducing the systemic level of the drug, keeping the individual calm and sedated, and preventing any of several severe adverse medical effects. It involves the following:

- Minimization of sensory inputs by placing the intoxicated individual in a quiet environment
- Oral administration of activated charcoal, which can bind any PCP present in the stomach and intestine and prevent its reabsorption

- Precautionary physical restraint to prevent self-injury
- Sedation with either a benzodiazepine (such as lorazepam) for agitation or an antipsychotic (such as haloperidol, clozapine, or olanzapine) for psychosis

Hyperthermia, hypertension, convulsions, renal failure, and other medical consequences should be treated as necessary by medical experts. PCP-induced psychotic states may be long-lasting, especially in individuals with a history of schizophrenia.

STUDY QUESTIONS

1. What is a psychedelic drug?
2. What differentiates a psychedelic drug from a behavioral stimulant? Discuss from both structural and behavioral viewpoints.
3. List the four classes of psychedelic drugs presented in this chapter.
4. Differentiate between mescaline and LSD.
5. How does LSD exert psychedelic actions?
6. What is the psychedelic syndrome?
7. What are some of the problems associated with LSD use?
8. How does phencyclidine work? Discuss the state of psychosis it produces.
9. What properties characterize the clinical usefulness of phencyclidine and ketamine?
10. Discuss MDMA and the problems and toxicities associated with its use.

REFERENCES

1. G. J. Marek and G. K. Aghajanian, "Indoleamine and the Phenethylamine Hallucinogens: Mechanisms of Psychotomimetic Action," *Drug and Alcohol Dependence* 51 (1998): 189–198.
2. G. K. Aghajanian and G. J. Marek, "Serotonin and Hallucinogens," *Neuropsychopharmacology* 21 (1999): 16S–23S.
3. T. A. Bowdie et al., "Psychedelic Effects of Ketamine in Healthy Volunteers: Relationship to Steady-state Plasma Concentrations," *Anesthesiology* 88 (1998): 82–88.
4. H. D. Abraham, A. M. Aldridge, and P. Gogia, "The Psychopharmacology of Hallucinogens," *Neuropsychopharmacology* 14 (1996): 285–298.

5. R. S. Holzman, "The Legacy of Atropos, the Fate Who Cut the Thread of Life," *Anesthesiology* 89 (1998): 241–249. See also letters and replies in *Anesthesiology* 90 (1999): 1794–1796.

6. E. Gouzoulis-Mayfrank et al., "Neurometabolic Effects of Psilocybin, 3,4-Methylenedioxyethylamphetamine (MDE) and d-Methamphetamine in Healthy Volunteers: A Double-blind, Placebo-controlled PET Study with [18F]FDG," *Neuropsychopharmacology* 20 (1999): 565–581.

7. A. P. Monte et al., "Dihydrobenzofuran Analogues of Hallucinogens. IV: Mescaline Derivatives," *Journal of Medicinal Chemistry* 40 (1997): 2997–3008.

8. L. Hermle, E. Gouzoulis, and M. Spitzer, "Blood Flow and Cerebral Laterality in the Mescaline Model of Psychosis," *Pharmacopsychiatry* 31, Suppl. 2 (1998): 85–91.

9. L. Hermle, M. Funfgeld, G. Oepen, et al., "Mescaline-induced Psychopathological, Neuropsychological, and Neurometabolic Effects in Normal Subjects: Experimental Psychosis as a Tool for Psychiatric Research," *Biological Psychiatry* 32 (1992): 976–991.

10. J. R. Coore, "A Fatal Trip with Ecstasy: A Case of 3,4-Methylene-dioxymethamphetamine/3,4-Methylenedioxy-amphetamine Toxicity," *Journal of the Royal Society of Medicine* 89 (1996): 51P–52P.

11. M. E. Molliver et al., "Neurotoxicity of MDMA and Related Compounds: Anatomic Studies," *Annals of the New York Academy of Sciences* 600 (1990): 640–661.

12. H. K. Kramer, J. C. Poblete, and E. C. Azmitia, "Characterization of the Translocation of Protein Kinase C (PKC) by 3,4–Methylene-dioxymethamphetamine (MDMA/Ecstasy) in Synaptosomes: Evidence for a Presynaptic Localization Involving the Serotonin Transporter (SERT)", *Neuropsychopharmacology* 19 (1998): 265–277.

13. U. D. McCann et al., "Cognitive Performance in 3,4-Methylene-dioxymethamphetamine (MDMA, 'Ecstasy') Users," *Psychopharmacology* 143 (1999): 417–425.

14. D. M. Semple et al., "Reduced In Vivo Binding to the Serotonin Transporter in the Cerebral Cortex of MDMA ('Ecstasy') Users," *British Journal of Psychiatry* 175 (1999): 63–69.

15. M. J. Morgan, "Recreational Use of 'Ecstasy' (MDMA) Is Associated with Elevated Impulsivity," *Neuropsychopharmacology* 19 (1998): 252–264.

16. H. Gijsman et al., "MDMA Study," *Neuropsychopharmacology* 21 (1999): 597.

17. F. X. Vollenweider, A. Gamma, M. Liechti, and T. Huber, "Is a Single Dose of MDMA Harmless?" *Neuropsychopharmacology* 21 (1999): 598–600.

18. F. X. Vollenweider, A. Gamma, M. Liechti, and T. Huber, "Psychological and Cardiovascular Effects and Short-term Sequelae of MDMA ('Ecstasy') in MDMA-naive Healthy Volunteers," *Neuropsychopharmacology* 19 (1998): 241–251.

19. L. Topp et al., "Ecstasy Use in Australia: Patterns of Use and Associated Harm," *Drug and Alcohol Dependence* 55 (1999): 105–115.

20. K. L. R. Jansen, "Ecstasy (MDMA) Dependence," *Drug and Alcohol Dependence* 55 (1999): 121–124.

21. M. Demirkiran, J. Jankovic, and J.M. Dean, "Ecstasy Intoxication: An Overlap Between Serotonin Syndrome and Neuroleptic Malignant Syndrome," *Clinical Neuropharmacology* 19 (1996): 157–164.

22. R. S. Cohen, "Adverse Symptomatology and Suicide Associated with the Use of Methylenedioxymethamphetamine (MDMA; 'Ecstasy')," *Biological Psychiatry* 39 (1996): 819–820.
23. J. E. Malberg, K. E. Sabol, and L. S. Seiden, "Co-administration of MDMA with Drugs that Protect Against MDMA Neurotoxicity Produces Different Effects on Body Temperature in the Rat," *Journal of Pharmacology and Experimental Therapeutics* 278 (1996): 258–267.
24. K. A. Zahn, R. L. Li, and R. A. Purssell, "Cardiovascular Toxicity After Ingestion of 'Herbal Ecstasy,'" *Journal of Emergency Medicine* 17 (1999): 289–291.
25. M. D. Schechter, "'Candyflipping': Synergistic Discriminative Effect of LSD and MDMA," *European Journal of Pharmacology* 341 (1998): 131–134.
26. M. K. Abernethy and L. B. Becker, "Acute Nutmeg Intoxication," *American Journal of Emergency Medicine* 10 (1992): 429–430.
27. M. A. Schuckit, "The Kitchen Condiment High: Nutmeg," *Drug Abuse and Alcoholism Newsletter* 26 (December, 1997): 1–4.
28. N. Almaula et al., "Mapping the Binding Site Pocket of the Serotonin 5-Hydroxytryptamine$_{2A}$ Receptor," *Journal of Biological Chemistry* 271 (1996): 14672–14675.
29. N. J. Penington and A. P. Fox, "Effects of LSD on Ca^{++} Currents in Central 5-HT-containing Neurons: 5-HT$_{1A}$ Receptors May Play a Role in Hallucinogenesis," *Journal of Pharmacology and Experimental Therapeutics* 269 (1994): 1160–1165.
30. C. T. Egan et al., "Agonist Activity of LSD and Lisuride at Cloned 5-HT$_{2A}$ and 5-HT$_{2C}$ Receptors," *Psychopharmacology* 136 (1998): 409–414.
31. K. Krebs-Thomson, M. P. Paulus, and M. A. Geyer, "Effects of Hallucinogens on Locomotor and Investigatory Activity and Patterns: Influence of 5-HT$_{2A}$ and 5-HT$_{2C}$ Receptors," *Neuropsychopharmacology* 18 (1998): 339–351.
32. R. Grailhe et al., "Increased Exploratory Activity and Altered Response to LSD in Mice Lacking the 5-HT$_{5A}$ Receptor," *Neuron* 22 (1999): 581–591.
33. S. Giacomelli et al., "Lysergic Acid Diethylamide (LSD) Is a Partial Agonist of D$_2$ Dopaminergic Receptors and It Potentiates Dopamine-mediated Prolactin Secretion in Lactrophs In Vivo," *Life Sciences* 63 (1998): 215–222.
34. N. J. Penington, "Actions of Methoxylated Amphetamine Hallucinogens on Serotonergic Neurons of the Brain," *Progress in Neuro-Psychopharmacology and Biological Psychiatry* 20 (1996): 951–965.
35. *Interim Drug Report of the Commission of Inquiry into the Nonmedical Use of Drugs* (Ottawa: Information Canada, 1970), 58–59.
36. A. Hofmann, "Notes and Documents Concerning the Discovery of LSD," *Agents and Actions* 43 (1994): 79–81.
37. D. Simpson et al., "Screening for Drugs of Abuse (II): Cannabinoids, Lysergic Acid Diethylamide, Buprenorphine, Methadone, Barbiturates, Benzodiazepines and Other Drugs," *Annals of Clinical Biochemistry* 34 (1997): 460–510.
38. G. G. Dimijian, "Contemporary Drug Abuse," in A. Goth, ed., *Medical Pharmacology*, 11th ed. (St. Louis: Mosby, 1984), 156.
39. W. Batzer, T. Ditzler and C. Brown, "LSD Use and Flashbacks in Alcoholic Patients," *Journal of Addictive Diseases* 18 (1999): 57–63.

40. J. H. Halpern and H. G. Pope, Jr., "Do Hallucinogens Cause Residual Neuropsychological Toxicity?" *Drug and Alcohol Dependence* 53 (1999): 247–256.

41. R. J. Strassman and C. R. Qualls, "Dose-response Study of N,N-dimethyltryptamine in Humans. I: Neuroendocrine, Autonomic, and Cardiovascular Effects," *Archives of General Psychiatry* 51 (1994): 85–97.

42. R. J. Strassman, C. R. Qualls, E. H. Uhlenhuth, and R. Kellner, "Dose-response Study of N,N-dimethyltryptamine in Humans. II: Subjective Effects and Preliminary Results of a New Rating Scale," *Archives of General Psychiatry* 51 (1994): 98–108.

43. R. W. Fuller, H. D. Snoddy, and K. W. Perry, "Tissue Distribution, Metabolism, and Effects of Bufotenine Administered to Rats," *Neuropharmacology* 34 (1995): 799–804.

44. N. Takeda, "Serotonin-degradative Pathways in the Toad (*Bufo bufo japonicus*) Brain: Clues to the Pharmacological Analysis of Human Psychiatric Disorders," *Comparative Biochemistry and Physiology. Pharmacology, Toxicology and Endocrinology* 107(1994): 275–281.

45. N. Takeda, R. Ikeda, K. Ohba, and M. Kondo, "Bufotenine Reconsidered as a Diagnostic Indicator of Psychiatric Disorders," *NeuroReport* 6 (1995): 2378–2380.

46. J. Karkkainen et al., "Urinary Excretion of Bufotenin (N,N-dimethyl-5-hydroxytryptamine) Is Increased in Suspicious Violent Offenders: A Confirmatory Study," *Psychiatry Research* 58 (1995): 145–152.

47. F. Hasler et al., "Determination of Psilocybin and 4-Hydroxyindole-3-acetic Acid in Plasma by HPLC-ECD and Pharmacokinetic Profiles of Oral and Intravenous Psilocybin in Man," *Pharmaceutica Acta Helvetiae* 72 (1997): 175–184.

48. M. E. Crahan, "God's Flesh and Other Pre-Columbian Phantastica," *Bulletin of the Los Angeles County Medical Association* 99 (1969): 17.

49. A. Weil, *The Marriage of the Sun and the Moon* (Boston: Houghton Mifflin, 1980), 73–79.

50. F. X. Vollenweider et al., "Positron Emission Tomography and Fluordeoxyglucose Studies of Metabolic Hyperfrontality and Psychopathology in the Psilocybin Model of Psychosis," *Neuropsychopharmacology* 16 (1997): 357–372.

51. F. X. Vollenweider et al., "Psilocybin Induces Schizophrenia-like Psychosis in Humans via a Serotonin-2 Agonist Action," *Neuroreport* 9 (1998): 3897–3902.

52. E. Gouzoulis-Mayfrank et al., "Effects of the Hallucinogen Psilocybin on Habituation and Prepulse Inhibition of the Startle Reflex in Humans," *Behavioral Pharmacology* 9 (1998): 561–566.

53. E. M. Brecher and Consumer Reports Editors, *Licit and Illicit Drugs* (Mt. Vernon, N.Y.: Consumers Union, 1972), 345.

54. C. S. Grob et al., "Human Psychopharmacology of Hoasca, a Plant Hallucinogen Used in Ritual Context in Brazil," *Journal of Nervous and Mental Disease* 184 (1996): 86–94.

55. M. Dobkin de Rios, "On 'Human Pharmacology of Hoasca': A Medical Anthropology Perspective," *Journal of Nervous and Mental Disease* 184 (1996): 95–98.

56. A. L. Halberstadt, "The Phencyclidine-glutamate Model of Schizophrenia," *Clinical Neuropharmacology* 18 (1995): 237–249.
57. S. A. Thornberg and S. R. Saklad, "A Review of NMDA Receptors and the Phencyclidine Model of Schizophrenia," *Pharmacotherapy* 16 (1996): 82–93.
58. J. D. Jentsch and R. H. Roth, "The Neuropharmacology of Phencyclidine: From NMDA Receptor Hypofunction to the Dopamine Hypothesis of Schizophrenia," *Neuropsychopharmacology* 20 (1999): 201–225.
59. J. W. Newcomer et al., "Ketamine-induced NMDA Receptor Hypofunction as a Model of Memory Impairment and Psychosis," *Neuropsychopharmacology* 20 (1999): 106–118.
60. S. R. Zukin, Z. Sloboda, and D. C. Javitt, "Phencyclidine (PCP)," in J. H. Lowinson, P. Ruiz, R. B. Millman, and J. G. Langrod, eds., *Substance Abuse: A Comprehensive Textbook*, 3rd ed. (Baltimore: Williams & Wilkins, 1997), 238–246.
61. A. F. Ikin, Y. Kloog, and M. Sokolovsky, "N-methyl-D-aspartate/ Phencyclidine Receptor Complex of Rat Forebrain: Purification and Biochemical Characterization," *Biochemistry* 29 (1990): 2290.
62. C. M. Adler et al., "Comparison of Ketamine-induced Thought Disorder in Healthy Volunteers and Thought Disorder in Schizophrenia," *American Journal of Psychiatry* 156 (1999): 1646–1649.
63. A. V. Ferrer-Montiel, W. Sun, and M. Montal, "Molecular Design of the N-methyl-D-aspartate Receptor Binding Site for Phencyclidine and Dizolcipine," *Proceedings of the National Academy of Science, USA* 92 (1995): 8021–8025.
64. K. R. Lees, "Cerestat and Other NMDA Antagonists in Ischemic Stroke," *Neurology* 49, Suppl 4, (1997): S66–S69.
65. M. A. Yenari et al., "Dose Escalation Safety and Tolerance Study of the Competitive NMDA Antagonist Selfotel (CGS 19755) in Neurosurgical Patients," *Clinical Neuropharmacology* 21 (1998): 28–34.
66. B. A. Orser, P. S. Pennefather, and J. F. MacDonald, "Multiple Mechanisms of Ketamine Blockade of N-methyl-D-aspartate Receptors," *Anesthesiology* 86 (1997): 903–917.
67. E. D. French, "Phencyclidine and the Midbrain Dopamine System: Electrophysiology and Behavior," *Neurotoxicology and Teratology* 16 (1994): 355–362.
68. W. A. Carlezon, Jr., and R. A. Wise, "Rewarding Actions of Phencyclidine and Related Drugs in Nucleus Accumbens Shell and Frontal Cortex," *Journal of Neuroscience* 16 (1996): 3112–3122.
69. K. Hirota et al., "Stereoselectivity Interaction of Ketamine with Recombinant Mu, Kappa, and Delta Opioid receptors Expressed in Chinese Hamster Ovary Cells," *Anesthesiology* 90 (1999): 174–182.
70. T. Kawamata and K. Omote, "Activation of Spinal N-methyl-D-aspartate Receptors Stimulates a Nitric Oxide/Cyclic Guanosine 3',5'-Monophasphare/ Glutamate Release Cascade in Nociceptive Signaling," *Anesthesiology* 91 (1999): 1415–1424.

Drug Abuse

Drug abuse has been a societal problem for thousands of years, ever since grain was fermented (ethyl alcohol) and natural substances were found that produced euphoria (cocaine) or altered states of consciousness (psychedelics). As history suggests, as long as these drugs persist in society (and they always will), their use will be associated with compulsive use and abuse as well as with dependency and addiction.

Chapter 13 reviews the mechanisms responsible for producing compulsive drug abuse and dependency. It also reviews the literature on the current concepts of treatment of dependency and abuse. The individual drugs discussed in their own chapters are brought together in a chapter devoted to general concepts that apply to all drugs of abuse.

Chapter 14 addresses the pharmacology of anabolic steroids, used by athletes to build muscle. These drugs are also used by young male and female nonathletes for cosmetic effects to "correct" body image problems. In addition to muscle-building properties, these drugs have profound psychological effects and significant long-term toxicities.

Chapter 13

Topics in Substance Use Disorders

Historical Perspective

In all of recorded history, every society has used drugs to produce alterations in mood, thought, feeling, or behavior or to provide temporary alterations in reality. Moreover, there have always been some people within societies who digressed from custom with respect to the time, the amount, and the situation in which drugs were used. Abuse of psychoactive drugs has always produced problems for the individual taking the drug, for those in direct contact with the user, and for society at large.

Alcohol is the classic psychoactive drug used throughout history primarily for recreational purposes, but it is not the only such agent. Naturally occurring substances are used to alleviate anxiety, produce relaxation, provide relief from boredom, alleviate pain, and/or increase strength or work tolerance. In most cultures, only very few naturally occurring substances were available, and their use was closely monitored, so just a relatively small minority of individuals abused them. Today, these patterns of abuse differ considerably from the traditional pattern:

- Available at one time are most of the naturally occurring psychoactive drugs ever identified.

- In most cases, the pharmacologically active ingredient in each natural product has been isolated, identified, and made available to those who desire it.

- Organic chemistry has made possible synthetic derivatives of naturally occurring drugs. In many cases, the synthetic derivatives magnify the psychoactive potency of the natural substance 100 times or more.

- Users have adopted new methods of drug delivery, starting with the invention of the hypodermic syringe in the 1860s, and new drugs, the most recent of which are crack cocaine, ICE methamphetamine, and "designer" derivatives of both fentanyl and mescaline. These developments have markedly increased the delivered dose, decreased the time to onset of drug action, and increased both the potency and the toxicity of these agents compared with their naturally occurring counterparts.

As in past decades, caffeine, nicotine, and ethyl alcohol are by far the addictive drugs used by the vast majority of people. Caffeine use is nearly universal; 90 percent of Americans over the age of 11 use the drug at least once weekly. Thankfully, little harm seems to follow. Nicotine and alcohol are the next most widely used and abused addictive drugs. The probability that an American living today has a drug abuse or dependence disorder is 36 percent for nicotine, 14 percent for alcohol, and 4 percent for marijuana.[1] The total economic costs of substance abuse are estimated at $428.1 billion in 1995: alcohol abuse at $175.9 billion, drug abuse at $114.2 billion, and smoking at $138 billion.[2]

A 1996 survey[3] notes that 11.7 million Americans had used an illicit drug during the month prior to the survey. "Hard-core" cocaine users now number close to 500,000. "Regular" marijuana users (weekly or more frequent use) number over 5 million. Gfroerer and Epstein[4] note that "the annual number of new marijuana users in 1995 was estimated to be 2.48 million, with the vast majority being under the age of 21 years" (Figure 13.1). One study in California[5] demonstrated that the yearly cost of treating 150,000 substance abusers was $200 million, but the financial benefits of treatment for these individuals was established at $1.5 billion, mostly as a function of reductions in crime. Thus, psychosocial treatments for drug abuse seem to yield substantial financial benefits and, hopefully, an increased quality of life for the abuser if treatment is long-term (6 months to a year).[3]

While on the topic of treatment, several important points need be remembered:

- Substantial heterogeneity exists among substance abusers in the nature and severity of their addiction-related problem.

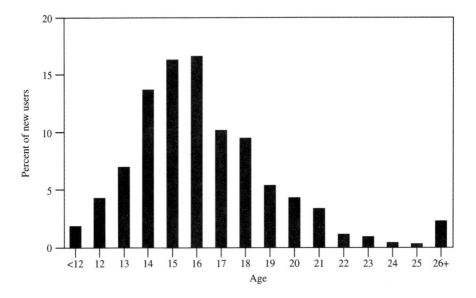

FIGURE 13.1 Percent distribution of annual marijuana initiates by age at which marijuana is first smoked. [From Gfroerer and Epstein.[4]]

- The majority of individuals with substance abuse problems have comorbid psychiatric disorders that require additional services,* such as pharmacotherapy or psychological therapies.

- Self-medication with potent psychoactive drugs in an attempt to, at least initially, treat underlying psychiatric symptoms may have led to the substance abuse disorder. Alternatively, a comorbid addiction vulnerability hypothesis[6] may account for the dual diagnoses of substance abuse and a psychiatric disorder.

- The potent behavior-reinforcing properties of certain psychoactive drugs sustain the attractiveness of and the need for these drugs, in addition to the ability of the drug to ameliorate the underlying psychological symptoms.

- Drug craving following withdrawal may represent the unmasking or worsening of preexisting psychiatric symptomatology, receptor dysfunction (now unmasked by drug removal), or any other unidentified causes, whether physiological, psychological, genetic, or environmental.

---

*Among persons with either alcohol abuse or alcohol dependence, 78 percent of men and 86 percent of women also have at least one other psychiatric disorder, such as conduct disorder, drug dependency, anxiety disorder, or affective disorder (depression, dysthymia, or mania).

As can be seen in Figure 13.1, initiation to marijuana use begins almost universally in individuals under the age of 21 years; most occurs in the 14-to-16-years range. The same holds true for initiation to both cigarette smoking and the ingestion of ethyl alcohol; early use of either is associated with an increased likelihood of progression to marijuana use.[7] While some individuals who develop a substance abuse disorder in adulthood did not expose themselves to recreational drugs until after the age of 21 years, this is an unusual occurrence. Furthermore, the age of first exposure (at least to marijuana) is an important predictor and estimate both of the likelihood of developing a substance abuse problem and of the number of people who eventually will need treatment for illicit drug abuse problems.[4] Based on current estimates of early-age drug exposure, substance abuse treatment needs will increase by 57 percent by the year 2020.[4] To stem this tide of substance dependence, early-age initiation to alcohol, cigarettes and marijuana must be curbed to minimize the progression to the eventual development of a substance abuse disorder.[7]

Nosology and Epidemiology of Substance Dependence and Abuse

Published in 1994 in its fourth edition, the *Diagnostic and Statistical Manual of Mental Disorder* (DSM-IV)[8] presents commonly accepted criteria for what constitutes substance dependence and substance abuse (Table 13.1). The two substance use disorders involve "maladaptive patterns of substance use, leading to clinically significant impairments or distress." The distinctions in DSM-IV between abuse and dependence are listed in the table and discussed by Bucholz.[9]

The prevalence of alcohol dependence or abuse is still the highest of that of all psychoactive drugs, with the lifetime prevalence varying (depending on criteria used) between 13 and 23 percent of the population.[9] The lifetime prevalence of nonalcohol drug dependence and abuse amounts to approximately 6 percent of the population.[10] Among young adults, alcohol and marijuana are the most commonly used drugs (90 percent and 53 percent, respectively, for lifetime use), followed by hallucinogens (16 percent ever used), inhalants (14 percent ever used), stimulants (14 percent ever used), cocaine (12 percent ever used), and opiates (9 percent ever used).[10] Cigarettes and smokeless tobacco have been used by 65 percent and 25 percent respectively of high school seniors.

Approximately one-third of individuals with a drug or alcohol addiction have a diagnosed *comorbid* (axis 1) psychiatric disorder, a situation covered by the term *dual diagnosis*. This term is one of convenience, used to capture the concept that some patients have a substance use disorder in addition to another psychiatric disorder.[11]

TABLE 13.1 DSM-IV criteria for substance dependence or abuse

CRITERIA FOR SUBSTANCE DEPENDENCE:

A maladaptive pattern of substance use, leading to clinically significant impairment or distress, as manifested by three (or more) of the following, occurring at any time in the same 12-month period:

(1) tolerance, as defined by either: (a) need for markedly increased amounts of the substance to achieve intoxication or desired effect; (b) markedly diminished effect with continued use of the same amount of substance

(2) withdrawal, as manifested by either: (a) the characteristic withdrawal syndrome for the substance; (b) the same (or a closely related) substance is taken to relieve or avoid withdrawal symptoms

(3) the substance is often taken in larger amounts or over a longer period than was intended

(4) there is a persistent desire or unsuccessful efforts to cut down or control substance use

(5) a great deal of time is spent in activities necessary to obtain the substance, use the substance, or recover from its effects

(6) important social, occupational, or recreational activities are given up or reduced because of substance use

(7) the substance use is continued despite knowledge of having a persistent or recurrent physical or psychological problem that is likely to have been caused or exacerbated by the substance

CRITERIA FOR SUBSTANCE ABUSE:

A. A maladaptive pattern of substance use leading to clinically significant impairment or distress, as manifested by one (or more) of the following occurring within a 12-month period:

(1) recurrent substance use resulting in a failure to fulfill major role obligations at work, school or home

(2) recurrent substance use in situations in which it is physically hazardous

(3) recurrent substance-related legal problems

(4) continued substance use despite having persistent or recurrent social or interpersonal problems caused or exacerbated by the effects of the substance

B. The symptoms have never met the criteria for Substance Dependence for this class of substance.

From American Psychiatric Association, *Diagnostic and Statistical Manual of Mental Disorders*, 4th ed. (Washington, D.C., American Psychiatric Association, 1994), pp. 181–183, with permission.

(The reverse is also true; many patients have a psychiatric disorder, often undiagnosed, in addition to a diagnosed substance use disorder.) The epidemiology of this comorbidity is striking. Of individuals with a lifetime diagnosis of schizophrenia or schizophreniform disorders, 47 percent have met criteria for substance abuse or dependence; of those with an anxiety disorder, 23.7 percent; obsessive-compulsive disorder, 32.8 percent; bipolar disorder, 50 percent; and depression, 32 percent, with distribution equal for males and females.[11] Skodol and co-workers[12] reported that close to 60 percent of subjects with substance abuse disorders had personality disorders, including borderline personality disorder, antisocial personality disorder, and conduct disorder.

Leshner[13] states:

> Comorbidity is reality! Estimates vary by disorder, but more than 50 percent of people with mental disorders have also been found to abuse drugs, including alcohol; there is also a widespread belief that many mentally ill people who abuse drugs may be actually attempting to medicate themselves. We do not know if this is actually true, but the sequence of onset between the mental disorder and substance use favors the hypothesis for many patients. . . . many of our causative models ignore the almost inevitability of comorbidity or at best treat it superficially. Worse, many of our treatment approaches ignore comorbidity or insist that mental and addictive disorders be treated separately.

There are serious deficiencies in the diagnosis and provision of services for patients with dual or comorbid illnesses. Making the correct diagnosis is a pivotal component in the successful treatment of dual diagnoses patients. It is important to maintain a high level of suspicion of dual disorders and gather information about the patient from multiple sources. A key clinical issue is that both the underlying psychiatric disorder and the substance use disorder must be treated concomitantly, and the dual diagnosis program should include pharmacotherapy, psychoeducation, behavioral intervention, skills training, and case management.[14] It is essential that both diseases be addressed simultaneously, with appropriate communication and coordination among the treatment providers and corroboration from significant others in the patient's environment.

Psychoactive Drugs as Behavioral Reinforcers

One of the newer areas of interest in the field of chemical dependencies is the biochemistry, neurophysiology, and neuropathology of behavioral reward as it pertains to dependency and addiction. Drugs that are prone to compulsive abuse activate brain mechanisms involved in reward and positive reinforcement. The systems and structures involved include (1) dopamine, serotonin, opioid, GABA, and cannabinoid neurons and/or receptors, and (2) the median forebrain bundle, ventral tegmentum, hippocampus, frontal cortex, and nucleus accumbens. Here we describe a neuroanatomical system that underlies the behavioral reinforcing actions of drugs.[15] Because conditioning and learning processes are of central importance in drug addiction, drug-seeking behavior can be visualized as an amalgam of positive reinforcement, discriminative effects, aversive effects, and stimuli associated with drug use.

Lessons from the Laboratory

Laboratory animals self-administer psychoactive drugs, and the degree to which an animal self-administers a particular drug closely parallels the degree of abuse exhibited by human users of the drug. If a drug is to maintain drug-seeking behavior, it must serve as a positive reinforcer. For example, cocaine is self-administered to excess by every species of animal that has been tested, including rats, squirrels, monkeys, rhesus monkeys, pigtail macaques, baboons, dogs, and humans. The reinforcing property of cocaine is probably the most important factor in its compulsive abuse by humans, and it plays a major role in its appeal to users. The self-administration of strongly reinforcing drugs by several species also dispels the notion that the drug abuser (compared to a casual user or a nonuser) must have some kind of inherent pathological condition (for example, a preexisting psychopathology) that creates a propensity for abusing drugs.

Mechanism of Reinforcement Action

In recent years, it has become apparent that there are specific circuits in the brain dedicated to the neural mediation of reward and pleasure.[15] The activation of this reward mechanism seems to be the single feature shared by most if not all abusable substances. Drugs subject to compulsive abuse act on these brain mechanisms to produce the subjective reward that constitutes the reinforcing "high," "rush," or "hit" sought by substance abusers. Specifically, abusable drugs stimulate the nucleus accumbens dopaminergic system that runs through the medial forebrain bundle. Drugs that have negative-reward effects (such as the phenothiazines) inhibit activity in or increase the thresholds of the same system.

Exactly what is this brain reward system, and how is it influenced by drugs of such varying classes and neurotransmitter actions? First, there are two major dopaminergic neuronal systems in the midbrain (Figure 13.2). A primary system comprises descending (caudally

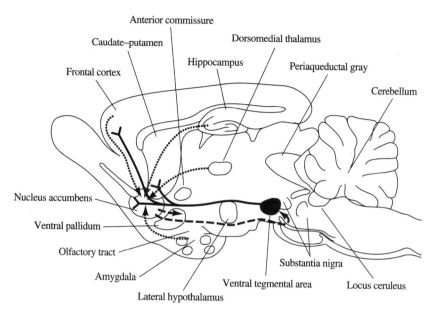

FIGURE 13.2 Sagittal rat brain section illustrating a cocaine and amphetamine neural reward circuit that includes a limbic-extrapyramidal motor interface. Dotted arrows indicate limbic afferents to the nucleus accumbens and dashed arrows represent efferents from the nucleus accumbens thought to be involved in psychomotor stimulant reward. Solid arrows indicate projections of the mesocorticolimbic dopamine system thought to be a critical substrate for psychomotor stimulant reward. This system originates in the ventral tegmental area and projects to the olfactory tubercle of the nucleus accumbens and the ventral striatal domains of the caudate putamen. [Adapted from G. F. Koob, "Drugs of Abuse: Anatomy, Pharmacology and Function of Reward Pathways," *Trends in Pharmacological Sciences* 13 (1992), 178.]

projecting) fibers of dopaminergic neurons whose cell bodies are located in the nucleus accumbens and several limbic structures. These fibers run within the medial forebrain bundle and synapse onto second-stage dopaminergic neurons whose cell bodies are located in the ventral tegmental area (VTA) of the midbrain. The second-stage fibers are the axons of these VTA cells, and they ascend (travel rostrally) in the medial forebrain bundle and project into neurons of the forebrain, largely in the nucleus accumbens, frontal cortex, amygdala, and septal area. In essence, this two-neuron system is a dopaminergic loop between the forebrain and the ventral tegmentum.

Cocaine and the amphetamines act on both the first- and the second-stage neuronal terminals; the drugs mimic the effects of direct electrical stimulation of these areas. Other behavior-reinforcing drugs act only on the second-stage neurons, probably through action on the endogenous opioid circuitry:

> Cell bodies, axons, and synaptic terminals of enkephalinergic and endorphinergic neurons are found in profusion throughout the extent of the reward-relevant mesotelencephalic dopamine circuitry. . . . Endogenous opioid peptide neurons synapse directly onto mesotelencephalic dopamine axon terminals, forming precisely the type of axoaxonic synapses one would expect of a system designed to modulate the flow of reward-relevant neural signals through the dopamine circuitry.[16]

Furthermore:

> The drug-sensitive dopamine "second stage" component of the reward circuitry is under the modulatory control of a wide variety of other neural systems, including the enkephalinergic mechanisms alluded to above, but also including GABAergic, seritonergic, noradrenergic, and neuropeptide neurotransmitter and neuromodulatory mechanisms.[16]

Koob[17] states:

> Dopamine forms a critical link for all reward, including opiates and sedative/hypnotics. While open to multiple neurotransmitter inputs and outputs, this view still holds a centrist position for dopamine in all reward. An emphasis on multiple independent neurochemical elements, . . . places the focus on the nucleus accumbens and its circuitry as an important, perhaps critical, substrate for drug reward.

Volkow and co-workers[18] expanded on this dopaminergic concept of reward by measuring dopamine$_2$ levels in 23 healthy males who had no drug abuse history; subjects were divided into those who liked and those who disliked the effects of intravenously administered methylphenidate (Ritalin). Subjects who liked the effects had significantly lower dopamine D_2 levels than subjects who disliked the effects. This was interpreted to mean that "low levels of D_2 receptors may contribute to psychostimulant abuse by favoring pleasant responses."*

Childress and colleagues[20] extended studies of brain circuitry underlying drug experiences, identifying limbic structures activated during cocaine craving. They point out that during craving, the user is gripped by a visceral emotional state, experiences a highly focused incentive to act, and is unencumbered by the memory of negative consequences of drug taking. Thus, drug abuse and dependence involves more than just the dopaminergic reward system.

---

*Interestingly, Winsberg and Comings[19] correlated lack of clinical response to the anti-ADHD drug methylphenidate with a genetically abnormal structure and functioning of the presynaptic dopamine transporter.

Stolerman[21] reviewed the complementary mechanisms that under-lie drug-seeking behavior. As shown in Figure 13.3, a drug's ability to serve as a positive reinforcer is the minimum requirement for a drug to maintain drug-seeking behavior. Positive reinforcement is main-tained by three influences:

1. The neural mechanisms previously discussed
2. Behavioral mechanisms, including drug-induced euphoria, relief from anxiety or depression, functional enhancement, and relief from withdrawal

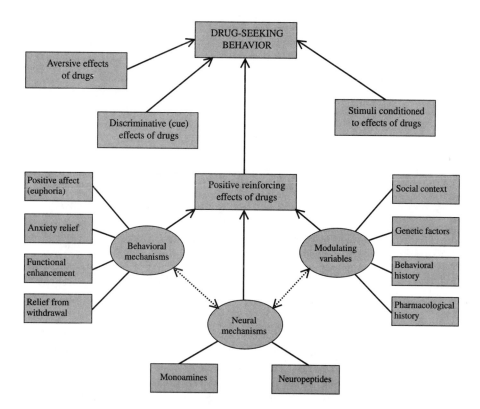

FIGURE 13.3 Psychopharmacological model of addiction as drug-seeking behavior controlled by four main processes: positive reinforcing effects of drugs, discriminative effects of drugs, stimuli conditioned to effects of drugs (which facilitate drug seeking), and aversive effects of drugs (which weaken the behavior). These four processes are common to drugs of many classes. A more detailed framework for analyzing positive reinforcing effects is shown (similar analyses could be made for discriminative and aversive effects); at this level it is envisaged that the relative importance of the different factors shown in the diagram will vary considerably between classes of drugs. [From Stolerman.[21]]

3. Multiple modulating variables, including the social context in which the drug is used, genetic factors, attitudes, expectations, and the history of previous reinforcement and reward

Cadoret and co-workers[22] studied the genetic pathways involved in the genesis of drug abuse and drug dependence in biological offspring who were separated at birth (eliminating social/environmental influences):

> Data . . . showed evidence of two genetic pathways to drug abuse/dependency. One pathway went directly from a biologic parent's alcoholism to drug abuse/dependency. The second pathway was more circuitous, and started with antisocial personality disorder in the biologic parent and proceeded through intervening variables of adoptee aggressivity, conduct disorder, antisocial personality disorder, and, eventually, ended in drug abuse/dependency. Environmental factors defined by psychiatric conditions in adoptive families independently predicted increased antisocial personality disorder in the adoptee. Adoptees born of alcohol-abusing mothers showed evidence of fetal alcohol syndrome, but controlling for this did not diminish the evidence for the direct genetic effect between an alcohol-abusing biologic parent and drug abuse/dependency in offspring.

Prescott and Kendler[23] extended these twin studies, demonstrating that genetic factors play a major role in the development of alcoholism among males. Environmental factors had little influence on the development of alcoholism. Similar levels of genetic loading have been suggested for addiction to virtually all other abusable substances as well.[24] Three articles in a recent issue of *Archives of General Psychiatry*[25-27] reinforce the developing concept that addictions are genetically influenced, complex disorders. "The hereditability of the addictions is substantial; the role of genotype accounts for about one-third of the overall variance in liability."[28]

The etiology of such genetic influence is unknown. It certainly may involve abnormalities in dopamine receptors, dopamine transporters, amino acid neurotransmitters, personality traits, comorbid psychopathology, or perhaps genetic variations in the hypothalamic-pituitary-adrenal axis resulting in elevations in secretion of the adrenal hormone cortisol. There is increased interest in the association between stress, cortisol levels, affective disorders (such as depression), and substance abuse. Rao and co-workers[29] studied adolescents with and without major depression and seven years later assessed their substance abuse history. Depressed adolescents had an earlier onset and higher frequency of substance abuse disorders than did nondepressed adolescents. Interestingly, the depressed group had more anxiety traits and a hyperactive hypothalamic-pituitary-adrenal axis with elevations in cortisol secretion (Figure 13.4). Piazza and

Le Moal[30] discuss this relationship and propose a model (Figure 13.5) to explain the mechanisms of the increase in drug self-administration induced by acute and chronic stress. Chapter 15 discusses the interaction among stress, depression, cortisol levels, and intracellular neurotropic factor alterations, leading to an explanation of why antidepressant medications remodel intracellular machinery, relieving stress, anxiety, depression, and thereby perhaps reducing substance use. This further ties together the relationship between substance use/abuse and psychological illnesses.

Drug Availability

Over the years, laws have been passed to limit the availability of drugs and to punish drug users deemed dangerous to themselves or to society. When these laws are strictly enforced, they can reduce drug use by persons who fear reprisal, but aggressive legislation does not control a person's craving for mind-altering drugs. This is true whether or not the person seeks the drug as self-medication for psychological distress, as pain relief for physical or psychological pain, or as anything else. Moreover, legislation often fails to address the legal drugs that cause the greatest amount of harm to individuals and society—ethanol and nicotine. Legalization of currently illegal drugs (e.g., tetrahydrocannabinol)

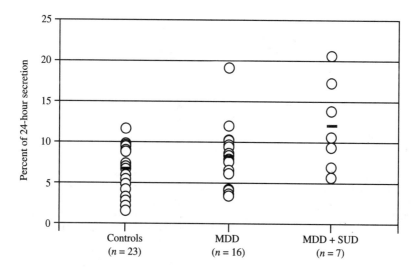

FIGURE 13.4 Percentage of 24-hour cortisol secreted near sleep onset in normal controls who remained free from psychopathology at 7-year follow-up (*left column*), in initially depressed (MDD) adolescents who had no substance use disorder (SUD) at the 7-year follow-up (*center column*), and in MDD adolescents who developed SUD by the end of the 7-year follow-up period. [From Rao et al.[29]]

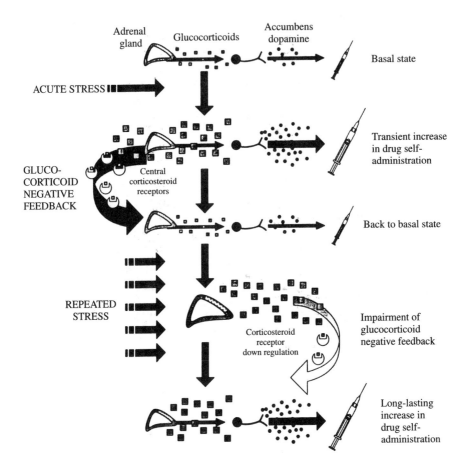

FIGURE 13.5 Possible pathophysiological mechanisms of the increase in drug self-administration induced by acute and repeated stress. In the basal state, glucocorticoids (cortisol) are released at physiological levels from the adrenal glands, and the nucleus accumbens releases dopamine at a basal rate, the concentrations of cortisol determining the rate of dopamine release. Under acute stress, cortisol secretion markedly increases and dopamine release is enhanced, resulting in increase in the sensitivity to the reinforcing effects of drugs of abuse, which can result in an increase in self-administration. However, activation by cortisol of a negative feedback that controls the secretion of these adrenal hormones returns the system to basal levels within 2 hours. Binding of cortisol to hippocampal corticosteroid receptors is a key step in the activation of this negative feedback. Repeated increase in glucocorticoids induced by repeated stress impairs the negative feedback system, resulting in prolonged increases in dopamine in the nucleus accumbens. These changes, in turn, produce a down regulation of hippocampal glucocorticoid receptors and determine a long-lasting increase in the sensitivity to the reinforcing effects of drugs of abuse. [From Piazza and Le Moal.[30]]

is not likely to solve drug abuse problems, and it certainly is politically unlikely. Simple legalization of the currently illegal drugs, if properly implemented, could solve much of the drug traffic-related crime problem. However, it would do nothing to solve the substance abuse problem, especially the major part of it caused by tobacco and alcohol.

Besides legislation, other traditional techniques for reducing drug abuse include education and developing negative attitudes toward drugs in both users and potential users. Such efforts have brought limited results, although the antianabolic steroid intervention (ATLAS program) described in Chapter 14 is encouraging. Perhaps it is time to take a public health approach to the problem of drug abuse, an approach that attempts to minimize danger to the individual and society. The primary goal of this approach is to reduce the use and abuse of all the recreational mood-altering drugs to a level of safe, pleasurable use consistent with centuries-old human experience, while minimizing to the greatest degree possible their harmful effects in individuals, the family, and society as a whole. A second major goal is the elimination of the use of alcohol, cigarettes, and marijuana by individuals under the age of 21 years. Given a historical perspective of human use of psychoactive drugs,[31] these are reasonable social goals. The first step is to agree on the need to implement them, and the second step is implementation of measures to achieve them.

Drug Education

Drug education and dependency treatment programs must consider the extent of a person's behavioral and physiological involvement with psychoactive drugs. Although educational programs may be useful approaches, formal treatment programs are necessary for persons who are compulsive abusers or addicts.

One approach to drug education is to teach the pharmacology of psychoactive drugs, as this text does. Even though this approach can be seen as providing directions for taking drugs, it can also be seen as providing accurate information for people to use in examining and modifying their own risk-taking behavior and thus making the informed decisions necessary to lead a healthy life in the community.

No program of drug education can guarantee to reduce the use of psychoactive drugs. A drug education program can, however, teach individuals the beneficial and harmful effects of a given drug (whether licit or illicit). Education may limit experimentation by some individuals. It will not dissuade those already involved in drugs, nor will it dissuade those who seek pharmacologic relief from their own psychiatric symptoms or disorders. In other words, it will not dissuade self-prescription for symptom relief. As stated in a White Paper[32] from the U.S. Office of National Drug Abuse Policy:

> Although [drug prevention] programs may not prevent someone from ever using drugs, they may well contribute toward a person ultimately leading a drug-free life. Furthermore, if a program can delay the onset of first use of a drug, while not the primary goal of prevention, it will decrease the likelihood of the user becoming addicted and a burden on society.

To alter the behavior of youths requires both education and examples set by teachers, peers, parents, and the whole community, including government officials. Three steps are necessary:

1. Basic information has to be imparted—truthful information—to generate motivation for behavior change. Only honest, straightforward, and full information about the health risks of the addictive drugs will meet this requirement.
2. The means for behavior change have to be provided. Here many techniques have proven effective, especially teaching children how to resist peer pressure. It is important to promote a redefinition of drug-using peers as not "cool."
3. Methods for reinforcing the new behaviors have to be employed. This means that children need recognition, praise, and other rewards for not using drugs. Emphasis on how drugs detract from a healthy body and an attractive appearance, for example, appeals to adolescents' interest in athletics as well as to their developing sexuality and their striving for intimate peer relationships.[33]

In essence, this approach is directed toward building self-esteem in a drug-free environment. While praiseworthy, the approach works best for those least likely to abuse drugs.

Prevention of drug abuse requires adults to be willing to set a consistent example by responsibly using or minimizing their own use of psychoactive drugs. In addition, legislation must be consistent and in agreement with accepted, documented scientific evidence. This action is particularly important regarding cigarettes and alcohol. The casualness with which these drugs are used and their promotion, distribution, and sale permitted demonstrates both ignorance and societal hypocrisy about the use of addicting drugs.

Treatment Issues

In past years, many people equated physical dependence with addiction. Indeed, in older views, the defining problem of addiction was physical dependence, implying that fear of withdrawal following drug removal was the "engine driving addictive substance use."[34] In such a view, detoxification was seen as the principle treatment for addiction. Free the addicted individual from the clutches of the drug by assisting him or her through withdrawal and the grip of the addiction was broken. Extending this concept to treatment, it is not surprising that treatment focused on detoxification, often in a clinical, residential, or hospital setting. Even today, detoxification is often still a primary goal of addiction treatment. That physical dependence (as defined by existence of a withdrawal syndrome with drug removal) is not equated with "addiction" is clear by study of the effects of the serotonin-type antidepressants. None would argue that these drug are prone to compulsive abuse or are "addicting," yet a well-characterized, multifaceted withdrawal syndrome can follow cessation of their use (Chapter 15).

A mid-1990s view of addiction treatment followed the observation that most individuals who go through detoxification eventually relapse to drug use. Focus was on drug-induced reward rather than on drug withdrawal as the engine driving addiction. Clearly, the positive aspects of the drug experience support drug self-administration. The reinforcing properties of drugs are powerful motivational forces that are preferred by the subjects to natural reinforcers. Thus, *drug reinforcement* becomes the unifying feature of drug abuse and dependence.[34,35] *Drug abstinence* can then be viewed as a behavioral and physical state induced by the absence of the drug of abuse to which the addict has adapted. It is behaviorally reinforcing to reverse the abstinence state by the readministration of a drug (i.e., relapse is behaviorally reinforcing). The state of abstinence is, therefore, not a return to "normal," as presumed by old models of addiction and withdrawal. Abstinence is characterized by a mental state of apathy, boredom, depression, malaise, anhedonia, and craving for relief. The individual needs the drug to feel normal. Thus, relapse is driven both by the negative reinforcement of abstinence and the positive reinforcement of the drug.

Now researchers are looking beyond the rather simplistic concepts of reward and withdrawal as the engines driving addiction. Not all individuals who experiment with drugs develop a substance abuse disorder; risk factors become an important predisposing variable to the expression of that genetically influenced, complex, chronic, and relapsing disease that we call "addiction" or "substance dependence." In adolescents,

> there are several broad classes of risk factors for the development of substance use disorders (SUDs), including parent and family risk factors, peer-related risk factors, individual risk factors (including biogenetic variables), and community risk factors. SUDs often are associated with other psychiatric diagnoses, such as disruptive behavior, mood and anxiety disorders; and problematic behaviors, including risk taking, aggression, and suicidal behavior.[36]

Just as focus cannot be solely on the drug of dependence and its rewarding and withdrawal effects as the principal factor involved in and driving abuse of the drug, neither can it be only on pharmacotherapy for treatment of the addiction. Focusing just on physical brain changes is not adequate; addicts will have to be able to handle later exposure to craving-eliciting cues in the environment and will need rehabilitation to either learn or relearn social skills or job skills. Moreover, it is likely that combined behavioral and pharmacological treatments will be truly synergistic, not just complementary in nature.

Comprehensive treatment does work,[37] and it can be provided in a cost-effective manner.[38] In general, regular outpatient treatment programs are the most cost-effective, while long-term residential treatment programs provide little extra benefit at a fivefold increase in expenses (Figure 13.6). Uniformly placing individuals in more intensive types of treatment is not the most cost-effective strategy, and incarceration as a treatment modality is prohibitively expensive. Any reasonable treatment strategy, even 5 to 10 minutes of physician counseling

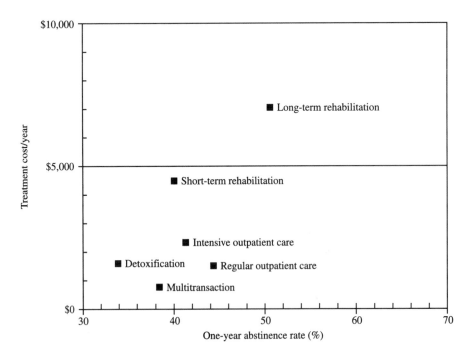

FIGURE 13.6 Cost-effect analysis comparing treatment costs of various modalities of treatment and one-year abstinence rates from substances of abuse. Not shown is the cost of incarceration at $25,900 per year. Regular outpatient treatment was the most effective treatment approach with more intensive interventions producing little additional reduction in the rates of relapse. [From Shepard, Larson, and Hoffmann.[38]]

on several visits, is more effective than no treatment.[39] Chappel and DuPont[40] describe the 12-step and mutual-help approaches used to treat addictive disorders. Monte and O'Leary[41] describe coping and social skills training techniques.

Friedmann, Saltz and Samet[39] summarize the techniques that can be used to manage adults recovering from substance abuse problems (Table 13.2). They present a practical approach to the support of a substance-free lifestyle, centering on patients who are early into recovery and at the highest risk of relapse, although many of the principles also apply to longer-term recovery.

Pharmacotherapy of Substance Use Disorders

It must be acknowledged that drugs have limited usefulness in most cases of substance use disorders; they should be used to augment psychosocial therapies. Despite this limitation, pharmacological treatment options for individuals with substance use disorders are many:

- Treatment to ameliorate withdrawal effects or syndromes
- Substituting a "legal," usually longer-acting drug for an illicit one to ameliorate some of the acute withdrawal effects
- Substituting a "legal" drug for an illicit one for long-term pharmacological maintenance
- Treating the substance abuse with a receptor antagonist
- Treating comorbid or underlying psychiatric disorders with nonaddicting, legally prescribed substitute medications

---

TABLE 13.2 Relapse prevention strategies in the primary care setting

Identify patients in recovery
Establish a supportive patient-physician relationship
Schedule regular follow-up
Mobilize family support
Facilitate involvement in 12-step recovery groups
Help recovering patients recognize and cope with relapse precipitants and craving
Advise recovering patients to develop a plan to manage early relapse
Facilitate positive lifestyle changes
Manage depression, anxiety, and other comorbid conditions
Consider adjunctive pharmacotherapy
Collaborate with addiction specialty professionals

From Friedman, Sailz, and Samet.[39]

The overall goals of pharmacologic therapy are twofold:

1. To reduce the intensity of withdrawal
2. To reduce the rate of relapse to future use of illicit drugs (so-called *relapse prevention pharmacology*)

These treatment goals were recently reviewed by Kranzler and co-workers.[42] Guidelines for the pharmacotherapy of substance use disorders in children and adolescents were detailed by Bukstein.[36]

Following is a summary of treatment options for specific drug dependencies. Complete details of the pharmacology of these and other drugs can be found in the chapters devoted to specific drugs of abuse.

Pharmacotherapy of Opioid Dependence

Detoxification and maintenance therapies (with opioid agonists, antagonists, or partial agonists) are the predominant approaches used to treat patients with opioid dependence (Chapter 9). In addition, underlying psychiatric comorbidities are treated with the appropriate psychopharmacologic medications. Comorbid pain syndromes are similarly treated with substitute analgesics of any of several types, including a variety of sophisticated techniques using opioid agonists and drugs that potentiate the actions of opioids.

Opioid detoxification is a process that enables individuals to withdraw from opioids safely, quickly, and comfortably. Medical detoxification relies on the substitution of a long-acting opioid agonist (methadone or LAAM; Chapter 9) for a shorter-acting one (e.g., heroin). Clonidine (an alpha-adrenergic agonist) with or without an opioid antagonist (e.g., naltrexone) can be used to reduce withdrawal symptoms during detoxification. The RAAD technique (Chapter 9) can be used to shorten the withdrawal period to 24 to 48 hours. Drawbacks to RAAD include its expense and the requirement for light general anesthesia. The major drawback to brief opioid detoxification is the extremely high rate of relapse to use of illicit opioids.

Maintenance treatment aims to provide stable abstinence from illicit opioids and improvement in overall health.[42] Methadone maintenance treatment programs are the most widely used long-term treatment approach for patients with opioid dependence: "All persons dependent on opioids should have access to methadone hydrochloride maintenance therapy under legal supervision."[43] Alternatives to methadone maintenance include LAAM (L-alpha-acetylmethadol) maintenance and buprenorphine (Buprenex); the latter is expected to be approved for this use in the near future. Alternatives to opioid agonists are drugs that act as opioid antagonists, naltrexone (Trexan, ReVia) is one such example. Generally unsuccessful, except in highly motivated patients, patients are poorly compliant with naltrexone therapy. Exceptions might be impaired professionals in whom therapy can be combined with contingency contracting to enhance compliance.

Pharmacotherapy of Nicotine Dependence

For each cigarette smoked, a bolus of about 1 mg to 3 mg of nicotine is delivered to the brain. Acute effects of nicotine include calmness, alertness, improved concentration, and elevation of mood, all of which can be behaviorally reinforcing. Moreover, smoking cessation produces withdrawal symptoms in most smokers (dysphoria, irritability, anxiety, frustration, poor concentration, increased appetite and drug craving). Both the primary reinforcing effects of smoking and the avoidance of withdrawal symptoms probably sustain tobacco use in most smokers.[42]

Nicotine-replacement therapies form the basis for treatment of cigarette dependence. Discussed at length in Chapter 8, these include gums, patches, nasal sprays, and inhalers. Kranzler and co-workers[42] reviewed these therapies.

As was discussed in Chapter 8, nicotine exerts a demonstrable antidepressant action. Therefore, antidepressants have been used as an adjunct to nicotine-replacement therapies. Most studied and most widely utilized for this purpose is the drug bupropion (Welbutrin, Zyban; Chapter 15). This drug appears to exert two actions: (1) an antidepressant action, efficacious in smokers with comorbid depression, and (2) an anticraving action that is independent of its antidepressant action.[44]

> Bupropion is believed to inhibit the neuronal reuptake of dopamine (which may play a role in the reinforcement of addictive drugs) and norepinephrine (which may affect nicotine withdrawal). Because nicotine also facilitates the release of dopamine, norepinephrine, and other neurotransmitters, the two drugs may have similar effects on brain chemistry.[42]

Comparative studies of bupropion and other antidepressants for use in smoking cessation have not been reported.

Pharmacotherapy of Alcohol Dependence

Drugs used in the treatment of alcohol dependence fall into the following categories:

- Drugs to ameliorate alcohol withdrawal (substitution therapy)
- Alcohol-sensitizing drugs (which make the ingestion of alcohol aversive or hazardous)

- Drugs that reduce the reinforcing effects of alcohol or the urge or craving to drink alcohol
- Drugs used to treat comorbid disorders, hopefully reducing the urge to ingest alcohol to treat psychiatric dysfunction

Alcohol-sensitizing drugs alter the body's response to alcohol. Disulfiram (Antabuse) is the only alcohol-sensitizing drug available in the United States. Calcium carbamide (Temposil), available in Canada and Europe, is a second agent.

Drugs to ameliorate withdrawal include the long-acting benzodi-azepines, such as chlordiazepoxide (Librium) and diazepam (Valium). They provide a substitute therapy, from which the dependent individual can later be withdrawn if such a therapeutic decision is made.

Drugs that reduce the reinforcing effects of alcohol or the urge or craving to drink alcohol all involve actions on neurotransmitter systems thought to be involved in the actions of alcohol. These transmitter systems include the opioid, the dopaminergic, the serotoninergic, and perhaps the glutamate. Presuming that some of the reinforcing effects of alcohol may be exerted through the opioid (endorphin) system, opioid antagonists, especially naltrexone, have been shown to be efficacious in the prevention of relapse to heavy drinking. As was discussed in Chapter 4, the long-term efficacy under less than laboratory conditions is open to debate.

The use of serotoninergic agents has been well studied. The SSRI-type antidepressants (Chapter 15) reduce alcohol consumption in both depressed and nondepressed alcoholics. Response rates are modest, usually affording a 15 to 20 percent reduction and usually only early in treatment. Combination therapy of naltrexone and SSRIs has not been reported, but the combination may be more effective than either alone.

As discussed in Chapter 4, *acamprosate*, available in many European countries, attenuates alcohol craving in laboratory animals and in humans who have been weaned from alcohol dependency.[45] It appears to have little effect on heroin self-administration.[46] Acamprosate is currently in clinical trials in the United States; study results are not yet available. Following oral administration, acamprosate is excreted unchanged (in the urine and the bile); therefore its kinetics are not affected by liver dysfunction seen in chronic alcoholism. Details of the kinetics of acamprosate are discussed by Saivin and co-workers.[47]

Mechanistically, acamprosate reduces calcium ion flows through NMDA-medicated glutamate neurotransmission; functioning as an NMDA-antagonist, especially in the nucleus accumbens.[48] Spanagel and Zieglgansberger[45] and Wilde and Wagstaff[49] review the anticraving actions of both acamprosate and naltrexone. Kranzler and colleagues[42] state:

> Studies of more than 3000 patients provide consistent evidence of the efficacy of acamprosate in alcoholism rehabilitation. Over the period of a year, the drug nearly doubled the rate of abstinence over the 11 percent observed among placebo patients. . . . As greater efforts are made to provide psychosocial therapies as a context for pharmacotherapy, the effects of adding medication may be greater . . . because [acamprosate] has a benign side effect profile, it seems to have a promising future for the treatment of patients with alcohol dependence.

A combination of acamprosate and disulfiram improved the clinical efficacy of either drug used alone.[50] It is quite likely that the drug will be approved for clinical use in the United States.

The drug *ibogaine*, a substance currently classified as a Schedule 1 "narcotic" because of its psychedelic properties, is an alkaloid obtained from the roots of a rain forest shrub, *Tabernanthe iboga*, indigenous to equatorial Africa. For centuries ibogaine has been used in low doses to combat fatigue and hunger and in higher doses as a sacrament in religious rituals.[51] Properties assigned to ibogaine include those of a stimulant, a performance enhancer, a hallucinogen, and an aphrodisiac.[52] Anecdotal reports attest that a single dose of ibogaine eliminates withdrawal symptoms, reduces drug cravings, and promotes long-term drug abstinence from addictive substances, including psychostimulants and alcohol.[51]

Isolated in 1901, the structure of ibogaine (Figure 13.7) closely resembles those of serotonin and harmine. In the late 1980s, it was noted that in animal experiments ibogaine reduced the self-administration of both cocaine and morphine and attenuated the symptoms of morphine withdrawal. Claims have been made that ibogaine "interrupts the dependency syndrome, allowing patients to maintain a drug-free lifestyle for at least six months."[52] Side effects in animals consist of ataxia, tremor, psychedelic-like mannerisms, and (in rats) damage to Purkinje cells in the cerebellum. In humans, ibogaine can cause hallucinations associated with severe anxiety, apprehension, and tremor. Cerebellar toxicity has not been demonstrated in humans.

Ibogaine attenuates alcohol intake in alcohol-preferring rats[53] (see Figure 13.7), and it decreases morphine and cocaine self-administration in rats. The mechanisms underlying this putative anticraving effect are unclear, but they may result from modulation of serotinergic systems,[54] and/or by activation of kappa-type opioid receptors and a PCP-like blockade of glutaminergic NMDA-type receptors.[55] These actions would ultimately modulate dopamine release.[56,57]

The claimed "antiaddictive" or "end abuse" properties of ibogaine require rigorous validation in humans, after careful assessment of its neurotoxic potential. The current federal regulations on ibogaine limit laboratory and clinical experimentation with the drug. Perhaps eventually analogues of ibogaine will be developed that retain the antiaddictive properties but spare its hallucinogenic and potential neurotoxic effects.[58]

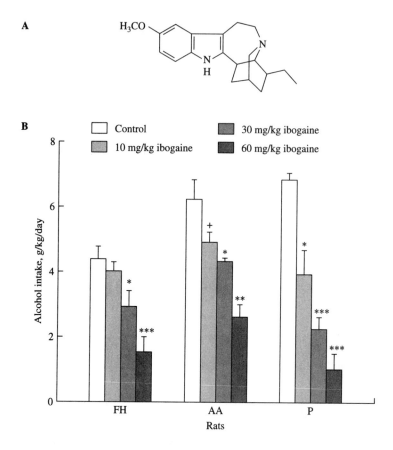

FIGURE 13.7 A. Structure of ibogaine. **B.** Effects of three doses of ibogaine and control vehicle (clear bars) on spontaneous intake of alcohol in three strains of alcohol-preferring rats (labeled FH, AA, and P). Data are means ± SEM. $*p < 0.05$, $**p < 0.002$, and $***p < 0.001$ compared with control. [From Rezvani, Overstreet, and Lee.[53]]

STUDY QUESTIONS

1. What is meant when a particular drug is called a "behavioral reinforcer"?

2. Why might the evaluation of drug-reinforcing properties in animals be valuable in the assessment of human experiences?

3. Is a propensity for abusing drugs caused by a psychopathological process in the user, or is it a property of the particular drug?

4. On a physiological level, what might explain the lack of self-reinforcing action of phenothiazines or antidepressants?

5. What is the mechanism that underlies the behavioral reinforcing properties of abused drugs?

6. List several key principles that underlie a positive approach toward drug education.

7. Where has drug education failed? How might drug education be used successfully?

8. What is the relationship between age of first use of drugs and development of a substance use disorder? What are the limitations to this relationship?

9. List, from most harmful to least harmful, the classes of psychoactive drugs presented in this book. Defend your choices.

10. Should certain drugs be more readily available? How should legislation be directed?

11. Are current efforts to limit cigarette smoking likely to prove successful? How should be change our approach?

12. Where should alcohol education be aimed? Defend your position.

REFERENCES

1. A. Goldstein, *Addiction: From Biology to Drug Policy* (New York: W. H. Freeman and Company, 1994), 9.
2. D. P. Rice, "Economic Costs of Substance Abuse, 1995," *Proceedings of the Association of American Physicians* 111 (1999): 119–125.
3. P. Crits-Christoph and L. Siqueland, "Psychosocial Treatment for Drug Abuse: Selected Review and Recommendations for National Health Care," *Archives of General Psychiatry* 53 (1996): 749–756.
4. J. C. Gfroerer and J. F. Epstein, "Marijuana Initiates and their Impact on Future Drug Abuse Treatment Need," *Drug and Alcohol Dependence* 54 (1999): 229–237.
5. D. R. Gerstein et al., "Evaluating Recovery Services: The California Drug and Alcohol Treatment Assessment General Report" (Sacramento, Calif.: California Department of Alcohol and Drug Programs, 1994).
6. J. H. Krystal, D. C. D'Souza, S. Madonick, and I. L. Petrakis, "Toward a Rational Pharmacotherapy of Comorbid Substance Abuse in Schizophrenic Patients," *Schizophrenia Research* 35, suppl. (1999): S35–S49.
7. J. C. Merrill et al., "Cigarettes, Alcohol, Marijuana, Other Risk Behaviors, and American Youth," *Drug and Alcohol Dependence* 56 (1999): 205–212.
8. American Psychiatric Association, *Diagnostic and Statistical Manual of Mental Disorders*, 4th ed (DSM-IV). Washington, D.C.: American Psychiatric Association, 1994.
9. K. K. Bucholz, "Nosology and Epidemiology of Addictive Disorders and Their Comorbidity," *Psychiatric Clinics of North America* 22 (1999): 221–240.

10. R. J. Goldsmith, "Overview of Psychiatric Comorbidity: Practical and Theoretical Considerations," *Psychiatric Clinics of North America* 22 (1999): 331–349.

11. E. F. McCance-Katz and T. R. Kosten, eds., *New Treatments for Chemical Addictions* (Washington, D.C.: American Psychiatric Press, 1998).

12. A. E. Skodol, J. M. Oldham, and P. E. Gallagher, "Axis II Comorbidity of Substance Use Disorders Among Patients Referred for treatment of Personality Disorders," *American Journal of Psychiatry* 156 (1999): 733–738.

13. A. I. Leshner, "Drug Abuse and Addiction Treatment Research: The Next Generation," *Archives of General Psychiatry* 54 (1997): 691–694.

14. J. S. Yongue, book review in *Journal of the American Medical Association* 281 (1999): 2145–2146.

15. R. A. Wise, "Drug Activation of Brain Reward Pathways," *Drug and Alcohol Dependence* 51 (1998): 13–22.

16. E. L. Gardner, "Brain Reward Mechanisms," in J. H. Lowinson, P. Ruiz, R. B. Millman, and J. G. Langrod, eds., *Substance Abuse: A Comprehensive Textbook*, 3rd ed. (Baltimore: Williams & Wilkins, 1997), 51–85.

17. G. F. Koob, "Drugs of Abuse: Anatomy, Pharmacology, and Function of Reward Pathways," *Trends in Pharmacologic Sciences* 13 (1992): 177–182.

18. N. D. Volkow et al., "Prediction of Reinforcing Responses to Psychostimulants in Humans by Brain Dopamine D_2 Receptor Levels," *American Journal of Psychiatry* 156 (1999): 1440–1443.

19. B. G. Winsberg and D. E. Comings, "Association of the Dopamine Transporter Gene (*DAT1*) with Poor Methylphenidate Response," *Journal of the American Academy of Child and Adolescent Psychiatry* 38 (1999): 1474–1477.

20. A. R. Childress et al., "Limbic Activation During Cue-induced Cocaine Craving," *American Journal of Psychiatry* 156 (1999): 11–18.

21. I. Stolerman, "Drugs of Abuse: Behavioral Principles, Methods, and Terms," *Trends in Pharmacological Sciences* 13 (1992): 170–176.

22. R. J. Cadoret et al., "Adoption Study Demonstrating Two Genetic Pathways to Drug Abuse," *Archives of General Psychiatry* 52 (1995): 42–52.

23. C. A. Prescott and K. S. Kendler, "Genetic and Environmental Contributions to Alcohol Abuse and Dependence in a Population-Based Sample of Male Twins," *American Journal of Psychiatry* 156 (1999): 34–40.

24. M. Van den Bree, E. O. Johnson, M. C. Neale, and R. W. Pickens, "Genetic and Environmental Influences on Drug Use and Abuse/Dependence in Male and Female Twins," *Drug and Alcohol Dependence* 52 (1998): 231–241.

25. M. T. Tsuang et al., "Co-occurrence of Abuse of Different Drugs in Men: The Role of Drug-specific and Shared Vulnerabilities," *Archives of General Psychiatry* 55 (1998): 967–972.

26. K. R. Merikanges et al., "Familial Transmission of Substance Abuse Disorders," *Archives of General Psychiatry* 55 (1998): 973–979.

27. L. J. Bierut et al., "Familial Transmission of Substance Dependence: Alcohol, Marijuana, Cocaine, and Habitual Smoking. A Report from the Collaborative Study on the Genetics of Alcoholism," *Archives of General Psychiatry* 55 (1998): 982–988.

28. D. Goldman and A. Bergen, "General and Specific Inheritance of Substance Abuse and Alcoholism," *Archives of General Psychiatry* 55 (1998): 964–965.
29. U. Rao et al., "Factors Associated with the Development of Substance Use Disorder in Depressed Adolescents," *Journal of the American Academy of Child and Adolescent Psychiatry* 38 (1999): 1109–1117.
30. P. V. Piazza and M. Le Moal, "The Role of Stress in Drug Self-administration," *Trends in Pharmacological Sciences* 19 (1998): 67–74.
31. R. Porter and M. Teich, eds., *Drugs and Narcotics in History* (New York: Cambridge University Press, 1995).
32. Office of National Drug Control Policy, Executive Office of the President, *Understanding Drug Prevention* (Washington, D.C.: U.S. Government Printing Office, 1992), 16.
33. A. Goldstein, *Addiction: From Biology to Drug Policy* (New York: W. H. Freeman and Company, 1994), 208–209.
34. M. S. Gold and D. H. Eaton, "Drugs in History," *Journal of the American Medical Association* 275 (1996): 1364–1365.
35. R. L. DuPont and M. S. Gold, "Withdrawal and Reward: Implications for Detoxification and Relapse Prevention," *Psychiatric Annals* 25 (1995): 663–668.
36. O. Bukstein and the Workgroup on Quality Issues, "Summary of the Practice Parameters for the Assessment and Treatment of Children and Adolescents with Substance Use Disorders," *Journal of the American Academy of Child and Adolescent Psychiatry* 37 (1998): 122–126.
37. C. Marwick, "Physician Leadership on National Drug Policy Finds Addiction Treatment Works," *Journal of the American Medical Association,* 279 (1998): 1149–1150.
38. D. S. Shepard, M. J. Larson, and N. G. Hoffman, "Cost-effectiveness of Substance Abuse Services: Implications for Public Policy," *Psychiatric Clinics of North America* 22 (1999): 385–400.
39. P. D. Friedman, R. Sailz, and J. H. Samet, "Management of Adults Recovering from Alcohol and Other Drug Problems," *Journal of the American Medical Association,* 279 (1998): 1227–1231.
40. J. N. Chappel and R. L. DuPont, "Twelve-step and Mutual-help Programs for Addictive Disorders," *Psychiatric Clinics of North America* 22 (1999): 425–446.
41. P. M. Monti and T. A. O'Leary, "Coping and Social Skills Training for Alcohol and Cocaine Dependence," *Psychiatric Clinics of North America* 22 (1999): 447–470.
42. H. R. Kransler, H. Amin, V. Modesto-Lowe, and C. Oncken, "Pharmacologic Treatments for Drug and Alcohol Dependence," *Psychiatric Clinics of North America* 22 (1999): 401–423.
43. National Consensus Development Panel on Effective Medical Treatment of Opiate Addiction, "Effective Medical Treatment of Opiate Addiction," *Journal of the American Medical Association* 280 (1998): 1936–1943.
44. R. D. Hurt et al., "A Comparison of Sustained-release Bupropion and Placebo for Smoking Cessation," *New England Journal of Medicine* 337 (1997): 1195–1202.
45. R. Spangel and W. Zieglgansberger, "Anti-craving Compounds for Ethanol: New Pharmacological Tools to Study Addictive Processes," *Trends in Pharmacological Sciences* 18 (1997): 54–59.

46. R. Spanagel et al., "Acamprosate Suppresses the Expression of Morphine-induced Sensitization in Rats but Does Not Affect Heroin Self-administration or Relapse Induced by Heroin or Stress," *Psychopharmacology* 139 (1998): 391–401.
47. S. Saivin et al., "Clinical Pharmacokinetics of Acamprosate," *Clinical Pharmacokinetics* 35 (1998): 331–345.
48. A. Dahchour et al., "Central Effects of Acamprosate. Part 1: Acamprosate Blocks the Glutamate Increase in the Nucleus Accumbens Microdialysate in Ethanol Withdrawn Rats," *Psychiatry Research* 82 (1998): 107–114.
49. M. I. Wilde and A. J. Wagstaff, "Acamprosate: A Review of Its Pharmacology and Clinical Potential in the Management of Alcohol Dependence after Detoxification," *Drugs* 53 (1997): 1038–1053.
50. J. Beeson et al., "Combined Efficacy of Acamprosate and Disulfiram in the Treatment of Alcoholism: A Controlled Study," *Alcoholism: Clinical and Experimental Research* 22 (1998): 573–579.
51. D. C. Mash et al., "Medication Development of Ibogaine as a Pharmacotherapy for Drug Dependence," *Annals of the New York Academy of Sciences* 844 (1998): 274–292.
52. P. Popik, R. T. Layer, and P. Skolnick, "100 Years of Ibogaine: Neurochemical and Pharmacological Actions of a Putative Anti-addictive Drug," *Pharmacological Reviews* 47 (1995): 235–253.
53. A. H. Rezvani, D. H. Overstreet, and Y.-W. Lee, "Attenuation of Alcohol Intake by Ibogaine in Three Strains of Alcohol-preferring Rats," *Pharmacology, Biochemistry, and Behavior* 52 (1995): 615–620.
54. G. B. Wells, M. C. Lopez, and J. C. Tanaka, "The Effects of Ibogaine on Dopamine and Serotonin Transport in Rat Brain Synaptosomes," *Brain Research Bulletin* 48 (1999): 641–647.
55. S. D. Glick and I. S. Maisonneuve, "Mechanisms of the Antiaddictive Actions of Ibogaine," *Annals of the New York Academy of Sciences* 844 (1998): 214–226.
56. E. D. French, K. Dillon, and S. F. Ali, "Effects of Ibogaine, and Cocaine and Morphine After Ibogaine, on Ventral Tegmental Dopamine Neurons," *Life Sciences* 59 (1996): 199–205.
57. H. Sershen, A. Hashim, and A. Lajtha, "Effect of Ibogaine on Cocaine-induced Efflux of [^{3}H]Dopamine and [^{3}H]Serotonin from Mouse Striatum," *Pharmacology, Biochemistry, and Behavior* 53 (1996): 863–869.
58. A. H. Rezvani et al., "Attenuation of Alcohol Consumption by a Novel Nontoxic Ibogaine Analogue (18-Methoxycoronaridine) in Alcohol-preferring Rats," *Pharmacology, Biochemistry, and Behavior* 58 (1997): 615–619.

Anabolic-Androgenic Steroids

Anabolic-androgenic steroids (hereafter referred to as *anabolic steroids*) are chemicals related to the male hormone *testosterone*. They have both muscle-building (anabolic) and masculinizing effects, and illicit use is a common practice among adolescents and adults, both male and female, athletes and nonathletes.[1,2] While it may not be surprising that 55 percent of 27-year-old male and 10 percent of 24-year-old female body builders use anabolic steroids, prevalence of anabolic steroid injection in college athletics may be as high as 20 percent, and anabolic steroid use in high schools has been estimated as high as 7 percent for males and 3 percent for females. Lifetime use is 4.9 percent for males and 2.4 percent for females, and the numbers are likely to increase.[3] Probably more than 1 million Americans have used these hormones illicitly to improve athletic performance or personal appearance.

In both athletes and nonathletes, anabolic steroids promote increased muscle mass and enhance physical strength, endurance, physical appearance, and athletic performance. The use of the testosterone precursor *androstenedione* by baseball home run record holder Mark McGwire focused even more attention on steroid use by athletes.

As well as illicit use, there is controversy over the role and use of anabolic steroids in prescription medicine.[4] Recent articles discuss the efficacy of these agents in preventing weight loss both in renal failure patients undergoing hemodialysis[5] and in males with HIV (AIDS)-related weight loss.[6] Rablin and co-workers[7] studied the effects of weekly injections of testosterone in 70 males with symptomatic HIV illness. The majority reported improved libido and energy, improvements in mood, and increases in muscle mass.

Much of the controversy over anabolic steroid use, medical and illicit, involves the documented health risks associated with steroid use as well as the "unfair advantage" a performance-enhancing drug offers the competitive athlete. Also, adolescent nonathletes who use steroids as cosmetic enhancers place themselves at risk for long-term health problems, and they also may suffer from serious body self-image problems that should be attended to.

Testosterone is the primary male sex hormone. Normally, the levels of testosterone in the body are tightly regulated by a negative feedback system involving the testes (where testosterone is synthesized), the hypothalamus, and the pituitary gland (Figure 14.1). When the plasma level of testosterone falls, cells in the hypothalamus (which has receptors sensitive to the circulating amount of testosterone) sense the decrease and begin producing a releasing factor called *gonadotropin-releasing factor* (GRF). GRF circulates in blood to the pituitary gland and stimulates the pituitary to produce and release *follicle-stimulating hormone* (FSH) and *luteinizing hormone* (LH). In turn, FSH and LH act on the testes to induce both spermatogenesis (the production of sperm) and synthesis and release of testosterone. (A similar process in the female regulates fertility.)

As testosterone levels in blood increase, the hypothalamus decreases its production of GRF, the pituitary decreases production of FSH and LH; the testes decrease production of testosterone and sperm; and the process repeats. Administering anabolic steroids overwhelms this system; abnormally high levels of steroids shut off production of GRF, FSH, LH and testosterone and shut off the process of spermatogenesis. Therefore, anabolic steroids (1) block the normal process that regulates testosterone, male fertility, and spermatogenesis, (2) exert peripheral hormone actions to increase muscle mass and produce a more masculine appearance, and (3) exert central effects that increase aggression.

Mechanism of Action and Effects

The anabolic steroids are a group of drugs that include testosterone and several synthetically produced structural derivatives with the same overall actions. Figure 14.2 illustrates the structures of these compounds. In addition, two other substances must be included: (1) androstenedione, a precursor to testosterone, and (2) dehydroepiandrosterone (DHEA), an androgen released by the adrenal glands. Androstenedione is discussed at the end of this chapter; DHEA is discussed in Chapter 15.

All anabolic steroids differ from each other not so much in structure as in their individual resistance to metabolic degradation by liver enzymes. After oral administration, testosterone is effectively absorbed from the intestine. Following absorption, it is rapidly transported in

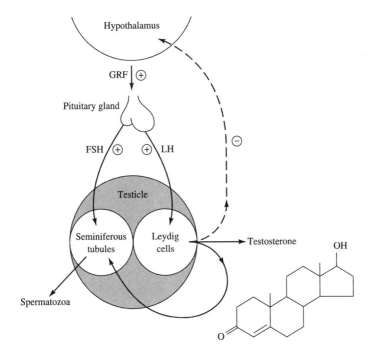

FIGURE 14.1 Hormonal regulation of male fertility. The brain (hypothalamus and pituitary gland) is involved in the control of fertility. However, fertility in the male is not subject to periodic cycling as it is in the female. The structure of naturally occurring testosterone is shown. GRF = gonadotropin-releasing factor; FSH = follicle-stimulating hormone; LH = luteinizing hormone. Solid arrows = stimulation; dashed arrows = inhibition.

the blood to the liver, where it is immediately metabolized. As a result, little testosterone reaches the systemic circulation.[8] Administered by injection, some of this first-pass metabolism is blunted, and it is the metabolic product, androstanolone, that is most active as an anabolic substance.[8] Structural modification of the testosterone molecule can reduce metabolic degradation and thus improve the effectiveness of both oral and intramuscular administration.

Not all these drugs are illicit substances. Eight synthetic A-AS substances (Table 14.1) are approved in the United States for therapeutic uses, including testosterone replacement in hypogonadal males,[7] the treatment of certain blood anemias and severe muscle loss following trauma, HIV, renal dialysis, and, in females, the treatment of endometriosis and fibrocystic disease of the breast. In malnourished males with severe pulmonary disease (chronic obstructive pulmonary disease), 27 weeks of oral androgen therapy increased lean body mass, and muscle mass even though endurance capacity was not changed.[9] Therefore, in

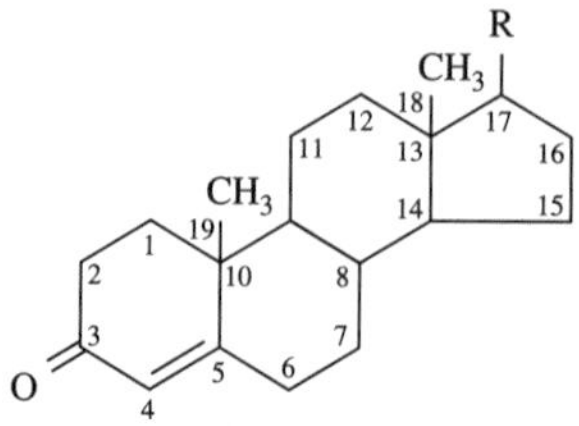

Compound	R
Testosterone	—OH
Testosterone propionate	—O—COCH$_2$CH$_3$
Testosterone enanthate	—O—CO(CH$_2$)$_5$CH$_3$
Testosterone cypionate	—O—COCH$_2$CH$_2$— (cyclopentyl) 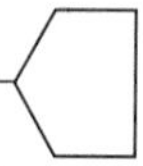
Nandrolone decanoate	—O—CO(CH$_2$)$_8$CH$_3$ (no methyl group at position 19)
Nandrolone phenpropionate	—O—CO(CH$_2$)$_2$— 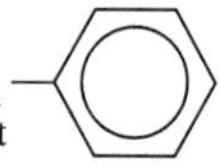 (phenyl) (no methyl group at position 19)

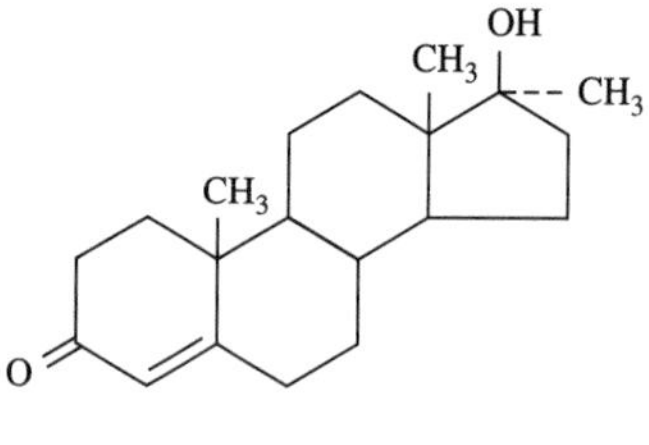

Methyltestosterone

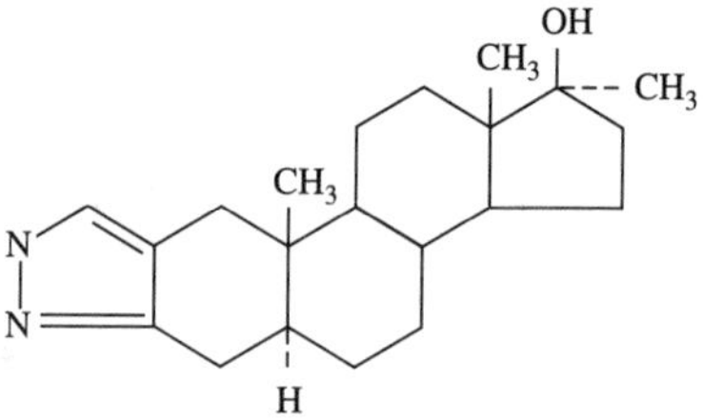

Stanozolol

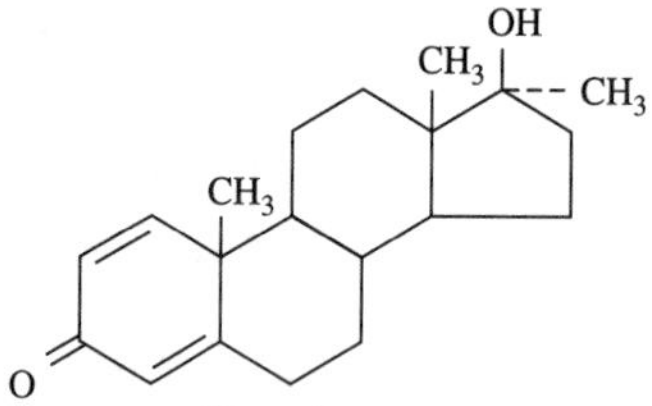

Metandienone

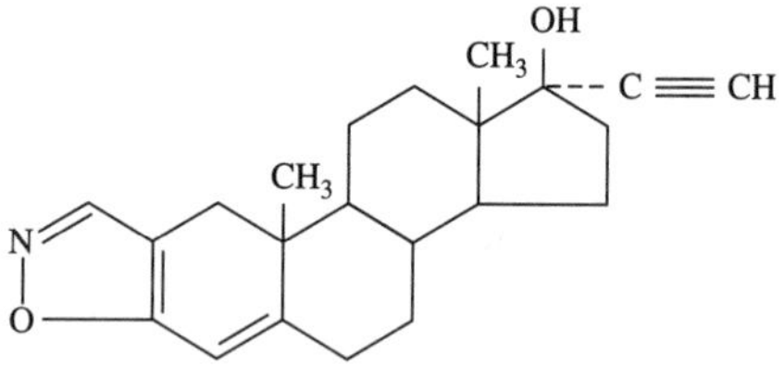

Danazol

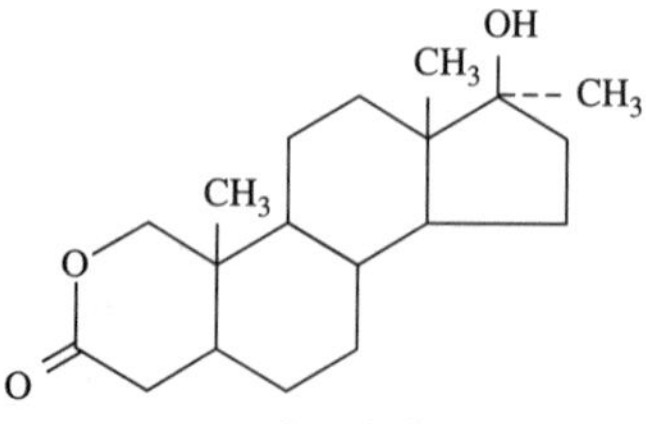

Oxandrolone

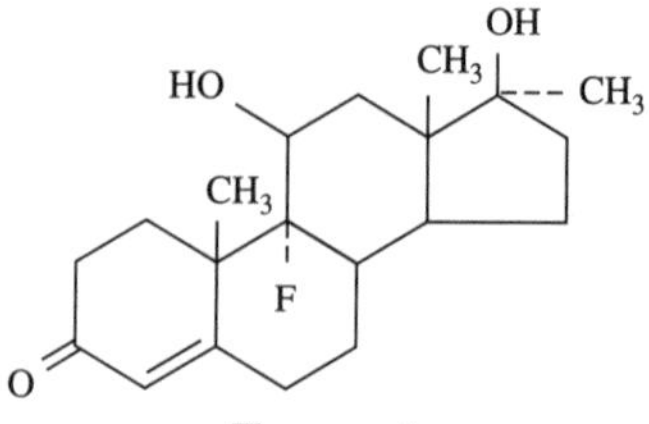

Fluoxymesterone

FIGURE 14.2 Structures of some common parenteral (*left*) and oral (*right*) anabolic-androgenic steroids. [From Lucas,[8] with permission.]

TABLE 14.1 Anabolic-androgenic steroids

Name	Route	Brand name
APPROVED IN UNITED STATES		
Testosterone cypionate	im	Depo-Testosterone, Virilon
Nandrolone phenpropionate	im	Durabolin
Nandrolone decanoate	im	Deca-Duraboli
Danazol	po	Danocrine
Fluoxymesterone	po	Halotestin
Methyltestosterone	po	Android, Metandren, Testred, Virilon
Oxymetholone	po	Anadrol-50
Slanozolol	po	Winstrol
APPROVED OUTSIDE UNITED STATES		
Testosterone enanthate	im	Delatestryl
Testosterone propionate	im	Testex, Oreton propionate
Methenolone enanthate	im	Primobolan Depot
Ethylestrenol	po	Maxibolan
Mesterolone	po	
Methandrostenolone	po	Dianabol
Methenolone	po	Primobolan
Norethandrolone	po	
Oxandrolone	po	Anavar
Oxymesterone	po	Oranabol
APPROVED FOR VETERINARY USE		
Bolasterone	im	Finiject 30
Boldenone undecylenate	im	Equipoise
Stanozolol	im	Winstrol
Mibolerone	po	

im = intramuscular; po = oral.

states of malnutrition, anabolic steroid therapy increases muscle mass, an effect that hopefully will reduce mortality and improve quality of life.

Mechanism of Action

The mechanism of action of testosterone and other A-AS drugs is quite well understood. The natural hormone is synthesized principally in a specialized type of cell (the Leydig cell) of the testes (Figure 14.1) under the influence of GRF released from the hypothalamus, which stimulates the synthesis and release of LH from the pituitary gland; LH acts on the Leydig cells to stimulate testosterone production.

Once in the bloodstream, testosterone (or an anabolic steroid) passes through the cell walls of its target tissues and attaches to steroid receptors in the cytoplasm of the cell[8] (Figure 14.3). This hormone-receptor complex is translocated into the nucleus of the cell and attaches to the nuclear material (the DNA). A process of genetic transcription follows, and new messenger RNA is produced. Translation of this RNA results in the production of specific new proteins that leave the cell and mediate the biological functions of the hormone. Thus, the effects of anabolic steroids on target cells are mediated by intracellular receptors and the synthesis of new proteins. The increased levels of circulating testosterone (or anabolic steroid) exert a negative feedback effect on the hypothalamus, inhibiting further stimulation of testosterone release.

Effects on Athletic Performance

Because testosterone and anabolic steroids increase protein synthesis, they increase muscle mass and strength and produce a more masculine appearance. The assumption that this is what happens has been around a long time, but the 1996 report by Bhasin and co-workers[10] was the first to demonstrate that supraphysiologic doses of testosterone, with or

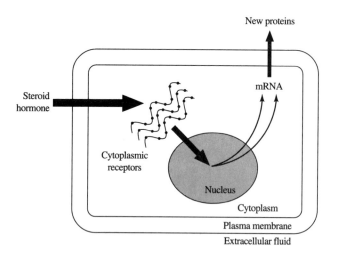

FIGURE 14.3 Mechanism of action of steroid hormones on cells. The hormone passes through the cell wall of its target tissue and binds to steroid receptors in the cytoplasm. The hormone-receptor complex moves into the nucleus and binds to sites on the chromatin, which is transcribed to give specific messenger RNA (mRNA). The mRNA is translated into specific new proteins that mediate the function of the hormone. [From Lucas,[8] with permission.]

without strength training, increase fat-free mass, muscle size, and strength in normal men. As shown in Figure 14.4, exercise alone or testosterone alone produced increases in strength, triceps and quadriceps size, and fat-free mass. The combination of testosterone

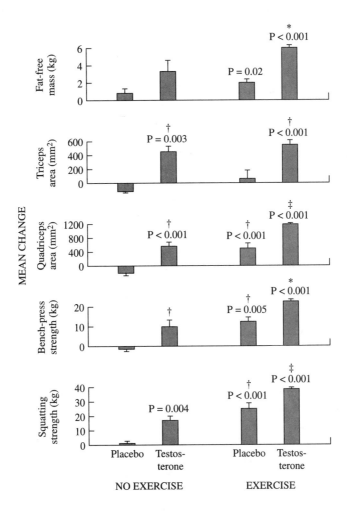

FIGURE 14.4 Changes from base line in mean (±SE) fat-free mass, triceps, and quadriceps cross-sectional areas, and muscle strength in the bench-press and squatting exercises over 10 weeks of treatment with testosterone. The P values shown are for the comparison between the change indicated and a change of zero. The asterisks indicate $P < 0.05$ for the comparison between the change indicated and that in either no-exercise group; the daggers indicate $P < 0.05$ for the comparison between the change indicated and that in the group assigned to placebo with no exercise; the double daggers indicate $P < 0.05$ for the comparison between the change indicated and the changes in all three other groups. [From Bhasin et al.,[10] with permission.]

and exercise produced additive increases. Despite these beneficial effects of testosterone, the authors concluded:

> Our results in no way justify the use of anabolic-androgenic steroids in sports, because, with extended use, such drugs have potentially serious adverse effects on the cardiovascular system, prostate, lipid metabolism, and insulin sensitivity. Moreover, the use of any performance-enhancing agent in sports raises serious ethical issues.[10]

Thus, anabolic steroids increase both the size and the strength of the athlete and thereby improve performance in athletic activities that require size and strength. They have no positive effects on aerobic performance.[11] Therefore, athletes who depend on aerobic energy expenditure (e.g., long-distance runners) benefit less from anabolic steroids than athletes who depend on bulk size and short bursts of energy expenditure (e.g., football players, sprint runners).

Anabolic steroids exert effects through anticatabolic, anabolic, and motivational effects on the athlete. Table 14.2 summarizes the constellation of effects and side effects. In the *anticatabolic effect*, the anabolic steroids block the action of natural cortisone, which normally functions to increase energy stores during periods of stress and training. Cortisone makes energy stores available by breaking down proteins into their constituent amino acids. Carried to excess, muscle wasting can occur. This action is blocked by the anabolic steroids. The anticatabolic action may be the major mechanism by which these drugs increase body mass.

The *anabolic effects* follow both the synthesis of new protein in muscle cells and steroid–induced release of endogenous growth hormone.[11] However, the doses commonly used by athletes are 10 to 200 times the therapeutic dosage for testosterone deficiency. This often involves the "stacking" or "pyramiding" of several drugs, even combining oral and injectable substances through cycles of several weeks' duration.[12]

The *motivational effects* are profound: athletes taking anabolic steroids often develop very aggressive personalities, a condition nicknamed "roid rage." For some sports, such as football, these steroids may serve the dual purpose of increasing strength and performance and enhancing combativeness.

In the female athlete, anabolic steroids exert the same anabolic and anticatabolic effects found in male athletes. However, these drugs also induce in females masculinizing and related effects, including increases in facial and body hair, lowered voice, enlarged clitoris, coarser skin, and menstrual cycle cessation or irregularity. Cessation of steroid use results in a variable and often incomplete return of the altered functions. Tuiten and colleagues[13] administered sublingual testosterone to 8 healthy females and evaluated its effects on sexual arousal. Testosterone achieved maximal plasma levels in 15 minutes, returning to baseline levels by

TABLE 14.2 Effects of anabolic-androgenic steroids

POSITIVE EFFECTS
   Transient increase in muscular size and strength
   Treatment of catabolic states
      Trauma
      Surgery
ADVERSE EFFECTS
   Cardiovascular
      Increase in cardiac risk factors
         Hypertension
         Altered lipoprotein fractions
         Increase in LDL/HDL ratio
      Reported strokes/myocardial infarctions
   Hepatic effects associated with oral compounds
      Elevated liver enzymes
      Peliosis hepatis (greater than 6 months' use)
      Liver tumors
         Benign
         Malignant (greater than 24 months' use)
   Reproductive system effects
      In males
         Decreased testosterone production
            Abnormal spermatogenesis
            Transient infertility
            Testicular atrophy
      In females
         Altered menstruation
   Endocrine effects
      Decreased thyroid function
   Immunologic effects
      Decreased immunoglobulins IgM/IgA/IgC
   Musculoskeletal effects
      Premature closure of bony growth centers
      Tendon degeneration
         Increased risk of tendon tears
   Cosmetic
      In males
         Gynecomastia
         Testicular atrophy
         Acne
         Acceleration of male pattern baldness
      In females
         Clittoral enlargement
         Acne
         Increased facial/body hair
         Coarsening of the skin
         Male pattern baldness
         Deepened voice
   Psychologic
      Risk of habituation
      Severe mood swings
      Aggressive tendencies
      Psychotic episodes
      Depression
      Reports of suicide
   Legislation
      Classified as Schedule III controlled substance

From Haupt,[11] with permission.

90 minutes. At about 4.5 hours, significant increases in arousal and genital responsiveness occurred. Alterations in "central" homonal mechanisms were postulated to account for the discrepancy between plasma levels and physiological responses.

Anabolic steroids are widely used (and abused) by young male (usually noncompetitive) athletes who take them to develop the muscular physique considered fashionable. As many as 250,000 to 500,000 young adult males may take steroids. Regardless of the exact number, a significant number of teenagers and young adults, primarily male, use supraphysiologic doses of anabolic steroids to give them more muscle strength and a more powerful, masculine appearance.[12] Unlike competitive athletes who may choose to terminate drug use when competition ends, nonathlete youths may continue to take steroids in order to maintain the cosmetic effect. As stated by Schwerin and co-workers:[14]

> Physique and physical appearance are ever important in how people are viewed in their social environment. With these come the spoils: social acceptance, admiration, and opportunity. To a certain extent, an attractive physique is related to enhanced self-esteem and perceived social competence. . . . Sometimes the drive reaches an unhealthy extreme . . . taking the form of anorexia, bulimia, and anabolic steroid use.

Furthermore:

> Anabolic steroid users present an appearance of healthfulness, strength, "sex appeal," and physical attractiveness. Other illicit drugs do not present such an image of healthfulness. . . . It may be this contradiction of increased steroid use leading to increased appearance of healthfulness and physical attractiveness which may allow the seriousness of steroid use to remain underappreciated. . . . Anabolic steroids are the only addictive substance over the short to middle term that enhances a user's physical appearance and whose purpose is to allow the user to work harder and longer (though stimulants share the latter characteristic).

Endocrine Effects

Males taking anabolic steroids experience a hypogonadal state, which is characterized by atrophy of the testicles, impaired production of sperm, and infertility, causing reduced libido and impotence.[15] These effects are usually reversible within a few months after cessation of drug use. As stated:

> Even when gonadal dysfunction occurs, persons often continue using the anabolic steroids, in part because of the neuropsychiatric effects, which include psychotic symptoms, affective syndromes, increased aggression, and psychological dependence.[15]

In addition, gynecomastia (enlargement of the breasts in males) may occur. Many users are quite sophisticated in their drug use, using such information sources as the *Underground Steroid Handbook* to guide therapy, which includes "the use of human chorionic gonadotropin, clomiphene citrate, and tamoxifen citrate, to counter the side effects of gynecomastia and reduced testicular volume."[14] The gynecomastia results from some of the anabolic steroid being metabolized to the female hormone estradiol.

Cardiovascular Effects

Adverse effects of anabolic steroids on the cardiovascular system have been of concern, and reports of fatal myocardial infarctions (heart attacks) occurring in users of anabolic steroids implicate atherosclerosis-induced coronary artery disease as a cause of death. Thus, analysis of the potential correlation between anabolic steroids and atherosclerosis is important. The effect of these steroids on blood cholesterol as a predisposing factor to atherosclerotic coronary artery disease must be considered. Cholesterol is of two types: "bad" cholesterol (low-density lipoprotein cholesterol, or LDL) and "good" cholesterol (high-density lipoprotein cholesterol, or HDL). Decreasing HDL and increasing LDL are strongly correlated with an increased risk of coronary artery disease.

All anabolic steroids induce a reduction in serum HDL cholesterol and an elevation in LDL cholesterol. This suggests that individuals taking these drugs are at greater risk of developing atheromatous plaques within arteries, which places such individuals at increased risk of coronary artery disease. This condition can be expressed as myocardial infarctions, thromboembolic disease (blood clots and emboli), strokes, and hypertension. The actual risk of cardiovascular disease is unknown, largely due to the young age of users, their relatively lean or muscular physiques, and the intermittent pattern of drug use. Once these users are adults, it can be determined whether they were harmed by using anabolic steroids during their earlier years. Melchert and Welder[16] and Sullivan and co-workers[17] review these adverse cardiovascular effects of the anabolic steroids and propose several models to explain this toxicity.

Effects on the Liver

The use of oral anabolic steroid preparations has been associated with a risk of liver disorders, especially jaundice and tumors. Increases in the blood levels of liver enzymes, indicative of possible liver dysfunction, are quite common among steroid users. Hepatitis is also common. Erlinger[18] reviews the effects of anabolic steroids on the movement of bile through the liver. In addition, several dozen cases of liver carcinomas of unusual types have been reported.[19] The incidence of developing these potentially fatal carcinomas is estimated to be 1 to 3 percent within 2 to 8 years of exposure to drugs.

Psychological Effects

Anabolic steroids are centrally acting drugs, involved in the regulation of sexuality, aggression, cognition, emotion, and personality.[20] Thus, drug-induced increases in aggression, competitiveness, and combativeness can be predicted in individuals using large doses of these drugs.[21] It is now well established that areas of the brain that influence mood and judgment contain steroid receptors and that sharp fluctuations in the levels of steroid hormones have profound psychological effects. Steroid receptors are widely distributed in the central nervous system, especially in the hypothalamus and the limbic regions. In the hypothalamus, they autoregulate their own reproductive actions through the negative feedback system discussed earlier. Hypothalamic actions also modulate other vegetative systems of the body, a matter of importance during steroid withdrawal. The limbic receptors appear to account for the effects of steroids on mood.

Pope and colleagues[22] conducted a six-week trial of testosterone in 56 males, increasing the weekly dose to 600 milligrams. Their goal was to assess drug effects on mood and aggression. Doses of up to 300 mg/week produced few psychiatric effects; doses of 500 to 600 mg/week produced prominent effects in some individuals. Under these "laboratory" conditions, 84 percent exhibited minimal psychiatric effects, 12 percent became mildly hypomanic, and 4 percent became markedly hypomanic or manic. Two participants withdrew when they became "alarmingly hypomanic and aggressive." From these results it appears that in small and unpredictable numbers of individuals, high doses of anabolic steroids may produce marked signs of mania and/or aggression. This report is perhaps the first to quantify these effects and provide statistics on the possible numbers of users who might be expected to display these symptoms. The authors of the study state that the statistics may understate the incidence in the real world: doses may be even higher and drug takers may have preexisting psychiatric conditions and/or may use other illicit drugs while using steroids. All these conditions would increase the probability of adverse reactions. Why some individuals were markedly and dangerously affected while the majority were not is unknown.

Thus, anabolic steroids administered in regular large doses are indeed mood-altering chemicals. They do, however, have a delayed onset of effect. This delay occurs because their mechanism of synthesizing new proteins takes days or weeks. Because their effects are not immediate, they may not be perceived as being a consequence of drug ingestion. Haupt[11] summarizes:

There are significant adverse psychological effects associated with the use of anabolic steroids although the effects are not easily measured by current psychological inventories. Athletes taking anabolic steroids suffer some degree of personality change that may range from simple mood swings to a psychosis requiring hospitalization for treatment. A Jekyll-and-Hyde personality is common, where even the slightest provocation can cause an exaggerated, violent, and often uncontrolled response. The users of anabolic steroids often suffer disturbed personality relationships that may include separations from family and friends and even divorce. Arrest records are not uncommon. Fortunately these psychological effects are reversible when the steroids are discontinued, but the social scars may be permanent.

Galloway[12] reviews these psychological effects at length, adding that about half of a small population of interviewed weightlifters experienced depression and an even higher percentage experienced paranoid thoughts and some psychotic features, experiences consistent with the recent study conducted by Pope and co-workers.[22]

Health Risk Behaviors

The use of anabolic steroids has been linked to other high-risk behaviors.[2] Used in combination with alcohol and cocaine, additive increases in aggressive behavior may be observed.[23] In addition:

The frequency of anabolic steroid use was significantly associated with the frequency of use of cocaine, the use of other drugs such as amphetamines and heroin, tobacco smoking, and alcohol use. . . . Students with self-perceived below-average academic performances and students reporting injected drug use also reported higher anabolic steroid use.[24]

Porcerelli and Sandler[25] administered psychological tests to 16 steroid-using weightlifters and body builders and 20 similar individuals who did not use steroids. They reported that steroid users had significantly higher scores on dimensions of pathological narcissism and significantly lower scores on clinical ratings of empathy. They were unable to assess whether narcissistic personality traits contributed to the initiation of steroid use or were the result of their use.

Physical Dependence

Physical dependence is characterized by withdrawal symptoms when the drug is removed. Withdrawal from large doses of anabolic steroids can be accompanied by psychological depression, fatigue, restlessness, insomnia, loss of appetite, and decreased libido. Other withdrawal symptoms that have been reported include drug craving, headache, dissatisfaction with body image, and (rarely) suicidal ideation. Despite these observations, no defined psychiatric withdrawal syndrome has been described; withdrawal psychosis or bipolar illness has not been reported, although depression is commonplace.

As with all other psychoactive drugs, treatment of steroid dependence requires drug abstinence, treatment of any signs of withdrawal, and maintenance of abstinence. Behavioral and cognitive approaches are possible treatment tools. Supportive therapy, including reassurance, education, and counseling, remains the mainstay of treatment. Antidepressants may be indicated when dependency is complicated by major depression. A physician trained in endocrinology can best prescribe other therapies for hormonal alterations.

Abuse and Treatment

The use of anabolic steroids for athletic or cosmetic purposes constitutes drug abuse, because the doses used far exceed those needed for medical indications. Such use persists despite recognized, unavoidable side effects and negative consequences for the physical and psychological health of the user. The mechanisms responsible for dependence are largely unknown and may be psychological and/or physiological.

> Testosterone is the most potent hormonal determinant of physical and behavioral masculinization. It has been implicated for decades in the stimulation of sexual behavior, as well as in the activation of dominance and aggressive behaviors in male primates, including humans.[26]

The attraction to the use of supraphysiologic doses of testosterone derivatives is strong, with significant numbers of young persons succumbing to their attractiveness.

One societal response to the use of anabolic steroids has been to ban their use in athletics. Since the beginning of organized competition, athletes have tried to gain every possible advantage over their competitors. Sometimes this competitive edge is gained fairly by training harder or developing new and improved methods. Sometimes, however, athletes seek an advantage by using substances that affect the body in ways that can improve athletic performance.

The National Collegiate Athletic Association (NCAA) and the United States Olympic Committee (USOC) have declared the use of anabolic steroids illegal, not only because of their ability to artificially increase muscle mass and competitiveness, but also because of their serious and sometimes permanent side effects.[27] Olivier[28] argues in favor of the ban, stating that these drugs not only harm the user but create a climate of subtle coercion toward their use by others, as well as placing others (e.g., partners of steroid users) at risk of violence from users while they are on the drug. Olivier concludes:

> I have argued that prohibition of harmful practices is justified by potential harm to others (rather than just to one's self). One must bear in mind the powerful effects of subtle coercion and influence and the consequent limitations placed on choice. So, on the grounds that it is wrong to harm others or to coerce them into potentially harmful situations, this paper takes issue with sports libertarians who claim that banning performance-enhancing substances is an unjustified paternalistic action that violates the principle of autonomy.

Education has to be the mainstay of anabolic steroid abuse prevention, especially since the drugs initially promote a more healthy, masculine appearance as well as increasing muscle mass and strength. Goldberg and co-workers[29] designed and tested a team-based, educational interventional program created to reduce the intent of adolescent athletes to use steroids. Conducted with 702 football players in 31 high schools, seven weekly classroom sessions, seven weekly weight-room sessions, and one evening parent session led to increased understanding of anabolic steroid effects, greater belief in personal vulnerability to the adverse consequences of steroids, improved drug refusal skills, less belief in steroid-promoting media messages, increased belief in the team as an information source, improved perception of athletic abilities and strength-training self-efficacy, improved nutritional and exercise behaviors, and reduced intentions to use steroids.*

The abuse of anabolic steroids by athletes, body builders, and body-conscious individuals poses a special challenge to society in general. Perhaps the desire of adolescents and young adults to take steroids has been fostered largely by our societal fixations on winning and on physical appearance. Thus, successful intervention must go beyond education, counseling, law enforcement, and drug testing: the social environment that subtly encourages steroid abuse may have to be changed.

Androstenedione

Androstenedione is promoted as a testosterone precursor and anabolic steroid and is available as a "dietary supplement," outside FDA regulation (see Chapter 20). It became prominent as a result of its use by Mark McGwire as a performance-enhancing substance.[30] As of the beginning of 2000, the drug is not outlawed in major league baseball,

---

*The title of the program is *The ATLAS Program*. It is available from its publisher, Jones and Bartlett, 40 Tall Pine Drive, Sudbury, MA 01776 (800–832–0034).

but it is banned by the International Olympic Committee, the National Football League, and the National Collegiate Athletic League. Adolescents, however, are drawn to the drug because of its availability (as a "natural" alternative to testosterone or synthetic anabolic steroids) and because of its popularization.

In 1999, King and co-workers[31] studied 30 young men not taking nutritional supplements, anabolic steroids, or engaging in resistance training. Twenty received intermittent schedules of androstenedione and 10 received placebo; all underwent 8 weeks of whole-body resistance training. Androstenedione supplementation did not increase serum testosterone concentrations and did not enhance skeletal muscle adaptations to resistance training. Interestingly, serum estrogens did increase while low-density cholesterol ("good" cholesterol) levels decreased; it was unclear whether or not these alterations might lead to long-term health consequences. The test doses given were 100 mg of androstenedione; it is unclear whether larger, massive doses would produce different results. This study, however, questions the efficacy of androstenedione as an anabolic substance and leaves open the question of possible long-term toxicity.

STUDY QUESTIONS

1. What are androgenic-anabolic steroids?

2. How do these substances affect body functions?

3. How do these agents increase muscle mass?

4. Describe the similarities and differences between dependence on anabolic steroids and on the more traditional drugs of abuse.

5. Describe the two groups of persons who are the most frequent users of these substances. How are they similar? How are they different?

6. Describe the anticatabolic, anabolic, and motivational effects of these drugs.

7. What are the side effects associated with use of these agents?

8. What are the psychological effects associated with use of these agents?

9. How might the misuse of these substances be prevented?

REFERENCES

1. J. H. Porcerelli and B. A. Sandler, "Anabolic-androgenic Steroid Abuse and Psychopathology," *Psychiatric Clinics of North America* 21 (1998): 829–833.

2. J. D. Rich et al., "Needle Exchange Program Participation by Anabolic Steroid Injectors, United States 1998," *Drug and Alcohol Dependence* 56 (1999): 157–160.

3. C. Yesalis, C. Barsukiewicz, A. Kopstein, and M. Bahrke, "Trends in Anabolic-androgenic Steroid Use Among Adolescents," *Archives of Pediatric and Adolescent Medicine* 151 (1997): 1197–1206.

4. A. S. Dobs, "Is There a Role for Androgenic Anabolic Steroids in Medical Practice?" *Journal of the American Medical Association* 281 (1999): 1326–1327.

5. K. L. Johansen, K. Mulligan, and M. Schambelan, "Anabolic Effects of Nandrolone Decanoate in Patients Receiving Dialysis: A Randomized Controlled Trial," *Journal of the American Medical Association* 281 (1999): 1275–1281.

6. A. Strawford et al., "Resistance Exercise and Supraphysiologic Androgen Therapy in Eugonadal Men with HIV-related Weight Loss," *Journal of the American Medical Association* 281 (1999): 1282–1290.

7. J. G. Rabkin, G. J. Wagner, and R. Rabkin, "A Double-blind, Placebo-controlled Trial of Testosterone Therapy for HIV-positive Men with Hypogonadal Symptoms," *Archives of General Psychiatry* 57 (2000): 141–147.

8. S. E. Lucas, "Current Perspectives on Anabolic-androgenic Steroid Abuse," *Trends in Pharmacological Sciences* 14 (1993): 61–68.

9. I. M. Ferreira et al., "The Influence of Six Months of Oral Anabolic Steroids on Body Mass and Respiratory Muscles in Undernourished COPD Patients," *Chest* 114 (1998): 19–28.

10. S. Bhasin et al., "The Effects of Supraphysiologic Doses of Testosterone on Muscle Size and Strength in Normal Men," *New England Journal of Medicine* 335 (1996): 1–7.

11. H. A. Haupt, "Anabolic Steroids and Growth Hormone," *American Journal of Sports Medicine* 21 (1993): 468–474.

12. G. P. Galloway, "Anabolic Steroids," in J. H. Lowinson, P. Ruiz, R. B. Millman, and J. G. Langrod, eds., *Substance Abuse: A Comprehensive Textbook*, 3rd ed. (Baltimore: Williams & Wilkins, 1997), 380–395.

13. A. Tuiten et al., "Time Course of Effects of Testosterone Administration on Sexual Arousal in Women," *Archives of General Pyschiatry* 57 (2000): 149–153.

14. M. J. Schwerin et al., "Social Physique Anxiety, Body Esteem, and Social Anxiety in Bodybuilders and Self-reported Anabolic Steroid Users," *Addictive Behaviors* 21 (1996): 1–8.

15. C. Bickelman, L. Ferries, and R. P. Eaton, "Impotence Related to Anabolic Steroid Use in a Body Builder: Response to Clomiphene Citrate," *Western Medical Journal* 162 (1995): 158–160.

16. R. B. Melchert and A. A. Welder, "Cardiovascular Effects of Androgenic-anabolic Steroids," *Medicine and Science in Sports and Exercise* 27 (1995): 1252–1262.

17. M. L. Sullivan, C. M. Martinez, P. Gennis, and E. J. Gallagher, "The Cardiac Toxicity of Anabolic Steroids," *Progress in Cardiovascular Diseases* 41 (1998): 1–15.

18. S. Erlinger, "Drug-induced Cholestasis," *Journal of Hepatology* 26, Suppl. 1 (1997): 1–4.

19. A. Kosaka et al., "Hepatocellular Carcinoma Associated with Anabolic Steroid Therapy: Report of a Case and Review of the Japanese Literature," *Journal of Gastroenterology* 31 (1996): 450–454.

20. D. R. Rubinow and P. J. Schmidt, "Androgens, Brain, and Behavior," *American Journal of Psychiatry* 153 (1996): 974–984.

21. E. M. Kouri, S. E. Lukas, H. G. Pope, Jr., and P. S. Oliva, "Increased Aggressive Responding in Male Volunteers Following the Administration of Gradually Increasing Doses of Testosterone Cypionate," *Drug and Alcohol Dependence* 40 (1995): 73–79.

22. H. C. Pope, Jr., E. M. Kouri, and J. I. Hudson, "Effects of Supraphysiologic Doses of Testosterone on Mood and Aggression in Normal Men: A Randomized Controlled Trial," *Archives of General Psychiatry* 57 (2000): 133–140.

23. S. E. Lukas, "CNS Effects and Abuse Liability of Anabolic-androgenic Steroids," *Annual Review of Pharmacology and Toxicology* 36 (1996): 333–357.

24. R. H. DuRant, L. G. Escobedo, and G. W. Heath, "Anabolic Steroid Use, Strength Training, and Multiple Drug Use Among Adolescents in the United States," *Pediatrics* 96 (1995): 23–28.

25. J. H. Porcerelli and B. A. Sandler, "Narcissism and Empathy in Steroid Users," *American Journal of Psychiatry* 152 (1995): 1672–1674.

26. B. Schaal, R. E. Tremblay, R. Soussignan, and E. J. Susman, "Male Testosterone Linked to High Social Dominance but Low Physical Aggression in Early Adolescence," *Journal of the American Academy of Child and Adolescent Psychiatry* 34 (1996): 1322–1330.

27. United States Pharmacopeial Convention, Inc., "Athletes Precautions," *USP DI Update* 1 (1996): 83–86.

28. S. Olivier, "Drugs in Sport: Justifying Paternalism on the Grounds of Harm," *American Journal of Sports Medicine* 24 (1996): S43–S45.

29. L. Goldberg et al., "Effects of a Multidimensional Anabolic Steroid Prevention Intervention: The Adolescents Training and Learning to Avoid Steroids (ATLAS) Program," *Journal of the American Medical Association* 276 (1996): 1555–1562.

30. C. E. Yesalis, "Medical, Legal, and Societal Implications of Androstenedione Use," *Journal of the American Medical Association* 281 (1999): 2043–2044.

31. D. S. King et al., "Effect of Oral Androstenedione on Serum Testosterone and Adaptations to Resistance Training in Young Men: A Randomized Controlled Trial," *Journal of the American Medical Association* 281 (1999): 2020–2028.

Drugs That Are Used to Treat Psychological Disorders

The chapters in this part introduce drugs that are used to treat psychological disorders, including depression and dysthymia (Chapter 15), bipolar disorder (Chapter 16), schizophrenia (Chapter 17), and Parkinsonism (Chapter 19). In the 1990s, remarkable advances were made in the pharmacotherapeutics of these disorders, allowing affected individuals to lead much more "normal" lives than they have ever been able to before in human history. These remarkable advances are continuing, with even more hope and promise of relief from frequently disabling disorders. Two goals of these chapters are to impart a sense of the historical development of therapeutics of each disorder and to convey a sense of excitement about the promise of even better drugs that will become available within the next few years.[1,2]

The drugs are neatly compartmentalized in these chapters under descriptive headings (antidepressants, mood stabilizers, antipsychotics, and antiparkinsonian agents), but the headings do not adequately describe or define the drugs. Besides relieving major depression, antidepressants are used as antianxiety drugs (perhaps better termed as anxiolytics), as analgesics, and as antidysthymic agents. Many of the mood stabilizers, besides being used to treat bipolar disorder, are used to treat epilepsy, chronic pain syndromes, and psychological disorders associated with agitation and aggression. Antipsychotic drugs, besides being used to treat schizophrenia, are now being used to treat bipolar disorder, explosive and aggressive disorders, and autism and other pervasive developmental disorders. One new antipsychotic agent has even been used to treat depression, and a yet-to-be-released antipsychotic has been successfully used to treat dysthymia!

Chapter 19 integrates pharmacological therapy of these disorders with psychological and behavioral interventions. In some situations (e.g., depression), behavioral therapies are as effective as drug therapies, and the combination offers additive clinical efficacy. In other situations (e.g., bipolar disorder and schizophrenia), pharmacological therapy is essential; psychological and behavioral therapies add to clinical efficacy and provide insights, behavioral changes, and support. Written in collaboration with a clinical psychologist (Donald Lange, Ph.D.), the chapter provides an important perspective both for medical practitioners and the nonprescribing therapists who need to understand the balance between drug and non-drug therapies.

REFERENCES

1. R. S. Duman, "Neuropharmacology in the Next Millennium: Promise for Breakthrough Discoveries," *Neuropharmacology* 20 (1999): 97–98.
2. J. F. Tallman, "Neuropharmacology at the Next Millennium: New Industry Directions," *Neuropharmacology* 20 (1999): 99–105.

Drugs Used to Treat Depression

Depression is an *affective disorder* characterized by loss of interest or pleasure in almost all of a person's usual activities or pastimes. Accompanying this condition are feelings of intense sadness and despair; diminished energy; decreased sexual drive; mental slowing and loss of concentration; pessimism; feelings of worthlessness or self-reproach; inappropriate guilt; recurrent thoughts of death, suicide, and hopelessness; blunted affect; fatigue; and insomnia. Depression is a common psychiatric disorder. About 5 percent of Americans (11 million people) suffer from a depressive disorder in any given year.[1] If left untreated, perhaps 25 to 30 percent of adult depressives attempt or commit suicide.

Antidepressant pharmacotherapy and psychological therapies are first-line options in the treatment of depressive disorders. Importantly, depression remains untreated in many individuals.[2,3] Segraves and co-workers[29] compared bupropion and sertraline (a SSRI) and concluded that "given the similar efficacy of the two drugs in treating depression, bupropion SR may be a more appropriate choice in patients for whom sexual dysfunction is a concern." Adherence to published guidelines for treatment increases therapeutic efficacy and reduces the probability of relapse or recurrence.[4] Nevertheless, there are significant differences in treatment and diagnosis rates among ethnic groups. Sclar and colleagues[5] compared rates of office visits, depression diagnosis, and antidepressant pharmacoloy among whites, African Americans, and Hispanics. Rates of diagnosis of a depressive disorder and prescription of an antidepressant were comparable among African Americans and Hispanics but less than half the rate for whites. Melfi and co-workers[6] recently reported similar data.

When antidepressant drugs were introduced 40 years ago, depression was the sole indication for their use. Today, several uses of antidepressants are recognized, such as the treatment of anxiety disorders,* dysthymia, violent and aggressive behavioral disorders, and certain chronic pain syndromes. Although many of the *anxiety disorders* have historically been treated with benzodiazepine anxiolytics (Chapter 6), they are today most often treated with antidepressants. The newer antidepressant-anxiolytic drugs are equally or more efficacious, they are less prone to compulsive abuse, and they impair learning, memory, and concentration to a lesser degree than do the benzodiazepines. Stahl[7] analyzes this largely historical progression of treatment of major depression and anxiety disorders (Figure 15.1).

In addition, individuals formerly regarded as having anxiety neurosis have now been reconceptualized as having *dysthymia,* an affective disorder responsive to antidepressant medication. The need for pharmacotherapy for dysthymia was articulated by Shelton and coworkers:

> Dysthymia . . . affects 3% to 6% of the adult population of the United States and as many as 36% of patients who seek treatment at psychiatric outpatient clinics. The symptoms of dysthymia are less severe than those observed in patients with major depression, and hence dysthymia is often considered to be a disorder of subsyndromal intensity. Nevertheless, patients with this disorder experience considerable social dysfunction and disability. Dysthymics . . . are more likely to take nonspecific psychotropic drugs, such as minor tranquilizers (benzodiazepines) and sedatives. . . . More than 75% of dysthymics have coexisting psychiatric disorders, including anxiety disorders and substance abuse. Approximately 40% of dysthymics have coexisting major depression—a combination termed *double depression.* Untreated dysthymia rarely improves spontaneously over time. Dysthymia has historically been underrecognized and undertreated.[8]

At the end of this chapter, the nutritional supplement DHEA is discussed as a treatment for dysthymia and depression. Also discussed is S-adenosyl-methionine (SAM; SAMe), an endogenous compound marketed as a "natural mood enhancer" to promote "emotional well-being."

Depression is a disease that results from biochemical changes in the brain, although these changes are just now being more clearly identified. Duman, Heninger, and Nestler proposed[9] that stress-induced vulnerability

---

*According to current diagnostic criteria, anxiety disorders include panic disorder (PD), obsessive-compulsive disorder (OCD), posttraumatic stress disorder (PTSD), social phobia, and generalized anxiety disorder (GAD), all of which are discussed in this chapter and in Chapter 19.

A. Treatment of Depression and Anxiety in the 1960s

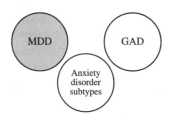

The earliest antidepressants were tricyclic anti-depressants (TCAs) and monoamine oxidase inhibitors (MAOIs) and were conceptualized as targeting an entirely different syndrome (major depressive disorder [MDD]) than did the earliest anxiolytics, namely, benzodiazepines. At that time, benzodiazepines targeted anxiety disorders as a whole including generalized anxiety disorder (GAD) or anxiety neurosis, which was much more broadly defined at that time, as well as anxiety disorder subtypes.

⬭ First-line treatments with antidepressants.
◯ First-line treatments with anxiolytics.

B. Treatment of Depression and Anxiety in the 1970s and 1980s

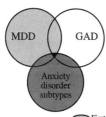

As the TCA/MAOI era matured, mixtures of anxiety and depression were increasingly recognized and treated both with these antidepressants and with buspirone as well as benzodiazepines. Benzodiazepines along with TCAs and MAOIs began to make inroads into treating anxiety disorder subtypes such as panic disorder, and in the case of the TCA clomipramine, obsessive-compulsive disorder (OCD).

⬭ First-line treatments with antidepressants.
◯ First-line treatments with anxiolytics.
⬤ First-line treatments with either antidepressants or anxiolytics.

C. Treatment of Depression and Anxiety in the 1990s

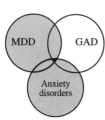

Once the serotonin-specific reuptake inhibitor (SRRI) era came into full swing, these agents eventually took over as first-line treatment choices not only of MDD but also of numerous anxiety disorder subtypes, from panic disorder and OCD to social phobia and posttraumatic stress disorder, but not GAD. Benzodiazepines became progressively second-line treatments of anxiety disorder, although buspirone continued as a first-line treatment of GAD.

⬭ First-line treatments with antidepressants.
◯ First-line treatments with anxiolytics.

D. Treatment of Depression and Anxiety in the Twenty-first Century

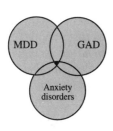

When is an antidepressant an antidepressant, and when is an antidepressant an anxiolytic? Recently, the first antidepressant was approved for the treatment of GAD, namely, venlafaxine XR. Venlafaxine XR, as well as nefazodone and mirtazapine, has preliminary evidence of efficacy for some anxiety disorder subtypes, such as panic disorder, social phobia, and posttraumatic stress disorder. SSRIs, nefazodone, and mirtazapine have preliminary evidence of efficacy in generalized anxiety disorder. Virtually all forms of anxiety can now be treated by an antidepressant, with the documentation of efficacy of some antidepressants better than that of others. Perhaps the distinction between an antidepressant and an anxiolytic will cease to exist in the twenty-first century.

⬭ First-line treatments with antidepressants.

FIGURE 15.1 Progression in the treatment of major depressive disorder (MDD), generalized anxiety disorder (GAD), and anxiety disorder subtypes from 1960 to 2000. [From Stahl.[7]]

to depression and other types of neuronal insult "occurs via intracellular mechanisms that decrease neurotropic factors necessary for the survival and function of particular neurons." Indeed, stress and other insults decrease the expression of "brain-derived neurotropic factors (BDNF) and leads to atrophy of vulnerable neurons in the hippocampus and cerebral cortex." Duman and co-workers[9] also proposed that the "transcription factor cyclic 3′, 5′-monophasphate response element-binding protein (CREB) is one intracellular target of long-term antidepressant drug treatment and that brain-derived neurotropic factor is one target gene of CREB" (Figures 15.2 and 15.3). Russo-Neustadt and co-workers[10] reported that, in rat studies, "combined antidepressant treatment (either a monoamine-oxidase inhibitor or a tricyclic agent) and physical activity have an additive, potentiating effect on BDNF mRNA expression within several areas of rat hippocampus." Brown and co-workers[11] expanded by evaluating the effects of stress and corticosteroids on hippocampal neurons. They conclude that "cumulative hippocampal changes by corticosteroids lead to abnormal neuroendocrine findings, cognitive impairment, and increased vulnerability to future episodes in people with mood disorders." Thus, stress-induced increases in corticosteroids lead to hippocampal neuronal damage and atrophy.[12] Antidepressant and other therapies reverse theatrophy-inducing effects of corticosteroids by "positively" remodeling the damage induced by stress.[13–14]

Evolution of Antidepressant Drug Therapy

Forty years ago, while investigating the potential antipsychotic efficacy of structural modifications of the phenothiazines (Figure 15.4), the antidepressant properties of *imipramine* were accidentally discovered. Imipramine lacked antipsychotic activity, but it possessed an antidepressant action. Today it is known that this occurs because antipsychotic drugs block postsynaptic dopamine receptors (Chapter 17), while antidepressants block the presynaptic transporter protein receptors for any of several neurotransmitters (dopamine, norepinephrine, and/or serotonin). Therefore, small structural changes between the antipsychotic drug and the antidepressant drug (Figure 15.4) alter the affinity of the drug from the postsynaptic receptor to the presynaptic receptor, in essence changing it from a dopamine antagonist to a potentiator of neurotransmission.

Imipramine belongs to a group of structurally related drugs called tricyclic antidepressants (TCAs), now expanded to include several commercially available products (Table 15.1). Note that *first-generation antidepressants* are defined by a commonality in basic *structure*, not by any perceived common mechanism of action. This is in contrast to other antidepressants, which are defined by their mechanism of action.

At about the same time the TCAs were discovered, a second class of first-generation antidepressant drugs called the monoamine oxidase

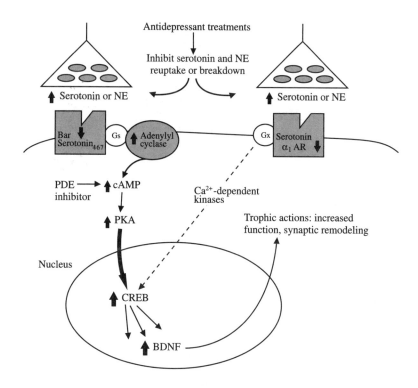

FIGURE 15.2 A model for the molecular mechanism of action of long-term antidepressant treatments. Antidepressants induce short-term increases in 5-HT and NE. Longer-term use decreases the function and expression of their receptors, but the cAMP signal transduction pathway is increased, including increased levels of adenyl cyclase and cAMP-dependent protein kinase (PKA), as well as translocation of PKA to the cell nucleus. Antidepressants increase expression and function of the transcription factor cAMP response element-binding protein (CREB), suggesting that CREB is a common postreceptor target for antidepressants. Brain-derived neurotrophic factor is also increased by antidepressant treatment; up regulation of CREB and BDNF could influence the function of hippocampal neurons or neurons innervating this brain region, increasing neuronal survival, function, and remodeling of synaptic or cellular architecture. [From Duman, Heninger, and Nestler.[9]]

inhibitors (MAOIs) were identified; three remain commercially available for the treatment of depression. Both the TCIs and the MAOIs are effective in the treatment of major depression, but both possess considerable disadvantages because of adverse effect profiles. TCAs carry a high incidence of anticholinergic effects and cardiotoxicity, extremely important in (suicidal) overdoses; MAOIs may cause hypertensive crises if sympathomimetic agents, e.g., certain other drugs or tyramine in foodstuffs, are additionally taken.

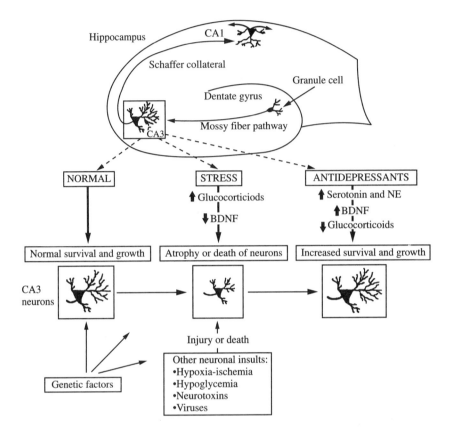

FIGURE 15.3 A molecular and cellular model for the action of antidepressants and the pathophysiology of stress-related disorders. Chronic stress decreases the expression of BDNF in the hippocampus, contributing to atrophy or death of neurons in the hippocampus. Elevated levels of glucocorticoids also decrease survival of these neurons, as do multiple other insults. Antidepressants increase the expression of BDNF and prevent the down regulation of BDNF elicited by stress, increasing neuronal survival or helping repair or protect neurons from further damage. See Figure 15.2. [From Duman, Heninger, and Nestler.[9]]

These problems precipitated the search for new antidepressants that were equally effective, better tolerated, and less toxic. First came development of several drugs that were slight modifications of the basic tricyclic structure but that still exhibited antidepressant efficacy. These drugs were termed *second-generation* or *atypical antidepressants*. Several are available clinically (Table 15.1).

During the late 1980s and continuing through the 1990s, the *serotonin-specific reuptake inhibitors* (SSRIs) were developed and

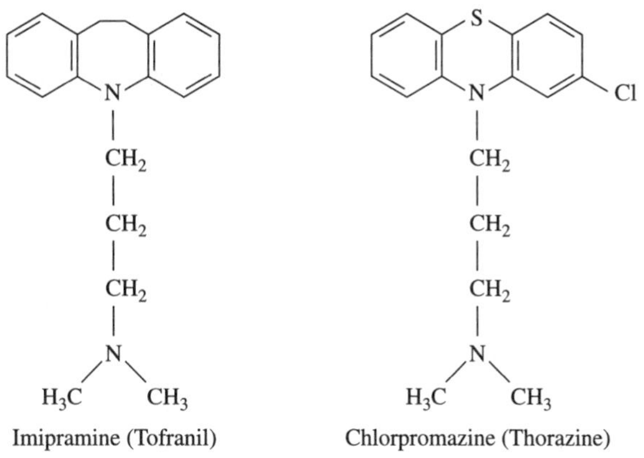

FIGURE 15.4 Chemical structures of imipramine (a tricyclic antidepressant) and chlorpromazine (an antipsychotic). Slight structural differences produce remarkably different receptor affinities: imipramine blocks the presynaptic catecholamine transporter, and chlorpromazine blocks postsynaptic dopamine$_2$ receptors.

introduced clinically; the first of these was fluoxetine (Prozac). Four additional agents are also clinically available (Table 15.1). Now, recognizing the limitations and side effects of the SSRIs, antidepressant drug research is progressing to identify compounds that combine SSRI activity with postsynaptic serotonin-type 2 receptor (5-HT$_2$) antagonism—e.g., nefazodone (Serzone) and mirtazapine (Remeron). These are not necessarily more clinically efficacious than the older TCAs, but they may have a more favorable profile of toxicity or side effects.

Availability of the newer drugs has not yet reduced the number of treatment-resistant individuals with major depression: the new drugs have only altered the profile of side effects, including a reduction in overdose cardiotoxicity. Three main therapeutic needs have still to be met: (1) superior efficacy to tricyclic antidepressants; (2) a faster onset of action; and (3) reliable effectiveness in the treatment of therapy-resistant depression.

Antidepressant drug research now underway is continuing to focus on the development of additional serotonin-acting, dual-action antidepressants; one investigational drug is sunepitron. Other serotonin-oriented research is evaluating the serotonin agonist flesinoxan, among other agents. Other research is focusing on specific norepinephrine reuptake inhibitors (SNRIs); an example is reboxetine (Vestra, Edronax). Finally, an altogether new class of drugs that block the neurokinin-1 receptors is in the early stages of development.

TABLE 15.1 Drugs used in affective disorders: Antidepressants

Drug name Generic (trade)	Sedative activity	Anticholinergic activity[a]	Elimination half-life (hr)	Reuptake inhibition		
				Norepinephrine	Serotonin	Dopamine
TRICYCLIC COMPOUNDS						
Imipramine (Tofranil)	Moderate	Moderate	10–20	++	++	0
Desipramine (Norpramin)	Low	Low	12–75	+++	+	0
Trimipramine (Surmontil)	High	Moderate	8–20	+	+	0
Protriptyline (Vivactil)	Low	Moderate	55–125	+++	+	0
Nortriptyline (Pamelor, Aventil)	Moderate	Low	15–35	++	++	0
Amitriptyline (Elavil)	High	High	20–35	++	++	0
Doxepin (Adapin, Sinequan)	High	High	8–24	++	++	0
Clomipramine (Anaframil)	Low	Low	19–37	++	+++	0
SECOND-GENERATION (ATYPICAL) COMPOUNDS						
Amoxapine (Asendin)[b]	Low	Moderate	8–10	++	+	0
Maprotiline (Ludiomil)	Moderate	Moderate	27–58	+++	0	0
Trazodone (Desyrel)	Moderate	Low	6–13	0	++	0
Bupropion (Wellbutrin)	Low	Low	8–14	0/+	0/+	++
Venlafaxine (Effexor)	None	None	3–11	++	+++	0

[a]Anticholinergic side effects include dry mouth, blurred vision, tachycardia, urinary retention, and constipation.
[b]Also has antipsychotic effects due to blockage of dopamine receptors (Chapter 7).
0 = no effect; + = mild effect; ++ = moderate effect; +++ = strong effect; ++++ = maximal effect.

TABLE 15.1 Drugs used in affective disorders: Antidepressants *(continued)*

Drug name Generic (trade)	Sedative activity	Anticholinergic activity[a]	Elimination half-life (hr)	Reuptake inhibition Norepinephrine	Reuptake inhibition Serotonin	Reuptake inhibition Dopamine
SEROTONIN-SPECIFIC REUPTAKE INHIBITORS						
Fluoxetine (Prozac)	None	None	24–96	0	++++	0
Sertraline (Zoloft)	None	None	26	0	++++	0
Paroxetine (Paxil)	None	None	24	+	++++	0
Citalopram (Celexa)	None	None	33	0	++++	0
Fluvoramine (Luvox)	None	None	15	0	++++	0
DUAL-ACTION ANTIDEPRESSANTS						
Nefazodone (Serzone)	Low	None	3–4	0	++++	0
Mirtazapine (Remeron)	High	Low	20–40	++	++++	0
MAO INHIBITORS: IRREVERSIBLE						
Phenelzine (Nardil)	Low	None	2–4[c]	0	0	0
Isocarboxazid (Marplan)	None	None	1–3[c]	0	0	0
Tranylcypromine (Parnate)	None	None	1–3[c]	0	0	0
MAO INHIBITOR: REVERSIBLE						
Moclobemide (Aurorix)[d]	None	Low	1–3[c]	0	0	0
NOREPINEPHRINE-SPECIFIC REUPTAKE INHIBITOR						
Reboxetine (Edronax)	None	Low	13	++++	0	0

[c]Half-life does not correlate with clinical effect (see text).
[d]Not available for use in the United States.
0 = no effect; + = mild effect; ++ = moderate effect; +++ = strong effect; ++++ = maximal effect.

Mechanism of Antidepressant Drug Action

The role of brain catecholamines (norepinephrine and dopamine) and serotonin in the mechanism of action of antidepressant drugs has been the subject of intensive research during the past three decades.[15] The *biological amine theory* of mania and depression was first postulated in the mid-1960s to explain the correlation between acute drug-induced increases in norepinephrine and serotonin and relief from depression. Thus, deficiency in these transmitters was thought to underlie major depressive episodes. Although reasonable correlations have been found between drug-induced increases in the levels of norepinephrine and serotonin and positive, mood-elevating effects in people who are depressed, several limitations and inconsistencies in this pattern have also been seen.

One major difficulty is that the time course of action is vastly different for the biochemical effect and the clinical response. Although neurotransmission of norepinephrine and serotonin is augmented soon after the drug is taken, the clinical antidepressant effect may not appear for three to six weeks. Thus, increasing the amounts of neurotransmitter may only be an initial step in relieving depression. The earlier discussion of drug-induced changes in BDNF would explain this discrepancy. Certainly, adaptive changes do take place. The emphasis of research has shifted from acute reuptake effects to the slower adaptive changes in NE and 5-HT receptor systems induced by chronic antidepressant therapy. Long-term antidepressant treatment produces complex changes in the sensitivity of both presynaptic and postsynaptic receptor sites.

Available antidepressant drugs may increase the sensitivity of postsynaptic catecholamine and serotonin receptors and may decrease the sensitivity of presynaptic receptor sites. The net effect is the correction (reregulation) of an abnormal receptor-neurotransmitter relationship. Clinically, this reregulatory action speeds up the patient's natural recovery process from the depressive episode by normalizing neurotransmitter efficacy. This certainly would be in agreement with the neurotropic enhancements postulated by Duman, Heninger, and Nestler:[9] "It is difficult to state with certainty that reuptake inhibition is the essential feature needed for antidepressant efficacy."

Regardless, and largely on a historical basis, attention continues to focus on acute effects on specific receptors, actions that allow classification of the antidepressive drugs and explain many of their side effects and toxicities. Table 15.2 compares how effectively various antidepressant drugs block the reuptake of norepinephrine, serotonin, and dopamine (in an experimental model) and calculates the selectivity for serotonin over norepinephrine. Most of the newer drugs have serotonin selectivity; bupropion does not, as it selectively blocks dopamine reuptake, and reboxetine selectively blocks norepinephrine reuptake. The TCAs block multiple receptors, accounting for both efficacy and toxicity.

Tricyclic Antidepressants

As stated, the term tricyclic antidepressant describes a class of drugs that all have a characteristic three-ring molecular core (Figure 15.5). TCAs effectively relieve depression in persons who experience major depressive illness. They also possess anxiolytic and analgesic actions.

TCAs exert four pharmacologic actions in varying degrees:

1. They block the presynaptic norepinephrine reuptake transporter.
2. They block the presynaptic serotonin reuptake transporter.
3. They block postsynaptic histamine receptors.
4. They block postsynaptic acetylcholine receptors.

These actions account for both the therapeutic actions and the side effects of these drugs. Historically, the TCAs are drugs of first choice for the treatment of major depression even though the SSRIs, which have become extremely popular, are no more effective and are considerably more expensive; they may, however, be less toxic. Indeed, the use of the

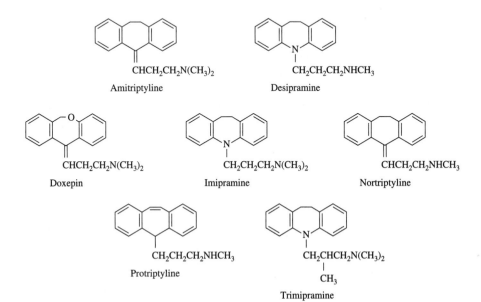

FIGURE 15.5 Chemical structures of seven tricyclic antidepressants.

TCAs is currently often overshadowed by the use of SSRIs and other, newer antidepressants. TCAs, however, remain the standard against which other antidepressants are compared;[16] no other group of antidepressants has yet been demonstrated to be either more clinically effective or capable of exerting a more rapid onset of antidepressant effect than the TCAs, although alternative agents may be better tolerated than the TCAs.[17]

As discussed earlier, antidepressants are now recognized for their anxiolytic action as well as their antidepressant action. TCAs, such as imipramine, are anxiolytic, for example, in the treatment of panic disorder with agoraphobia.[18] Since most of these older drugs are available in less expensive generic form, manufacturers are less willing to fund research or seek FDA approval for this new use. Therefore, despite efficacy, TCAs are not likely to be promoted for use as anxiolytics.*

Imipramine (Tofranil) is the prototype TCA, but another clinically available TCA, *desipramine* (Norpramin), is the pharmacologically active intermediate metabolite of imipramine. Likewise, *amitriptyline* (Elavil) has an active intermediate metabolite, *nortriptyline* (Pamelor, Aventil). In fact, these active intermediates may actually be responsible for much of the antidepressant effect of both imipramine and amitriptyline.

All the TCAs attach to and inhibit (to varying degrees) the presynaptic transporter proteins for both norepinephrine and serotonin (Table 15.2). The traditional TCAs, however, have three clinical limitations. First, they are claimed to have a slow onset of action, although overall, TCAs seem to start acting as fast as other available compounds, provided that comparable dosage strategies can be tolerated. Second, the TCAs exert a wide variety of effects on the CNS, causing a variety of bothersome side effects not shared with use of the SSRIs. Third, in overdosage (as in suicide attempts), TCAs are cardiotoxic and potentially fatal. Nelson and co-workers[19] studied 81 patients with depression and ischemic heart disease. The authors administered either a TCA (nortriptyline) or an SSRI (paroxetine); the two drugs were equally effective

---

*FDA approval does not necessarily mean that a drug is any more effective than any other drug for the treatment of a given medical symptom or disorder. It means that the manufacturer submitted sufficient research data, applied for approval to advertise the indication, and demonstrated sufficient efficacy and safety to justify the formal approval by the FDA. If a similar drug is not approved for a use that another drug is approved for, it does not necessarily mean that the nonapproved drug is ineffective; the manufacturer just had not conducted the research and applied for approval. If any drug is over about 17 years old, it goes "generic" and any other manufacturer can sell that drug. Therefore, one manufacturer probably will not spend the money to conduct the research and go through the approval process when anyone can then sell the drug for that use. Therefore, a new use for an old drug will be "off label," meaning that there is no FDA approval for that specific use. Off-label use is not illegal, but it must be defensible by the prescribing physician.

TABLE 15.2 Potency and selectivity of various antidepressants

Drug	Potency[a]			Selectivity[b]
	Norepinephrine	Serotonin	Dopamine	
Amitriptyline	4.2	1.5	0.043	0.36[c]
Amoxapine	23	0.21	0.053	0.0091
Bupropion	0.043	0.0064	0.16	0.15
Clomipramine	3.6	18	0.057	5.3[d]
Desipramine	110	0.29	0.019	0.0026
Doxepin	5.3	0.36	0.018	0.067
Fluoxetine	0.36	8.3	0.063	23
Imipramine	7.7	2.4	0.020	0.31
Maprotiline	14	0.030	0.034	0.0021
Nortriptyline	25	0.38	0.059	0.015
Paroxetine	3.0	136	0.059	45
Protriptyline	100	0.36	0.054	0.0036
Sertraline	0.46	29	0.38	64
Trazodone	0.020	0.53	0.0070	26
Trimipramine	0.20	0.040	0.029	0.20
REFERENCE COMPOUND				
d-Amphetamine[e]	2.00	—	1.2	

From E. Richelson "Treatment of Acute Depression," *Psychiatric Clinics of North America* 16 (1993): 468.
Note: The higher the number, the more potent the reuptake blockade.
[a]10^{27} 3 $1/K_i$, where K_i = inhibitor constant in molarity.
[b]Ratio of potency of serotonin uptake blockade to potency of norephinephrine uptake blockade.
[c]Indicates that amitriptyline as about 2.8 (1/0.36) times more potent at blocking uptake of norepinephrine than uptake of serotonin.
[d]Indicates that clomipramine is about 5 times more potent at blocking uptake of serotonin than uptake of norepinephrine.
[e]This is not an antidepressant but is shown here for comparison.

(averaging a 50% improvement in the Hamilton Depression Rating Scale), but paroxetine was "better tolerated than nortriptyline and less likely to produce cardiovascular side effects."

Because TCAs do not produce euphoria in normal individuals, they have no recreational or behavior-reinforcing value. Therefore, abuse and psychological dependence are not concerns. Similarly, in contrast to withdrawal from SSRIs, withdrawal from TCAs is not usually a cause for undue concern. The clinical choice of TCA is determined by effectiveness, tolerance of side effects, and duration of action of the particular TCA.

In depressed patients, TCAs elevate mood, increase physical activity, improve appetite and sleep patterns, and reduce morbid preoccupation.

They are useful in treating acute episodes of major depression as well as in preventing relapses. In addition, they are clinically effective in the long-term therapy of dysthymia, although SSRIs may be equally effective and better tolerated.[7,8] In children and adolescents, TCAs have been used in the treatment of behavioral disorders accompanied by depression, as well as in a variety of anxiety states. In general, TCAs are not indicated for the treatment of depression in children and adolescents because they lack demonstrable efficacy and are potentially quite toxic in this population.

Wilens and co-workers[20] evaluated protriptyline in a small study of attention-deficit/hyperactivity disorder (ADHD) children and reported the drug effective in only 45 percent of patients; half the children discontinued the drug because of adverse effects. In a related study, Wilens and co-workers[21] reviewed the effectiveness of TCAs in the treatment of adult ADHD. In a group of 37 patients receiving either desipramine or nortriptyline, the TCA relieved ADHD symptoms in 25. Positive responders received "robust doses" of the TCA, and most patients also received adjunctive agents, especially behavioral stimulants such as methylphenidate. This survey concluded that additional evaluations of TCAs in adult ADHD are warranted.

Pharmacokinetics

The TCAs are well absorbed when they are administered orally. Because most of them have relatively long half-lives (Table 15.1), they should be taken only once a day at bedtime to minimize unwanted side effects, especially persistent sedation. The TCAs are metabolized in the liver, and, as discussed earlier, two TCAs are converted into pharmacologically active intermediates that are detoxified later (Figure 15.6). This combination of a pharmacologically active drug and active metabolite results in a clinical effect lasting up to 4 days, even longer in elderly patients.

TCAs readily cross the placental barrier. However, in utero exposure does not affect global IQ, language development, or behavioral development in preschool children.[22] No fetal abnormalities from these drugs have yet been reported. Wisner and co-workers[23] recently reviewed the pharmacologic treatment of depression during pregnancy.

Pharmacological Effects

Central Nervous System. The therapeutic effects of the TCAs result from drug-induced blockade of presynaptic serotonin, dopamine, and norepinephrine receptors (Table 15.3); the down regulation of these receptors accounts for therapeutic effectiveness. Blockade of acetylcholine receptors results in dry mouth, confusion, memory impairments, and blurred vision. Blockade of histamine receptors results in

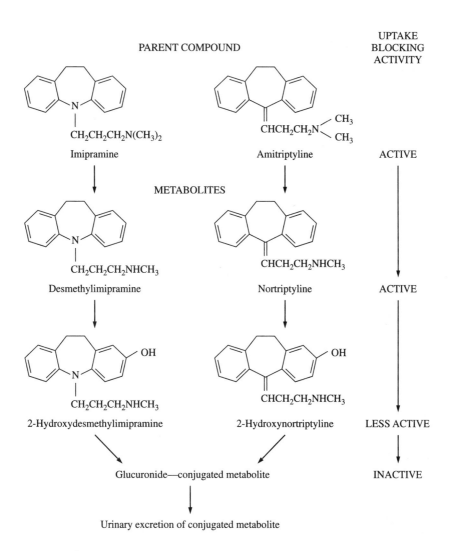

FIGURE 15.6 Metabolism of imipramine and amitriptyline. Note that the two active intermediates are marketed commercially.

drowsiness and sedation, an effect similar to the sedation seen after administration of the classic antihistamine diphenhydramine (Benadryl). In general, nortriptyline and desipramine are preferred TCAs in a patient without a history of favorable response to a specific antidepressant (in other words, they are good drugs of first choice for initial treatment of depression). These two TCAs cause less sedation and cognitive impairment and exert fewer anticholinergic side effects than most other TCAs.

TABLE 15.3 Affinity of antidepressants for neurotransmitter receptors of human brain

Drug	Histamine (H₁)ᵃ	Acetylcholine (Muscarinic)	Norepinephrine (α₁-Adrenoceptor)	Dopamine (D₂)
Amitriptyline	91	5.6	3.7	0.10
Amoxapine	4.0	0.10	2.00	0.62
Bupropion	0.015	0.0021	0.022	0.00048
Clomipramine	3.2	2.7	2.63	0.53
Desipramine	0.91	0.50	0.77	0.030
Doxepin	420	1.2	4.2	0.042
Fluoxetine	0.016	0.050	0.0169	0.015
Imipramine	9.1	1.1	1.1	0.050
Maprotiline	50	0.018	1.1	0.29
Nortriptyline	10	0.7	1.7	0.083
Paroxetine	0.0045	0.93	0.029	0.0031
Protriptyline	4.0	4.0	0.77	0.043
Sertraline	0.0041	0.16	0.27	0.0093
Trazodone	0.29	0.00031	2.8	0.026
Trimipramine	370	1.7	4.2	0.56
REFERENCE COMPOUNDSᵇ				
Diphenhydramine	7.1	—	—	—
Atropine	—	42	—	—
Phentolamine	—	—	6.7	—
Haloperidol	—	—	—	26

From E. Richelson, "Treatment of Acute Depression," *Psychiatric Clinics of North America* 16 (1993): 469.
Note: Higher numbers mean greater blockade of that given receptor (e.g., doxepine exerts the most histamine receptor blockade).
ᵃ10^{27} 3 $1/K_d$, where K_d = equilibrium dissociation constant in molarity.
ᵇThese are not antidepressants but are shown here for comparison.

In the patient on long-term therapy with TCAs, tolerance develops to most of these side effects, but choosing a particular drug with an awareness of its side effects can turn a disadvantage into a therapeutic advantage. For example, amitriptyline and doxepin are the most sedating of the TCAs, making them useful in treating individuals with agitation as well as depression or where improved sleep is desirable. Administering one of these drugs at bedtime would provide both the antidepressant effect as well as the needed sedation. Table 15.4 lists the clinical consequences that can follow blockade of each type of receptor.

TABLE 15.4 Pharmacological properties of antidepressants and possible clinical consequences

Property	Possible clinical consequences
Blockade of presynaptic norepinephrine reuptake at nerve endings	Tremors, Tachycardia Erectile and ejaculatory dysfunction Augmentation of pressor effects of sympathomimetic amines
Blockade of presynaptic serotonin reuptake at nerve endings	Gastrointestinal disturbances Increase in anxiety Sexual dysfunction Extrapyramidal side effects Multiple drug interactions
Blockade of presynaptic dopamine reuptake at nerve endings	Psychomotor activation Antiparkinson effect Aggravation of psychosis
Blockade of postsynaptic histamine receptors (antihistaminic)	Potentiation of central depressant drugs Sedation, drowsiness Weight gain, Hypotension
Blockade of postsynaptic acetylcholine receptors (anticholinergic)	Blurred vision, Dry mouth Sinus tachycardia Constipation, Urinary retention
Blockade of postsynaptic dopamine D_2 receptors	Extrapyramidal movement disorders Endocrine changes Sexual dysfunction (males)

Of additional importance are the effects of TCAs on memory and cognitive function. Here, one must distinguish between the direct adverse effects on cognition, which are related to their intrinsic properties, and more positive, indirect effects, which result from the improvement in mood. TCAs with either sedative (antihistamine) effects or anticholinergic effects can directly impair attention, motor speed, dexterity, and memory. Relatively nonsedating compounds with low degrees of anticholinergic side effects cause very little direct impairment of psychomotor or memory functions. The young and the elderly may be more susceptible to the anticholinergic-induced impairment of memory. Individuals at the extremes of age, if treated with TCAs, should probably receive a drug with low degrees of antihistaminic and anticholinergic effects.

TCAs, as well as other antidepressant drugs, are effective analgesics in a variety of clinical pain syndromes, TCAs consistently superior to a placebo in the treatment of chronic pain.[24] Analgesia follows from a direct spinal cord mechanism, explained in Chapter 9. The antidepressant action no doubt adds a feeling of well-being to the analgesic action, improving the affect as well as reducing physical discomfort.

Peripheral Nervous System. The TCAs exert a variety of effects on the peripheral nervous system. The effects of TCAs on the heart deserve special mention, since TCAs cause both cardiac depression and increased electrical irritability (as shown by cardiac arrhythmias). Cardiac depression can be life threatening when an overdose is taken, as in suicide attempts. In such a situation, the patient commonly exhibits excitement, delirium, and convulsions, followed by respiratory depression and coma, which can persist for several days. Cardiac arrhythmias can lead to ventricular fibrillation, cardiac arrest, and death. Arrhythmias are extremely difficult to treat. Thus, all TCAs can be lethal in doses that are commonly available to depressed patients. For this reason, it is unwise to dispense more than a week's supply of an antidepressant to an acutely depressed patient.

There have been reports of about 12 cases of sudden death in children receiving desipramine for the treatment of ADHD or depression.[25] These deaths are certainly cause for concern in using TCAs to treat depression in children, and the therapeutic efficacy of TCAs in treating major depression in children is questionable anyway. In cases where efficacy is more demonstrable—e.g., enuresis (bed-wetting), obsessive-compulsive disorder (OCD), and ADHD—use is appropriate, but caution is warranted.

Second-Generation (Atypical) Antidepressants

Efforts from the late 1970s to the mid-1980s to find structurally different agents that might overcome some of the disadvantages of the TCAs (slow onset of action, limited efficacy, and significant side effects) produced the so-called second-generation (or atypical) antidepressants (Figure 15.7). Their pharmacokinetic data and a comparison with standard TCAs are listed in Tables 15.1 and 15.5.

Maprotiline (Ludiomil) was one of the first clinically available antidepressants (other than the MAOIs) that modified the basic tricyclic structure (Figure 15.7). It has a long half-life, blocks norepinephrine reuptake, and is as efficacious as imipramine (the "gold standard" of

TCAs). However, it offers few, if any, therapeutic advantages. A major limitation of maprotiline is that it tends (albeit rarely) to cause seizures, presumably because of the accumulation of active metabolites that excite the CNS. Maprotiline does not appear to cause deterioration in cognitive functions. It is generally not an antidepressant of first choice, but it may be useful in individuals in whom other antidepressants have not proven effective.

Amoxapine (Asendin) was another atypical antidepressant, structurally different from the TCAs (Figure 15.7). Amoxapine is primarily a norepinephrine reuptake inhibitor, clinically as effective an antidepressant as imipramine, although it may be slightly more effective in relieving accompanying anxiety and agitation. The use of amoxapine can be associated with parkinsonian-like neuroleptic side effects (it blocks postsynaptic dopamine receptors). The drug is metabolized to an active intermediate, 8-hydroxy-amoxapine, which may be responsible for the dopamine-receptor blockade and neuroleptic effects. Like TCAs, overdosage can result in fatalities.

Trazodone (Desyrel) is yet another chemically unique antidepressant (Figure 15.7), therapeutically as efficacious as the TCAs. Its mechanism of antidepressant action is unclear, because it is not a potent reuptake blocker of either norepinephrine or serotonin. However, it (or its active metabolite) does block a subclass of serotonin receptors (the

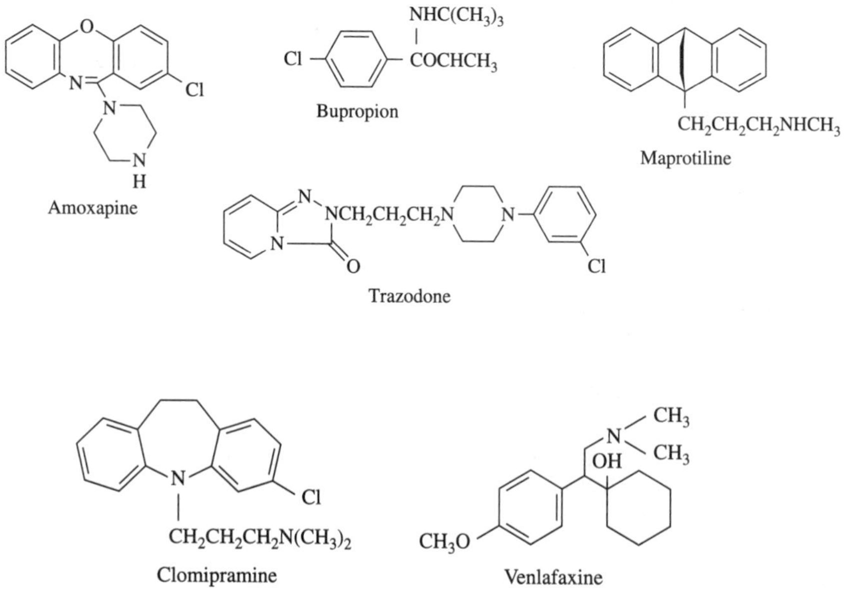

FIGURE 15.7 Chemical structures of six second-generation "atypical" antidepressants.

TABLE 15.5 Advantages and disadvantages of second-generation antidepressants compared to tricyclic antidepressants

Drug	Advantages	Disadvantages
Maprotiline	Sedating and may be useful for agitation Does not antagonize antihypertensive effects of clonidine Minimal cognitive impairment	Increased incidence of seizures Increased lethality in overdose Has long half-life, therefore accumulates Increased incidence of rashes
Amoxapine	Low in sedative effects Low in anticholinergic effects Possibly effective for monotherapy for psychotic depression Has possible rapid onset Relieves anxiety and agitation Toxic in overdose	Can promote parkinsonian side effects and tardive dyskinesia Cannot separate antidepressant from "antipsychotic" effect Increased lethality in overdose
Trazodone	Relatively safe in overdose Sedating (may be useful in controlling agitation and hostility in geriatric patients) Useful as a hypnotic in conjunction with MAO inhibitors	Efficacy not clearly established May induce or exacerbate ventricular arrhythmia Can promote priapism Drowsiness is common
Bupropion	Low in sedative, hypotensive, and anticholinergic side effects Does not promote weight gain Lack of ECG changes May assist with weight loss May be "anticraving"	Tends to "overstimulate," with insomnia, terror Not effective for panic; unknown effectiveness for obsessive-compulsive disorders Increased incidence of seizures in bulimia May induce perceptual abnormalities and psychosis Causes increase in prolactin
Venlafaxine	Low in anticholinergic and antihistaminic effects Improves psychomotor and cognitive function Few drug interactions	Can increase blood pressure May cause anxiety, nervousness, and insomnia
Clomipramine	Indicated in OCD Long half-life	Toxicity limits therapy Increased risk of seizures May increase risk of psychotic episodes May activate mania/hypomania Can promote weight gain Can decrease libido

serotonin$_2$, or 5-HT$_2$, receptor), and it appears to down regulate serotonin receptors. Trazodone has a short onset of action (about a week), but two to five weeks are required to produce an optimal effect. Drowsiness, its most common side effect, occurs in about 20 percent of all patients. In rare instances, priapism (prolonged and painful penile erections) limits its use in males. The detrimental effects of trazodone on cognitive functioning appear modest. Trazadone has less anticholinergic activity than the TCAs and causes fewer problems than TCAs when taken in overdose.

Bupropion (Welbutrin, Zyban; Figure 15.7) is an effective antidepressant that is used both for its antidepressant action and for an anti-craving action in the treatment of nicotine and other drug dependencies. Bupropion differs mechanistically from the other antidepressants in that it selectively inhibits dopamine reuptake, a cocaine-like action, but unlike cocaine, it does not seem to exert a reinforcing or dependency-inducing action.[26] Because of its potentiation of dopamine, it has been used to treat children with ADHD[27] (Chapter 7). Side effects include anxiety, restlessness, tremor, and insomnia. More serious side effects include the induction of psychosis de novo and generalized seizures. Bupropion is not effective in the treatment of panic disorder, and it may even exacerbate or precipitate panic in susceptible individuals.

Bupropion has a special place as a substitute for SSRIs in the treatment of patients who suffer sexual dysfunction as a side effect of SSRIs. While perhaps 40 to 70 percent of patients treated with SSRIs report sexual dysfunction as a side effect,[28] few bupropion-treated patients report sexual dysfunction as a result of drug therapy, and most report significant increases in libido, level of arousal, and intensity of orgasm. Segraves and co-workers[29] compared bupropion and sertraline (a SSRI) and concluded that "given the similar efficacy of the two drugs in treating depression, bupropion SR may be a more appropriate choice in patients for whom sexual dysfunction is a concern." Because of its relative lack of effect in treating anxiety disorders, bupropion is generally not a first-line drug in treating depression. It is often used in patients resistant to other antidepressants, in patients who suffer the sexual side effects of SSRIs, and perhaps in patients with comorbid depression and a substance dependency disorder. Short-term treatment with long-acting bupropion (Wellbutrin SR) can result in weight loss, an advantage in individuals in whom weight gain is a problem.

Clomipramine (Anafranil) is structurally a TCA (Figure 15.7); but unlike TCAs, it exerts inhibitory effects on serotonin reuptake. In addition, it and its active metabolite, *desmethylclomipramine*, also inhibit norepinephrine reuptake. Thus, it is classified as a mixed serotonin-norepineprine reuptake inhibitor, similar to venlafaxine (discussed next). Clomipramine has been used for many years to treat OCD; about 40 to 75 percent of patients with OCD respond favorably. The drug has also been used in the treatment of depression, panic disorder, and phobic disorders. Clomipramine is approximately equal to the TCAs in both its efficacy and its profile of side effects.

Clinically, clomipramine is one of the older antidepressants. It has strong antidepressant and anti-panic efficacy, equaling or surpassing that of many other antidepressants.[30] Its efficacy, however, is limited by a high dropout rate due to adverse side effects. Papp and co-workers[31] concluded that "clomipramine should not be used as a first-line antipanic medication."

Venlafaxine (Effexor, Figure 15.7) is also classified as a mixed *serotonin-norepinephrine reuptake inhibitor*. To a far lesser degree, it also inhibits the reuptake of dopamine. Venlafaxine differs from the TCAs in that it lacks anticholinergic or antihistaminic effects, a distinct advantage. The primary metabolite of venlafaxine is pharmacologically active; the half-lives of the parent compound and the primary metabolite are 5 hours and 11 hours, respectively. Its clinical effectiveness compares favorably with that of SSRIs, even in depressed patients with psychotic features (delusional depression). Venlafaxine produces improvements in psychomotor and cognitive function, probably because of the relief of depression and the absence of detrimental sedative and anticholinergic effects. In high doses, venlafaxine can cause unwanted increases in blood pressure.

Khan and co-workers[33] studied venlafaxine in 384 patients with major depression with and without anxiety. Beneficial effects on both anxiety and depression were observed within 1 to 2 weeks, continuing through the 12 weeks of study. Side effects were modest and tolerable. Venlafaxine also appears to have only minimal effects on drug-metabolizing enzymes and drug interactions are few. Einarson and co-workers[34] conducted a meta-analysis review of venlafaxine, SSRIs, and TCAs in the treatment of depression, concluding that "venlafaxine may be clinically superior to other classes of antidepressants in treating adults with major depression." An extended-release form of venlafaxine (Effexor XR) was approved in 1999 for the treatment of generalized anxiety disorder.

Serotonin-Specific Reuptake Inhibitors (SSRIs)

Selective serotonin reuptake inhibitors have been used to treat depression for more than 15 years.[35] Five SSRIs are currently available: fluoxetine (Prozac), paroxetine (Paxil), sertraline (Zoloft), fluvoxamine (Luvox), and citalopram (Celexa). These drugs all block the function of the presynaptic transporter for serotonin reuptake; they do not appear to block reuptake of other neurotransmitters to any significant degree, nor do they block postsynaptic serotonin receptors of any subtype. Therefore, more serotonin is available to stimulate any or all of the many postsynaptic receptors for serotonin. Such "purity" of effect has led to both the popularity and the side effects of SSRIs.

> The only known common final effect of antidepressant treatments is an enhancement of 5-HT neurotransmission in the CNS upon their long-term administration. . . . Stimulation of 5-HT$_1$ type receptors is probably associated with antidepressant and anxiolytic effects, while stimulation of 5-HT$_2$ and 5-HT$_3$ type receptors is related to adverse effects. Stimulation of 5-HT$_2$ receptors is associated with insomnia, anxiety, agitation, and sexual dysfunction, whereas stimulation of 5-HT$_3$ receptors is associated with nausea.[36]

As a general statement, there appear to be few differences in efficacy in individual SSRIs; all appear to be equivalent in effectiveness.[16] However, they are not necessarily interchangeable, because patients who discontinue one SSRI for lack of tolerability or response can generally be treated effectively with another.[37] Differences may lie in individual pharmacokinetics and in effects on drug-metabolizing enzymes.[35,38] Therapeutic indications for SSRI therapy include major depression, anxiety disorders (e.g., panic disorder, OCD, PTSD, anorexia, bulemia, and generalized anxiety disorder), childhood anxiety disorders, ADHD, morbid obesity, alcohol abuse and others.

Serotonin Syndrome

At high doses or when combined with other drugs, a potentially life-threatening serotonin syndrome can occur. Increased central accumulation of serotonin leads to an exaggerated response, characterized by alterations in cognition (disorientation, confusion, hypomania), behavior (agitation, restlessness), autonomic nervous system functions (fever, shivering, chills, sweating, diarrhea, hypertension, tachycardia), and neuromuscular activity (ataxia, increased reflexes, myoclonus).[39] In theory, any drug that has a net effect of increasing serotonin function can produce a this syndrome; usually, however, it results from the combination of an SSRI and other serotoninergic drugs, especially since these drugs can inhibit each other's metabolic detoxification and potentiate each other's effects.[40,41] This can even apply to herbal substances such as valerian (Chapter 20). Once drugs are discontinued, the syndrome usually resolves within 24 to 48 hours; during this time, support is the primary treatment. Table 15.6 lists some drugs that can potentiate serotonin activity and that can interact with each other to produce the serotonin syndrome.

Serotonin Withdrawal Syndrome

If drug dependence is defined as a change in physiology or behavior following drug discontinuation, a person can become dependent on

---

TABLE 15.6 Drugs that act through serotoninergic mechanisms or that potentiate serotoninergic drugs

---

Inhibitors of serotonin reuptake

Amitriptyline	(a TCA)	Imipramine	(a TCA)
Amphetamine	(a psychostimulant)	Meperidine	(a narcotic)
Citalopram	(a SSRI)	Nefazodone	(dual action)
Clomipramine	(an atypical)	Paroxetine	(a SSRI)
Cocaine	(a psychostimulant)	Sertraline	(a SSRI)
Dextromethorphan	(non-narcotic)	Trazodone	(an atypical)
Fluoxetine	(a SSRI)	Venlafaxine	(an atypical)
Fluvoxamine	(a SSRI)		

Inhibitors of serotonin metabolism

Isocarboxazid	(a MAOI)	Selegiline	(Eldepryl)
Moclobemide	(a MAOI)	Tranylcypromine	(a MAOI)
Phenelzine	(a MAOI)		

Increased serotonin release

Amphetamines	(psychostimulant)	Cocaine	(psychostimulant)

Increased serotonin synthesis

L-Tryptophan

Serotonin receptor agonists (direct)

Buspirone	(Buspar)	Sumatriptan	(Imitrex)
Dihydroergotamine	(D.H.E.)		

Increased serotonin activity (nonspecific)

Electroconvulsive therapy		Lithium	(a mood stabilizer)

Modified from Lane and Baldwin,[39] with permission.

SSRIs. A serotonin withdrawal syndrome occurs in perhaps 60 percent of SSRI-treated patients following drug removal.[42] Originally associated with withdrawal from paroxetine, the syndrome can occur following discontinuation of any SSRI. Onset is usually within a few days and persists perhaps three to four weeks. The exception is fluoxetine, whose long half-life results in a slow onset of symptomatology (perhaps one to two weeks) with persistence for several weeks thereafter.

Schatzberg and co-workers[43] describe five core somatic sets of symptoms:

• Disequilibrium (dizziness, vertigo, ataxia)
• Gastrointestinal symptoms (nausea, vomiting, diarrhea)
• Flu-like symptoms (fatigue, lethargy, myalgia, chills)

- Sensory disturbances (paresthesia, sensation of electric shocks)
- Sleep disturbances (insomnia, vivid dreams)

Psychological symptoms include anxiety, agitation, crying spells, and irritability. Other less frequently reported symptoms include overactivity, depersonalization, depressed mood, memory problems, confusion, decreased concentration and slowed thinking.[43] All these somatic and psychological phenomena abate over time and rapidly disappear when the SSRI is reintroduced. It is felt that the syndrome results from a relative deficiency of serotonin when the SSRI is stopped; however, the etiology of the exact mechanism may be more complex.

Specific Agents

Fluoxetine. Fluoxetine (Prozac; Figure 15.8) became clinically available in the United States in 1988 as the first SSRI-type antidepressant and the first non-TCA that could be considered a first-line antidepressant (not just for patients who have failed therapy with TCAs). Fluoxetine's efficacy is comparable to that of the TCAs; more important, it is not fatal in overdosage, because it is devoid of the TCA-caused cardiac toxicity (as are all SSRIs). Because of its long half-life, it can be administered as infrequently as once a week.[44]

Fluoxetine has an intermediate-duration half-life (2 to 4 days), but its active metabolite (norfluoxetine, which is even a stronger reuptake inhibitor than fluoxetine) has a half-life of about 7 to 15 days. This prolonged action distinguishes fluoxetine from other SSRIs, which have half-lives of about 1 day and no active intermediates. Fluoxetine's antidepressant action is of slow onset (about 4 to 6 weeks), and the drug and its metabolite thus tend to build with repeated doses over about 2 months, presumably because both compounds continue to accumulate. This can explain the slow onset of peak therapeutic effect, the late onset of side effects, and the prolonged duration of action following drug discontinuation. As a result of the long half-lives of fluoxetine and norfluoxetine, a 5-week drug-free interval is recommended between cessation of fluoxetine administration and the initiation of another drug therapy.

Because of their selectivity, fluoxetine and other SSRIs demonstrate few anticholinergic or antihistaminic side effects. Thus, they cause little or no sedation and little impairment of learning, memory, or cognition. Significant and important side effects include anxiety, agitation, and insomnia, which at the extreme can result in the serotonin syndrome.

Sexual dysfunction can also be a significant problem; it occurs in about 60 percent of patients taking fluoxetine or other SSRIs. Sexual dysfunction may contribute significantly to noncompliance with drug therapy and may significantly impair the patient's quality of life.

Attempts at a "drug holiday," during which drug is not taken so that sexual function may return, frequently results in onset of the SSRI withdrawal syndrome, offsetting any return of libido. Some have attempted to ameliorate SSRI-induced sexual dysfunction by adding a drug such as buspirone or amantadine; some authors report that combinations are effective,[45] but others report that the therapy is ineffective.[46] More frequently, patients are switched to antidepressants with fewer adverse effects on sexual function (e.g., buproprion[29] or one of the "dual-action" antidepressants discussed later).

During initial therapy (perhaps the first month), depressed patients respond to fluoxetine with modest weight loss.[47] During continued treatment, as depression resolves, the lost weight is regained and further weight gains are no different than that seen during placebo therapy.[48]

Sertraline. Sertraline (Zoloft; Figure 15.8) was the second SSRI approved for clinical use in the United States. Clinically, like all SRIs, it is as effective as TCAs in the treatment of major depression.[49] In one of the first demonstrations of the superiority of an SSRI over a TCA, Hoehn-Saric and co-workers,[50] in a study of 166 patients with major depression or OCD, concluded that "the SSRI sertraline was more effective in reducing major depressive disorder and OCD symptoms than the primary norepinephrine reuptake inhibitor desipramine for patients with concurrent OCD and MDD." Further, "more patients receiving desipramine than sertraline discontinued treatment because of adverse effects."

Sertraline is four to five times more potent than fluoxetine in blocking serotonin reuptake and is more selective. Steady-state levels of the drug in plasma are achieved within 4 to 7 days, and its metabolites are less cumulative and less pharmacologically active. Like all SSRIs, sertraline has few anticholinergic, antihistaminic, and adverse cardiovascular effects, as well as a low risk of toxicity in overdose. Sertraline is notable for having few clinically significant drug interactions at usual doses. Like all SSRIs, sertraline is effective in the treatment of anxiety disorders such as panic disorder[51,52] and OCD.[50,53]

Memmen and co-workers[54] documented the presence of sertraline in infants of breast-feeding mothers, and no adverse consequences resulted. Similar results have been obtained with fluoxetine[55] and paroxetine.[56] One SSRI, citalopram, may affect nursing infants. Taken during pregnancy, no SSRI introduced through 1998 (fluoxetine, fluvoxamine, paroxetine, or sertraline) increased the incidence of major malformations, live births, teratogenicity, low birth weights, or higher rates of miscarriage, stillbirths, or prematurity.[57] Again, this may be a problem with citalopram.

Paroxetine. Paroxetine (Paxil) was the third SSRI available for clinical use in treating major depression. Therapeutically, it is comparable to the TCAs in efficacy, clearly superior to placebo. It is highly effective

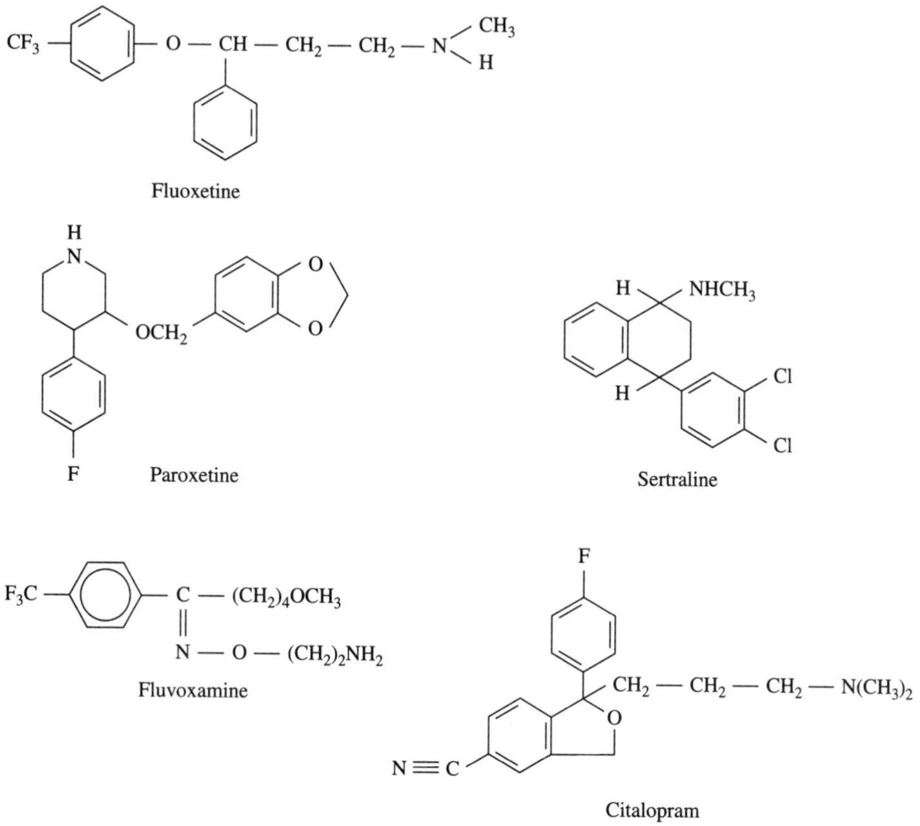

FIGURE 15.8 Chemical structures of five serotonin-specific reuptake inhibitor (SSRI) antidepressants.

in reducing anxiety, a common symptom in depressive illness. It has also been reported effective in posttraumatic stress syndrome (PTSD),[58] and data indicate usefulness in OCD, panic disorder, social phobia, premenstrual dysphoric disorder, and chronic headache.[59] It is FDA-approved for the treatment of social anxiety disorder. Like sertraline, paroxetine is more selective than fluoxetine in blocking serotonin re-uptake. Also, paroxetine's metabolites are relatively inactive, and steady state is achieved within about 7 days. The metabolic half-life is about 24 hours.

Fluvoxamine. In 1995 fluvoxamine (Luvox), a structural derivative of fluoxetine (Figure 15.8), became available for the treatment of OCD.[60] Like all SSRIs, fluvoxamine has well-described antidepressant properties, comparable in efficacy to the TCA imipramine, but it is devoid of adverse cardiac effects. Fluvoxamine, like all SSRIs, has a variety of clinical uses, including treatment of PTSD, dysphoria, panic disorder, and social phobia.[61]

Citalopram. Citalopram (Celexa; Figure 15.8) is an SSRI available in Europe since 1989 and introduced into the United States in 1998. It is promoted for the treatment of major depression, social phobia, panic disorder, and OCD.

Citalopram is well absorbed orally; peak plasma levels are reached in about 4 hours. Steady state is achieved in about 1 week, and maximal effects are seen in about 5 to 6 weeks. Citalopram is metabolized in the liver to three metabolites with SSRI activity; however, these metabolites are less selective and less potent than the parent drug and they are present in only low levels in plasma. The elimination half-life is about 33 hours, enabling once-per-day dosing. The elderly have a reduced ability to metabolize citalopram and a 33 to 50 percent reduction in dose is necessary. Citalopram appears to have less inhibitory effect on drug metabolizing enzymes in the liver than fluoxetine; therefore, it appears to cause fewer drug interactions.[62]

Citalopram exerts antidepressant effects comparable to those exerted by other SSRIs.[63] Citalopram has been reported to moderately reduce alcohol consumption in problem alcoholics. It would be expected that citalopram would exert anxiolytic effects similar to those exerted by other SSRIs. Adverse effects of citalopram resemble those of other SSRIs. Teratogenic effects have been observed after large doses in animals, and the drug is excreted in human breast milk, causing somnolence, decreased feeding, and weight loss in breast-fed infants.[64] Large doses have caused ECK abnormalities, convulsions, and rare fatalities. The *Medical Letter*[64] concluded that "citalopram (Celexa) offers no advantage over other SSRIs for treatment of depression."

SSRIs in Children and Adolescents

DeVane and Sallie[65] and Leonard and co-workers[66] reviewed the use of SSRIs in children and adolescents. While SSRIs have been reported to be useful for the treatment of at least 13 different conditions (e.g., autism, anorexia, bulimia, ADHD), clinical evidence of efficacy is strongest in support of their use in depression and OCD.[67] Birmaher and co-workers[68] review the pharmacotherapy of childhood and adolescent depression and arrive at a different conclusion. They state that in this disorder, 40 percent to 70 percent of children and adolescents respond to placebo therapy:

> Taken together, these studies suggest that TCAs are no more effective than placebo for the treatment of major depressive disorder in children and adolescents. . . . [While] open studies have reported 70% to

90% response to fluoxetine for the treatment of adolescents with major depressive disorder . . . a double-blind, placebo-controlled study . . . did not find significant differences between placebo and fluoxetine. . . . Despite the successful response to fluoxetine, many patients had only partial improvement, suggesting that the ideal treatment may involve variation in dose or length of treatment, or a combination of pharmacological and psychosocial treatments.

Controlled studies are not yet available to support widespread use of SSRIs for other disorders of childhood. Popper[69] cautions:

SSRIs appear to be changing the treatment philosophy of child and adolescent psychiatrists. Almost as quickly as these new drugs became available, psychiatrists began to prescribe them in adolescents and children for a variety of presumed indications. In contrast to the caution characteristic of the past, children and adolescents in large numbers have been exposed to these new agents—despite the lack of a lengthy track record to demonstrate their safety in adults. . . Whatever their merits and liabilities may turn out to be, SSRIs have led many psychiatrists to feel comfortable in prescribing newly developed medications in children, although long-term and even many short-term issues were still largely unclear. By breaking this barrier, psychiatrists have perhaps become blasé about playing with newly found fire.

Zito and colleagues[70] note in preschool children (ages 2 through 4 years) enrolled in either Medicaid or health management organization (HMO) programs that "antidepressants were the second most commonly prescribed psychotropic class of drugs for preschoolers, and their use increased substantially from 1991–1995." Tricyclic antidepressants still represented the bulk of early childhood antidepressant use, although use of SSRIs was increasing. It is likely that SSRI use in the year 2000 would be even higher, as would the continuing increase in drug prescription for this population of children. In an editorial accompanying the Zito article, Coyle[71] states:

Given that there is no empirical evidence to support psychotropic drug treatment in very young children and that there are valid concerns that such treatment could have deleterious effects on the developing brain, the reasons for these troubling changes in practice need to be identified. . . . It appears that behaviorally disturbed children are now increasingly subjected to quick and inexpensive pharmacologic fixes as opposed to informed, multimodal therapy associated with optimal outcomes. These disturbing prescription practices suggest a growing crisis in mental health services to children and demand more thorough investigation.

Dual-Action Antidepressants

Nefazodone (Serzone)

Nefazodone (Figure 15.9) is a unique antidepressant, differing from the SSRIs by a *dual action* on the serotonin synapse. Nefazodone's strongest pharmacological action is 5-HT$_{2A}$ receptor blockade, an action that distinguishes it from the SSRIs. Nefazodone resembles the TCAs as an inhibitor of both serotonin and norepinephrine reuptake at its therapeutic dose. With chronic administration, nefazedone ultimately down regulates both norepinephrine and serotonin receptors. Blockade of reuptake is thought to be responsible for its antidepressant activity, and the 5-HT$_{2A}$ blockade is thought to be responsible for nefazodone's lack of SSRI-type side effects as well as its particular benefit on sleep disturbances[72] and comorbid anxiety symptoms[73] often seen in depressed patients. Serotonin 5-HT$_2$ receptor blockade also accounts for the relative lack of drug-induced sexual dysfunction with ongoing treatment.

Sedation can be bothersome, as can nausea, dry mouth, dizziness, and light-headedness. Nefazodone is effective in the treatment of depression-related insomnia and nighttime awakenings. Wilens and co-workers[74] reported successful treatment of juvenile mood disorders. In treating depression, nefazodone has not been shown to have therapeutic superiority over TCAs or SSRIs or faster onset of action. Davis, Whittington, and Bryson[75] reviewed the pharmacology and efficacy of nefazodone.

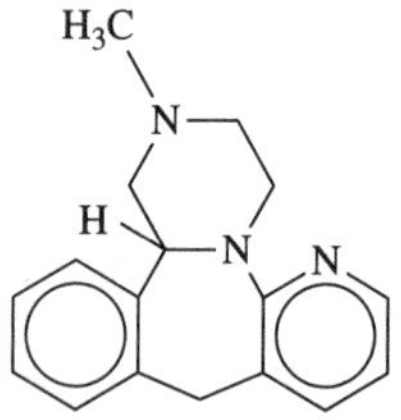

Mirtazapine (Remeron)

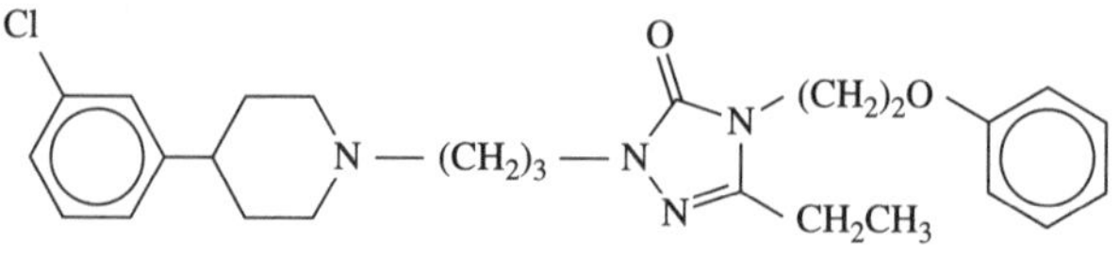

Nefazodone (Serzone)

FIGURE 15.9 Chemical structures of two dual-action antidepressants.

Newly reported uses of nefazodone include use in alcoholics with comorbid depression (relieving depression but not reducing alcohol consumption) [75A] and use in relieving the distress of PTSD in treatment resistant combat veterans.[75B,75C]

Mirtazapine (Remeron)

Mirtazapine (Figure 15.9) was introduced into clinical use in the United States in 1997. Wheatley and co-workers[76] compared mirtazepine to fluoxetine and found mirtazepine to be "as well tolerated as fluoxetine and significantly more effective after 3 and 4 weeks of therapy." According to Kasper:[77]

> In line with the concept that severe depression may respond better to drugs with a dual rather than a single mode of action, mirtazapine is a noradrenergic and specific serotonergic antidepressant. It has a different mode of action from TCAs, SSRIs, and MAOIs, because it increases noradrenergic and serotonergic neurotransmission via a blockade of the central alpha$_2$-autoreceptors and heteroreceptors. The increased release of serotonin, via increased cell firings of 5-HT neurons, stimulates only the 5-HT$_1$ type receptors, because 5-HT$_2$ and 5-HT$_3$ type receptors are specifically blocked by mirtazapine.

Stated differently, mirtazapine is not a reuptake blocker like SSRIs or TCAs. It is an antagonist of both alpha$_2$ autoreceptors (the receptors located on noradrenergic terminals by which NE controls its own release) and alpha$_2$ heteroreceptors (receptors located on serotoninergic nerve terminals by which NE controls the release of serotonin). This antagonism explains how mirtazapine enhances both NE and serotonin neurotransmission and ultimately down regulates receptor activity. Holm and Markham[78] reviewed the pharmacology of mirtazepine.

Mirtazapine is a potent antagonist of postsynaptic 5-HT$_2$ and 5-HT$_3$ receptors (Figure 15.10), precluding the side effects of SSRIs (especially anxiety, insomnia, agitation, nausea, and sexual dysfunction). Mirtazapine is also a potent blocker of histamine receptors, and drowsiness can be a prominent side effect. Sedation may be advantageous in depressed patients with symptoms of anxiety and insomnia, a common occurrence. Because of this drowsiness, the drug should not be combined with alcohol or other CNS depressants. Other side effects of mirtazapine include increased appetite and weight gain.

Mirtazapine is rapidly absorbed orally, with peak blood levels occurring 2 hours after administration. The elimination half-life is 20 to 40 hours, allowing once-a-day administration, usually at bedtime to maximize sleep and minimize daytime sedation.

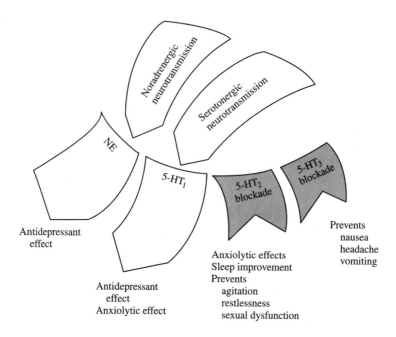

FIGURE 15.10 Pharmacological profile of mirtazapine. Note that the drug potentiates noradrenergic and serotoninergic neurotransmission and blocks serotonin 5-HT$_2$ and 5-HT$_3$ receptors. The consequences of each action are shown at the bottom of the figure. [From R. M. Pinder, *Journal of Clinical Psychiatry* 58 (1997): 501–507.]

Monoamine Oxidase Inhibitors (MAOIs)

Long-acting, irreversible monoamine oxidase (MAO) inhibitors have been used since the 1950s for treating major depressive illnesses. Their use is, however, limited by serious side effects that include potentially fatal interactions when taken with certain foods and medicines. The drugs included adrenaline-like drugs found in nasal sprays, antiasthma medications, cold medicines, and cocaine. The foods included those that contain tyramine, a by-product of fermentation, such as many cheeses, wines, beers, liver, and some beans. As a result of the interaction, blood pressure increases severely, occasionally enough to be fatal. During their checkered and controversial history, it was learned that, although they are potentially dangerous, they can be used safely with strict dietary restrictions. Gardner and colleagues[79] discuss the MAOI diet and its appropriate presentation to patients (Tables 15.7 and 15.8). Today, the MAOIs are experiencing a resurgence in use for several reasons:

TABLE 15.7 Relative restrictions of food and beverages with MAOI use

Restriction	Foods
Absolute	Aged cheeses; aged and cured meats; banana peel; broad bean pods; improperly stored or spoiled meats, poultry, and fish; Marmite; sauerkraut; soy sauce and other soybean condiments; tap beer
Moderate	Red or white wine; bottled or canned beer (including nonalcoholic varieties)
Unnecessary	Avocados; bananas; beef/chicken bouillon; chocolate; fresh and mild cheeses, e.g., ricotta, cottage, cream cheese, processed slices; fresh meat, poultry, or fish; gravy (fresh); monosodium glutamate; peanuts; properly stored pickled or smoked fish, e.g., herring; raspberries; soy milk; yeast extracts (except Marmite)

Reproduced with permission from Gardner et al.[79]

- With appropriate dietary restrictions, they can be as safe or safer than TCAs.
- They can work in many patients who respond poorly to both TCAs and SSRIs.
- They are excellent drugs for the treatment of atypical depression, which presents primarily with anxiety and phobic symptoms, masked depression (such as hypochondriasis), anorexia nervosa, bulimia, bipolar depression, dysthymia, depression in the elderly, panic disorder, and phobias.

Monoamine oxidase (MAO) is one of two enzymes that break down normal neurotransmitters in the body, including norepinephrine and serotonin. There are two types of the enzyme: MAO-A ("good" MAO) is found in norepinephrine and serotonin nerve terminals; MAO-B ("bad" MAO) is found in dopamine-secreting neurons. Pharmacologically, drug-induced inhibition of MAO-A is presumably responsible for the antidepressant activity, while inhibition of MAO-B is responsible for the side effects, including serious drug interactions.

Drug-induced blockade of MAO (especially MAO-A) allows large amounts of transmitters to accumulate in the nerve terminals. As a result, more transmitter is released when the neurons are stimulated. Three MAO inhibitors have been available for many years, and all three are both nonselective and irreversible in their inhibition of both

TABLE 15.8 Sunnybrook Health Science Center MAOI diet

Several foods and beverages contain tyramine and may interact with medication. The patient must follow the dietary instructions below from the day taking the medication begins until 2 weeks after you start stopping it.
Note: All foods must be fresh or properly frozen. Patients should avoid foods if storage conditions are not known.

	Food to avoid	Food allowed
Cheese	All matured or aged cheese All casseroles made with these cheeses, i.e., pizza, lasagna, etc. Note: All cheeses are considered matured or aged except those listed opposite	Fresh cottage cheese, cream cheese, ricotta cheese, and processed cheese slices. All fresh milk products that have been stored properly (e.g., sour cream, yogurt, ice cream)
Meat, fish, and poultry	Fermented/dry sausage: pepperoni, salami, mortadella, summer sausage, etc. Improperly stored meat, fish, or poultry Improperly stored pickled herring	All fresh packaged or processed meat (e.g., chicken loaf, hot dogs), fish, or poultry Store in refrigerator immediately and eat as soon as possible
Fruits and vegetables	Fava or broad bean pods (not beans) Banana peel	Banana pulp All others except those listed opposite
Alcoholic beverages	All tap beers	Alcohol: No more than two domestic bottled or canned beers or 4-fl.-oz. glasses of red or white wine per day; this also applies to nonalcoholic beer; note that red wine may produce headache unrelated to a rise in blood pressure
Miscellaneous foods	Marmite concentrated yeast extract Sauerkraut Soy sauce and other soybean condiments	Other yeast extracts (e.g., brewer's yeast) Soy milk

Reproduced with permission from Gardner et al. (1996).[79]

MAO-A and MAO-B. Short-acting, reversible MAO-A inhibitors are newer and as yet clinically unavailable in the United States, although one (moclobemide) is available in Canada and Europe.

Irreversible MAOIs

The three MAO inhibitors currently available—*phenelzine* (Nardil), *tranylcypromine* (Parnate), and *isocarboxazid* (Marplan)—irreversibly block both MAO-A and MAO-B. Irreversible effects are unusual in pharmacology; most drugs exert reversible actions, usually by competing for receptors with naturally occurring neurotransmitters. The irreversible MAO inhibitors form a chemical bond with part of the MAO enzyme, a bond that cannot be broken; enzyme function returns only as new enzyme is biosynthesized.

Pharmacokinetics and Mechanism of Action. As shown in Figure 15.11, the elimination half-life of tranylcypromine (a prototype MAOI) is about two hours. This rapid rate of elimination results in a rapid decline in plasma levels of the drug (Figure 15.11A) but not in the degree of MAO inhibition (Figure 15.11B). The reason for this lack of correlation is that after tranylcypromine is absorbed, it is metabolized to a reactive intermediate compound. This compound then binds irreversibly with MAO-A and MAO-B in a tight covalent bond. Excess drug that is not converted to the intermediate compound is rapidly metabolized and then excreted. This course of events is illustrated in Figure 15.11B. The upper graph reflects the rapid rise and fall in the blood (plasma) levels of tranylcypromine given orally three times a day for seven days. There is little drug accumulation because the liver rapidly metabolizes the drug. The irreversible inhibition of MAO occurs slowly; a level of 70 percent inhibition is reached by day 7. After the patient stops taking the drug, MAO activity returns very slowly, reflecting the synthesis of new, biologically active enzyme.

Efficacy. The nonselective, irreversible MAO inhibitors were the first clinically effective drugs for treating major depression, preceding the TCAs by about ten years. Their fall from favor was not from lack of efficacy—their efficacy is comparable to that of the TCAs[80]—but from fear of adverse reactions. MAO inhibitors can be effective in patients in whom therapy with TCAs and SSRIs has failed.[81] Therefore, when administered with dietary counseling, these drugs can be used relatively safely. Needed, however, are MAO inhibitors with shorter durations of clinical action, more specificity, and an increased margin of safety.

Reversible MAOIs

Several short-acting, selective, reversible MAO inhibitors have been developed, but they are not available in the United States. Reversible

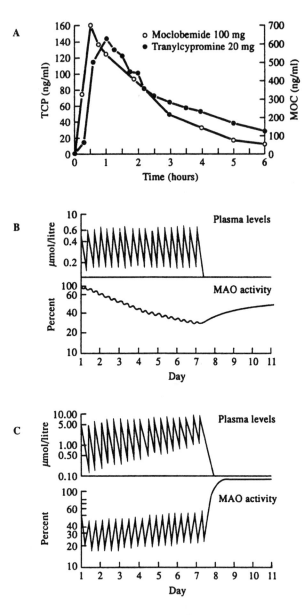

FIGURE 15.11 A. Concentration profiles of moclobemide (MOC) and tranylcypromine (TCP) after an oral dose. **B.** Tranylcypromine (10 mg three times a day) plasma levels and MAO activity. **C.** Moclobemide (150 mg three times a day) plasma levels and MAO activity. [From R. Amrien et al., "The Pharmacology of Reversible Monoamine Oxidase Inhibitors," *British Journal of Psychiatry* Suppl. 6 (1989), 66–71.]

MAOIs include *brofaromine, pirlindole, toloxatone,* and *moclobemide.* These drugs are highly selective in their ability to reversibly inhibit MAO-A. Thus, they are much safer than the irreversible MAO inhibitors because they have minimal interaction with the tyramine in food. Fulton and Benfield[82] noted that moclobemide is as effective as the TCAs, with similar onset of antidepressant action and (reportedly) with fewer side effects.

Figure 15.11 demonstrates that the half-lives and plasma decay curves of moclobemide and tranylcypromine are virtually identical. With moclobemide (administered orally three times a day for seven days), however, the inhibition of MAO is correlated with the plasma concentration of the drug (Figure 15.11C). With each dose, MAO activity fell and then returned as the drug was metabolized and its plasma level fell. When therapy ended, MAO activity rapidly returned to normal. This pattern is like that of most drugs; unlike tranylcypromine, moclobemide does not form an irreversible covalent bond. Figure 15.11C shows that MAO inhibition is at a maximum after a single dose of moclobemide. Drug effects can be controlled easily, plasma concentration parallels pharmacological effects, and the effect has a short duration with no aftereffects. Because of the specificity of enzyme blockade, side effects are minimal.

Moclobemide does not cause deterioration in cognitive functions; rather, it improves vigilance, attention, and some crucial components of memory. These improvements may be related to inhibition of MAO-A as well as to the lack of any anticholinergic or antihistaminic actions. Fulton and Benfield[82] review its superior efficacy in the treatment of social phobias.

In conclusion, the newer, selective, reversible MAO-A inhibitors offer distinct advantages over the older MAOIs. It is hoped that one or more of these reversible MAO-A inhibitors will become available in the United States.

COMT Inhibitors

COMT (catechol-o-methyltransferae) is the second of the two enzymes that catalyse the inactivation of catecholamine neurotransmitters (dopamine and norepinephrine) in both the liver and the brain (the other catabolic enzyme is MAO). As with MAO inhibition, COMT inhibition increases the levels of NE and DA in the brain and the periphery.

Tolcapone (Tasmar) is a potent and specific inhibitor of COMT, markedly increasing brain DA and NE. Currently, it is marketed for use in the treatment of Parkinsonism, being especially effective when administered together with L-dopa (Chapter 18). In an open study, Fava and co-workers[83] administered tolcapone to 21 adults with major depression for 8 weeks. The authors reported significant improvements in about 50 percent of patients; however, 8 patients (38 percent) dropped out of the study because of side effects (diarrhea, elevated liver function tests, increased anxiety) and noncompliance. These early results are encouraging for a new concept in the treatment of depression.

Specific Norepinephrine Reuptake Inhibitor (SNRI)

Until recently, no antidepressant exhibited specific NE reuptake blockade in the absence of dopamine or serotonin reuptake blockade. *Reboxetine* (Vestra, Edronax) appears to be such an agent. Versiani and co-workers[84,85] document the superiority of reboxetine over placebo therapy in severely depressed patients. Massana and co-workers[86] compared reboxetine with fluoxetine and reported that "reboxetine is an effective and well-tolerated antidepressant, being more effective than fluoxetine in patients with severe depression, and more effective in terms of social functioning in those patients who achieved remission." Side effects were mild and primarily caused by an anticholinergic action (dry mouth, sweating, blurred vision, constipation, tachycardia). A recent symposium[87] discusses reboxetine and the role of norepinephrine in the treatment of depression. It is expected that reboxetine will soon become available for clinical use.

Serotonin 5-HT$_1$ Agonists*

Chapter 6 introduced *buspirone* (BuSpar) as an anxiolytic agent and noted that it exerts its effects secondary to weak stimulation of serotonin 5-HT$_{1A}$ receptors. It was also noted that its poor absorption after oral administration could be greatly augmented by administering the drug with grapefruit juice, an inhibitor of gastric CYP3A4 enzyme, and that stimulation of 5-HT$_1$ receptors appears to be responsible for the acute antidepressant effects of several antidepressant drugs, such as SSRIs. It would therefore appear logical that specific stimulation of 5-HT$_1$ receptors would provide antidepressant efficacy without production of side effects resulting from 5-HT$_2$ and 5-HT$_3$ receptor stimulation. Indeed, buspirone and related agents, such as *ipsapirone*, have

*The structure of the 5-HT$_{1A}$ receptor is illustrated in Figure 2.2.

demonstrable antidepressant efficacy.[88,89] Further investigation in this area is indicated.

Dehydroepiandrosterone (DHEA)

DHEA is a major glucocorticoid hormone secreted by the adrenal glands, but its physiological role is unclear. Sold as a food supplement in nutrition centers, DHEA is a precursor of both estrogen and testosterone. Secretion of the hormone peaks at 20 to 25 years of age and declines by about 90 percent by age 70. Low levels of DHEA have been associated with increased incidence of cardiovascular disease and death in middle-aged men but not in women. DHEA has been promoted (with minimal evidence) to prevent heart disease, cancer, diabetes, obesity, dementia, aging, multiple sclerosis, and lupus; it increases feelings of physical and psychological well-being. There probably is some truth and much exaggeration in these claims of efficacy.

Perhaps the most enduring claim has been that DHEA may delay the aging process, improve mood, and delay the cognitive decline that occurs with age. Bloch and co-workers[90] and Wolkowitz and co-workers[91] conducted double-blind, randomized studies of DHEA on objective measurements of depression, dysthymia, and cognitive functioning. DHEA, but not placebo, exerted a robust effect on mood, improving depression ratings on all measurement scales (Figure 15.12). "Symptoms that improved after six weeks of DHEA compared with baseline or placebo were as follows: low energy, anhedonia, lack of motivation, emotional flattening (numbness), sadness, excessive worry, and inability to cope."[90] Response rates (60 percent) were comparable to those seen with standard antidepressants. DHEA had no effect on cognitive function or sleep disturbances. Wolkowitz and co-workers state:

> DHEA had statistically significant antidepressant effects; nearly half of the DHEA-treated subjects showed clinically meaningful improvement. . . . This finding adds to the growing literature indicating that hormonal dysregulation may be causally related to depressive illness and that certain hormonal treatments can have antidepressant effects. Larger scale controlled trials with DHEA are clearly warranted.

The mechanism of action is unclear, but Bloch and co-workers speculate on competitive blockade of $GABA_A$ receptors or augmentation of glutamate/NMDA activity in the hippocampus. They conclude by stating that "DHEA may represent a new therapeutic option for mid-life dysthymia." Commenting on this report, Young[92] stated that "these exciting new findings will likely stimulate a flurry of use of DHEA and hopefully a flurry of placebo-controlled clinical trials."

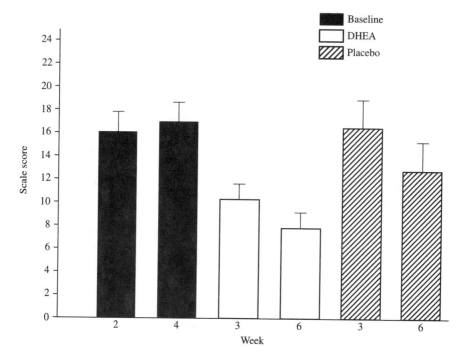

FIGURE 15.12 Reduction of Beck Depression Inventory (BDI) scores during DHEA, but not placebo, in mid-life-onset dysthymia. Fifteen men and women with mid-life dysthymia experienced significant reduction in BDI during DHEA treatment compared to both their baseline scores and their scores after placebo treatment. [From Bloch et al.[89]]

DHEA is usually classified as an androgen, because one of its metabolites is testosterone. Therefore, it would not be surprising to see its use accompanied by a potential for side effects characteristic of androgens: acne, male-pattern baldness, hirsutism, voice changes, and so on. More serious effects include the theoretical potential for causing breast or prostate cancer and liver damage. The degree to which this might happen is unknown.

S-adenosy-methionine (SAM; SAMe)

SAMe is a ubiquitous molecule located throughout the body. It plays a key intermediary role in numerous metabolic reactions that involve the transfer of methyl groups between molecules. It is not commonly present in the diet, but it is formed in the body by the combination of the amino acid methionine and adenosine triphosphate (ATP). SAMe functions by donating its methyl group to any of a wide range of molecules and is subsequently transformed to homocysteine. Ultimately, the homocysteine is transformed to methionine and the process repeats.

SAMe became available in oral formulation in the United States in 1999. It is marketed as a dietary supplement or natural mood enhancer, promoting emotional well-being. In European countries, SAMe is used for the treatment of arthritis, liver disease, and depression, among other disorders. The mechanism by which SAMe works with any of these disorders is a mystery.

Orally administered, SAMe is very poorly absorbed into the body, with less than 1 percent of the ingested drug ever reaching the bloodstream. This is important since almost all European trials of the drug have involved parenteral administration. Administered in this form, the drug appears to be effective in reducing depression. Trials utilizing oral SAMe have produced equivocal and inconclusive results. With such poor oral absorption, efficacy by that route is unlikely; it is not valid to extrapolate data from studies that used the parenteral formulation of SAMe to the oral formulations that are available in the United States.

The *Medical Letter*[93] reviewed the reported clinical trials with SAMe and reported that in short-term trials (usually less than three weeks), SAMe (about 200 mg/day parenterally) was more effective than placebo in relieving depression and about as effective as several comparison tricyclic antidepressants. Adversely, the *Medical Letter* noted that many different formulations are available in the United States, all of which are oral, none of which are FDA regulated, and many of which contain no SAMe at all. Despite the myriad claims of efficacy, the *Medical Letter* concluded:

> There is no convincing evidence that SAMe, a dietary supplement, is effective or safe for treatment of depression. The few clinical trials finding it as effective as proven antidepressants were too small or too short to be useful. As with other dietary supplements, the potency and purity of SAMe preparations sold in the USA are unknown. According to *Medical Letter* consultants, dietary supplements sold here should not be assumed to be identical to drugs sold in other countries, even if they are produced under the same name by the same manufacturer.

Side effects of SAMe appear to be modest. The primary adverse effect associated with the use of parenteral SAMe has been mania, manifest as pressured speech and grandiosity. SAMe is therefore contraindicated in patients with a history of mania or bipolar disorder and perhaps in those with anxiety disorders. Since SAMe is metabolized to homocysteine and because elevated homocysteine levels have been associated with early onset of atherosclerosis and coronary artery disease, there is concern that overuse of SAMe may predispose to these diseases. It is not known whether SAMe raises homocysteine levels in blood or whether SAMe has any adverse effects on coronary artery disease, although caution is certainly advised. No reports of safety in pregnancy or breast feeding are available.

Promoters of SAMe advise oral doses of 400 to 800 mg/day (two to four tablets daily); clinical studies demonstrating modest antidepressant effects with oral doses of SAMe have utilized doses of up to 1600 mg/day. Given its expense, poor oral absorption, and its potential for causing mania and atherosclerosis, SAMe cannot be recommended for the treatment of depression. As with many other dietary supplements (Chapter 20), time will tell whether SAMe is effective.

STUDY QUESTIONS

1. Differentiate between major depression and bipolar disorder.

2. What is the correlation between depression and the biological amine transmitters in the brain?

3. Describe the probable mechanism of both acute and ultimate effects of antidepressant drugs. What might account for the delay in clinical effect?

4. Differentiate cocaine and the amphetamines from clinical antidepressants. Include acute effects, psychological effects, and liabilities for misuse.

5. What are the seven or eight major classes of antidepressants?

6. Compare and contrast imipramine and fluoxetine.

7. Discuss what happens when a patient overdoses on a tricyclic antidepressant. Who is at risk?

8. Discuss the side effects of SSRIs. What is the serotonin syndrome? What is the serotonin withdrawal syndrome? Discuss the effects of these drugs on sexual function.

9. Discuss the use of antidepressants in children and adolescents.

10. Which drug or class of drugs do you think is the "best" antidepressant? Defend your position.

11. Which antidepressants are used in the treatment of anxiety disorders? Why? How do these drugs differ from the benzodiazepine-type anxiolytics?

12. What can be done if a formerly depressed patient becomes manic on antidepressant medication? Which antidepressants are most

likely to bring on such an effect? To which drug can the patient be switched? Why?

13. What is DHEA? What is its therapeutic potential? Its potential complications?

REFERENCES

1. J. M. Murphy et al., "A 40-Year Perspective on the Prevalence of Depression: The Stirling County Study," *Archives of General Psychiatry* 57 (2000): 209–215.
2. R. M. A. Hirschfeld et al., "The National Depressive and Manic-depressive Association Consensus Statement on the Undertreatment of Depression," *Journal of the American Medical Association* 227 (1997): 333–340.
3. B. G. Druss, R. A. Hoff and R. A. Rosenheck, "Underuse of Antidepressants in Major Depression: Prevalence and Correlates in a National Sample of Young Adults," *Journal of Clinical Psychiatry* 61 (2000): 234–237.
4. C. A. Melfi et al., "The Effects of Adherence to Antidepressant Treatment Guidelines on Relapse and Recurrence of Depression," *Archives of General Psychiatry* 55 (1998): 1128–1132.
5. D. A. Sclar, L. M. Robison, T. L. Skaer, and R. S. Galin, "Ethnicity and the Prescribing of Antidepressant Pharmacotherapy: 1992–1995," *Harvard Reviews of Psychiatry* 7 (1999): 29–36.
6. C. A. Melfi, T. W. Croghan, M. P. Hanna, and R. L. Robinson, "Racial Variation in Antidepressant Treatment in a Medicaid Population," *Journal of Clinical Psychiatry* 61 (2000): 16–21.
7. S. M. Stahl, "Mergers and Acquisitions Among Psychotropics: Antidepressant Takeover of Anxiety May Now Be Complete," *Journal of Clinical Psychiatry* 60 (1999): 282–283. Also "Antidepressants: The Blue-Chip Psychotropic for the Modern Treatment of Anxiety Disorders," *Journal of Clinical Psychiatry* 60 (1999): 356–357.
8. R. C. Shelton et al., "The Undertreatment of Dysthymia," *Journal of Clinical Psychiatry* 58 (1997): 59–65.
9. R. S. Duman, G. R. Heninger, and E. J. Nestler, "A Molecular and Cellular Theory of Depression," *Archives of General Psychiatry* 54 (1997): 597–606.
10. A. Russo-Neustadt, R. C. Beard, and C. W. Cotman, "Exercise, Antidepressant Medications, and Enhanced Brain-derived Neurotropic Factor Expression," *Neuropsychopharmacology* 21 (1999): 679–682.
11. E. S. Brown, A. J. Rush, and B. S. McEwen, "Hippocampal Remodeling and Damage by Corticosteroids: Implications for Mood Disorders," *Neuropsychopharmacology* 21 (1999): 474–484.
12. S. E. Lindley et al., "Glucocorticoid Effects on Mesotelencephalic Dopamine Neurotransmission," *Neuropsychopharmacology* 21 (1999): 399–407.
13. R. S. Duman, J. Malberg and J. Thome, "Neural Plasticity and Antidepressant Treatment," *Biological Psychiatry* 46 (1999): 1181–1191.

14. K. Fujimaki, S. Morinobu and R. S. Duman, "Administration of a cAMP Phosphodiesterase-4 Inhibitor Enhances Antidepressant-Induction of BDNF mRNA in Rat Hippocampus," *Neuropsychopharmacology* 22 (2000): 42–51.

15. N. Bonhomme and E. Esposito, "Involvement of Serotonin and Dopamine in the Mechanism of Action of Novel Antidepressant Drugs," *Journal of Clinical Psychopharmacology* 18 (1998): 447–454.

16. R. M. A. Hirschfeld, "Efficacy of SSRIs and Newer Antidepressants in Severe Depression: Comparison with TCAs," *Journal of Clinical Psychiatry* 60 (1999): 326–335.

17. P. J. McGrath et al., "A Placebo-Controlled Study of Fluoxetine Versus Imipramine in the Acute Treatment of Atypical Depression," *American Journal of Psychiatry* 157 (2000): 344–350.

18. M. R. Mavissakalian and J. M. Perel, "Long-term Maintenance and Discontinuation of Imipramine in Panic Disorder With Agoraphobia," *Archives of General Psychiatry* 56 (1999): 821–827.

19. J. C. Nelson et al., "Treatment of Major Depression with Nortriptyline and Paroxetine in Patients with Ischemic Heart Disease," *American Journal of Psychiatry* 156 (1999): 1024–1028.

20. T. E. Wilens, J. Biederman, A. M. Abantes, and T. J. Spencer, "A Naturalistic Assessment of Protriptyline for Attention-Deficit Hyperactivity Disorder," *Journal of the American Academy of Child and Adolescent Psychiatry* 35 (1996): 1485–1490.

21. T. E. Wilens, J. Biederman, E. Mick, and T. J. Spencer, "A Systematic Assessment of Tricyclic Antidepressants in the Treatment of Adult Attention-Deficit Hyperactivity Disorder," *Journal of Nervous and Mental Diseases* 183 (1995): 48–50.

22. I. Nulman et al., "Neurodevelopment of Children Exposed in Utero to Anti-depressant Drugs," *New England Journal of Medicine* 336 (1997): 258–262.

23. K. L. Wisner, "Pharmacologic Treatment of Depression During Pregnancy," *Journal of the American Medical Association* 282 (1999): 1264–1269.

24. R. G. Godfrey, "A Guide to the Understanding and Use of Tricyclic Antidepressants in the Overall Management of Fibromyalgia and Other Chronic Pain Syndromes," *Archives of Internal Medicine* 156 (1996): 1047–1052.

25. C. K. Varley and J. McClellan, "Case Study: Two Additional Sudden Deaths With Tricyclic Antidepressants," *Journal of the American Academy of Child and Adolescent Psychiatry* 36 (1997): 390–394.

26. J. A. Ascher et al., "Bupropion: A Review of Its Mechanism of Antidepressant Action," *Journal of Clinical Psychiatry* 56 (1995): 395–401.

27. L. L. Barrickman et al., Bupropion versus Methylphenidate in the Treatment of Attention-Deficit Hyperactivity Disorder," *Journal of the American Academy of Child and Adolescent Psychiatry* 34 (1995): 649–657.

28. J. G. Modell, C. R. Katholi, J. D. Modell, and R. L. DePalma, "Comparative Sexual Side Effects of Bupropion, Fluoxetine, Paroxetine, and Sertraline," *Clinical Pharmacology and Therapeutics* 61 (1997): 476–487.

29. R. T. Segraves et al., "Evaluation of Sexual Functioning in Depressed Outpatients: A Double-Blind Comparison of Sustained-Release Bupropion and Sertraline Treatment," *Journal of Clinical Psychopharmacology* 20 (2000): 122–128.

30. Danish University Antidepressant Group, "Clomipramine Dose-effect Study in Patients with Depression: Clinical End Points and Pharmacokinetics," *Clinical Pharmacology and Therapeutics* 66 (1999): 152–165.

31. L. A. Papp et al., "Clomipramine Treatment of Panic Disorder: Pros and Cons," *Journal of Clinical Psychiatry* 58 (1997): 423–425.

32. R. Zanardi et al., "Venlafaxine Versus Fluvoxamine in the Treatment of Delusional Depression: A Pilot Double-blind Controlled Study," *Journal of Clinical Psychiatry* 61 (2000): 26–29.

33. A. Khan et al., "The Use of Venlafaxine in the Treatment of Major Depression and Major Depression Associated with Anxiety: A Dose-Response Study," *Journal of Clinical Psychopharmacology* 18 (1998): 19–25.

34. T. Einarson et al., "Meta-analysis of Venlafaxine, SSRIs, and TCAs in the Treatment of Major Depressive Disorder," *Canadian Journal of Clinical Pharmacology* 5 (1999): 205–216.

35. J. G. Edwards and I. Anderson, "Systematic Review and Guide to Selection of Selective Serotonin Reuptake Inhibitors," *Drugs* 57 (1999): 507–533.

36. C. DeMontigny, "The Pharmacological Profile of Mirtazapine," in "Controversies in the Treatment and Diagnosis of Severe Depression," *Journal of Clinical Psychiatry* 57 (1996): 554–561.

37. H. G. Nurnberg, P. M. Thompson, and P. L. Hensley, "Antidepressant Medication Change in a Clinical Treatment Setting: A Comparison of the Effectiveness of Selective Serotonin Reuptake Inhibitors," *Journal of Clinical Psychiatry* 60 (1999): 574–579.

38. S. H. Preskorn, "Clinically Relevant Pharmacology of Selective Serotonin Reuptake Inhibitors: An Overview with Emphasis on Pharmacokinetics and Effects on Oxidative Drug Metabolism," *Clinical Pharmacokinetics* 32, Suppl. 1 (1997): 1–21.

39. R. Lane and D. Baldwin, "Selective Serotonin Reuptake Inhibitor-induced Serotonin Syndrome: Review," *Journal of Clinical Psychopharmacology* 17 (1997): 208–221.

40. P. I. Rosebush and P. Margetts, "Serotonin Syndrome as a Result of Clomipramine Monotherapy," *Journal of Clinical Psychopharmacology* 19 (1999): 285–287.

41. G. L. Birbeck and P. W. Kaplan, "Serotonin Syndrome: A Frequently Missed Diagnosis? Let the Neurologist Beware," *The Neurologist* 5 (1999): 279–285.

42. J. Zajecka, K. A. Tracy, and S. Mitchell, "Discontinuation Symptoms After Treatment with Serotonin Reuptake Inhibitors: A Literature Review," *Journal of Clinical Psychiatry* 58 (1997): 291–297.

43. A. F. Schatzberg et al., "Serotonin Reuptake Inhibitor Discontinuation Syndrome: A Hypothetical Definition," *Journal of Clinical Psychiatry* 58, Suppl. 7 (1997): 5–10. (See also the other articles in Supplement 7.)

44. N. P. Emmanuel et al., "Once-Weekly Dosing of Fluoxetine in the Maintenance of Remission in Panic Disorder," *Journal of Clinical Psychiatry* 60 (1999): 299–301.

45. M. Landen, E. Eriksson, H. Agren, and T. Fahlen, "Effect of Buspirone on Sexual Dysfunction in Depressed Patients Treated with Selective Serotonin Reuptake Inhibitors," *Journal of Clinical Psychopharmacology* 19 (1999): 268–271.

46. D. Michelson et al., "Female Sexual Dysfunction Associated with Antidepressant Administration: A Randomized, Placebo-controlled Study of Pharmacologic Intervention," *American Journal of Psychiatry* 157 (2000): 239–243.

47. R. G. Robinson et al., "Nortriptyline Versus Fluoxetine in the Treatment of Depression and in Short-Term Recovery After Stroke: A Placebo-Controlled, Double-Blind Study," *American Journal of Psychiatry* 157 (2000): 351–359.

48. D. Michelson et al., "Changes in Weight During a One-year Trial of Fluoxetine," *American Journal of Psychiatry* 156 (1999): 1170–1176.

49. R. B. Lydiard, S. M. Stahl, M. Hertzman, and W. M. Harrison, "A Double-blind, Placebo-controlled Study Comparing the Effects of Sertraline Versus Amitriptyline in the Treatment of Major Depression," *Journal of Clinical Psychiatry* 58 (1997): 484–491.

50. R. Hoehn-Saric et al., "Multicenter Double-blind Comparison of Sertraline and Desipramine for Concurrent Obsessive-Compulsive and Major Depressive Disorders," *Archives of General Psychiatry* 57 (2000); 76–82.

51. R. B. Pohl, R. M. Wolkow, and C. M. Clary, "Sertraline in the Treatment of Panic Disorder: A Double-blind Multicenter Trial," *American Journal of Psychiatry* 155 (1998): 1189–1195.

52. M. H. Pollack et al., "Sertraline in the Treatment of Panic Disorder: A Flexible-dose Multicenter Trial," *Archives of General Psychiatry* 55 (1998): 1010–1016.

53. M. H. Kronig et al., "Placebo-controlled, Multicenter Study of Sertraline Treatment for Obsessive-Compulsive Disorder," *Journal of Clinical Psychopharmacology* 19 (1999): 172–176.

54. O. K. Memmen, J. M. Perel, G. Randolph, et al., "Sertraline and Norsertraline Levels in Three Breastfed Infants," *Journal of Clinical Psychiatry* 58 (1997): 100–103.

55. M. E. Moretti et al., "Fluoxetine and Its Effects on the Nursing Infant: A Prospective Cohort Study," *Clinical Pharmacology and Therapeutics* 65 (1999): 141.

56. Z. N. Stowe et al., "Paroxetine in Human Breast Milk and Nursing Infants," *American Journal of Psychiatry* 157 (2000): 185–189.

57. N. A. Kulin et al., "Pregnancy Outcome Following Maternal Use of the New Selective Serotonin Reuptake Inhibitors: A Prospective Controlled Multicenter Study," *Journal of the American Medical Association* 279 (1998): 609–610.

58. R. D. Marshall et al., "An Open Trial of Paroxetine in Patients with Noncombat-related, Chronic Posttraumatic Stress Disorder," *Journal of Clinical Psychopharmacology* 18 (1998): 10–18.

59. N. S. Gunasekara, S. Noble, and P. Benfield, "Paroxetine: An Update of its Pharmacology and Therapeutic Use in Depression and a Review of Its Use in Other Disorders," *Drugs* 55 (1998): 85–120.

60. L. M. Koran et al., "Fluvoxamine Versus Clomipramine for Obsessive-Compulsive Disorder: A Double-blind Comparison," *Journal of Clinical Psychopharmacology* 16 (1996): 121–129.

61. M. B. Stein et al., "Fluvoxamine Treatment of Social Phobia (Social Anxiety Disorder): A Double-blind, Placebo-Controlled Study," *American Journal of Psychiatry* 156 (1999): 756–760.

62. D. J. Greenblatt,"Drug Interactions with Newer Antidepressants: Role of Human Cytochromes P450s," *Journal of Clinical Psychiatry* 59 (1998): 19–27.

63. L. Ekselius, L. von Knorring, and G. Eberhard, "A Double-blind Multicenter Trial Comparing Sertraline and Citalopram in Patients with Major Depression Treated in General Practice," *International Clinical Psychopharmacology* 12 (1997): 323–331.

64. "Citalopram for Depression," *Medical Letter on Drugs and Therapeutics* 40 (Dec. 4, 1998): 113–114.

65. C. L. DeVane and F. R. Sallee, "Serotonin-selective Reuptake Inhibitors in Child and Adolescent Psychopharmacology: A Review of Published Experience," *Journal of Clinical Psychiatry* 57 (1996): 55–66.

66. H. L. Leonard, J. March, K. C. Rickler, and A. J. Allen, "Pharmacology of the Selective Serotonin Reuptake Inhibitors in Children and Adolescents," *Journal of the American Academy of Child and Adolescent Psychiatry* 36 (1997): 725–736.

67. D. R. Rosenberg et al., "Paroxetine Open-label Treatment of Pediatric Outpatients with Obsessive-Compulsive Disorder," *Journal of the American Academy of Child and Adolescent Psychiatry* 38 (1999): 1180–1185.

68. B. Birmaher et al., "Childhood and Adolescent Depression: A Review of the Past Ten Years, Part II," *Journal of the American Academy of Child and Adolescent Psychiatry* 35 (1996): 1575–1583.

69. C. W. Popper, "Balancing Knowledge and Judgment," *Child and Adolescent Psychiatry Clinics of North America* 4 (1995): 483–513.

70. J. M. Zito et al., "Trends in the Prescribing of Psychotropic Medications to Preschoolers," *Journal of the American Medical Association* 283 (2000): 1025–1030.

71. J. T. Coyle, "Psychotropic Drug Use in Very Young Children," *Journal of the American Medical Association* 283 (2000): 1059–1060.

72. J. C. Gillin et al., "A Comparison of Nefazodone and Fluoxetine on Mood and on Objective, Subjective, and Clinician-rated Measures of Sleep in Depressed Patients: A Double-blind, Eight-week Clinical Trial," *Journal of Clinical Psychiatry* 58 (1997): 185–192.

73. J. M. Zajecka, "The Effect of Nefazodone on Comorbid Anxiety Symptoms Associated with Depression: Experience in Family Practice and Psychiatric Outpatient Settings," *Journal of Clinical Psychiatry* 57, Suppl. 2 (1996): 10–14.

74. T. E. Wilens, T. J. Spencer, J. Biederman, and D. Schleifer, "Case Study: Nefazodone for Juvenile Mood Disorders," *Journal of the American Academy of Child and Adolescent Psychiatry* 36 (1997): 481–485.

75. R. Davis, R. Whittington, and H. M. Bryson, "Nefazodone: A Review of Its Pharmacology and Clinical Efficacy in the Management of Major Depression," *Drugs* 53 (1997): 608–636.

75A. P. P. Roy-Byrne et al., "Nefazodone Treatment of Major Depression in Alcohol-Dependent Patients: A Double-Blind, Placebo-Controlled Trial," *Journal of Clinical Psychopharmacology* 20 (2000): 129–136.

75B. L. L. Davis et al., "Nefazodone Treatment for Chronic Posttraumatic Stress Disorder: An Open Trial," *Journal of Clinical Psychopharmacology* 20 (2000): 159–164.

75C. S. Zisook et al., "Nefazodone in Patients with Treatment-Refractory Posttraumatic Stress Disorder," *Journal of Clinical Psychiatry* 61 (2000): 203–208.

76. D. P. Wheatley et al., "Mirtazapine: Efficacy and Tolerability in Comparison with Fluoxetine in Patients with Moderate to Severe Major Depressive Disorder," *Journal of Clinical Psychiatry* 59 (1998): 306–312.

77. S. Kasper, "Treatment Options in Severe Depression," in "Controversies in the Diagnosis and Treatment of Severe Depression," *Journal of Clinical Psychiatry* 57 (1996): 554–561 (556–558).

78. K. J. Holm and A. Markham, "Mirtazapine: A Review of Its Use in Major Depression," *Drugs* 57 (1999): 607–631.

79. D. M. Gardner, K. I. Shulman, S. E. Walker, and S. Tailor, "The Making of a User-friendly MAOI Diet," *Journal of Clinical Psychiatry* 57 (1996): 99–104.

80. A. C. Swann et al., "Desipramine Versus Phenelzine in Recurrent Unipolar Depression: Clinical Characteristics and Treatment Response," *Journal of Clinical Psychopharmacology* 17 (1997): 78–83.

81. R. I. Shader and D. J. Greenblatt, "The Reappearance of a Monoamine Oxidase Inhibitor (Isocarboxazid)," *Journal of Clinical Psychopharmacology* 19 (1999): 105–106.

82. B. Fulton and P. Benfield, "Moclobemide: An Update of Its Pharmacological Properties," *Drugs* 52 (1996): 450–474.

83. M. Fava et al., "Open Study of the Catechol-o-methyltransferase Inhibitor Tolcapone in Major Depressive Disorder," *Journal of Clinical Psychopharmacology* 19 (1999): 329–335.

84. M. Versiani et al., "Reboxetine, a Unique Selective NRI, Prevents Relapse and Recurrence in Long-Term Treatment of Major Depressive Disorder," *Journal of Clinical Psychiatry* 60 (1999): 400–406.

85. M. Versiani, M. Amin and G. Chouinard, "Double-Blind, Placebo-Controlled Study with Reboxetine in Inpatients with Severe Major Depressive Disorder," *Journal of Clinical Psychopharmacology* 20 (2000): 28–34.

86. J. Massana, H. J. Moller, G. D. Burrows, and R.M. Montenegro, "Reboxetine: A Double-blind Comparison with Fluoxetine in Major Depressive Disorder," *International Clinical Psychopharmacology* 14 (1999): 73–80.

87. Symposium, "The Role of Norepinephrine in the Treatment of Depression," *Journal of Clinical Psychiatry* 60 (1999): 623–631.

88. Y. D. Lapierre et al., "A Canadian Multicenter Study of Three Fixed Doses of Controlled-release Ipsapirone in Outpatients with Moderate to Severe Major Depression," *Journal of Clinical Psychopharmacology* 18 (1998): 268–273.

89. M. Landen et al., "A Randomized, Double-blind, Placebo-controlled Trial of Buspirone in Combination with an SSRI in Patients with Treatment-refractory Depression," *Journal of Clinical Psychiatry* 59 (1998): 664–668.

90. M. Bloch et al., "Dehydroepiandrosterone Treatment of Midlife Dysthymia," *Biological Psychiatry* 45 (1999): 1533–1541.

91. O. M. Wolkowitz et al., "Double-blind Treatment of Major Depression with Dehydroepiandrosterone," *American Journal of Psychiatry* 156 (1999): 646–649.

92. E. A. Young, "DHEA: Mood, Memory, and Aging," *Biological Psychiatry* 45 (1999): 1531–1532.

93. "SAMe for Depression," *The Medical Letter* 41 (November 5, 1999): 107–108.

Chapter 16

Drugs Used to Treat Bipolar Disorder

Bipolar disorder (manic-depressive disorder) is characterized by recurrent episodes of mania and depression. The disorder requires therapeutic intervention when the mood changes are severe enough to disrupt the patient's life or the lives of people associated with the patient. It is a major medical disorder, occurring in up to 4 percent of the population; a patient is defined as having suffered at least one manic, hypomanic, or mixed episode. If the episode was severe enough to require hospitalization or to seriously interfere with normal functioning, the disorder is classified as bipolar I; if the manic episode was less severe, the disorder is classified as bipolar II. *Cyclothymia* is defined as recurrent mood swings between depression and elation but of lower severity than bipolar II. Cyclothymia is therefore a part of a continuum from normal to bipolar and can be termed a bipolar spectrum disorder.[1]

Bipolar patients who have had four illness episodes in a 12-month period are termed "rapid cyclers." Rapid cycling may not be permanent; it may appear and disappear during the course of the illness:

> Bipolar I disorder can lead to the destruction of a patient's livelihood, marriage, social relationships, or even life. The course of the illness is usually episodic, with periods of mania and/or depression alternating with intervening well periods of varying duration. The great majority of patients experience several episodes during the course of their lives and the risk of recurrence remains ever present.[1]

A person who experiences onset of bipolar disorder at age 25 and remains untreated will lose about 9 years of life, 14 years of effective activity, and 12 years of normal health. It is estimated that one of every four or five untreated or inadequately treated patients commits suicide during the course of the illness. An increase in deaths secondary to accidents or intercurrent illnesses (especially substance abuse) also contributes to the greater mortality rate seen in this disorder. Unfortunately, epidemiological studies have indicated that only one-third of bipolar patients are in active treatment despite the availability of effective therapies. It is generally agreed that a patient who exhibits at least two episodes of mania is a candidate for long-term (i.e., lifetime) treatment with an antimanic (mood stabilizing) drug.

A patient with bipolar disorder can present initially with either mania or depression. If the patient presents with depression, reduction of depressive symptoms may require the temporary co-administration of an antidepressant drug.[2] If the patient presents in a manic state, the initial goal is to reduce manic symptoms, a situation that may require either a benzodiazepine or an antipsychotic drug such as olanzapine (Zyprexa). Successful long-term management of bipolar disorder is best accomplished by use of a mood stabilizer, the subject of this chapter. The classic mood stabilizer is lithium. In refractory cases, several other drugs are available, including any of four antiepileptic drugs: carbamazepine (Tegretol), valproic acid (Depakote), gabapentin (Neurontin), and lamotrigine (Lamictal).

In 1996, the American Psychiatric Association published a practice guideline for the treatment of patients with bipolar disorder.[3] In 1997, the American Academy of Child and Adolescent Psychiatry published practice parameters for the assessment and treatment of children and adolescents with bipolar disorder.[4]

The major objectives of pharmacologic intervention are to treat acute episodes of mania and to reduce the frequency of recurrence of these episodes. Additional goals of therapy are to maintain compliance with therapy, treat accompanying depression, psychosis, and substance abuse, and institute psychosocial treatments appropriate to the patient's needs.[*]

Lithium

Lithium has historically been the most recommended drug for treating bipolar disorder and reducing its rate of relapse.[†] Unfortunately, its

---

[*]A recent issue of *The Psychiatric Clinics of North America* discusses changing views of bipolar illness, its variations, age spectrum, and psychosocial interventions ("Bipolarity: Beyond Classic Mania," H. S. Akisal, guest editor), Vol. 22, number 3, Sept., 1999).

[†]For a historical overview of lithium therapy and commentaries on lithium, see four related letters by M. Schou, by D. J. Kupfer and E. Frank, by S. Gershon and J. C. Soares, and by M. J. Gitlin and L. L. Altshuler in *Archives of General Psychiatry* 54 (1997): 9–23.

clinical effectiveness is less than that predicted by clinical trials; relapse often occurs because of patient noncompliance with therapy. Therefore, the pharmacology of lithium and reasons for patient noncompliance with lithium therapy must be clearly understood and alternative drug therapies closely examined.

Lithium (Li+) is the lightest of the alkali metals (Figure 16.1) and shares some characteristics with sodium (Na+). In nature, lithium is abundant in some alkaline mineral spring waters. Devoid of psychotropic effects in normal individuals, lithium is effective in treating 60 to 80 percent of acute hypomanic and manic episodes, although in recent years, the limitations, side effects, relapse, and the compliance issues associated with its use have become increasingly appreciated.

History

Lithium was used in the 1920s as a sedative-hypnotic compound and as an anticonvulsant drug. During the late 1940s, lithium chloride was employed as a salt substitute for patients with heart disease. Wide use for this purpose resulted in cases of severe toxicity and death, causing medicine to abandon use of the drug. In 1949, however, an Australian scientist (J. Cade) noted that when lithium was administered to guinea pigs, the animals became lethargic. Taking an intuitive leap, Cade administered lithium to patients with acute mania, noting somewhat remarkable improvement. However, because of the earlier problems with lithium as a salt substitute, the medical community took more than 20 years to accept this agent as an effective treatment for mania. Clinical research in the 1970s found lithium to be clearly superior to placebo in the prophylaxis of bipolar disorder; fewer than a third of lithium-treated patients relapsed, compared with 80 percent of placebo-treated patients.

Today, lithium's efficacy is again being questioned. On the one hand, Maj and co-workers[5] conclude that long-term studies are reporting

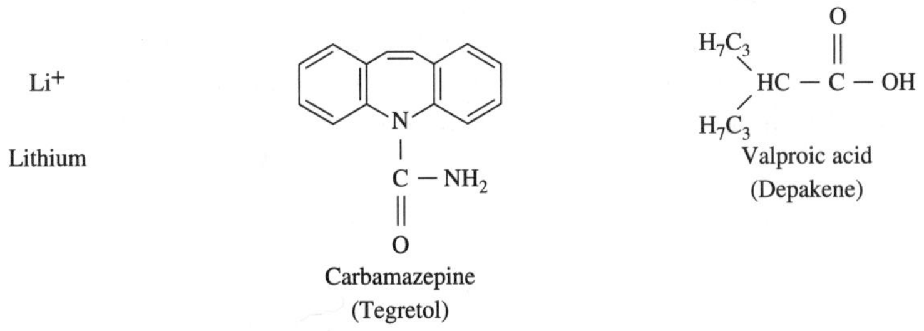

FIGURE 16.1 Drugs used in the treatment of bipolar disorder. Structures of other anticonvulsants used in bipolar disorder are shown in Figure 5.6.

poorer results than expected; 28 percent of patients discontinue the drug, 38 percent take the drug but experience recurrences of the disorder, and only 23 percent taking the drug did not have recurrent episodes.[5] On the other hand, Baldessarini and Tondo[6] still recommend lithium as a drug of first choice for both the treatment of acute manic attacks and the long-term management of bipolar disorder:

> We suggest that the growing American urge to abandon lithium maintenance therapy as ineffective, excessively toxic, or complicated is unwarranted. No other proposed mood-stabilizing treatment has such substantial research evidence of long-term efficacy in both type I and type II bipolar disorders, as well as yielding a substantial reduction of mortality risk.

Pharmacokinetics

Lithium is absorbed rapidly and completely when it is administered orally. Peak blood levels are reached within 3 hours, complete absorption by 8 hours. The therapeutic efficacy of lithium is directly correlated to its level in the blood. Lithium crosses the blood-brain barrier slowly and incompletely. There also can be a twofold variation in the concentration of lithium in the brain when compared with its concentration in plasma.[7] The clinical significance of this observation is unclear.

Lithium is not metabolized before excretion; most is excreted unchanged by the kidneys, with only small amounts excreted through the skin. About half an oral dose is excreted within 18 to 24 hours and the rest (which represents the amount of lithium that is taken up by body's cells) is excreted over the next 1 to 2 weeks. Thus, when therapy is initiated, lithium accumulates slowly over about 2 weeks until a steady state is reached. With this long half-life, once-daily dosage is appropriate for many individuals.

The therapeutic dose of lithium is determined by closely monitoring blood levels of the drug. Lithium has a very narrow therapeutic range, below which the drug fails to have therapeutic effect and above which side effects and toxicity dominate. In the 1980s and early 1990s, a therapeutic goal was to maintain a plasma level of lithium between 0.75 to 1.0 milliequivalents per liter (mEq/L) of blood, because toxicity becomes more severe at levels above 2 mEq/L. Today, levels of about 0.5 to 0.7 mEq/L are recommended,[8] although many patients do not receive appropriate testing.[9]

> A level much below this is likely to be associated with a greater likelihood of relapse, while a higher one is frequently accompanied by more adverse effects, leading to an increased risk of noncompliance.[1]

Because lithium closely resembles table salt, when a patient lowers his or her salt intake or loses excessive amounts of salt (such as through sweating), lithium blood levels rise and intoxication may inadvertently follow. Consequently, patients taking lithium should avoid marked changes in sodium intake or excretion.

Pharmacodynamics

In therapeutic concentrations, lithium has almost no discernible psychotropic effect in normal persons. It does not induce sedation, depression, or euphoria, which differentiates it from other psychoactive drugs. Indeed, it exhibits few effects on the brain other than its specific action on mania. The mechanism through which lithium exerts its antimanic effect is a matter of speculation and ongoing research.[10] A basic problem is to explain how a simple ion could exert complex effects on multiple transmitter systems and, in particular, have mood-stabilizing effects in the treatment of both manic and depressive aspects of bipolar illness. Lithium has been shown to affect nerve membranes, multiple receptor systems, and intracellular second-messenger impulse transduction systems. The latter effect would reduce a neuron's responsiveness to synaptic input, resulting in a membrane-stabilizing effect. In 1996, these membrane-stabilizing effects were described in more detail;[11,12] one study concluded:

> Signal transduction pathways are targets for the actions of mood stabilizing agents; given their key roles in the amplification and integration of signals in the central nervous system, these findings have clear implications not only for research into the etiology/pathophysiology of manic-depressive illness, but also for the development of innovative treatment strategies.[12]

In 1999, Ikonomov and Manji[10] extended this conclusion to include a drug-induced alteration in the expression of specific genes in critical neuronal circuits. Thus, lithium has the potential to regulate CNS gene expression, stabilizing neurons through "underappreciated neurotrophic/neuroprotective effects" with associated changes in the expression of multiple genes. Massot and colleagues[13] described a specific interaction of lithium with serotonin 5-HT$_{1B}$ receptors, an action that can account at least for lithium's efficacy against the negative component of bipolar disorder.

Side Effects and Toxicity

Because lithium has an extremely narrow therapeutic range, blood levels of the drug must be closely monitored. The occurrence and intensity of side effects are, in most cases, directly related to plasma concentrations of lithium. When levels in plasma fall below 0.5 to 0.6 mEq/L, side effects are usually minimal; they become much more bothersome at levels of 1.0 mEq/L or higher. At levels above 2.0 mEq/L, toxicity becomes severe and potentially fatal.

The main toxic effects involve the gastrointestinal tract, the kidneys, the thyroid, the cardiovascular system, the skin, and the nervous system. At plasma levels of 1.5 to 2.0 mEq/L (and sometimes at lower levels), most reactions involve the gastrointestinal tract, resulting in nausea, vomiting, diarrhea, and abdominal pain. Neurological side effects commonly seen at this level of lithium include a slight tremor, lethargy, impaired concentration, dizziness, slurred speech, ataxia, muscle weakness, and nystagmus. Difficulty with memory is another frequent complaint, as is weight gain with continued treatment. In long-term therapy, "up to 30 percent of patients became frankly obese, a prevalence of obesity three times greater than in the general population."[1] Elmslie and co-workers[14] recently reviewed the subject of drug-induced obesity in treating bipolar illness.

With long-term lithium therapy, the thyroid may become enlarged; rashes or some other kind of skin eruption may occur. In addition, about 60 percent of patients taking lithium experience an increase in urine output (due to an impairment of renal concentrating ability), along with increased thirst and water intake. Although kidney function should be assessed periodically, permanent damage is rare.

Chronic lithium therapy is accompanied by adverse effects on memory and cognitive functioning. Some researchers report improvements in motor performance, cognition, and creative ability after lithium withdrawal, implying detrimental effects of lithium in these areas during drug therapy.[15] Hypotheses have been offered to explain these deficits; however, compensatory mechanisms appear to develop, preventing many of the severe memory impairments that can occur during lithium treatment.[16]

At plasma levels of lithium above 2.0 mEq/L, more severe side effects include fatigue, muscle weakness, slurred speech, and worsening tremors. Thyroid gland function becomes depressed, and the thyroid gland may enlarge further, resulting in goiter. Muscle fasciculations, increased reflexes, abnormal motor movements, and even seizures, psychosis, and stupor may occur. At plasma levels exceeding 2.5 mEq/L, toxic effects include muscle rigidity, coma, renal failure, cardiac arrhythmias, and death.

Treatment of poisoning or overdosage is nonspecific; there is no antidote to lithium. Usually drug administration is halted and sodium-containing fluids are infused immediately. If toxic signs are serious, hemodialysis, gastric lavage, diuretic therapy, antiepileptic medication, and other supports may be urgently needed. Complete recovery from intoxication may be prolonged, with full renal and neurological recovery taking weeks or months.

Lithium possesses a degree of teratogenic potential, especially to the heart of the developing fetus.[17] In general, lithium is not advised during pregnancy, particularly in the first trimester, as the risk of fetal malformation involving the cardiovascular system is increased. If mood stabilization treatment is necessary during pregnancy, other agents should be employed if possible. When a pregnant woman is on lithium therapy, the drug should be discontinued for several days before delivery, because the newborn will have difficulty excreting the drug. On the other hand, restarting lithium within 24 hours of delivery is important to reduce the risk of relapse. Viguera and co-workers[18] addressed this issue in a study of 42 pregnant and 59 nonpregnant females with bipolar disorder. Discontinuation of lithium during pregnancy was followed by a recurrence rate similar to that seen in nonpregnant females. However, following delivery, postpartum females demonstrated a threefold increase in the rate of recurrence compared with that in nonpregnant females. The authors concluded:

> Treatment planning for potentially pregnant women with bipolar disorder should consider the relative risks of fetal exposure to mood stabilizers versus the high recurrence risks after discontinuing lithium.

Noncompliance

In clinical use, up to 50 percent of patients taking lithium stop taking the drug against medical advice. Noncompliance is associated with significant morbidity, recurrent manic episodes, and greatly increased suicide risk.[19] It is felt that the illness course after stopping lithium treatment can actually be worse than would be predicted from the natural history of bipolar disease. Thus, treatment of only a few years followed by drug withdrawal might "actually be harmful to bipolar patients,"[20] although "discontinuation of lithium therapy does not appear to result in treatment resistance when therapy is resumed."[21]

Noncompliance seems to result largely from intolerance of side effects, particularly memory impairment and cognitive slowing, weight gain, and the subjective feeling of reduced energy and productivity.[1] Other reasons include missing the manic "highs," feelings that the disorder has resolved and the drug is unnecessary, and feelings of stigmatism of chronic illness. Psychological support, family therapy, and other treatments and encouragements can help the patient stay on the drug.

Baldessarini and co-workers[19] studied the rate of relapse following acute and gradual withdrawal of lithium. Although they concluded that gradual withdrawal reduced early relapse, the great majority of patients under either protocol did relapse, especially those classified as bipolar I (Figure 16.2). This finding appears to reinforce the notion that once mood stabilization therapy is started, it may be a lifelong necessity.

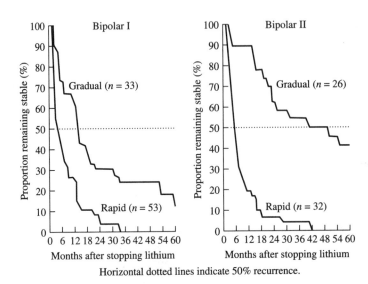

FIGURE 16.2 Proportion of bipolar I patients (*left*) and bipolar II patients (*right*) who remained stable after stopping lithium therapy either rapidly (*lower lines*) or gradually (*upper lines*). [From Baldessarini et al.[19]]

In another study, the Baldessarini group[22] reported that lithium therapy in bipolar patients reduced suicidal behaviors by 77 percent. Unfortunately, when patients stopped taking lithium, the rate of suicide attempts increased fourteenfold, and the rate of completed suicides was increased thirteenfold. This data reinforces the necessity for long-term, even lifelong therapy once the decision is made to initiate drug therapy. It is currently not known whether or not this same decision-making process applies to other antimanic drugs.

Combination Therapy

Peselow and co-workers[23] first conjectured that combination therapy (lithium plus an antiepileptic drug) might afford both greater therapeutic efficacy and greater protection against relapse than lithium therapy alone. One example of the increased effectiveness achieved with combination therapy (in the Peselow study, lithium plus carbamazepine) is shown in Figure 16.3. Many additional studies have supported this claim, and combination therapy has become the rule rather than the exception.[24-26]

Substance Abuse

It is disturbing to note that more than 55 percent of bipolar patients have a history of substance abuse.[27] Substances involved include

ANTICONVULSANTS **469**

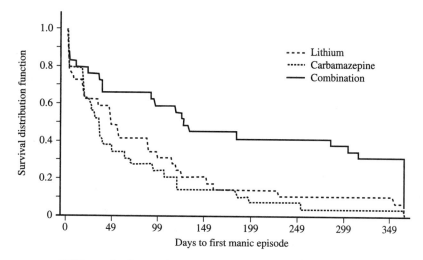

*Lithium and carbamazepine mean survival time = 179.3 days, lithium mean
survival time = 89.8 days, and carbamazepine mean survival time = 66.2 days.

FIGURE 16.3 Mean time to first recurrent manic episode in 29 patients to whom
either lithium (*dashed line*), carbamazepine (*dotted line*), or a combination of both
drugs (*black line*). Lithium and carbamazepine combination time to first recurrence was
180 days; lithium time to first recurrence was 90 days; carbamazepine time to
recurrence was 66 days. Thus, the rank order of efficacy was (1) combination therapy,
(2) lithium monotherapy, and (3) carbamazepine monotherapy. [From Denicoff et al.[25]]

alcohol (82 percent), cocaine (30 percent), marijuana (29 percent),
sedatives or amphetamines (21 percent), and opioid (13 percent).[28] In
some individuals, substance abuse predated the first bipolar episode,
and in others the abuse postdated the affective diagnosis.[29] Perhaps in
both instances, it may, at least initially, represent an attempt at self-
medication for the symptoms accompanying the affective disorder.
Regardless, this comorbidity of disease complicates treatment and outcomes[28] and needs to be recognized and addressed during treatment.

In children and adolescents, bipolar disorder (and its close correlates of aggressive and explosive behaviors) is becoming increasingly
recognized,[4] along with the associated substance abuse problems.
Early recognition of bipolar disorder and early treatment with antimanic drugs can reduce the severity of both disorders.[30,31]

Anticonvulsants

Heterogeneity does exist within bipolar disorder. Persons with mania differ in family history of affective illness, their age at the onset of illness,

sex, and organic cause and course of the illness. In addition, since many individuals with explosive behavioral disorders respond to antimanic drugs, such disorders may also represent a different spectrum of bipolar disorder. Also, since several antimanic drugs were originally developed as antiepileptic drugs, it is interesting to speculate whether there is a relationship between epilepsy, bipolar disorder, and explosive behavioral disorders.

As in all areas of psychopharmacology, not all individuals with a disorder respond identically—or at all—to a single drug. About 40 percent of bipolar patients either are resistant to lithium treatment or develop side effects that limit its effectiveness. Only about 60 percent to 70 percent of patients with bipolar disorder can be adequately controlled on lithium alone (for maintenance/prevention therapy), and the drug is even less effective in controlling episodes of acute or rapid cycling mania. Therefore, there is a need for alternative agents, effective in patients for whom lithium is inadequate, patients who are noncompliant with lithium therapy, and patients who are intolerant of lithium's side effects.[32]

Carbamazepine

Studies conducted in the early 1990s indicated that carbamazepine (Tegretol; Figure 16.1) might be as effective as lithium in preventing the recurrence of mania. In addition, some patients who did not respond adequately to either lithium or carbamazepine alone responded to the two drugs used together. Also, carbamazepine was superior to lithium in correcting rapid-cycling bipolar disorder, a condition for which lithium is quite ineffective.

Dardennes and co-workers[33] reviewed the comparative studies of lithium and carbamazepine and concluded that the therapeutic efficacy of carbamazepine was more questionable than earlier thought. This pessimistic view of carbamazepine was challenged by Silverstone and Romans.[1] Current algorithms generally regard carbamazepine as a second-line treatment for mania, used primarily in combination with lithium.[25] Greil and co-workers[34] concluded that while "lithium seems to be superior to carbamazepine in treating classical bipolar cases, . . . patients with nonclassical features might profit more from prophylaxis with carbamazepine, which seems to have a broader spectrum of activity."

It is important to note that patients who fail to respond to carbamazepine often have taken an amount of the drug that is inadequate in plasma. There is correlation between therapeutic effectiveness and the plasma level of the drug; the therapeutic level of carbamazepine is estimated to be between 5 and 10 micrograms per milliliter,[35] the same as the range for antiepileptic effectiveness.

Adverse effects of carbamazepine include gastrointestinal upset, sedation, ataxia, visual disturbances, and dermatological reactions. Carbamazepine may also have modest detrimental effects on cognitive functioning, but any negative effect on higher-order cognitive functioning appears rather limited.[36] Nevertheless, some patients may be particularly sensitive to the cognitive side effects of the drug. More serious reactions involve the blood, ranging from a relatively benign reduction in white blood cell count (leukopenia) to, on rare occasions, severe aplastic anemia. For this reason blood should be analyzed periodically.

Drug interactions involving carbamazepine are common and result from drug-induced stimulation of drug-metabolizing enzymes (especially CYP-3A4) in the liver.[37] As a result, tolerance to the drug develops and more drug is needed to maintain a therapeutic blood level; this tolerance also extends to other drugs metabolized by the same enzyme family.

Because carbamazepine is potentially teratogenic (it produces a neural tube defect in 1 percent of offspring[38]), it should not be administered during pregnancy if possible. It is thought that supplemental administration of folic acid may reduce the risk in pregnant women who decide to continue carbamazepine during pregnancy.

Woolston[39] studied carbamazepine in a small case series of adolescents with juvenile-onset bipolar I disorder. He noted the drug to be both safe and effective therapy for this disorder, concluding that more controlled studies appear warranted.

Valproic Acid

Valproate (valproic acid, divalproex, Depakene, Depakote; Figure 16.1) is the second antiepileptic drug systematically studied for use in bipolar illness. Indeed, from 1994 to 1996, the use of valproate to treat bipolar disease more than doubled, and the progression continues today: valproate is now the most widely used antimanic drug. It is felt that valproate acts by augmenting the postsynaptic action of GABA at its receptors, although the mechanisms through which this is accomplished are complicated:

> Valproate increases GABA synthesis and release and thereby potentiates GABAergic functions in some brain regions . . . Furthermore, valproate seems to reduce the release of the epileptogenic amino acid gamma-hydroxybutyric acid and to attenuate neuronal excitation induced by NMDA-type glutamate receptors. In addition to effects on amino acidergic neurotransmission, valproate exerts direct effects on excitable membranes, although the importance of this action is equivocal."[40]

Chen and co-workers[41] studied the effects of valproate on gene expression in vitro and concluded that valproate-induced mediation of gene expression in critical brain circuits may underlie its antiepileptic, antimanic, and antiaggression effectiveness.

Valproate is particularly effective in the treatment of acute mania, mixed states, schizo-affective disorder, and rapid-cycling bipolar disorder.[42] It is as effective as and less toxic than lithium when used in low doses as an alternative to lithium in the treatment of cyclothymia.[43] It is also more effective than lithium in patients with comorbid depression.[44] Recently, the added efficacy of valproate and antipsychotics in reducing acute mania was demonstrated.[45]

In acute mania in lithium-resistant patients, valproate therapy results in positive response rates of up to 71 percent of patients. Also, the therapeutic combination of valproate and lithium may provide an effective treatment for both bipolar I and rapid-cycling bipolar disorders.[24] Therapeutic blood levels of valproate range between 50 and 100 micrograms per milliliter. Grunze and co-workers[46] describe an intravenous loading technique with valproate to control acute mania; this was the first reported use of an intravenously administered antimanic drug. It overcomes the slow (3- to 10-day) period normally required to control manic symptoms with orally administered drug. It may also reduce the need for the use of benzodiazepine sedatives and phenothiazine or butyrophenone antipsychotics to control the manic behavior until the mood stabilizer cuts in. Intravenous valproate loading was also effective in patients formerly unresponsive to orally administered valproate.

Side effects associated with valproate include GI upset, sedation, lethargy, hand tremor, alopecia (loss of hair), and some metabolic changes in the liver. In females starting valproate before the age of 20 years, the drug has been associated with an 8 percent prevalence of marked obesity, polycystic ovaries, and markedly increased levels of serum androgens (increased testosterone levels).[47] Valproate may be slightly more detrimental to cognitive function than is carbamazepine. Like lithium and carbamazepine, valproate can be teratogenic, and caution must be exercised in using this agent in women who might become pregnant during drug therapy.[1] Unlike lithium, little valproate is secreted in breast milk.[48] Valproate therefore may be a preferred drug for use by nursing mothers who must take an antimanic drug.

In addition to its uses as an antiepileptic and an antimanic drug, valproate has been used in the treatment of borderline personality disorder and disorders associated with behavioral dyscontrol (agitation, aggression, temper outbursts).[31] Davis and co-workers[49] reviewed the psychiatric use of valproate and concluded: "Valproate shows the most promising efficacy in treating mood and anxiety disorders, with possible efficacy in the treatment of agitation and impulsive aggression, and less convincing therapeutic response in treating psychosis and alcohol withdrawal or dependence." Furthermore, "Valproate is useful in reducing aggression, anxiety, irritability, and agitation in patients with personality disorders." It may be effective in the treatment of depression, but data are currently insufficient to draw conclusions. The same holds true for use in treating posttraumatic stress disorder, panic disorder, and borderline personality disorder.

Gabapentin

The efficacy in bipolar disorder of other anticonvulsants has been investigated. Two anticonvulsants (gabapentin and lamotrigine) are now being used clinically, and others (topiramate and tiagabine) are under evaluation.

Gabapentin (Neurontin; Figure 16.1) was introduced in the United States in 1993 for use as an anticonvulsant. In addition to this use, it is used "off label" (without formal FDA approval) for the treatment of bipolar disorder, anxiety disorders, behavioral dyscontrol disorders, and substance dependency disorders.[50] Its use in bipolar disorder was based on the fact that it is a GABA analogue and may have some effects on GABA neurotransmission.[51] In addition, it has an excellent pharmacokinetic profile: it is not bound to plasma proteins (Chapter 1), is not metabolized, is excreted unchanged through the kidneys, and has few pharmacokinetic drug interactions.[51] Its elimination half-life is 5 to 7 hours. Gabapentin is absorbed by a saturable active transport mechanism from intestine to plasma, so doses to only 1500 mg can be given at any one time. Gabapentin does not alter the kinetics of lithium, implying that it may turn out to be an excellent choice for combination therapy with lithium (Figure 16.4).[52]

Until 1999, only case reports had been published concerning the efficacy of gabapentin. In 1999, McElroy and co-workers[51] conducted an open trial in nine patients unresponsive to lithium therapy. Doses were advanced to as much as 4800 mg/day, usually in divided doses. Of the nine patients studied, seven were moderately or markedly improved after one month of treatment and an eighth was improved at 3 months. Side effects were tolerable, consisting of sleepiness, dizziness, ataxia, nystagmus, and double vision. In other case reports, therapeutic doses averaged about 600 mg/day, but some patients required doses of up to 5000 mg/day. Gabapentin has been inadequately studied in either pregnant or breast-feeding females.

No doubt much will be written about gabapentin, and it is likely that it will emerge as a drug of choice for augmentation of lithium therapy as well as a single-drug therapy for several other disorders. For example, Pande and co-workers[53] noted positive results of gabapentin on 69 patients with social phobia. Side effects included dizziness, dry mouth, somnolence, nausea, flatulence, and reduced libido. Preliminary data with gabapentin indicate that it improves depression and anxiety in female patients with borderline personality disorder. Finally, gabapentin (as well as lamotrigine and carbamazepine) holds a special place for the treatment of certain pain states, including peripheral neuropathy (as occurs with diabetes), sympathetic dystrophy

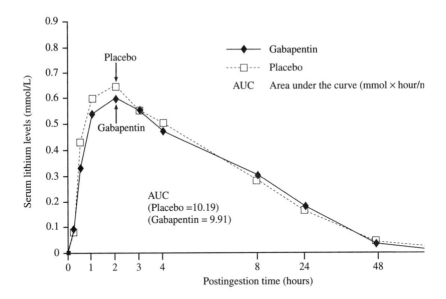

FIGURE 16.4 Mean plasma concentrations over time following administration of lithium plus placebo (*dashed line*) or lithium plus gabapentin (*solid line*). Note that gabapentin does not affect the plasma time-concentration pharmacokinetics of lithium. [From Frye et al.[52]]

(as follows peripheral nerve injury), post-radiation myopathy, phantom limb pain, and other difficult-to-treat pain syndromes.[54,55] Such analgesic action occurs secondary to a direct spinal cord action of gabapentin on pain-processing circuits involving glutamate and substance P neurotransmission.[55,56]

At this time, the manufacturer of gabapentin is not seeking FDA approval for indication for use in bipolar disorder. Instead, the manufacturer is developing *pregabalin*, which is essentially an "improved" gabapentin molecule. Clinical trials of pregabalin are underway and approval may be sought for use in pain, epilepsy, and psychiatric disorders.

Lamotrigine

Several recent clinical studies have reported the effectiveness of the anticonvulsant drug lamotrigine (Lamictal; Figure 16.1) as a treatment for bipolar disorder (Figure 16.5).[57–59] Lamotrigine has also been reported to be effective in the treatment of borderline personality disorder,[60] post-traumatic stress disorder, and schizoaffective disorder.

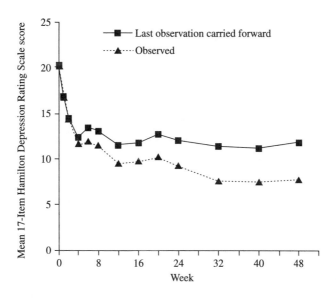

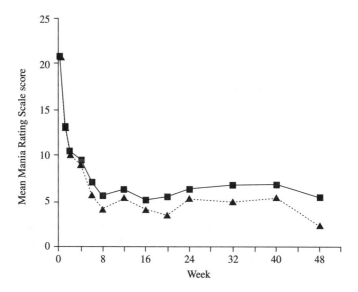

FIGURE 16.5 *Top:* Mean scores on the Hamilton Depression Rating Scale (HDRS) for the reduction in depression in 40 patients with bipolar disorder who presented with depression. Among them, 48 percent exhibited a marked response and 20 percent exhibited a moderate response to lamotrigine as measured by the HDRS. *Bottom:* Mean scores on the Mania Rating Scale of 31 patients with bipolar disorder presenting in hypomanic, manic, or mixed states during lamotrigine treatment. Of the patients, 81 percent exhibited a marked response and 3 percent exhibited a moderate response on the mania rating scale. [From Calabrese et al.[57]]

Following oral administration, lamotrigine is rapidly and completely absorbed, with little first-pass metabolism. Ninety-eight percent of administered drug reaches plasma. Peak plasma concentrations occur in 1 to 5 hours, and it is about 55 percent protein bound. Lamotrigine is metabolized before excretion and its half-life is about 26 hours.

While full understanding of the action of lamotrigine is unclear, the drug is known to inhibit the release of the excitatory neurotransmitter glutamate in the cortex and hippocampus, an action that accounts for antiepileptic, antimanic, and analgesic actions of the drug.[61,62] It therefore inhibits neuronal excitability and modifies synaptic plasticity.

Lamotrigine appears to be more of an activating drug than is gabapentin. Side effects include dizziness, tremor, somnolence, headache, nausea, and rash. The most serious of these is rash, which occurs in about 10 percent of patients and can be so severe that hospitalization is necessary; rash has been fatal in some cases. Adolescents may be more prone to serious rashes, so lamotrigine probably should be withheld in this population of patients. Despite this toxicity, the effectiveness of the drug may warrant its use in individuals refractory to other drugs.[57] Its effects on reproduction remain to be delineated. Its effects on cognition (glutaminergic neurons are involved in learning and memory) are subtle and less than the adverse cognitive effects of topiramate.[63] Drug interactions involving lamotrigine are common: for example, valproate markedly increases (even doubles!) the half-life of lamotrigine (requiring cutting the required dose of lamotrigine in half). Conversely, carbamazepine shortens lamotrigine's half-life, necessitating increased doses of lamotrigine.

As with gabapentin, there is a special place for lamotrigine in the treatment of pain states, probably due to its action in reducing glutaminergic neurotransmission.[64]

Topiramate and Tiagabine

Recently, open-label studies of these two recently marketed anticonvulsants (Figure 16.1) have indicated efficacy in the treatment of bipolar disorder, particularly as adjunctive agents. The use of topiramate (Topamax) is associated with weight loss as a side effect, possibly making the drug useful to offset the weight gain associated with use of other antimanic drugs, such as lithium and valproate. It may be useful as a mood stabilizer in obese patients with bipolar disorder who want to lose weight. Longer-term studies, however, indicate that the lost weight may be regained after 12 to 18 months of therapy.[65] Unfortunately, its cognitive depressant effects are greater than those of gabapentin or lamotrigine.[63] Side effects include tingling in the extremities, irritability, anxiety, and depression.[66]

Tiagabine (Gabitril) is a novel GABA reuptake inhibitor that, in three patients, effectively treated both bipolar disorder and schizoaffective disorder. Side effects were minimal.[67] In contrast to the positive results in three patients, Grunze and co-workers,[68] in a two-week study of eight patients, reported that none of the eight showed clear-cut relief from manic symptoms. Side effects were more prominent. They concluded that tiagabine seemed to have no pronounced efficacy compared with standard treatments such as valproate or lithium.

Mechanistically, tiagabine inhibits GABA reuptake into neurons and glia, potentiating GABAergic activity. These negative results with tiagabine call into question the exclusive GABAergic mechanism in bipolar disorder and the action of anticonvulsant-antimanic drugs.

Atypical Antipsychotics

For decades, traditional antipsychotic drugs, such as haloperidol, have been used to help control the symptoms and behaviors associated with acute mania. Such therapy was not without problems, including the production of extrapyramidal signs that included akathesia and tardive dyskinesia. Brotman and colleagues[69] concluded that "the majority of even treatment-resistant bipolar patients can be stabilized without neuroleptics" and "the routine intermittent use of typical neuroleptics to treat patients with bipolar disorder should be minimized." There are now two classes of neuroleptic (antipsychotic) drugs: the "typical" and the "atypical" (Chapter 17). While the typical neuroleptics are of little efficacy, the newer atypical agents require examination. Three of these drugs are clozapine, risperidone, and olanzapine.

Frye and co-workers[70] reviewed the use of these three antipsychotics in bipolar disorder. Clozapine appeared more antimanic than antidepressant. Risperidone (Risperdol) appeared more antidepressant than antimanic, potentially aggravating mania. Olanzapine (Zyprexa) and sertindole (Serlect) were too new in 1998 to evaluate. With clozapine, many open-label studies have verified its efficacy; about 70 percent do well on therapy. If it were not for the potential for serious side effects (Chapter 17), clozapine might well be a drug of first choice for the treatment of bipolar disorder.

Olanzapine has now been evaluated in several studies. Sharma and Pistor[71] and McElroy and co-workers[72] documented the efficacy and safety of olanzapine. Zarate and co-workers[73] reported clinical predictors for therapeutic success with olanzapine: these include younger age, female sex, and short duration of illness. They concluded that olanzapine "may be a useful alternative or adjunctive treatment for patients with bipolar illness." Ghaemi and Goodwin[74] reviewed the use of olanzapine and other atypical antipsychotic agents in bipolar disorder. In May 2000, the FDA formally approved olanzapine for the short-term treatment of acute mania, the first such approval for an antipsychotic drug. Data for long-term use is encouraging, but are insufficient for FDA approval.

Frazier and co-workers[75] studied *risperidone* in 28 youths with bipolar disorder and concluded that the drug is effective, mimicking earlier reports in adults, and warrants further investigation in juveniles.

Anticholinesterase Inhibitors

Despite best efforts, many patients are unresponsive to or intolerant of the antimanic drugs heretofore discussed. Therefore, a need exists for additional alternative agents, especially those with unique mechanisms of action. One such drug is *donepezil* (Aricept), an acetylcholinesterase inhibitor used in the treatment of Alzheimer's disease.

Study of the psychedelic drug *scopolamine* (Chapter 12) reveals that blockade of the action of acetylcholine produces clinical effects that include euphoria, talkativeness, difficulties in concentration, and flight of ideas, all resembling symptoms seen in manic disorder. Therefore, perhaps potentiating the action of acetylcholine might exert the opposite effect: relief from mania. *Donepezil* inhibits the enzyme acetylcholine esterase (Chapter 3) and therefore can be postulated to be therapeutically effective in bipolar disorder.

Burt, Sachs, and Demopulos[76] administered donepezil to eleven patients with bipolar disorder who were treatment resistant to other medications. Six patients demonstrated marked improvement, while three additional patients demonstrated slight improvement. Side effects were minor. While this unusual paper indicates efficacy in treatment-resistant patients, it is too early to tell whether or not donepezil will become a useful alternative or adjunctive therapy.

Omega-3 Fatty Acids

The mechanisms of action of antimanic drugs involve inhibitory effects on neuronal signaling transduction systems. Omega-3 fatty acids, obtained from marine or plant sources, are known to damp these signal transduction pathways in a variety of cell systems. Stoll and co-workers[77] hypothesized that these fatty acids might be therapeutically useful in bipolar disorder. They administered the omega-3 fatty acids (under double-blind, placebo-controlled conditions) to 30 patients with bipolar disorder for 4 months. Patients received the fatty acids in addition to their normal antimanic medications (if any). The authors concluded that the omega-3 fatty acid patient group had a much longer period of remission than the placebo group (Figure 16.6). Results were impressive even for individuals who were not taking concurrent medication for their disorder (Figure 16.7). In addition, "for nearly every other outcome measure, the omega-3 group performed better than the placebo group" (which also received their normal medications). These

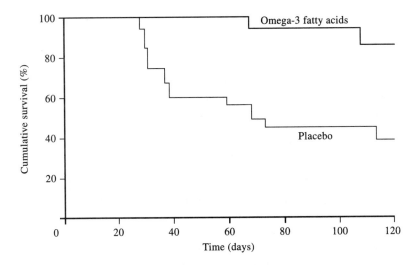

FIGURE 16.6 The effect of omega-3 fatty acids on mean time to recurrence of a bipolar episode compared to placebo (olive oil) therapy. Note the 50 percent recurrence rate at about 75 days with placebo therapy and the prolonged efficacy observed in omega-3-treated patients. [From Stoll et al.[77]]

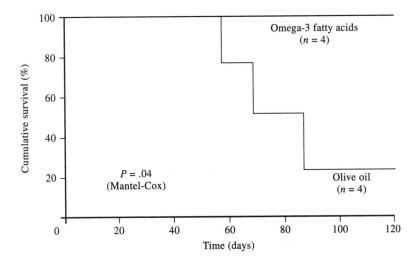

FIGURE 16.7 The effect of omega-3 fatty acids on mean time to recurrence of a bipolar episode. Four patients received only omega-3 fatty acids monotherapy (no other antimanic drugs were taken). These four had no recurrences over the 120-day study period. Four patients received only placebo therapy (olive oil) and no other antimanic drugs: recurrences began at 60 days and all had a recurrence by 90 days. [From Stoll et al.[77]]

pilot results are certainly intriguing and merit further study. The authors concluded:

> If further studies confirm their efficacy in bipolar disorder, omega-3 fatty acids may represent a new class of membrane-active psychotropic compounds, and may herald the advent of a new class of rationally designed mood-stabilizing drugs.[77]

Miscellaneous Agents

In Chapter 6, the pharmacology of the *benzodiazepines* was presented. Two such drugs (*clonazepam* and *lorazepam*) can be used to treat symptoms and behaviors associated with acute mania, although intravenous loading with injectable valproate may be superior.[47]

The pharmacology of *antidepressant drugs* was presented in Chapter 15. Some patients with bipolar disorder with recurrent depressive episodes may require continuous treatment with one of these agents. However, therapy with antidepressants is undertaken with the knowledge that antidepressants may precipitate a manic episode. The practice guidelines of the American Psychiatric Association state:

> As some bipolar patients continue to develop depression despite optimal use of mood stabilizers, antidepressants are often necessary for acute and/or prophylactic treatment. Patients who require antidepressant treatment should receive the lowest effective dose for the shortest time necessary.[3]

Because lithium interferes with membrane ion function, *verapamil* and other *calcium channel blockers* have been tried in the treatment of bipolar disorder. Despite early reports of impressive improvements, their effectiveness remains questionable.

Clonidine is an antihypertensive drug that has been tried in treatment-refractory patients with bipolar disorder. Because clonidine decreases the release of norepinephrine, it was hypothesized that such action might lead to a reduction in manic episodes. Despite initial positive results, effectiveness remains unproven.

Psychotherapeutic and Psychosocial Treatments

A combination of drug therapy and psychotherapeutic interventions is the most effective treatment modality for bipolar illness. Patients with bipolar disorder suffer from the psychosocial consequences of past episodes, the ongoing vulnerability to future episodes, and the burdens of adhering to a long-term treatment plan that may involve some unpleasant side effects. In addition, many patients have clinically significant mood instability between episodes. Goals of psychotherapeutic treatments are to reduce distress and improve functioning between episodes and to decrease the frequency and intensity of future episodes. Successful treatment involves a social network primed to recognize the early symptoms of an episode, to seek help for individuals who lack insight into their condition, and to assist with recognition of side effects and toxicities, thus aiding in compliance with therapy. Issues of importance include the following:

- Emotional consequences of periods of major mood disorder and diagnosis of a chronic mental illness
- Developmental deviations and delays caused by past episodes
- Problems associated with stigmatization
- Problems regulating self-esteem
- Fears of recurrence and consequent inhibition of normal psychosocial functioning
- Interpersonal difficulties
- Marriage, family, childbearing, and parenting issues
- Academic and occupational problems
- Other legal, social, and emotional problems that arise from reckless, violent, withdrawn, or bizarre behavior that may occur during episodes

It is also important to ensure that the manic state is not being caused by medications, such as antidepressants, caffeine, herbals containing ephedrine, behavioral stimulants (including illegal drugs such as cocaine), corticosteroids (cortisone), anabolic steroids, antiparkinsonian drugs, over-the-counter cough and cold preparations, and diet aids. One must also rule out diseases known to cause or exacerbate mania, notably thyroid disease, because mania secondary to thyroid hyperactivity is common.

Psychotherapy interventions used with pharmacotherapy include cognitive-behavioral therapy, psychodynamically oriented therapy, family therapy, couples therapy, interpersonal psychotherapy, and self-help groups. For complete treatment, a practitioner well versed in the pharmacological management of poorly responsive bipolar patients is necessary. Other personnel are required to monitor the effectiveness of treatment, side effects, other causative factors, and compliance with therapy. The American Psychiatric Association[3] and Callahan and Bauer[78] review these psychosocial and psychotherapeutic modalities.

STUDY QUESTIONS

1. Outline the pharmacological agents useful in the treatment of bipolar disorder. What are the major drugs in each category?

2. List the clinical uses of lithium.

3. Describe the correlations between plasma levels of lithium and the therapeutic and side effects of the drug.

4. How does lithium exert its antimanic effect?

5. List the major organ systems affected by lithium. What are the drug's major side effects on each system?

6. Discuss the effects of the various antimanic drugs on memory and cognitive behaviors.

7. Discuss the use of antimanic drugs in pregnancy and in the potentially pregnant female with bipolar disorder.

8. Discuss the comorbidity of bipolar disorder with other psychological disorders.

9. Which antiepileptic drugs are used in the treatment of bipolar disorder? List the advantages and disadvantages of each.

10. What intrudes on patient compliance with antibipolar medication? What can be done to improve compliance?

11. What medications or diseases might precipitate or worsen bipolar illness?

12. How can a health care professional who is not the prescribing physician contribute to the well-being of the bipolar patient?

13. Describe the possible role of omega-3 fatty acids in bipolar illness.

REFERENCES

1. T. Silverstone and S. Romans, "Long-term Treatment of Bipolar Disorder," *Drugs* 51 (1996): 367–382.

2. L. T. Young et al., "Double-blind Comparison of Addition of a Second Mood Stabilizer Versus an Antidepressant to an Initial Mood Stabilizer for Treatment of Patients with Bipolar Depression," *American Journal of Psychiatry* 157 (2000): 124–126.

3. American Psychiatric Association, *Practice Guidelines* (Washington, D.C.: American Psychiatric Association, 1996).

4. J. McClellan and J. Werry, principal authors, "Practice Parameters for the Assessment and Treatment of Children and Adolescents with Bipolar Disorder," *Journal of the American Academy of Child and Adolescent Psychiatry* 36 (1997): 138–157.

5. M. Maj, R. Pirozzi, L. Magliano, and L. Bartoli, "Long-term Outcome of Lithium Prophylaxis in Bipolar Disorder: A Five-year Prospective Study of 402 Patients at a Lithium Clinic," *American Journal of Psychiatry* 155 (1998): 30–35.

6. R. J. Baldessarini and L. Tondo, "Does Lithium Treatment Still Work? Evidence of Stable Responses over Three Decades," *Archives of General Psychiatry* 57 (2000): 187–190.

7. G. Sachs et al., "Variability of Brain Lithium Levels During Maintenance Treatment: A Magnetic Resonance Spectroscopy Study," *Biological Psychiatry* 38 (1995): 422–428.

8. W. Greil et al., "Differential Response to Lithium and Carbamazepine in the Prophylaxis of Bipolar Disorder," *Journal of Clinical Psychopharmacology* 18 (1998): 455–460.

9. S. C. Marcus et al., "Therapeutic Drug Monitoring of Mood Stabilizers in Medicaid Patients with Bipolar Disorder," *American Journal of Psychiatry* 156 (1999): 1014–1018.

10. O. C. Ikonomov and H. K. Manji, "Molecular Mechanisms Underlying Mood Stabilization in Manic-depressive Illness: The Phenotype Challenge," *American Journal of Psychiatry* 156 (1999): 1506–1514.

11. R. H. Lenox, R. K. McNamara, J. M. Watterson, and D. G. Watson, "Myristoylated Alanine-rich C Kinase Substrate (MARCKS): A Molecular Target for the Therapeutic Action of Mood Stabilizers in the Brain?" *Journal of Clinical Psychiatry* 57, Suppl. 13 (1996): 23–31.

12. H. K. Manji et al., "Regulation of Signal Transduction Pathways by Mood-Stabilizing Agents: Implications for the Delayed Onset of Therapeutic Efficacy," *Journal of Clinical Psychiatry* 57, Suppl. 13 (1996): 34–46.

13. O. Massot et al., "5-HT1B Receptors: A Novel Target for Lithium: Possible Involvement in Mood Disorders," *Neuropsychopharmacology* 21 (1999): 530–541.

14. J. L. Elmslie et al., "Prevalence of Overweight and Obesity in Bipolar Patients," *Journal of Clinical Psychiatry* 61 (2000): 179–184.

15. J. H. Kocis et al., "Neuropsychological Effects of Lithium Discontinuation," *Journal of Clinical Psychopharmacology* 13 (1993): 268–275.

16. G. Richter-Leven, H. Markram, and M. Segal, "Spontaneous Recovery of Deficits in Spatial Memory and Cholinergic Potentiation of NMDA in CA-1 Neurons During Chronic Lithium Treatment," *Hippocampus* 2 (1992): 279–286.

17. S. M. Ramin, L. C. Gilstrap, and B. B. Little, "Psychotropics in Pregnancy," in L. C. Gilstrap and B. B. Little, eds., *Drugs and Pregnancy*, 2nd ed. New York: Chapman & Hall, 1998: 171.

18. A. C. Viguera et al., "Risk of Recurrence of Bipolar Disorder in Pregnant and Nonpregnant Women After Discontinuing Lithium Maintenance," *American Journal of Psychiatry* 157 (2000): 179–184.

19. R. J. Baldessarini et al., "Effects of the Rate of Discontinuing Lithium Maintenance Treatment in Bipolar Disorders," *Journal of Clinical Psychiatry* 57 (1996): 441–448.

20. G. Goodwin, "Recurrence of Mania After Lithium Withdrawal," *British Journal of Psychiatry* 164 (1994): 149–152.

21. W. Coryell et al., "Lithium Discontinuation and Subsequent Effectiveness," *American Journal of Psychiatry* 155 (1998): 895–898.

22. R. J. Baldessarini, L. Tondo, and J. Hennen, "Effects of Lithium Treatment and its Discontinuation on Suicidal Behavior in Bipolar Manic Depressive Disorders," *Journal of Clinical Psychiatry* 60, Suppl. 2 (1999): 77–84.

23. E. D. Peselow, R. R. Fieve, C. Difiglia, and M. P. Sanfilipo, "Lithium Prophylaxis of Bipolar Illness: The Value of Combination Treatment," *British Journal of Psychiatry* 164 (1994): 208–214.

24. D. A. Solomon, G. I. Keitner, C. E. Ryan, and I. W. Miller, "Lithium Plus Valproate as Maintenance Polypharmacy for Patients with Bipolar I Disorder: A Review," *Journal of Clinical Psychopharmacology* 18 (1998): 38–49.

25. K. D. Denicoff et al., "Comparative Prophylactic Efficacy of Lithium, Carbamazepine, and the Combination in Bipolar Disorder," *Journal of Clinical Psychiatry* 58 (1997): 470–478.

26. M. P. Freeman and A. L. Stoll, "Mood Stabilizer Combinations: A Review of Safety and Efficacy," *American Journal of Psychiatry* 155 (1998): 12–21.

27. S. C. Sonne and K. T. Brady, "Substance Abuse and Bipolar Comorbidity," *Psychiatric Clinics of North America* 22 (1999): 609–627.

28. J. F. Goldberg et al., "A History of Substance Abuse Complicates Remission From Acute Mania in Bipolar Disorder," *Journal of Clinical Psychiatry* 60 (1999): 733–740.

29. M. Tohen et al., "The Effect of Comorbid Substance Abuse Disorders on the Course of Bipolar Disorder: A Review," *Harvard Review of Psychiatry* 6 (1998): 133–141.

30. B. Geller et al., "Double-blind and Placebo-controlled Study of Lithium for Adolescent Bipolar Disorders with Secondary Substance Dependency," *Journal of the American Academy of Child and Adolescent Psychiatry* 37 (1998): 171–178.

31. M. Fava, "Psychopharmacologic Treatment of Pathologic Aggression," *Psychiatric Clinics of North America* 20 (1997): 427–451.

32. R. M. Post et al., "Beyond Lithium in the Treatment of Bipolar Illness," *Neuropsychopharmacology* 19 (1998): 206–219.

33. R. Dardennes, C. Even, F. Bange, and A. Heim, "Comparison of Carbamazepine and Lithium in the Prophylaxis of Bipolar Disorders. A Meta-analysis," *British Journal of Psychiatry* 166 (1995): 378–381.

34. W. Greil et al., "Differential Response to Lithium and Carbamazepine in the Prophylaxis of Bipolar Disorder," *Journal of Clinical Psychopharmacology* 18 (1998): 455–460.

35. P. Petit et al., "Carbamazepine and Its 10,11-Epoxide Metabolite in Acute Mania: Clinical and Pharmacokinetic Correlates," *European Journal of Clinical Pharmacology* 41 (1991): 541–546.

36. A. P. Aldenkamp et al., "Withdrawal of Antiepileptic Medication in Children—Effects on Cognitive Function: The Multicenter Holmfrid Study," *Neurology* 43 (1993): 41–50.

37. E. Spina, F. Pisani, and E. Perucca, "Clinically Significant Pharmacokinetic Drug Interactions with Carbamazepine: An Update," *Clinical Pharmacokinetics* 31 (1996): 198–214.

38. F. W. Rosa, "Spina Bifida in Infants of Women Treated with Carbamazepine During Pregnancy," *New England Journal of Medicine* 324 (1991): 674–677.

39. J. L. Woolston, "Case Study: Carbamazepine Treatment of Juvenile-onset Bipolar Disorder," *Journal of the American Academy of Child and Adolescent Psychiatry* 38 (1999): 335–338.

40. W. Loscher, "Valproate: A Reappraisal of its Pharmacologic Properties and Mechanisms of Action," *Progress in Neurobiology* 58 (1999): 31–59.

41. G. Chen et al., "Valproate Robustly Enhances AP-1 Mediated Gene Expression," *Brain Research: Molecular Brain Research* 64 (1999): 52–58.

42. J. R. Calabrese, S. H. Fatemim, and M. J. Woyshville, "Predictors of Response to Mood Stabilizers," *Journal of Clinical Psychopharmacology* 16 (1996): 24–31.

43. F. M. Jacobsen, "Low-dose Valproate: A New Treatment for Cyclothymia, Mild Rapid Cycling Disorders, and Premenstrual Syndrome," *Journal of Clinical Psychiatry* 54 (1993): 229–234.

44. A. C. Swann et al., "Depression During Mania: Treatment Response to Lithium or Divalproex," *Archives of General Psychiatry* 54 (1997): 37–42.

45. B. Muller-Oerlinghausen et al., "Valproate as an Adjunct to Neuroleptic Medication for the treatment of Acute Episodes of Mania: A Prospective, Randomized, Double-Blind, Placebo-Controlled, Multicenter Study," *Journal of Clinical Psychopharmacology* 20 (2000): 195–203.

46. H. Grunze et al., "Intravenous Valproate Loading in Acutely Manic and Depressed Bipolar I Patients," *Journal of Clinical Psychopharmacology* 19 (1999): 303–309.

47. L. K. Vainionpaa et al., "Valproate-Induced Hyperandrogenism during Pubertal Maturation in Girls with Epilepsy," *Annals of Neurology* 45 (1999): 444–450.

48. C. M. Piontek, S. Baab, K. S. Peindl and K. L. Wisner, "Serum Valproate Levels in 6 Breastfeeding Mother-Infant Pairs," *Journal of Clinical Psychiatry* 61 (2000): 170–172.

49. L. L. Davis, W. Ryan, B. Adinoff, and F. Petty, "Comprehensive Review of the Psychiatric Uses of Valproate," *Journal of Clinical Psychopharmacology* 20, Supplement 1 (2000): 1S–17S.

50. L. Letterman and J. S. Markowitz, "Gabapentin: A Review of Published Experience in the Treatment of Bipolar Disorder and Other Psychiatric Conditions," *Pharmacotherapy* 19 (1999): 565–572.

51. S. L. McElroy, C. A. Soutullo, P. E. Keck, and G. F. Kmetz, "A Pilot Trial of Adjunctive Gabapentin in the Treatment of Bipolar Disorder," *Annals of Clinical Psychiatry* 9 (1997): 99–103.

52. M. A. Frye et al., "Gabapentin Does Not Alter Single-dose Lithium Pharmacokinetics," *Journal of Clinical Psychopharmacology* 18 (1998): 461–464.

53. A.C. Pande et al., "Treatment of Social Phobia with Gabapentin: A Placebo-controlled Study," *Journal of Clinical Psychopharmacology* 19 (1999): 341–348.

54. M. W. Neville, "Gabapentin in the Management of Neuropathic Pain," *American Journal of Pain Management* 10 (2000): 6–12.

55. S. Chen, J. C. Eisenach, P. P. McCaslin, and H. Pan, "Synergistic Effect Between Intrathecal Non-NMDA Antagonist and Gabapentin on Allodynia Induced by Spinal Nerve Ligation in Rats," *Anesthesiology* 92 (2000): 500–506.

56. B. J. Partgidge, S. R. Chaplan, E. Sakamoto, and T. L. Yaksh, "Characterization of the Effects of Gabapentin and 3-Isobutyl-gamma-

aminobutyric acid on Substance P-induced Thermal Hyperalgesia," *Anesthesiology* 88 (1998): 196–205.

57. J. R. Calabrese et al., "Spectrum of Activity of Lamotrigine in Treatment-refractory Bipolar Disorder," *American Journal of Psychiatry* 156 (1999): 1019–1023.

58. C. L. Bowden et al., "The Efficacy of Lamotrigine in Rapid Cycling and Non-rapid Cycling Patients with Bipolar Disorder," *Biological Psychiatry* 45 (1999): 953–958.

59. I. N. Ferrier, "Lamotrigine and Gabapentin. Alternative in the Treatment of Bipolar Disorder," *Neuropsychobiology* 38 (1998): 192–197.

60. O. C. Pinto and H. S. Akiskal, "Lamotrigine as a Promising Approach to Borderline Personality: An Open Case Series Without Concurrent DSM-IV Major Mood Disorder," *Journal of Affective Disorders* 51 (1998): 333–343.

61. X. Xie and R. M. Hagen, "Cellular and Molecular Actions of Lamotrigine: Possible Mechanisms of Efficacy in Bipolar Disorder," *Neuropsychobiology* 38 (1998): 119–130.

62. J. G. Klamt, "Effects of Intrathecally Administered Lamotrigine, a Glutamate-release Inhibitor, on Short- and Long-term Models of Hyperalgesia in Rats," *Anesthesiology* 88 (1998): 487–494.

63. R. Martin et al., "Cognitive Effects of Topiramate, Gabapentin, and Lamotrigine in Healthy Young Adults," *Neurology* 52 (1999): 321–327.

64. G. Lunardi et al., "Clinical Effectiveness of Lamotrigine and Plasma Levels in Essential and Symptomatic Trigeminal Neuralgia," *Neurology* 48 (1997): 1714–1717.

65. A. Gordon and L. H. Price, "Mood Stabilizers and Weight Loss with Topiramate," *American Journal of Psychiatry* 156 (1999): 968–969.

66. M. W. Kellet et al., "Topiramate in Clinical Practice: First Year's Postlicensing Experience in a Specialist Epilepsy Clinic," *Journal of Neurology and Neurosurgical Psychiatry* 66 (1999): 759–763.

67. K. R. Kaufman, "Adjunctive Tiagabine Treatment of Psychiatric Disorders: Three Cases," *Annals of Clinical Psychiatry* 10 (1998): 181–184.

68. H. Grunze et a., "Tiagabine Appears Not to Be Efficacious in the Treatment of Acute Mania," *Journal of Clinical Psychiatry* 60 (1999): 759–762.

69. M. A. Brotman, E. L. Feregus, R. M. Post, and S. G. Leverich, "High Exposure to Neuroleptics in Bipolar Patients: A Retrospective Review," *Journal of Clinical Psychiatry* 61 (2000): 68–72.

70. M. A. Frye et al., "Clozapine in Bipolar Disorder: Treatment Implications for Other Atypical Antipsychotics," *Journal of Affective Disorders* 48 (1998): 91–104.

71. V. Sharma and L. Pistor, "Treatment of Bipolar Mixed State with Olanzapine," *Journal of Psychiatry and Neuroscience* 24 (1999): 40–44.

72. S. L. McElroy et al., "Olanzapine in Treatment-Resistant Bipolar Disorder," *Journal of Affective Disorders* 49 (1998): 119–122.

73. C. A. Zarate et al., "Clinical Predictors of Acute Response with Olanzapine in Psychotic Mood Disorders," *Journal of Clinical Psychiatry* 59 (1998): 24–28.

74. S. N. Ghaema and F. K. Goodwin, "Use of Atypical Antipsychotic Agents in Bipolar and Schizoaffective Disorders: Review of the Empirical Literature," *Journal of Clinical Psychopharmacology* 19 (1999): 354–361.

75. J. A. Frazier et al., "Risperidone Treatment for Juvenile Bipolar Disorder: A Retrospective Chart Review," *Journal of the American Academy of Child and Adolescent Psychiatry* 38 (1999): 960–965.

76. T. Burt, G. S. Sachs, and C. Demopulos, "Donepezil in Treatment-resistant Bipolar Disorder," *Biological Psychiatry* 45 (1999): 959–964.

77. A. L. Stoll et al., "Omega-3 Fatty Acids in Bipolar Disorder: A Preliminary Double-blind, Placebo-controlled Trial," *Archives of General Psychiatry* 56 (1999): 407–412.

78. A. M. Callahan and M. S. Bauer, "Psychosocial Interventions for Bipolar Disorder," *Psychiatric Clinics of North America* 22 (1999): 675–688.

Chapter 17

Drugs Used to Treat Schizophrenia: Antipsychotic Drugs

Schizophrenia is a debilitating psychiatric illness that typically strikes young people just when they are maturing into adulthood.[1] The disorder is associated with marked social or occupational dysfunction, and its course and outcome vary greatly. Approximately 1 percent of the population suffer from schizophrenia; a majority are unemployed, and family costs (e.g., lost work time and treatment expenses) are enormous. Schizophrenia is associated with an increased risk of suicide; approximately 10 to 15 percent of individuals with schizophrenia take their own lives, usually within the first 10 years of developing the disorder.

Until recently, antipsychotics have been reserved for seriously ill patients because of the numerous adverse effects associated with their use. The development of new agents, however, has revolutionized antipsychotic drug use. There is now hope of raising patients' functioning to levels that truly can facilitate reintegration into the community. In the late 1990s, pharmacologic breakthroughs occurred that offered patients a real chance of leading more normal lives. This revolution, however, occurred in an atmosphere of reduced social services and support. The challenge of the new millennium may not be so much the discovery of additional agents to improve functional levels but the preparation of social services, family, and counselors to help patients develop their newly found skills and abilities.[2] Only through multilevel interventions can patients with severe and persistent mental illness successfully reintegrate into the community.[3] While continuous drug therapy is indispensible in most cases to achieve social integration, other (nondrug) therapeutic interventions, the cooperation of several professions, and regard for the views of patients and relatives are essential. In this chapter, of course, the focus is on the pharmacology of the medications used to treat schizophrenia.

Etiology of Schizophrenia

> Schizophrenia is a disease of the brain that is expressed clinically as a disease of the mind. It is a disease of neural connectivity caused by multiple factors that affect brain development.[4]

Schizophrenia is a misconnection syndrome that reflects a basic disorder in neural circuits:

> The underlying disruption in functional circuitry is presumed to be a final common pathway produced by the convergence of multiple etiological and pathophysiological factors: e.g., inherited DNA, regulation of gene expression, or the influence of "environmental factors" (ranging from viruses to amphetamine-induced dopamine upregulation to academic failures) on a "plastic brain" (Figure 17.1).[5]

> Schizophrenia is a disruption of thought; a mental process that is poorly localized in brain and influenced by multiple neural systems. . . . It implies a pathologically heterogenous group of diseases. . . . Schizophrenia may result from a perinatal insult in a genetically predisposed individual that produces neuronal alterations during final synaptic reorganization and myelination of early adulthood.[6]

> Despite a hundred years' research, the neuropathology of schizophrenia remain obscure. . . . In general, the relationship between neurochemical findings (which center upon dopamine, 5-hydroxytryptamine, glutamate and GABA systems) and the neuropathology of schizophrenia is unclear.[7]

Despite familial and environmental diversity,[8] however, a final common pathway defines the illness: schizophrenia is a misregulation of information processing in the brain.[4] The signs and symptoms encompass the entire range of human mental activity and include abnormalities in perception (hallucinations), inferential thinking (delusions), language (disorganized speech), social and motor behavior (disorganized behavior and abnormal or stereotyped movements), and initiation of goal-directed activity (avolition), as well as impoverishment of speech and mental

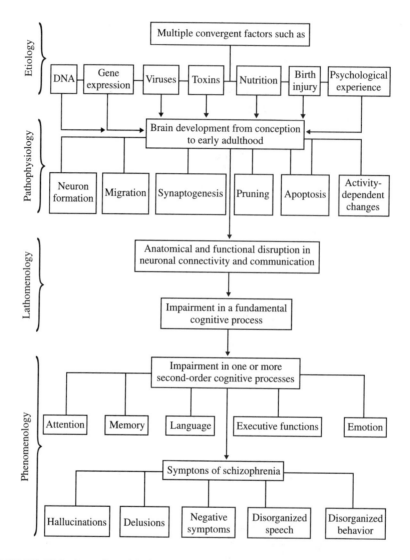

FIGURE 17.1 General model of the development of schizophrenia. [From Andreasen.[5]]

creativity (alogia), blunting of emotional expression (flattened affect), and loss of the ability to experience pleasure (anhedonia). Patients with schizophrenia also have impairments in many different cognitive systems such as memory, attention, and executive function.

Classically, the symptoms of schizophrenia have been classified as positive and negative. The positive symptoms are those typical of psychosis and include delusions and hallucinations, bizarre behaviors, dissociated or fragmented thoughts, incoherence, and illogicality. The negative symptoms include blunted affect, impaired emotional responsiveness, apathy, loss of motivation and interest, and social withdrawal. This differentiation of symptomatology is important in the pharmacology of antipsychotic drugs because the classic agents affect primarily the positive symptoms, while the atypical antipsychotic drugs relieve both the positive and the negative symptoms.

Dopaminergic Involvement

In the 1970s, scientific evidence favored a *dopamine theory* of schizophrenia: the disorder arises from dysregulation in certain brain regions of the dopamine system, and antipsychotic drugs work by being pharmacological antagonists of the neurotransmitter dopamine. In the 1990s, molecular cloning studies identified several genes coding for dopamine receptors. There are now at least two dopamine$_1$-like receptors (D_{1A} and D_{1B}, also called D_5) and three dopamine$_2$-like receptors (D_2, D_3, and D_4). The D_1-like and D_2-like receptors exert opposite effects on intracellular mechanisms. The traditional view of antipsychotic drug activity (at least against positive symptomatology) involves antagonism of D_2-like receptors, some drugs blocking D_2 receptors and some blocking D_4 receptors (Table 17.1). Yang, Seamans, and Gorelova[9] review these dopaminergic theories of schizophrenia, two issues of *Biological Psychiatry*[10] and a volume of *Neuropsychopharmacology*[11] are devoted to this topic.

Until the 1990s, dopamine receptor blockade was the mainstay of drug treatment for schizophrenia (traditional antipsychotics). These drugs, however, cause acute drug-induced parkinsonian symptoms, persistent (even permanent) residual motor dysfunction (tardive dyskinesias), and they may worsen the negative symptomatology of schizophrenia. Given these limitations, alternative (atypical) antipsychotics were, and continue to be, developed; they exhibit antipsychotic efficacy with fewer undesirable side effects.

There is no consensus concerning the biological mechanisms that might impart and define an atypical antipsychotic.[11,12] Most are antagonists at D_2 receptors and have a second action; perhaps D_1, 5-HT$_2$, or adrenergic receptor blockade. Some have selectivity for other D_2-like receptors (D_3 or D_4), shown by a preferential distribution of these receptors in mesocorticolimbic areas of the brain. The D_2 receptor blockade is thought to be associated with extrapyramidal side effects and is thus considered to be an undesirable property for an antipsychotic,[13] although there is strong correlation between D_2 blockade and clinical potency and efficacy (Figure 17.2).

Investigation into alternative mechanisms besides dopamine receptor blockade has followed from observations on the actions of psychedelic drugs:[14]

TABLE 17.1 Pharmacology of antipsychotic drugs

Compound	Target receptor populations	Developer
CLASSIC AND EARLY ATYPICAL DRUGS		
Chlorpromazine	D_2, D_3, D_4, D_1, α_1, H_1, mACh	SmithKine
Haloperidol	D_2, D_3, D_4, α_1, H_1	Janssen
Thioridazine	D_2, D_3, D_4, D_1, mACh, α_1, H_1	Novartis (Sandoz)
Sulpiride	D_2, D_3, D_4, H_1	Astra (Bristol-Meyer Squibb)
NOVEL ATYPICAL DRUGS		
Clozapine	D_2, D_1, 5-HT_{2A}, α_1, α_2, H_1, ACH	Novartis (Sandoz)
Olanzapine	D_1, D_2, D_4, 5-HT_{2A}, 5-HT_{2C}, α_1, H_1, (5-HT_1, $GABA_A$, β)	Lilly
Risperidone	5-HT_{2A}, D_2, α_1, α_2, H_1, (5-HT_{1C}, 5-HT_{1D}, 5-HT_{1A}, D_1)	Janssen
Quetiapine	5-HT_{2A}, D_2, H_1, α_1, α_2, (D_1, ACH)	Zeneca
Sertindole	5-HT_{2A}, α_1, D_2, D_1, (5-HT_{1A}, α_2, β, H_1)	Abbott

D_1, D_2, D_3, D_4 = dopamine receptors; 5-HT_{1C}, 5-HT_{2A}, 5-HT_{2C} = serotonin isoforms; α_1, β = adrenergic isoforms; H_1 = histamine isoform; $GABA_A$ = γ-aminobutyric acid isoform. Parentheses indicate lower binding affinities.
From C. Anderson et al., "Emerging Roles for Novel Antipsychotic Medications in the Treatment of Schizophrenia," *Psychiatric Clinics of North America* 21 (1998): 151–179.

- The serotonin psychedelic drugs psilocybin and LSD produce a state similar to schizophrenia and these drugs are thought to be agonists of 5-HT_2 receptors (Chapter 12). Thus 5-HT_2 antagonism may be beneficial in antipsychotic efficacy.

- The dissociative psychedelics phencyclidine and ketamine (Chapter 12) likewise produce a schizophrenic-like state, and they are potent blockers of NMDA-type glutamate receptors. Thus, there may be an involvement of glutamate receptor dysfunction in the etiology of schizophrenia. In other words, NMDA antagonism results in schizophrenic-like behaviors.

A brief review of the roles of serotonin and glutamate in the etiology of schizophrenia follows.

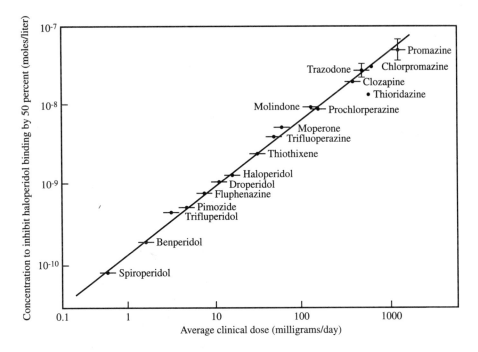

FIGURE 17.2 Correlation between the clinical potency and receptor-binding activities of neuroleptic drugs. Clinical potency is expressed as the daily dose used in treating schizophrenia, and binding activity is expressed as the concentration needed to produce 50 percent inhibition of haloperidol binding. Haloperidol binds to dopamine$_2$ receptors; other antipsychotic drugs compete for the same receptors. Thus, measuring the competitive inhibition of haloperidol binding correlates with potency as an antipsychotic drug.

Serotonin Involvement

In 1996, Richelson[15] stated: "Serotonergic receptor blockade may also be the underlying mechanism for the efficacy of an atypical neuroleptic to treat the negative symptoms of schizophrenia." The exact serotonin mechanisms involved have been elusive. Autopsy studies in deceased patients with schizophrenia showed reduced 5-HT$_2$ receptors in the prefrontal cortex, consistent with the serotonin psychedelic hypothesis. However, Lewis and co-workers[16] were unable to replicate this finding in PET studies in patients with schizophrenia.

Sprouse and co-workers[17] studied ziprasidone (an atypical antipsychotic) and noted that it functions as an agonist at 5-HT$_{1A}$ receptors and an antagonist at 5-HT$_{1D}$, 5-HT$_2$, and D$_2$ receptors. The 5-HT$_{1A}$ agonist action distinguishes this atypical agent, possibly endowing it with an antidepressant-anxiolytic action similar to that exerted by buspirone (BuSpar; Chapter 6), the prototype 5-HT$_{1A}$ agonist. Thus, serotoninergic activity may be a complementary action to dopaminergic blockade, reducing negative symptomatology and blocking the production of abnormal drug-induced motor problems. Finally, Aghajanian and Marek[18] propose that atypical antipsychotics are capable of blocking serotonin 5-HT$_{2A}$ receptors and that the physiological role of these receptors is to induce the release of glutamate. Thus, there may be a serotonin-glutamate interaction whereby drug-induced serotonin blockade functions to limit glutamate release.

Glutamate Involvement

Olney and Farber[19] studied the dysfunction of dopaminergic and N-methyl-D-aspartate-glutamate receptors, noting:

> A unified hypothesis pertaining to combined dysfunction of dopamine and N-methyl-D-aspartate-glutamate receptors that highlights N-methyl-D-aspartate-glutamate receptor hypofunction as a key mechanism that can help explain major clinical and pathophysiological aspects of schizophrenia. . . . We propose that since N-methyl-D-aspartate-glutamate receptor hypofunction can cause psychosis in humans and corticolimbic neurodegenerative changes in the rat brain, and since these changes are prevented by certain antipsychotic drugs, including atypical neuroleptic agents (clozapine, olanzapine, fluperlapine), a better understanding of the N-methyl-D-aspartate-glutamate receptor hypofunction and ways of preventing its neurodegenerative consequences in the rat brain may lead to improved pharmacotherapy in schizophrenia.

Bachus and Kleinman[20] concluded:

> Increasingly, focus is shifting to a role for glutaminergic dysfunction in schizophrenia, opening the possibility that drugs that act upon glutamate function, either directly or indirectly via comodulators of glutamate transmission, could potentially be developed as adjunctive or primary novel pharmacotherapeutic strategies. . . . Although there are a number of drugs that can regulate the psychotic symptoms associated with the subcortical dopamine system, there are essentially no drugs to date that successfully target the cortical glutamate system and cognitive deficits.

Thus, increasingly, there is a glutamate-NMDA receptor hypofunction hypothesis of schizophrenia.[21-23] This NMDA-hypofunction is proposed to result in excessive release of excitatory neurotransmitters (glutamate and acetylcholine) in frontal cortex, damaging cortical neurons and triggering the deterioration seen in patients with schizophrenia. A protracted NMDA-hypofunctional state could trigger neuronal injury throughout many corticolimbic brain regions.

Thus, as an integrated hypothesis, hyperdopaminergic activity could be relevant for positive symptoms, whereas a glutamate-NMDA receptor deficiency could explain the negative symptoms and cognitive dysfunction seen in the disease. Indeed, two atypical antipsychotic drugs (clozapine and quetiapine) reduce the mRNA expression for NMDA-forming subunits in the nucleus accumbens.[24] Quetiapine also increased the mRNA expression of a second type of glutamate receptor, the AMPA-receptor (Chapter 3).[24] This provides further evidence that glutamate receptors can be a target for antipsychotic drug action as well as a potential site of receptor dysfunction in schizophrenia.

As further evidence that glutaminergic NMDA dysfunction may be involved in schizophrenia, Mohn and colleagues[25] developed genetically engineered mice in which NMDA receptors were reduced by 95 percent. These mice exhibited behavioral homologies remarkably similar to schizophrenia, unrelated to dopaminergic dysfunction and sensitive to antipsychotic drugs. Once again, this finding is consistent with a glutaminergic rather than a dopaminergic dysfunction in schizophrenic symptomatology.

Overview of Antipsychotic Drugs

Mechanism of Action

The clinical efficacy of traditional antipsychotic drugs is, as stated, highly correlated with their ability to competitively block dopamine receptors (Figure 17.2). It is thus the purity of action of the traditional agents that accounts for efficacy against positive symptoms as well as many of the undesirable side effects. With the atypical agents, dopaminergic blockade is balanced by other actions on serotonin and glutamate neurons, adding beneficial effects against negative symptoms and cognitive deficits while reducing the incidence of abnormal movement-generating side effects.

The extent of binding to dopamine$_2$ receptors predicts efficacy, daily dosage, and likelihood of causing extrapyramidal side effects.[15] Studies demonstrate that the therapeutic effects of neuroleptics,* with the exception of clozapine, are achieved beginning at about 70 percent

---

*The word neuroleptic means "to take control of the neuron." Some 70 years ago, the antipsychotic and extrapyramidal (motor) effects of classical antipsychotics (e.g., chlorpromazine) were thought to be linked and inseparable. This led to the *neuroleptic threshold concept* that held that the neuroleptic dose was gradually increased to the level that produced extrapyramidal side effects. Thus, the "right" dose was the one that caused some degree of motor side effects. Atypical antipsychotics, in general, have a better therapeutic ratio, with antipsychotic effects seen at doses that do not produce motor side effects (Figure 17.3B).

dopamine D_2 receptor occupancy, while extrapyramidal side effects are generally seen at higher D_2 receptor occupancies.

As Figure 17.3 illustrates, it is now possible to separate antipsychotic efficacy from extrapyramidal side effects. Drugs that exhibit this pattern do so through a variety of receptor mechanisms, but, in general, this separation is vitally important. The antipsychotic compounds being developed today all have demonstrable antipsychotic efficacy combined with encouragingly low extrapyramidal profiles and a low liability to produce tardive dyskinesia at therapeutic doses. Improvements in negative symptomatology and cognitive deficits are added benefits.

Thus, while the terms "classical," "traditional," or "neuroleptic" antipsychotic apply to the drugs with inseparable therapeutic and extrapyramidal effects (Figure 17.3A), the term "atypical" applies to agents that do separate the two. These new drugs were as revolutionary in the 1990s as chlorpromazine and other "phenothiazines" were in the 1950s.

Clozapine (Clozaril) was the first of the new-generation antipsychotics (early 1990s), and it was followed by *risperidone* (Risperdal). Clozapine is a relatively weak blocker of dopamine D_2 receptors; it is a much more effective blocker of serotonin $5\text{-}HT_2$ receptors. Risperidone exhibits high levels of dopamine$_2$ receptor blockade and a very high affinity for $5\text{-}HT_2$ receptors. Table 17.2 lists the therapeutic and adverse effects that follow receptor blockade by antipsychotic drugs.

Olanzapine (Zyprexa), introduced in late 1996, acts much like clozapine, except for a higher affinity for D_2 receptors and a slightly

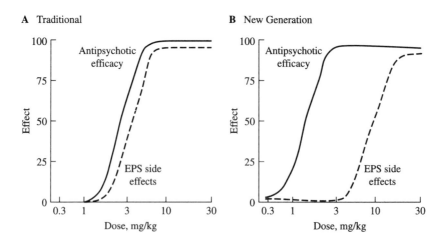

FIGURE 17.3 Dose-response curves for antipsychotic efficacy (*solid lines*) and extrapyramidal symptoms (*dashed lines*) for (**A**) traditional antipsychotic neuroleptics and (**B**) new-generation antipsychotics. [From D. E. Casey, "Motor and Mental Aspects of EPS," *International Journal of Psychopharmacology* 10 (1995): 105–114.]

TABLE 17.2 Possible therapeutic and adverse effects of receptor blockade by neuroleptics

---

Blockade of dopamine D_2 receptors
  Therapeutic effects
    Amelioration of the positive signs and symptoms of psychosis
  Adverse effects
    Extrapyramidal movement disorders: dystonia, parkinsonism, akathisia, tardive dyskinesia, rabbit syndrome
    Endocrine effects: prolactin elevation (galactorrhea, gynecomastia, menstrual changes, sexual dysfunction in males)
Blockade of muscarinic receptors
  Therapeutic effects
    Mitigation of extrapyramidal side effects
  Adverse effects
    Blurred vision
    Attack or exacerbation of narrow angle glaucoma
    Dry mouth
    Sinus tachycardia
    Constipation
    Urinary retention
    Memory dysfunction
Blockade of serotonin $5\text{-}HT_{2A}$ receptors
  Therapeutic effects
    Amelioration of the negative signs and symptoms of psychosis
    Mitigation of extrapyramidal side effects
  Adverse effects
    Unknown
Blockade of histamine H_1 receptors
  Therapeutic effects
    Sedation
  Adverse effects
    Sedation
    Drowsiness
    Weight gain
    Potentiation of central depressant drugs
Blockade of α_1-adrenoceptors
  Therapeutic effects
    Unknown
  Adverse effects
    Potentiation of the antihypertensive effects of prazosin, terazosin, doxazosin, and labetalol
    Postural hypotension, dizziness
    Reflex tachycardia
Blockade of α_2-adrenoceptors
  Therapeutic effects
    Unknown
  Adverse effects
    Blockade of the antihypertensive effects of clonidine and methyldopa

---

From Richelson,[15] p. 8.

lower affinity for 5-HT$_2$ receptors. Only about 40 percent of dopamine$_2$ receptors are blocked by either clozapine or olanzapine. A fourth atypical antipsychotic, *sertindole* (Serlect), was introduced in 1997. It affects a variety of dopamine receptors as well as serotonin receptors. The fifth and sixth atypical antipsychotics, *quetiapine* (Seroquel) and *ziprasidone* (Zeldox), were introduced in 1999 and 2000; they also serve as antagonists at several neurotransmitter receptors including 5-HT$_{1A}$, 5-HT$_2$, D$_1$, D$_2$, histamine, and adrenergic. The combination of D$_2$ and 5-HT$_2$ blockade probably underlies most of quetiapine's and ziprasidone's therapeutic action. Table 17.3 summarizes the binding of several antipsychotic drugs to various receptors in the CNS.

Historical Background

Prior to 1950, effective drugs for treating psychotic patients were virtually nonexistent, and psychotic patients were usually permanently or semipermanently hospitalized; by 1955, more than half a million psychotic persons in the United States were residing in mental hospitals. In 1956, a dramatic and steady reversal in this trend began (Figure 17.4). By 1983, fewer than 220,000 were institutionalized. This decline occurred despite a doubling in the numbers of admissions to state hospitals. Until the early 1990s, people with schizophrenia were routinely stabilized on medication and discharged from institutions

TABLE 17.3 Relative in-vitro binding profiles of one traditional antipsychotic neuroleptic (haloperidol) and four new-generation antipsychotic drugs

Receptor	Sertindole	Clozapine	Haloperidol	Olanzapine	Risperidone
D$_1$	28.0	130.0	36.0	25.0	50.0
D$_2$	4.1	410.0	7.5	19.0	4.0
D$_3$	1.6	83.0	2.7	?	6.7
D$_4$	14.0	21.0	23.0	27.0	7.0
5-HT$_{2A}$	0.4	7.8	55.0	3.7	0.76
5-HT$_{2C}$	1.2	15.0	2100.0	6.1	14.0
α_1	3.4	9.2	18.0	18.0	1.7
α_2	350.0	64.0	2000.0	180.0	2.3
H$_1$	600.0	23.0	>1000.0	7.7	110.0
Muscarinic	2500.0	9.4	5500.0	20.0	6500.0

D$_1$, D$_2$, D$_3$, D$_4$ = dopamine receptors; 5-HT$_{2A}$, 5-HT$_{2C}$ = serotonin receptors; α_1, α_2 = adrenergic receptors; Muscarinic = cholinergic receptor; H$_1$ = histamine receptor.

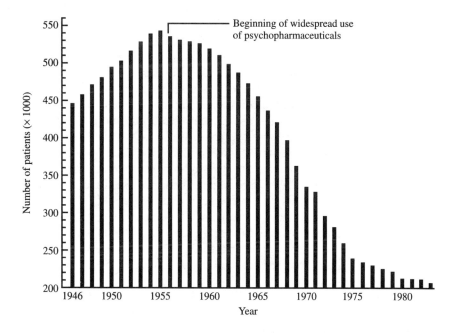

FIGURE 17.4 Numbers of resident patients in state and local government mental hospitals in the United States from 1946 through 1983. Note the dramatic change that began in 1956 with the introduction of psychoactive drugs into therapy.

quite rapidly.* What accounted for the dramatic shift resided in a class of drugs called the *phenothiazines*.

In 1952, French researcher H. Laborit used *promethazine* (the first of the phenothiazines) to deepen anesthesia. Later that year, other French researchers studied a second phenothiazine, *chlorpromazine* (Thorazine). This drug was administered in a "cocktail" to patients the night before surgery to allay their fears and anxieties. Chlorpromazine (Figure 17.5) was found to lower the amount of anesthetic drugs that a patient needed without making the patient unconscious; instead, treatment with chlorpromazine produced a state characterized by calmness, conscious sedation, and disinterest in and detachment from external stimuli. This condition was termed a *neuroleptic state,* and chlorpromazine was the first neuroleptic drug. Because of these behavioral effects, chlorpromazine was found to be remarkably effective in

---

*Although the discharge rate of schizophrenics from institutions is high, there is concern about their ultimate functioning in society. Many patients who were discharged on phenothiazines failed to continue their medication, and they functioned poorly as a result. It has been estimated that about 50 percent of the adult homeless population in the United States may suffer from inadequately controlled schizophrenia.

alleviating the clinical manifestations of the psychotic process. Although chlorpromazine did not provide a permanent cure, its use in conjunction with supportive therapy allowed thousands of patients who otherwise would have been hospitalized permanently to return to their communities, although in a less than satisfactory state.

In the continuing search for more effective and less bothersome drugs, alternatives to the phenothiazines have been (and are continuing to be) developed. *Reserpine* (Serpasil) was a late 1950s alternative, but significant side effects have today rendered the drug obsolete. The second class of alternative agents was the *butyrophenones*, developed in Belgium in the mid-1960s. Two butyrophenones are currently available—*haloperidol* (Haldol; Figure 17.5) and *droperidol* (Inapsine). Neither drug seems to have significant advantages over the phenothiazines, but haloperidol is occasionally used for patients who cannot tolerate the phenothiazines. During the 1970s, other agents became available, including *loxapine* (Loxitane) and *molindone* (Moban).

The early twenty-first century has ushered in a new era of treatment goals for the patient with schizophrenia. Treatment of the positive symptoms of schizophrenia may make a patient more manageable, but it leads to an important question: how do these changes actually benefit

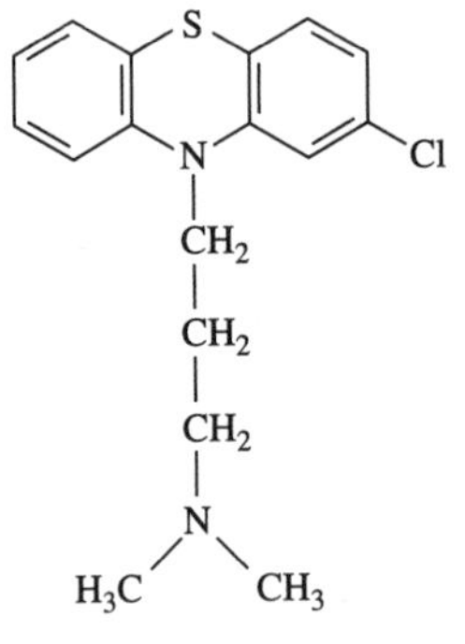

Chlorpromazine (Thorazine)

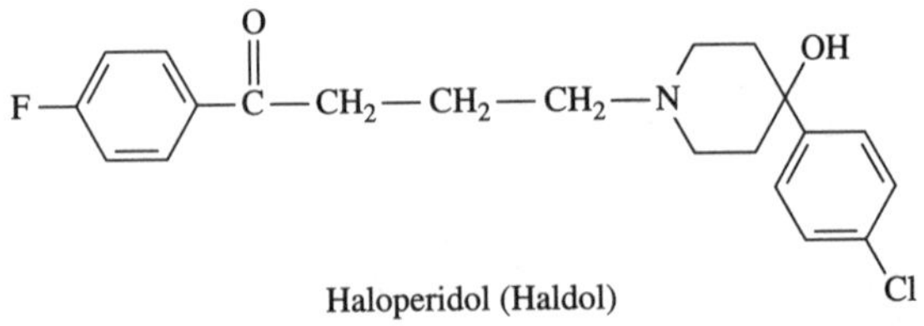

Haloperidol (Haldol)

FIGURE 17.5 Structural formulas of a phenothiazine (chlorpromazine) and a butyrophenone (haloperidol).

the person with schizophrenia? Previously peripheral concerns, such as quality of life, are now being addressed. The new-generation atypical antipsychotics—clozapine, risperidone, olanzapine, sertindole, and quetiapine—are providing the means to address these vital issues. In addition, they are providing tools with which researchers can explore the mechanisms underlying the genesis of the illness. These new drugs have vast implications for how health care is delivered to patients with schizophrenia, challenging the "system" as never before.[2,3,26,27] The documented savings in hospitalization (and rehospitalization) costs associated with the new-generation drugs can occur only by committing increased funds for the new drugs as well as increased commitment to social and community services for outpatient treatment of patients who may "waken" from their prior incapacitation.

Major Versus Minor Tranquilizers

The benzodiazepines (Chapter 6) are often called tranquilizers because they reduce anxiety states and neurotic behavior and produce a state of calmness or tranquility. They are, however, not effective in treating psychosis. The antipsychotic drugs discussed in this chapter are sometimes also referred to as tranquilizers. To distinguish these two very different classes of drugs, the benzodiazepines are sometimes called minor tranquilizers and the antipsychotic drugs major tranquilizers. Although these terms are less commonly used today, they are occasionally encountered. Thus, the terms "major tranquilizer," "neuroleptic," "antipsychotic," and "antischizophrenic" can all be used interchangeably.

Note that the word tranquilizer implies an agent that induces a peaceful, tranquil, calm, or pleasant state. Such a state can be produced by a minor tranquilizer, such as diazepam. However, the psychological effects produced by the major tranquilizers are seldom pleasant or euphoric. Indeed, they may cause unpleasant or dysphoric feelings, especially when administered to nonpsychotic persons. Hence, these drugs do not cause positive behavioral reinforcement and are not encountered as drugs of abuse.

Classification

Antipsychotic drugs can be broadly classified into two groups: (1) standard, classical, or traditional agents, and (2) new-generation, atypical agents. The phenothiazines are the prototypical agents of the first class, while clozapine, risperidone, olanzapine, sertindole, quetiapine, and ziprazadone are the currently available agents of the second class. With the traditional antipsychotics, it has not been possible to separate the therapeutic effects on the positive symptoms from their prominent side effects involving the extrapyramidal motor system. These side effects closely resemble the motor alterations observed in patients who

502 CHAPTER 17 DRUGS USED TO TREAT SCHIZOPHRENIA

have Parkinson's disease: rigidity, tremor, slowed movements, and restlessness (discussed in Chapter 18). Some of these symptoms disappear when the medication is discontinued, but persistent or permanent motor disorders (e.g., tardive dyskinesia) also occur. Atypical agents have two advantages: (1) They may be therapeutically effective without causing this neuroleptic syndrome, and (2) they help relieve the negative symptoms and cognitive dysfunctions associated with schizophrenia.

Phenothiazines

The phenothiazines are the most widely used and least expensive drugs for treating psychosis. They are also used extensively for other purposes, such as to treat nausea and vomiting, to sedate patients before anesthesia, to delay ejaculation, to relieve severe itching, to manage the psychotic component that may accompany acute manic attacks, to treat alcoholic hallucinosis, and to manage the hallucinations caused by psychedelic agents. Table 17.4 lists the 10 phenothiazines currently available for clinical use.

Pharmacokinetics

The phenothiazines are absorbed erratically and unpredictably from the gastrointestinal tract. However, because patients usually take these drugs for long periods of time (even for a lifetime), the oral route of administration is still effective and commonly used. Intramuscular injection of phenothiazines is also quite effective; it increases the effectiveness of the drug to about four to ten times that achieved with oral administration. Once these drugs are in the bloodstream, they are rapidly distributed throughout the body. The levels of phenothiazines that are found in the brain are low compared with the levels found in other body tissues; the highest concentrations are found in the lungs, liver, adrenal glands, and spleen.

The phenothiazines have half-lives of 24 to 48 hours, and they are slowly metabolized in the liver. The clinical effects of a single dose persist for at least 24 hours. Thus, taking the daily dose at bedtime often minimizes certain side effects (such as excessive sedation). The phenothiazines become extensively bound to body tissues, which partially accounts for their slow rate of elimination. Indeed, metabolites of some of the phenothiazines can be detected for several months after the drug has been discontinued. Such slow elimination may also contribute to the slow rate of recurrence of psychotic episodes following the cessation of drug therapy.

To date, therapeutic drug monitoring and correlation of plasma levels of neuroleptics with clinical response and toxicity have not been widely utilized; most dosage decisions are made on a trial-and-error

TABLE 17.4 Antipsychotic drugs

Chemical classification	Drug name: Generic (Trade)	Dose equivalent (mg)	Sedation	Autonomic side effects[a]	Involuntary movement
Phenothiazine	Chlorpromazine (Thorazine)	100	High	High	Moderate
	Prochlorperazine (Compazine)	15	Moderate	Low	High
	Fluphenazine (Prolixin)	2	Low	Low	High
	Trifluoperazine (Stelazine)	5	Moderate	Low	High
	Perphenazine (Trilafon)	8	Low	Low	High
	Acetophenazine (Tindal)	20	Moderate	Low	High
	Carphenazine (Proketazine)	25	Moderate	Low	High
	Triflupromazine (Vesprin)	25	High	Moderate	Moderate
	Mesoridazine (Serentil)	50	High	Moderate	Low
	Thioridazine (Mellaril)	100	High	Moderate	Low
Thioxanthene	Thiothixene (Navane)	4	Low	Low	High
	Chlorprothixene (Taractan)	100	High	High	Moderate
Butyrophenone	Haloperidol (Haldol)	2	Low	Low	Very High
Miscellaneous	Loxapine (Loxitane)	10	Moderate	Low	Moderate
	Molindone (Moban)	10	Moderate	Moderate	Moderate
	Pimozide (Orap)	2	Low	Low	Moderate
New generation	Clozapine (Clozapil)	50	Moderate	Moderate	Low
	Risperidone (Risperdal)	1	Low	Low	Low-Moderate
	Olanzapine (Zyprexa)	1.5	Moderate	Low	Low
	Sertindole (Serlect)	NA[b]	NA	NA	Low

[a]Autonomic side effects include dry mouth, blurred vision, constipation, urinary retention, and reduced blood pressure.
[b]Not available

basis. Studies have shown, however, that the plasma concentrations vary widely among patients given similar amounts of orally administered neuroleptics. These differences probably result from large variations in drug absorption and metabolism.

Pharmacological Effects

In addition to blocking the dopamine$_2$ receptors, the phenothiazines also block acetylcholine, serotonin, histamine, and norepinephrine receptors. The consequences of such blockade are summarized in Table 17.3. Blockade of acetylcholine receptors results in dry mouth, dilated pupils, blurred vision, constipation, urinary retention, and tachycardia. Blockade of norepinephrine receptors can result in hypotension and sedation. Blockade of histamine receptors has sedating as well as antiemetic effects. Indeed, phenothiazines are used in medicine for their antinausea effect.

Limbic System Dopamine-secreting neurons located in the central midbrain portion of the brain stem send axonal projections to those parts of the limbic system that regulate emotional expression as well as to the limbic forebrain areas, where thought and emotions are integrated. Indeed, an increased sensitivity of dopamine receptors in those areas may be responsible for the positive symptomatology of schizophrenia. Thus, chlorpromazine decreases paranoia, fear, hostility, and agitation; it also reduces the intensity of schizophrenic delusions and hallucinations. In addition, chlorpromazine dramatically relieves the agitation, restlessness, and hyperactivity associated with an acute schizophrenic attack. The delusions and hallucinations are particularly sensitive to treatment.

Brain Stem Through actions on the brain stem, phenothiazines suppress the centers involved in behavioral arousal (the ascending reticular activating center) and vomiting (the chemoreceptor trigger zone). By suppressing activity in the reticular formation, the phenothiazines induce an indifference to external stimuli, reducing the inflow of sensory stimuli that would otherwise reach higher brain centers.

Basal Ganglia Neuroleptic drugs produce two main kinds of motor disturbances, which comprise both the most bothersome and the most serious side effects associated with the use of these agents. The two syndromes are (1) acute extrapyramidal reactions, which develop early in treatment in up to 90 percent of patients, and (2) tardive (late) dyskinesia, which occurs much later, during and even after cessation of chronic neuroleptic therapy. Acute extrapyramidal side effects are threefold:

1. Akathesia, a syndrome of the subjective feeling of anxiety, accompanied by restlessness, pacing, constant rocking back and forth, and other repetitive, purposeless actions

2. Dystonia, characterized by involuntary muscle spasms and sustained abnormal, bizarre postures of the limbs, trunk, face, and tongue

3. Neuroleptic-induced parkinsonism, which resembles idiopathic (of unknown etiology) Parkinson's disease (drugs used to treat parkinsonism are discussed in Chapter 18)

Neuroleptic-induced parkinsonism is characterized by tremor at rest, rigidity of the limbs, and slowing of movement with a reduction in spontaneous activity. In idiopathic parkinsonism, these symptoms occur when the concentration of dopamine in the nuclei of the basal ganglia (caudate nucleus, putamen, and globus pallidus) decreases to about 20 percent of normal. Here neuroleptic drug-induced blockade of dopamine receptors in excess of 80 percent occupancy produces the parkinsonism-like symptoms.

Tardive dyskinesia is a much more puzzling and serious form of movement disorder. Victims exhibit involuntary hyperkinetic movements, often of the face and tongue but also of the trunk and limbs, which can be severely disabling. More characteristic are sucking and smacking of the lips, lateral jaw movements, and darting, pushing, or twisting of the tongue. Choreiform movements of the extremities are frequent. The syndrome appears a few months to several years after the beginning of neuroleptic treatment (hence the description "tardive") and is often irreversible. The incidence of tardive dyskinesia has been estimated at more than 10 percent of patients who are treated with traditional neuroleptic drugs, but this side effect depends greatly on the dosage, the age of the patient (it is most common in patients older than 50), and the particular drug used. Adequately controlling dyskinesia may necessitate restarting the neuroleptic medication or increasing the dosage, which is a problem if parkinsonian side effects are troublesome. Baldessarini[28] reviews these effects at length.

Hypothalamus-Pituitary   Pathways of dopamine-secreting neurons extend from the hypothalamus to the pituitary gland. The hypothalamus is intimately involved in the emotions, eating and drinking, sexual behavior, and the secretion of some pituitary hormones. By suppressing the function of the hypothalamus, phenothiazines interrupt these functions. By suppressing the appetite, food intake may be reduced. By suppressing the temperature-regulating centers of the hypothalamus, body temperature fluctuates widely with changes in room temperature. In addition, several body hormones are affected. Dopamine is probably the hormone that inhibits the release of prolactin in the hypothalamus. Thus, when dopamine receptors are blocked, the hormone prolactin is released, which often causes breast enlargement in males and lactation in females. Phenothiazines also reduce the release of hormones from the pituitary gland, which regulate the secretions of sex hormones. Thus, in men ejaculation may be blocked; in women libido may be decreased, ovulation may be blocked, and normal menstrual cycles may be suppressed, resulting in infertility.

Side Effects and Toxicity

The therapeutic use of the phenothiazines invariably leads to many side effects. Indeed, much of the art of managing patients with schizophrenia is in the diagnosis and management of side effects. Specific phenothiazines are chosen not so much because of differences in therapeutic efficacy but because of the relative intensities of their side effects.

In general, the high-potency phenothiazines (e.g., fluphenazine, trifluoperazine, and perphenazine; see Table 17.4) cause less sedation, fewer anticholinergic side effects, less postural hypotension, and more extrapyramidal side effects than the low-potency phenothiazines (e.g., chlorpromazine and thioridazine). Where sedation is desirable, either a low-potency phenothiazine used alone or a high-potency drug combined with a benzodiazepine has the desired therapeutic effect. Where the anticholinergic side effects limit drug compliance, a high-potency drug is desirable, and the drug-induced movement disorders can often be controlled with other medications (anticholinergic, antihistaminic, antiadrenergic, or antiparkinsonian drugs), discussed in Chapter 18.

In patients who are at risk for developing extrapyramidal side effects, who cannot tolerate phenothiazines, or who are treatment resistant, two options are available: (1) they can be prophylactically medicated with anticholinergic, antiparkinsonian, or antiadrenergic drugs, or (2) they can receive a trial of an atypical antipsychotic as a replacement for the phenothiazine. Marder[29] states that there are three categories of treatment-resistant patients:

> The first category includes patients who continue to demonstrate positive psychotic symptoms when they receive adequate trials of an antipsychotic. . . . The second category of poor responders consists of patients who are unable to tolerate the side effects of antipsychotics. . . . The third category includes patients who have persistent negative symptoms while they are treated with an antipsychotic.

Marder concludes this review by stating:

> There is substantial evidence that these patients will demonstrate improvement . . . when they receive clozapine and risperidone as well as newer antipsychotics including olanzapine, sertindole, and quetiapine.

Other potentially serious, but much less common, side effects of phenothiazines include altered pigmentation of the skin, pigment deposits in the retina, permanently impaired vision, decreased pituitary function, menstrual dysfunction, and allergic (hypersensitivity) reactions, which include liver dysfunction and blood disorders.

It has long been recognized that cognitive disturbances are evident in 40 to 60 percent of patients with schizophrenia. Tests show deficits in attention, language, memory, problem solving, judgment, concentration, planning, concept formation, and other "executive functions." Servan-Schreiber and co-workers[30] proposed that "a single deficit in the processing of context information* may underlie various cognitive impairments observed in schizophrenia" and that "such an impairment is associated with positive rather than negative symptoms, and that it may worsen with the course of the illness." Neurochemical assays suggest that serotonin, dopamine, and glutamate all play significant roles in schizophrenia-induced cognitive impairments. These impairments impede psychosocial performance and eventual reintegration into society and are especially relevant targets for new therapeutic modalities.

Goldberg and Weinberger[31] reviewed the effects of traditional neuroleptics and clozapine on cognitive function and concluded that these drugs have few predictable effects on cognition. Phenothiazines with anticholinergic and/or sedative side effects may even have additional detriments. Depressingly, their review of clozapine studies led Goldberg and Weinberger to conclude that few if any cognitive measures improved with this new-generation agent. Any improvements in symptom status did not translate into markedly improved quality of life, living arrangements, or occupational status:

> Taken in toto, these results suggest the need for new pharmacological agents that specifically target cognitive dysfunction in schizophrenia, i.e., *nootropics*, as neither typical nor atypical neuroleptics appear capable of normalizing key impaired cognitive functions in schizophrenia.

This statement is in agreement with the results reported by Meltzer and co-workers,[32] who demonstrated minor improvements in cognitive function in animals, results that will probably translate into only minimal changes in patients. Recently, Purdon and co-workers[33] reported cognitive improvements in 65 patients treated with olanzapine, an encouraging result.

---

*The Servan-Schreiber group[30] defines context information as "information that has to be held actively in mind in such a form that it can be used to mediate an appropriate behavioral response." It can be the "result of processing a sequence of previous stimuli, a specific previous stimulus, or even a set of task instructions. . . . It is relevant to the performance of almost all cognitive tasks."

Tolerance and Dependence

One of the positive attributes of the phenothiazines is that they are not prone to compulsive abuse. They do not produce tolerance, physical dependence, or psychological dependence. Psychotic patients may take phenothiazines for years without increasing their dose because of tolerance; if a dose is increased, it is usually done to increase the control of psychotic episodes.

Despite the fact that discontinuation of a phenothiazine is not followed by symptoms of drug withdrawal, possibly because of the long half-lives of the antipsychotic drugs and their metabolites, the therapeutic dilemmas associated with neuroleptic withdrawal are considerable.[34] In general, since neuroleptic treatment does not cure schizophrenia and long-term use is associated with risk of serious side effects (especially tardive dyskinesia), at some point consideration is often given to reducing or discontinuing medication. Neuroleptic withdrawal can be followed by psychotic exacerbation or relapse, although not all patients relapse after medication withdrawal. Adverse effects of withdrawal other than relapse are mild and transient. In considering drug withdrawal, "The clinician and the patient have to choose between two unwelcome risks: relapse (with drug withdrawal) and adverse effects of continued treatment."[34]

Haloperidol

In 1967, haloperidol (Haldol) was introduced as the first therapeutic alternative to the phenothiazines. A related compound, *droperidol,* was subsequently introduced into anesthesia for the treatment of postoperative nausea and vomiting.

Pharmacologically, haloperidol is remarkably similar to the phenothiazines. It produces sedation and an indifference to external stimuli and reduces initiative, anxiety, and activity. It is well absorbed orally and has a moderately slow rate of metabolism and excretion. Indeed, stable blood levels can be seen for up to three days following discontinuation of the drug. It takes approximately five days for 40 percent of a single dose to be excreted by the kidneys.

The mechanism of the antipsychotic action of haloperidol is like that of the phenothiazines—it occupies and competitively blocks dopamine$_2$ receptors. Haloperidol does not produce many of the serious side effects occasionally observed in patients who are taking phenothiazines (jaundice, blood abnormalities, and so on), but it causes parkinsonian motor movements that are of the same or greater intensity as those induced by the high-potency phenothiazines. Prophylactic antiparkinsonian medication may be needed. Sedation is unusual. In general, however, haloperidol is an effective drug for treating psychotic patients, offering an alternative for patients who do not respond to the phenothiazines.

Atypical Antipsychotics

Until the 1990s most attempts at finding alternative agents to the phenothiazines and haloperidol met with little success. Two alternative medications (molindone and loxapine) were introduced in the early 1970s, but these were not widely successful. From 1975 to 1990, not a single new antipsychotic was marketed in the United States. Since 1990, clozapine (1990), risperidone (1994), pimozide (1996), olanzapine (1996), sertindole (1997), quetiapine (1999), and ziprazadone (2000) have been introduced, and others are on the horizon. Each of these alternatives to the phenothiazines is unique in action.

Molindone

Molindone (Moban) was an early attempt at developing a structurally unique molecule with antipsychotic properties (see Figure 17.6): it resembles the neurotransmitter serotonin. Whether this resemblance is related to its antipsychotic action is unknown. Molindone resembles the traditional antipsychotic drugs in therapeutic efficacy, occupancy of dopamine receptors, and side effects. It produces moderate sedation, increased motor activity, and possibly euphoria. It can also lead to abnormal motor (parkinsonian) movements that resemble those observed in patients taking phenothiazines. Molindone is rapidly absorbed when it is taken orally, and it is metabolized before it is excreted. Clinical effects following a single dose of molindone persist for about 24 to 36 hours. Interestingly, it is also a blocker of the enzyme monoamine oxidase (Chapter 15), and its use is infrequently associated with tardive dyskinesia.

Loxapine

Loxapine (Loxitane) is a traditional antipsychotic drug that is structurally somewhat related to the atypical antipsychotic clozapine (Figure 17.6).[35] Despite this resemblance, its actions differ little from those of the traditional antipsychotic drugs. It has antipsychotic, antiemetic, and sedative properties and causes abnormal motor movements. It lowers convulsive thresholds somewhat more than the phenothiazines. Taken orally, loxapine is well absorbed, and it is metabolized and excreted within about 24 hours.

Loxapine binds strongly to both dopaminergic and serotoninergic receptors; it exhibits negligible binding to NMDA receptors. Singh and co-workers[35] demonstrated that loxapine binds to D_4 and $5\text{-}HT_2$ receptors (as does clozapine); but loxapine also binds strongly to

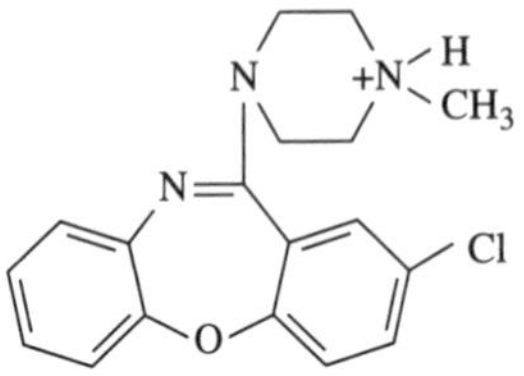

Loxapine (Loxitane)

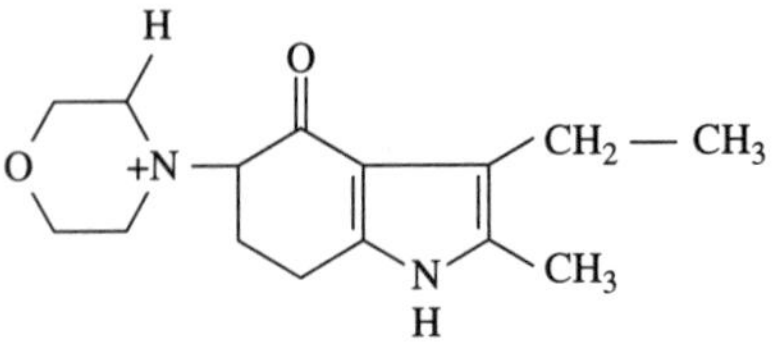

Molindone (Moban)

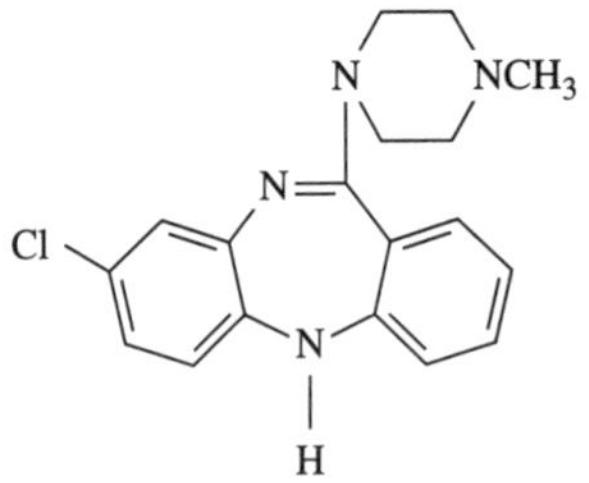

Clozapine (Clozaril)

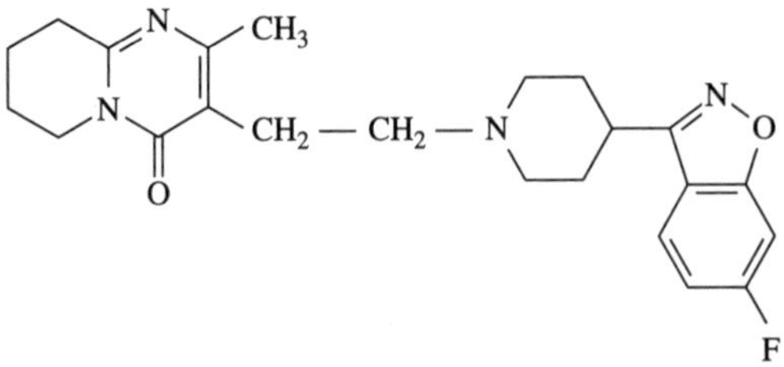

Risperidone (Risperdal)

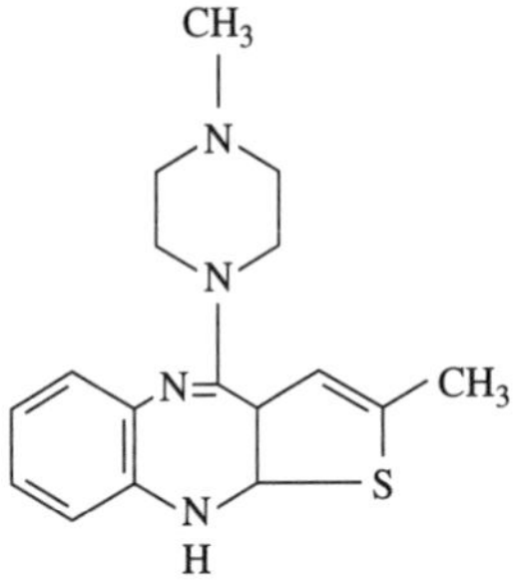

Olanzapine (Zyprexa)

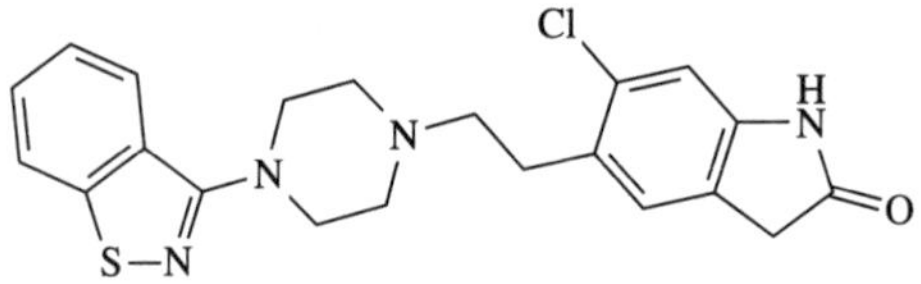

Ziprasidone (Zeldox)

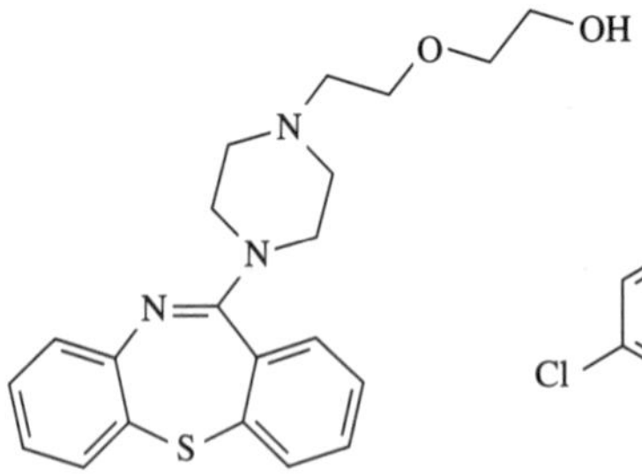

Quetiapine (Seroquel)

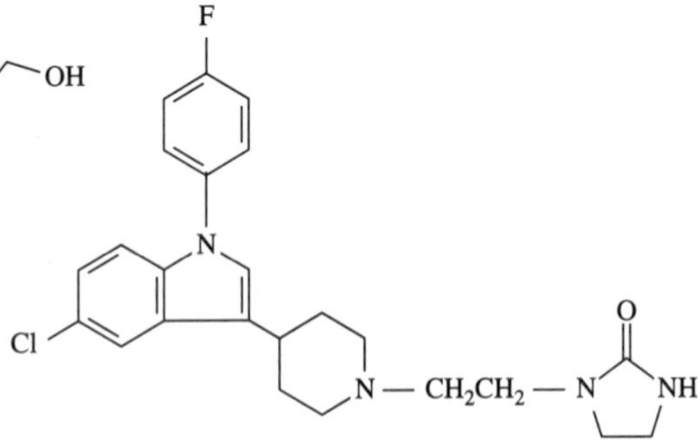

Sertindole (Serlect)

FIGURE 17.6 Structural formulas of new-generation atypical antipsychotic drugs.

D_2 receptors, accounting for its extrapyramidal side effects. Kapur and co-workers[36] explained loxapine's unique status as a clozapine-like but traditional neuroleptic drug. It differs from traditional antipsychotics in that it has a high degree of 5-HT_2 receptor occupancy and blockade; it is not atypical since its 5-HT_2 occupancy is not higher than its D_2 occupancy and blockade (Figure 17.7):

> A high level of 5-HT_2 occupancy is not a sufficient condition for atypicality. If atypical antipsychotic action is predicated on a combination of 5-HT_2 and D_2 effects, then it requires >80% 5-HT_2 occupancy in conjunction with <80% D_2 occupancy.[36]

Pimozide

Pimozide (Orap) is an antipsychotic drug that also blocks dopamine receptors. Currently, the drug is marketed in the United States as an alternative drug for the treatment of motor and phonic tics in patients with Tourette's disorder who are unresponsive to other medications. (Recently, Sallee and co-workers[37] reported that ziprasidone, discussed later, has similar efficacy in Tourette's Syndrome.) In Europe and South America, however, pimozide is a widely used neuroleptic antipsychotic drug, which may ameliorate some of the negative symptomatology of schizophrenia.

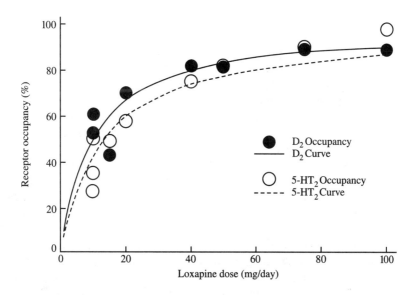

FIGURE 17.7 Dopamine D_2 receptor occupancy and serotonin 5-HT_2 occupancy in PET studies of 10 subjects taking loxapine. Fifty percent of D_2 receptors were occupied at a dose of 9.6 mg/day and 50% of the 5-HT_2 receptors were occupied at a dose of 13.6 mg/day. See text for details. [From Kapur, Zipursky, and Remington.[52]]

Interestingly, pimozide may also have a somewhat unique role in the pharmacologic treatment of delusional disorder,[38] although some authors dispute this use.[39] The side effects that most limit use of pimozide (besides the usual movement disorders and tardive dyskinesia) are electrocardiographic abnormalities that are potentially serious and can even be fatal.[40]

Clozapine

Clozapine (Clozaril) was the first atypical antipsychotic introduced into medicine, approved for marketing in 1989. Its structure is closely related to that of loxapine (Figure 17.6). Clozapine is the only antipsychotic drug that is effective in treating treatment-resistant schizophrenics.[41] It is clinically superior to traditional antipsychotics; it relieves much of the negative symptomatology of schizophrenia, lacks many of the extrapyramidal side effects associated with the standard neuroleptics, and is much less of a cognitive inhibitor.[42-44] "There is evidence that clozapine may improve the core deficit of schizophrenia," improving psychomotor speed, verbal fluency, verbal learning, and memory.[45] In addition, patients with primary parkinsonism can demonstrate psychotic symptoms (such as visual hallucinations and delusions). Traditional neuroleptics worsen the parkinsonism, whereas clozapine can effectively treat the psychosis in parkinsonian patients without aggravating the movement disorder.[46] Despite all this, clozapine is relatively underutilized.[41]

Background Synthesized in 1959, clozapine was introduced into clinical practice in Europe in the early 1970s. Its lack of extrapyramidal side effects was appreciated immediately. However, in 1975 several schizophrenic patients in Finland died of severe infectious diseases after developing agranulocytosis (loss of white cells in the blood) while taking clozapine. As a result, clinical testing ceased, and the drug was withdrawn from unrestricted use in Europe. Later, clozapine was reexamined for two major reasons: (1) the agranulocytosis was found to be reversible when the drug was discontinued, and (2) the drug was found to be therapeutically beneficial in patients with schizophrenia who failed to respond to the traditional neuroleptic compounds.

In 1986 a large, multicenter trial of the drug in the United States found a 30 percent improvement among 318 severely psychotic patients with schizophrenia who were unresponsive to other drugs; only 1 to 2 percent developed agranulocytosis. More recent studies show that the rate of improvement may approach 60 percent with longer therapy. In some patients who appear hopelessly lost in a psychotic world, the improvements in both positive and negative symptoms result in striking changes; the patients emerge as individuals who can be discharged from hospitals or participate meaningfully in rehabilitation programs. The phenomenon has been called "wakening."

Other clozapine responders do not improve substantially in their positive symptoms but report that their mood and sense of well-being are much improved; the deficits associated with schizophrenia do not improve, but the quality of life is better. Wahlbech and colleagues[42] are not as optimistic:

> Scores on symptom rating scales showed greater improvement among clozapine-treated patients (compared with a conventional neuroleptic), who were also more satisfied with their treatment. However, there was no evidence that the superior clinical effect is reflected in levels of functioning.

Meltzer[47] stated that clozapine is particularly effective against a third type of psychotic symptomatology (besides the positive and negative symptoms), which he calls *disorganization*. This set of symptoms consists of loose association, inappropriate affect, incoherence, and reduction in rational thought processes.

Finally and importantly, while clozapine can occasionally be fatal because of serious effects on white blood cells, it actually reduces mortality in patients with severe schizophrenia, mostly by decreasing suicide rates.[48] The reduction in suicide rate must be balanced against the possibility of developing toxic side effects; equal attention must be paid to preventing suicide by continuing therapy and monitoring against potentially fatal agranulocytosis.

Pharmacokinetics   The pharmacokinetics of clozapine varies significantly among patients. The drug is well absorbed orally, and significant metabolism takes place as the drug reaches plasma and is carried to the liver, before it is distributed throughout the body.[49] Plasma levels of the drug peak in about 1 to 4 hours, and its distribution in the body appears to vary: some patients sequester significant quantities of drug. Clozapine is metabolized in the liver into two major metabolites, both of which are fairly inactive pharmacologically. The metabolic half-life of clozapine varies from 9 to 30 hours.

Conley[41] states that "in some patients, monitoring blood levels of clozapine may aid in optimizing treatment. The optimal plasma level of clozapine is 200 to 350 ng/mL, corresponding to a daily dose of 200 to 400 mg, although dosage must be individualized." Monitoring might be useful, for example, when psychotic symptoms recur during clozapine therapy, indicating either noncompliance with therapy or abrupt discontinuation of the drug.[50]

Pharmacodynamics   This chapter earlier introduced theories regarding both the etiology of schizophrenia and the mechanisms of action of antipsychotic drugs, including clozapine. As reviewed by Brunello and co-workers[51]:

> If schizophrenia is in some way related to morphological abnormalities, it becomes hard to believe that a *curative* treatment will ever be possible. Considering this scenario, treatment of schizophrenia will be restricted to symptomatic and preventive therapy and therefore, more effective and better tolerated antipsychotics are necessary. . . . Clozapine constitutes a major advance in particular for patients not responding to conventional neuroleptics.

Clozapine has high binding affinity for dopamine$_4$, serotonin$_{1C}$, serotonin$_2$, alpha$_1$ (an adrenergic receptor), muscarinic (an acetylcholine receptor), and histamine receptors; moderate affinity is seen for many other receptor subtypes:

> Clozapine, differently from all other conventional neuroleptics, is a mixed but weak D_1/D_2 antagonist. This observation has prompted speculation that the synergism between D_1 and D_2 receptors might allow antipsychotic effects to be achieved below the threshold for unwanted motor side effects.[51]

As noted, clozapine has a low rate of binding to D_2 receptors and has greater 5-HT$_2$ blockade at therapeutic doses.[52] Also as noted earlier, this binding ratio defines an atypical antipsychotic.

Side Effects and Toxicity   As stated, despite clozapine's efficacy, it is underutilized therapeutically. The reason for this is a constellation of side effects, some extremely bothersome and some serious. Side effects to be discussed include sedation, weight gain, withdrawal, constipation, and agranulocytosis. Other side effects include urinary incontinence, hypotension, esophagitis, seizures, and excessive drooling.

Sedation occurs in about 40 percent of patients taking clozapine; it may be dose-limiting and have a negative impact on compliance. It appears to be due to an antihistaminic effect of the drug. Taking the drug at bedtime may help improve compliance.

Weight gain is a problem for up to 80 percent of patients; it can be severe, with gains of 20 pounds or more not unusual. Again, it can seriously affect drug compliance.[53] Clozapine and olanzapine seem to cause more of a problem than risperidone or sertindole; the weight gain with clozapine appears to persist for a longer period of time than the weight gain with other antipsychotics.[54,55] The mechanism responsible for this effect is unknown. Education and dietary assistance may help.

Discontinuation of clozapine is followed by a syndrome characterized by delusions, hallucinations, hostility, and paranoid reaction. Other less severe signs include nausea, vomiting, diarrhea, headache, restlessness, agitation, confusion and sweating.[50] Olanzapine has a structure and receptor-blocking profile similar to that of clozapine, so it has been tried in efforts to block this withdrawal syndrome: direct substitution appears to greatly minimize the syndrome, and olanzapine is the only other atypical antipsychotic that does so.[50] Gradual tapering of the dose may also be beneficial.

Constipation occurs in about 30 percent of patients and can be quite bothersome. The anticholinergic and serotonin receptor antagonism could contribute to this effect. Education and stool softeners can help.

As discussed, the major concern with clozapine is the risk of developing severe, life-threatening (although reversible) *agranulocytosis.* White blood cell counts must be monitored weekly or biweekly for the first four to five months of therapy and monthly thereafter, with more frequent monitoring if the white blood cell count decreases. Other drugs that can cause reductions in white blood cell count (most notably carbamazepine; see Chapter 16) should not be taken concomitantly. The incidence of this side effect has been estimated to be as low as 0.38 percent,[41] more commonly estimated at 1 percent to 2 percent;[56] some state that altered white blood cell counts occur in up to 7 percent of patients on continued therapy.[42]

The etiology of clozapine-induced agranulocytosis appears to involve a cellular-toxic mechanism.[56] Eutrecht[57] first reported that clozapine can be metabolized not only in the liver but by the white blood cells themselves. An intermediate compound in this metabolic process is reactive and is postulated to be toxic to the cell, possibly killing the white cells that formed the metabolite.

Cost Concerns   Clozapine therapy is much more expensive than therapy with any of the conventional antipsychotic drugs; it is also more expensive than other atypical antipsychotics (Table 17.5).[58] Adding the costs of the necessary blood monitoring increases total costs even further.

TABLE 17.5 Monthly cost for three new antipsychotic agents relative to a conventional product

Drug name	Daily dose range (mg)	Usual daily dose (mg)	Monthly cost*	Relative cost
Clozapine	300–900	300	317.03	180 : 1
Risperidone	6–16	6	241.62	137 : 1
Olanzapine	10–20	10	232.00	132 : 1
Haloperidol	6–20	10	1.76	—

*Monthly costs based on AWP (average wholesale price) for March 1997.
From J. M. Zito.[58]

Currently, the annual cost of taking clozapine totals about $6,000. To justify these costs, they must be accompanied by lowered health resource utilization expenses (cost offsets) and improved quality of life.

Zito[58] and Revicki[59] applied pharmacoeconomic theory to clozapine and other atypical antipsychotics and found that the costs of drug therapy and monitoring are more than offset by savings in health care costs (primarily reduced rates of relapse and hospitalizations in clozapine-taking patients). These statistical data are often clouded by individual biases and sources of support for individual studies. The high costs of the new drugs make mental health agencies and health care organization workers reluctant to prescribe the drug more, despite the reduced rate of rehospitalization and improved quality of life. A recent symposium reviews the side effects of clozapine and newer atypical antipsychotics.[60]

Risperidone

Risperidone (Risperdal; Figure 17.6) was marketed in 1993 as the second new-generation, atypical antipsychotic drug. Risperidone was first administered to schizophrenic patients in 1986; since then it has been used in Europe and its pharmacology has been studied extensively. Risperidone acts as a potent inhibitor of both D_2 and 5-HT_2 receptors, particularly the latter. As discussed earlier, the serotonin antagonism can result in improved control of psychotic symptoms with only minimal neuroleptic-induced extrapyramidal side effects.

> From the distribution of 5-HT_2 receptors, one would expect dopaminergic transmission to be enhanced in the basal ganglia, resulting in diminished extrapyramidal symptoms. . . . Improved frontal cortical function results in the normalization of descending GABA and NMDA neuronal function . . . systems also implicated in the pathogenesis of positive and negative symptoms.[61]

Pharmacokinetics   The pharmacokinetics of risperidone have been well studied.[49,62] The drug is well absorbed when administered orally and is highly bound to plasma proteins. It is metabolized to an active intermediate (9-hydroxy-risperidone), but the rate of metabolism varies because of genetic differences. The metabolic half-life of risperidone is about 3 hours, that of the metabolite (which accounts for much of the action of risperidone) about 22 hours.

Pharmacodynamics   Several studies and reviews have concluded that risperidone is as effective as haloperidol in reducing the positive symptomatology of schizophrenia without producing a high incidence of extrapyramidal side effects (at least at low to moderate therapeutic doses). Risperidone is however not as effective as clozapine for relieving the positive symptoms of schizophrenia and the parkinsonian side effects, but it is equal to clozapine in relieving negative symptoms.[63] Risperidone can be considered a first-line agent in treating schizophrenia because of its efficacy and safety profile. Risperidone has significant advantages over neuroleptic antipsychotics, and it is comparable to clozapine and olanzapine, with few detrimental effects on memory and minimal extrapyramidal side effects at moderate doses.[7]

Risperidone is effective in treating symptoms of autism and other pervasive developmental disorders both in children[64] and adults[65] (Figure 17.8). It also reduces aggression in youths with conduct disorder.[66]

Side Effects   Common side effects of risperidone include somnolence, agitation, anxiety, insomnia, headache, extrapyramidal effects (at high doses), and nausea. Weight gain is observed but is not quite as severe as that seen with either clozapine or olanzapine.[55] Extrapyramidal symptoms are minimal at doses below 8 mg/day and increase with doses above 8 mg/day.[67] However, in newly diagnosed patients with

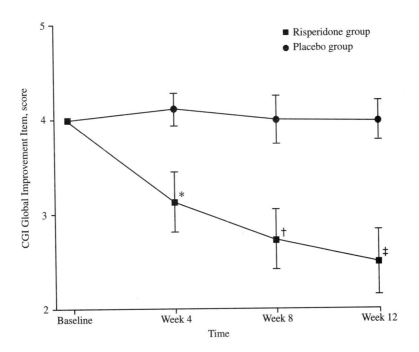

FIGURE 17.8 Global improvement in patients with autism or pervasive development disorder who were given risperidone or placebo for 12 weeks, as measured on the Clinical Global Impression Scale global improvement item. * = <.006; † = <.004; ‡ = <.001 (risperidone vs placebo). [From McDougle.[66]]

schizophrenia with no previous exposure to antipsychotic drugs, extrapyramidal symptoms were identical to those produced by haloperidol, even at low doses of risperidone (mean daily dose was 3.2 mg).[68] This disturbing result implies that risperidone may not be an ideal alternative to traditional antipsychotic drugs for newly diagnosed patients with schizophrenia.

Olanzapine

Introduced in 1996, olanzapine (Zyprexa) is structurally related to clozapine (Figure 17.6). Olanzapine is a blocker of different receptor types in the CNS,[7] but therapeutically its blockade of dopamine and serotonin receptors is of most interest. Kapur and colleagues[69] found that in vivo olanzapine completely blocked $5\text{-}HT_2$ receptors at low doses (5 mg/day); D_2 blockade increased (43 to 80 percent) with increasing doses (5 to 20 mg/day; see Figure 17.9). The greater serotonin blockade accounts for a low incidence of extrapyramidal side effects. The dopamine blockade is higher than that of clozapine and similar to that of risperidone.

Pharmacokinetics   Olanzapine is well absorbed orally. Peak plasma levels occur in about 5 to 8 hours. Metabolized in the liver, olanzapine has an elimination half-life in a range of 27 to 38 hours. This half-life is similar in both adults and children.[70]

Pharmacodynamics   The clinical efficacy of olanzapine in comparison with haloperidol was reported by Beasley and co-workers,[71] by Tollefson and co-workers,[72] by Breier and Hamilton,[73] and by Sanger and co-workers[74]. Improvements in both positive and negative symptoms were impressive in all four studies. Extrapyramidal side effects are only rarely observed. As noted by Marder,[75] however, these four reports were from the manufacturer of the drug: "Until data become available from independent investigators, clinicians should carefully scrutinize these studies for sources of bias." For example, Conley and co-workers[76] reported less impressive results in a population of more severely impaired patients. These differing results suggest that olanzapine may be more effective and better tolerated than traditional antipsychotics in less severely impaired patients. Marder[75] outlines a reasonable medication strategy for treatment-resistant patients. Contradicting efficacy comparisons between clozapine, risperidone, olanzapine, and even newer atypical antipsychotics are likely to continue. Biases and funding sources for the research will certainly cloud the issue.[77]

Other Uses   As was discussed in Chapter 16, there is evidence for the use of olanzapine in the treatment of *bipolar disorder.* Tohen and co-workers[78] compared olanzapine with placebo in 139 patients with acute mania. Olanzapine therapy resulted in at least 50 percent improvement in 48 percent of patients compared with a 24 percent response rate in placebo-

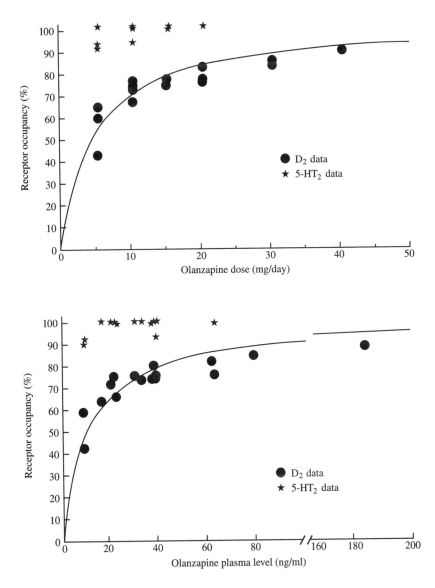

FIGURE 17.9 Relationship between dopamine D_2 and serotonin 5-HT$_2$ receptor occupancy and olanzapine dose and plasma level. [From Kapur et al.[69]]

treated patients. Somnolence, dizziness, dry mouth, and weight gain were the major side effects. Potenza and co-workers[79] studied olanzapine in four adolescents and four adults with *pervasive developmental disorder*. Seven of the eight demonstrated marked improvement in most of the symptoms associated with their disorder. Increased appetite and weight gain (almost 20 pounds per patient) were the major side effects. Buckley[80] reviewed the use of loxapine (a typical antipsychotic) and olanzapine, clozapine, and other atypical antipsychotic drugs in the management of *agitation* and *aggression*. The latter agents are less effective for acute agitation but more appropriate when aggression in psychosis persists and/or is repetitive. More investigation into the use of both mood stabilizers (Chapter 16) and atypical antipsychotics in agitation and aggressive disorders is warranted.

Side Effects   The major side effects induced by olanzapine are weight gain, sedation, orthostatic hypotension, and dizziness. The weight gain is greater than that seen with risperidone but less than that seen with clozapine.[54] Cognitive function is minimally impaired.[31] In contrast to clozapine, there have been no reports of agranulocytosis or reduced white blood cell count with olanzapine.[81]

Sertindole

Sertindole (Serlect, Figure 17.6), introduced in 1997, the fourth introduced atypical antipsychotic, is primarily a $5-HT_2$ antagonist, binding (in decreasing order of affinity) to serotonin $5-HT_2$, $alpha_1$-adrenoreceptors, and dopamine D_2 receptors. It therefore possesses the requisite dual action of blocking D_2 and $5-HT_2$, thought to define the new-generation antipsychotics. This dual action is predicted to be therapeutically useful in ameliorating both the positive and the negative symptoms of schizophrenia, with a low incidence of extrapyramidal side effects. Unlike risperidone and clozapine, sertindole has no affinity for histamine receptors; therefore it is much less sedative.

The metabolic half-life of sertindole varies from about 60 hours to 95 hours and is relatively unaffected by either age or renal function. This half-life value is considerably longer than that of clozapine or risperidone, allowing once-daily or even every-other-day dosing.

Several studies have demonstrated the efficacy and relative lack of extrapyramidal side effects of sertindole.[7,82] Time and experience will define the role of sertindole, its efficacy, and its side effects in comparison with those induced by other atypical antipsychotics. At this point, however, it compares favorably with other atypical agents. One possible complication is that the drug can adversely affect the electrocardiogram, prolonging the Q-T interval, an effect that can lead to severe cardiac arrhythmias. The drug is probably contraindicated in patients with underlying heart disease.[83]

Quetiapine

Quetiapine (Seroquel), the fifth atypical, $5-HT_2/D_2$ receptor blocking agent, was introduced in 1998. It is structurally related to both loxapine and clozapine (Figure 17.6). Like clozapine, quetiapine has greater affinity for 5-HT$_2$ receptors than for D$_2$ receptors, separating antipsychotic action from extrapyramidal side effects. Arvanitis and Miller[84] note that quetiapine is effective, superior to placebo, and comparable to haloperidol in reducing positive symptoms; relief from negative symptoms was less consistent; extrapyramidal symptoms were few. Quetiapine, in its pharmacology, appears to closely resemble clozapine (without the hemodynamic problems with white blood cells). Like clozapine, quetiapine reduces the expression of glutamate receptor mRNA.

The half-life of quetiapine is about 7 hours, necessitating twice (or three times) daily dosage.[85] Quetiapine is also reported to be useful in treating drug-induced psychosis in Parkinson's disease,[86,87] as well as in patients with bipolar and schizoaffective disorders.[88]

Ziprasidone

Ziprasidone (Zeldox; Figure 17.6) is the sixth and newest of the available atypical antipsychotic agents. The drug is more effective than placebo and as effective as haloperidol in treating schizophrenia, with low liability for causing extrapyramidal side effects. One clinical advantage is that unwanted weight gain is negligible.[54,89,90] Ziprasidone is poorly absorbed orally, but the drug that is absorbed is extensively metabolized to a variety of inactive byproducts. Its half-life appears to be short, in the range of 6 hours.[91]

The receptor actions of ziprasidone are unique. In addition to blocking 5-HT$_2$ and D$_2$ receptors, it is an agonist at 5-HT$_{1A}$ receptors, a buspirone-like action (Chapter 6).[16] It is possible that this may confer an antidepressant action on the drug, a potentially advantageous effect. It is, at present, unclear what contribution the 5-HT$_{1A}$ agonist action contributes to its pharmacologic actions. Future publications should help clarify the role of ziprasidone as an atypical antipsychotic agent.

Amisulpride

A yet-to-be-released atypical antipsychotic drug that deserves review is amisulpride. This drug has a unique and interesting neurochemical and psychopharmacological profile: it has high selectivity for blocking dopamine D$_2$ and D$_3$ receptor subtypes in the limbic system (but not the basal ganglia), and it blocks functional responses mediated by those receptors.[92]

As a dopamine blocker, one would predict that it would exert actions similar to those of the traditional antipsychotics. However, that is not the case. Amisulpride is twice as selective for D$_3$ receptors than for D$_2$ receptors; at low doses it blocks presynaptic dopamine autoreceptors (increasing dopamine release), while postsynaptic dopamine receptor (D$_2$) antagonism becomes apparent at higher doses.[93,94] This dual action results in increased dopamine activity in the mesolimbic system at low doses and an antipsychotic action at higher doses, with a low incidence of extrapyramidal side effects.[95] The drug does not bind to serotonin 5-HT$_2$ receptors, an unusual situation for an atypical antipsychotic drug.

Clinically, amisulpride, at low doses, has been shown to be effective in the treatment of dysthymia and depression.[96,97,98] In higher doses, it relieves psychosis, with perhaps more efficacy against negative symptoms than positive ones.[93,99] In nonpsychotic volunteers, amisulpride was well tolerated, exhibited few extrapyramidal side effects, and had half-lives of 12 hours in young people and 16 hours in the elderly.[100,101]

Conclusion: What Makes an Antipsychotic Atypical?

The first revolution in the treatment of schizophrenia started in the 1950s with the introduction of the phenothiazines and haloperidol (now called traditional antipsychotics). The second revolution started in 1989 with the introduction of the atypical antipsychotics. Stahl[102] answers the question, What makes an antipsychotic atypical?

> "Atypical" as applied to an antipsychotic can mean different things to different experts. To clinicians it can connote "low extrapyramidal side effects" or "good for negative symptoms"; to a pharmacologist, "5-HT$_2$ and D$_2$ receptor antagonism"; to a marketer, "new and different"; and, to an economist, "expensive."

As is now apparent, all new and old antipsychotics improve positive symptoms and are also D$_2$ antagonists. Atypical antipsychotics also block 5-HT$_2$ receptors (amisulpride is an exception) and have fewer extrapyramidal side effects. Interestingly, a couple of traditional antipsychotics also display some binding to 5-HT$_2$ receptors, although at lower levels than they block D$_2$ receptors. Some atypicals have greater efficacy than does haloperidol for negative symptoms. Most have less of a detrimental effect on memory and cognition. Many have associated weight gain; ziprasidone has less than most. Are other receptors involved? Quite likely, but this is as yet unclear; no two drugs have the same profile of receptor blockade. Research on the atypical drugs is proceeding rapidly, and a new drug is added to the roster almost yearly. The future of research in this area will be most interesting and, hopefully, of benefit to patients.[103]

Antipsychotic Drugs in the Young and the Elderly

The treatment of schizophrenia in children has received scant attention. Traditional neuroleptics are prescribed with caution and trepidation because of the severity of side effects and the potential for inducing tardive dyskinesia, which may eventually develop in up to half of patients. The use of clozapine in children is limited by the risk of agranulocytosis, necessitating weekly or biweekly blood tests, which makes this treatment unappealing to most adolescents.

Research into the use of the newer atypical antipsychotics introduced in the 1990s in children and adolescents is increasing rapidly. Toren and co-workers[104] reviewed the use of the drugs through 1998. Some (if not most) of these agents were found to be efficacious in the treatment of schizophrenia, bipolar disorders, and pervasive developmental disorders. Their role in treating OCD was unclear. Several of these agents are untested in children and adolescents. The Toren group concluded that some of the atypical neuroleptics may become the first-line treatment for childhood schizophrenia, pervasive developmental disorders, and aggression in conduct disorder.

The use of traditional neuroleptics in the elderly, especially the debilitated nursing-home population, has always been both widespread and controversial. In an effort to use these drugs more appropriately in the elderly nursing-home population, federal legislation was passed in 1987 intended to block overtreatment of elderly individuals with neuroleptic medications. Indeed, it is well recognized that neuroleptics probably can be stopped or the dose lowered in the vast majority of nonschizophrenic nursing home elderly to whom these drugs are inappropriately administered for behavioral control (i.e., restlessness, anxiety, agitation, insomnia).

STUDY QUESTIONS

1. What are the positive and negative symptoms of schizophrenia? Why are these symptoms important in drug therapy and in rehabilitation?

2. Which neurotransmitters are most involved in the pathogenesis of schizophrenia?

3. Are all antipsychotics neuroleptic? Are all neuroleptics antipsychotic?

4. What are the primary clinical differences between traditional and atypical antipsychotic drugs?

5. Discuss the meaning of the word "tranquilizer."

6. Discuss the mechanisms of action of traditional antipsychotics and atypical antipsychotics.

7. Discuss the side effects of phenothiazines.

8. Discuss the consequences of reducing the numbers of institutionalized schizophrenic patients.

9. Compare and contrast clozapine and chlorpromazine, and clozapine and olanzapine.

10. Name the currently available atypical antipsychotic drugs. How are they alike? How do they differ?

11. What appears unique about the drug amisulpride?

REFERENCES

1. J. M. Kane, "Schizophrenia," *New England Journal of Medicine* 334 (1996): 34–41.
2. A. F. Lehman, "Public Health Policy, Community Services, and Outcomes for Patients with Schizophrenia," *Psychiatric Clinics of North America* 21 (1998): 221–231.
3. F. J. Frese, "Advocacy, Recovery, and the Challenges of Consumerism for Schizophrenia," *Psychiatric Clinics of North America* 21 (1998): 233–249.
4. N. C. Andreasen, "Understanding the Causes of Schizophrenia," *New England Journal of Medicine* 340 (1999): 645–647.
5. N. C. Andreasen, "A Unitary Model of Schizophrenia: Bleuler's 'Fragmented Phrene' as Schizencephaly," *Archives of General Psychiatry* 56 (1999): 781–787.
6. R. E. Powers, "The Neuropathology of Schizophrenia," *Journal of Neuropathology and Experimental Neurology* 58 (1999): 679–690.
7. P. J. Harrison, "The Neuropathology of Schizophrenia: A Critical Review of the Data and Their Interpretation," *Brain* 122 (1999): 593–624.
8. P. B. Mortensen et al., "Effects of Family History and Place and Season of Birth on the Risk of Schizophrenia," *The New England Journal of Medicine* 340 (1999): 603–608.
9. C. R. Yang, J. K. Seamans, and N. Gorelova, "Developing a Neuronal Model for the Pathophysiology of Schizophrenia Based on the Nature of Electrophysiological Actions of Dopamine in the Prefrontal Cortex," *Neuropsychopharmacology* 21 (1999): 161–194.
10. *Biological Psychiatry* 46, nos. 1 and 2 (July 1, 1999, and August 1, 1999).
11. S. R. Marder and P. S. Goldman-Rakic, editors, "Special Supplement Issue: Is D_2 antagonism required for Antipsychotic Activity?" *Neuropsychopharmacology* 21, Supplement 6 (December, 1999): S117–S224.
12. J. Arnt and T. Skarsfeldt, "Do Novel Antipsychotics Have Similar Pharmacological Characteristics? A Review of the Evidence," *Neuropsycopharmacology* 18 (1998): 63–101.
13. C. P. Lawler et al., "Interactions of the Novel Antipsychotic Aripiprazole (OPC-14597) with Dopamine and Serotonin Receptor Subtypes," *Neuropsychopharmacology* 20 (1999): 612–627.
14. F. X. Vollenweider, "Advances and Pathophysiological Models of Hallucinogenic Drug Actions in Humans: A Preamble to Schizophrenia Research," *Pharmacopsychiatry* 31, Suppl. 2 (1998): 92–103.

15. E. Richelson, "Preclinical Pharmacology of Neuroleptics: Focus on New-generation Compounds," *Journal of Clinical Psychiatry* 57, Suppl. 11 (1996): 4–11.

16. R. Lewis, et al., "Serotonin 5-HT$_2$ Receptors in Schizophrenia: A PET Study Using [^{18}F]Setoperone in Neuroleptic-naive Patients and Normal Subjects," *American Journal of Psychiatry* 156 (1999): 72–78.

17. J. S. Sprouse et al., "Comparison of the Novel Antipsychotic Ziprasidone with Clozapine and Olanzapine: Inhibition of Dorsal Raphe Cell Firing and the Role of 5-HT$_{1A}$ Receptor Activation," *Neuropsychopharmacology* 21 (1999): 622–631.

18. G. K. Aghajanian and G. J. Marek, "Serotonin-glutamate Interactions: A New Target for Antipsychotic Drugs," *Neuropsychopharmcology* 21 (1999): S122–S133.

19. J. W. Olney and N. B. Farber, "Glutamate Receptor Dysfunction and Schizophrenia," *Archives of General Psychiatry* 52 (1995): 998–1007.

20. S. E. Bachus and J. E. Kleinman, "The Neuropathology of Schizophrenia," *Journal of Clinical Psychiatry* 57, Suppl. 11 (1996): 72–83.

21. C. M. Adler et al., "Comparison of Ketamine-Induced Thought Disorder in Healthy Volunteers and Thought Disorder in Schizophrenia," *American Journal of Psychiatry* 156 (1999): 1646–1649.

22. D. W. Volk et al., "Decreased Glutamic Acid Decarboxylase$_{67}$ Messenger RNA Expression in a Subset of Prefrontal Cortical gamma-Aminobutyric Acid Neurons in Subjects with Schizophrenia," *Archives of General Psychiatry* 57 (2000): 237–245.

23. A. C. Lahti, H. H. Holcomb, X. Gao, and C. A. Tamminga, "NMDA-sensitive Glutamate Antagonism: A Human Model for Psychosis," *Neuropsychopharmacology* 21 (1999): S158–S169.

24. F. Tascedda et al., "Regulation of Ionotropic Glutamate Receptors in the Rat Brain in Response to the Atypical Antipsychotic Seroquel (Quetiapine Fumarate)," *Neuropsychopharmacology* 221 (1999): 211–217.

25 A. R. Mohn et al., "Mice with Reduced NMDA Receptor Expression Display Behaviors Related to Schizophrenia," *Cell* 98 (1999): 427–436.

26. P. S. Albright et al., "Reduction of Healthcare Resource Utilization and Costs Following the Use of Risperidone for Patients with Schizophrenia Previously Treated with Standard Antipsychotic Therapy," *Clinical Drug Investigation* 11 (1996): 289–299.

27. J. M. Zito, "Pharmacoeconomics of the New Antipsychotics for the Treatment of Schizophrenia," *Psychiatric Clinics of North America* 21 (1998): 181–202.

28. R. J. Baldessarini, "Drugs and the Treatment of Psychiatric Disorders: Psychosis and Anxiety," in J. G. Hardman, L. E. Limbird, P. B. Molinoff, R. W. Ruddon, and A. G. Gilman, eds., *Goodman and Gilman's The Pharmacological Basis of Therapeutics*, 9th ed. (New York: McGraw-Hill, 1995), 399–430.

29. S. R. Marder, "Management of Treatment-resistant Patients with Schizophrenia," *Journal of Clinical Psychiatry* 57, Suppl. 11 (1996): 26–30.

30. D. Servan-Schreiber, J. D. Cohen, and S. Steingard, "Schizophrenic Deficits in the Processing of Context: A Test of a Theoretical Model," *Archives of General Psychiatry* 53 (1996): 1105–1112.

31. T. E. Goldberg and D. R. Weinberger, "Effects of Neuroleptic Medications on the Cognition of Patients with Schizophrenia: A Review of Recent Studies," *Journal of Clinical Psychiatry* 57, Suppl. 9 (1996): 62–65.

32. H. Y. Meltzer et al., "Neuropsychologic Deficits in Schizophrenia: Relation to Function and Effects of Antipsychotic Drug Treatment," *Neuropsychopharmacology* 14 (1996): S27–S33.

33. S. E. Purdon et al., "Neuropsychological Changes in Early Phase Schizophrenia During 12 Months of Treatment with Olanzapine, Risperidone, or Haloperidol," *Archives of General Psychiatry* 57 (2000): 249–258.

34. P. L. Gilbert, M. J. Harris, L. A. McAdams, and D. V. Jeste, "Neuroleptic Withdrawal in Schizophrenic Patients," *Archives of General Psychiatry* 52 (1995): 173–188.

35. A. N. Sinh et al., "A Neurochemical Basis for the Antipsychotic Activity of Loxapine: Interactions with Dopamine D_1, D_2, D_4 and Serotonin 5-HT_2 Receptor Subtypes," *Journal of Psychiatry and Neuroscience* 21 (1996): 29–35.

36. S. Kapur et al., "PET Evidence That Loxapine Is an Equipotent Blocker of 5-HT_2 and D_2 Receptors: Implications for the Therapeutics of Schizophrenia," *American Journal of Psychiatry* 154 (1997): 1525–1529.

37. F. R. Sallee et al., "Ziprasidone Treatment of Children and Adolescents With Tourette's Syndrome: A Pilot Study," *Journal of the American Academy of Child and Adolescent Psychiatry* 39 (2000): 292–299.

38. L. A. Opler, D. M. Klahr, and P. M. Ramirez, "Pharmacologic Treatment of Delusions," *Psychiatric Clinics of North America* 18 (1995): 379–391.

39. H. Silva et al., "Effects of Pimozide on the Psychopathology of Delusional Disorder," *Progress in Neuro-psychopharmacology and Biological Psychiatry* 22 (1998): 331–340.

40. Z. Desta, T. Kerbusch, and D. A. Flockhart, "Effect of Clarithromycin on the Pharmacokinetics and Pharmacodynamics of Pimozide in Health-poor and Extensive Metabolizers of Cytochrome P450 2D6 (CYP2D6)," *Clinical Pharmacology and Therapeutics* 65 (1999): 10–20.

41. R. R. Conley, "Optimizing Treatment with Clozapine," *Journal of Clinical Psychiatry* 59, Suppl. 3 (1998): 44–48.

42. K. Wahlbeck et al., "Evidence of Clozapine's Effectiveness in Schizophrenia: A Systematic Review and Meta-analysis of Randomized Trials," *American Journal of Psychiatry* 156 (1999): 990–999.

43. R. Rosenheck et al., "Impact of Clozapine on Negative Symptoms and on the Deficit Syndrome in Refractory Schizophrenia," *American Journal of Psychiatry* 156 (1999): 88–93.

44. V. Kumari, W. Soni, and T. Sharma, "Normalization of Information-processing Deficits in Schizophrenia with Clozapine," *American Journal of Psychiatry* 156 (1999): 1046–1051.

45. S. R. McGurk, "The Effects of Clozapine on Cognitive Functioning in Schizophrenia," *Journal of Clinical Psychiatry* 60, Suppl. 12 (1999): 24–29.

46. The Parkinson Study Group, "Low-dose Clozapine for the Treatment of Drug-induced Psychosis in Parkinson's Disease," *New England Journal of Medicine* 340 (1999): 757–763.

47. H. Y. Meltzer," New Drugs for the Treatment of Schizophrenia," *Psychiatric Clinics of North America* 16 (1993): 365–385.

48. A. M. Walker, L. L. Lanza, F. Arellano, and K. J. Rothman, "Mortality in Current and Former Users of Clozapine," *Epidemiology* 8 (1997): 671–677.
49. M. J. Byerly and C. L. DeVane, "Pharmacokinetics of Clozapine and Risperidone: A Review of Recent Literature," *Journal of Clinical Psychopharmacology* 16 (1996): 177–187.
50. G. D. Tollefson et al., "Controlled, Double-blind Investigation of the Clozapine Discontinuation Symptoms with Conversion to Either Olanzapine or Placebo," *Journal of Clinical Psychopharmacology* 19 (1999): 435–443.
51. N. Brunello, C. Masotto, L. Steardo, R. Markstein, and G. Racagni, "New Insights into the Biology of Schizophrenia Through the Mechanism of Action of Clozapine," *Neuropsychopharmacology* 13 (1995): 177–213.
52. S. Kapur, R. B. Zipursky, and G. Remington, "Clinical and Theoretical Implications of 5-HT$_2$ and D$_2$ Receptor Occupancy of Clozapine, Risperidone, and Olanzapine in Schizophrenia," *American Journal of Psychiatry* 156 (1999): 286–293.
53. T. Wetterling and H. E. Mugigbrodt, "Weight Gain: Side Effects of Atypical Neuroleptics?" *Journal of Clinical Psychopharmacology* 19 (1999): 316–321.
54. D. B. Allison et al., "Antipsychotic-induced Weight Gain: A Comprehensive Research Synthesis," *American Journal of Psychiatry* 156 (1999): 1686–1696.
55. D. A. Wirshing et al., "Novel Antipsychotics: Comparison of Weight Gain Liabilities," *Journal of Clinical Psychiatry* 60 (1999): 358–363.
56. A. C. Tschen, M. J. Rieder, K. Oyewumi, and D. J. Freeman, "The Cytotoxicity of Clozapine Metabolites: Implications for Predicting Clozapine-induced Agranulocytosis," *Clinical Pharmacology and Therapeutics* 65 (1999): 526–532.
57. J. P. Eutrecht, "Metabolism of Clozapine by Neutrophils: Possible Implications for Clozapine-induced Agranulocytosis," *Drug Safety* 7, Suppl. 1 (1992): 51–56.
58. J. M. Zito, "Pharmacoeconomics for the New Antipsychotics for the Treatment of Schizophrenia," *Psychiatric Clinics of North America* 21 (1998): 181–202.
59. D. A. Revicki, "Pharmacoeconomic Studies of Atypical Antipsychotic Drugs for the Treatment of Schizophrenia," *Schizophrenia Research* 35, Suppl. (1999): S101–S109.
60. H. Y. Meltzer, editor, "Side Effects of Antipsychotic Medications," *Journal of Clinical Psychiatry* 61, Supplement 8 (2000): 3–66.
61. A. Megens, "Survey on the Pharmacodynamics of the New Antipsychotic Risperidone," *Psychopharmacology* 114 (1994): 9–23.
62. G. Mannens et al., "Absorption, Metabolism, and Excretion of Risperidone in Humans," *Drug Metabolism and Disposition* 21 (1993): 1134–1141.
63. A. F. Breier et al, "Clozapine and Risperidone in Chronic Schizophrenia: Effects on Symptoms, Parkinsonian Side Effects, and Neuroendocrine Response," *American Journal of Psychiatry* 156 (1999): 294–298.
64. R. Nicolson, G. Awad, and L. Sloman, "An Open Trial of Risperidone in Young Autistic Children," *Journal of the American Academy of Child and Adolescent Psychiatry* 37 (1998): 372–376.
65. C. J. McDougle, "A Double-blind, Placebo-controlled Study of Risperidone in Adults with Autistic Disorder and Other Pervasive Developmental Disorders," *Archives of General Psychiatry* 55 (1998): 633–641.

66. R. L. Findling et al., "A Double-Blind Pilot Study of Risperidone in the Treatment of Conduct Disorder," *Journal of the American Academy of Child and Adolescent Psychiatry* 39 (2000): 509–516.

67. P. Lemmens, M. Brecher, and B. Van Baelen, "A Combined Analysis of Double-blind Studies with Risperidone vs. Placebo and Other Antipsychotic Agents: Factors Associated with Extrapyramidal Symptoms," *Acta Psychiatrica Scandinavia* 99 (1999): 160–170.

68. P. I. Rosebush and M. F. Mazurek, "Neurologic Side Effects in Neuroleptic-naive Patients Treated with Haloperidol or Risperidone," *Neurology* 52 (1999): 782–785.

69. S. Kapur et al., "5-HT$_2$ and D$_2$ Receptor Occupancy of Olanzapine in Schizophrenia: A PET Investigation," *American Journal of Psychiatry* 155 (1998): 921–928.

70. D. R. Grothe et al., "Olanzapine Pharmacokinetics in Pediatric and Adolescent Inpatients with Schizophrenia," *Journal of Clinical Psychopharmacology* 20 (2000): 220–225.

71. C. M. Beasley, G. D. Tollefson, and P. V. Tran, "Efficacy of Olanzapine: An Overview of Pivotal Clinical trials," *Journal of Clinical Psychiatry* 58, Suppl. 10 (1997): 7–12.

72. G. D. Tollefson, T. M. Sanger, and M. E. Thieme, "Depressive Signs and Symptoms in Schizophrenia: A Prospective Blinded Trial of Olanzapine and Haloperidol," *Archives of General Psychiatry* 55 (1998): 250–258.

73. A. Breier and S. H. Hamilton, "Comparative Efficacy of Olanzapine and Haloperidol for Patients with Treatment-resistant Schizophrenia," *Biological Psychiatry* 45 (1999): 403–411.

74. T. M. Sanger et al., "Olanzapine Versus Haloperidol Treatment in First-episode Psychosis," *American Journal of Psychiatry* 156 (1999): 79–87.

75. S. M. Marder, "New Antipsychotics in Treatment-Resistant Schizophrenia," *Biological Psychiatry* 45 (1999): 383–384.

76. R. R. Conley et al., "Olanzapine Compared with Chlorpromazine in Treatment-Resistant Schizophrenia," *American Journal of Psychiatry* 155 (1998): 914–920.

77 P. V. Tran et al., "Double-blind Comparison of Olanzapine Versus Risperidone in the Treatment of Schizophrenia and Other Psychotic Disorders," *Journal of Clinical Psychiatry* 17 (1997): 407–418. See also replies to this research, published in *Journal of Clinical Psychiatry* 18 (1998): 174–176, 176–179, and 353–356.

78. M. Tohen et al., "Olanzapine Versus Placebo in the Treatment of Acute Mania," *American Journal of Psychiatry* 156 (1999): 702–709.

79. M. N. Potenza, J. P. Holmes, S. J. Kanes, and C. McDougle, "Olanzapine Treatment of Children, Adolescents, and Adults with Pervasive Developmental Disorders: An Open-label Pilot Study," *Journal of Clinical Psychopharmacology* 19 (1999): 37–44.

80. P. F. Buckley, "The Role of Typical and Atypical Antipsychotic Medications in the Management of Agitation and Aggression," *Journal of Clinical Psychiatry* 60, Suppl. 10 (1999): 52–60.

81. D. E. Casey, "Side Effect Profiles of New Antipsychotic Agents," *Journal of Clinical Psychiatry* 57, Suppl. 11 (1996): 40–45.

82. A. M. Lee, J. L. Knoll, and T. Suppes, "The Atypical Antipsychotic Sertindole: A Case Series," *Journal of Clinical Psychiatry* 58 (1997): 410–416.

83. A. S. Hale, "A Review of the Safety and Tolerability of Sertindole," *International Clinical Psychopharmacology* 13, Suppl. 3 (1998): S65–S70.
84. L. A. Arvanitis and B. G. Miller, "Multiple Fixed Doses of "Seroquel" (Quetiapine) in Patients with Acute Exacerbation of Schizophrenia: A Comparison with Haloperidol and Placebo. The Seroquel Trial 13 Study Group," *Biological Psychiatry* 42 (1997): 233–246.
85. D. J. King, C. G. Link, and B. Kowalcyk, "A Comparison of bid and tid Dose Regimens of Quetiapine (Seroquel) in the Treatment of Schizophrenia," *Psychopharmacology* 137 (1998): 139–146.
86. H. H. Fernandez, J. H. Friedman, C. Jacques, and M. Rosenfeld, "Quetiapine for the Treatment of Drug-Induced Psychosis in Parkinson's Disease," *Movement Disorders* 14 (1999): 484–487.
87. S. D. Targum and J. L. Abbott, "Efficacy of Quetiapine in Parkinson's Patients With Psychosis," *Journal of Clinical Psychopharmacology* 20 (2000): 54–60.
88. C. A. Zarate et al., "Clinical Predictors of Acute Response With Quetiapine in Psychotic Mood Disorders," *Journal of Clinical Psychiatry* 61 (2000): 185–189.
89. D. G. Daniel et al., "Ziprasidone 80 mg/day and 160 mg/day in the Acute Exacerbation of Schizophrenia and Schizoaffective Disorder: A 6-week, Placebo-controlled Trial. Ziprasidone Study Group," *Neuropsychopharmacology* 20 (1999): 491–505.
90. P. Keck, Jr., et al., "Ziprasidone 40 and 120 mg/day in the Acute Exacerbation of Schizophrenia and Schizoaffective Disorder: a 4-week, Placebo-controlled Trial," *Psychopharmacology* 140 (1998): 173–184.
91. C. Prakash, A. Kamel, J. Gummerus, and K. Wilner, "Metabolism and Excretion of a New Antipsychotic Drug, Ziprasidone, in Humans," *Drug Metabolism and Disposition* 25 (1997): 863–872.
92. J.-M. Danion, W. Rein, O. Fleurot, and the Amisulpride Study Group, "Improvement of Schizophrenic Patients with Primary Negative Symptoms Treated with Amisulpride," *American Journal of Psychiatry* 156 (1999): 610–616.
93. B. Scatton et al., "Amisulpride: From Animal Pharmacology to Therapeutic Action," *International Clinical Psychopharmacology* 12, Suppl. 2 (1997): S29–S36.
94. G. Perrault et al., "Psychopharmacological Profile of Amisulpride: An Antipsychotic Drug with Presynaptic D_2/D_3 Dopamine Receptor Antagonist Activity and Limbic Sensitivity," *Journal of Pharmacology and Experimental Therapeutics* 280 (1997): 73–82.
95. G. Di Giovanni, M. Di Mascio, V. Di Matteo, and E. Esposito, "Effects of Acute and Repeated Administration of Amisulpride, a Dopamine D_2/D_3 Receptor Antagonist, on the Electrical Activity of Midbrain Dopaminergic Neurons," *Journal of Pharmacology & Experimental Therapeutics* 287 (1998): 51–57.
96. E. Smeraldi, "Amisulpride versus Fluoxetine in Patients with Dysthymia or Major Depression in Partial Remission: A Double-blind Comparative Study," *Journal of Affective Disorders* 48 (1998): 47–56.
97. P. Boyer, Y. Lecrubier, A. Stalla-Bourdillon, and O. Fleurot, "Amisulpride versus Amineptine and Placebo for the Treatment of Dysthymia," *Neuropsychobiology* 39 (1999): 25–32.

98. Y. Lecrubier, P. Boyer, S. Turjanski and W. Rein, "Amisulpride Versus Imipramine and Placebo in Dysthymia and Major Depression. Amisulpride Study Group," *Journal of Affective Disorders* 43 (1997): 95–103.

99. J-M. Danion et al., "Improvement of Schizophrenic Patients With Primary Negative Symptoms Treated with Amisulpride," *American Journal of Psychiatry* 156 (2000): 610–616.

100. J. G. Ramaekers et al., "Psychomotor, Cognitive, Extrapyramidal, and Affective Functions of Healthy Volunteers During Treatment with an Atypical (Amisulpride) and a Classic (Haloperidol) Antipsychotic," *Journal of Clinical Psychopharmacology* 19 (1999): 209–221.

101. B. Hamon-Vilcot et al., "Safety and Pharmacokinetics of a Single Oral Dose of Amisulpride in Healthy Elderly Volunteers," *European Journal of Clinical Pharmacology* 54 (1998): 405–409.

102. S. M. Stahl, "What Makes an Antipsychotic Atypical?" *Journal of Clinical Psychiatry* 59 (1998): 403–404.

103. R. R. Murray and N. R. Schooler, chairs., "Novel Antipsychotic Use in Schizophrenia," (Academic Highlights) *Journal of Clinical Psychiatry* 61 (2000): 223–232.

104. P. Toren, N. Laor, and A. Weizman, "Use of Atypical Neuroleptics in Child and Adolescent Psychiatry," *Journal of Clinical Psychiatry* 59 (1998): 644–656.

Chapter 18

Drugs Used to Treat Parkinsonism

Chapter 17 discussed the classical neuroleptic agents that are used to treat schizophrenia. The most prominent side effects of those drugs are movement disorders that resemble those seen in idiopathic Parkinson's disease (parkinsonism). Mechanistically, these side effects result from drug-induced blockade of dopamine$_2$ receptors, resulting in a hypodopaminergic state. Parkinson's disease is similarly associated with a hypodopaminergic state, characterized by a loss of dopamine neurons, most prominently in the extrapyramidal motor areas of the basal ganglia (caudate and putamen).[1] Thus, the symptomatology of parkinsonism resembles the side effects seen with use of neuroleptics; the goals of therapy are to replace the lost dopaminergic function and (hopefully) reverse the loss of dopamine neurons.

Parkinson's disease is a neurodegenerative disease that occurs in about 1 percent of all adults over the age of 65. Although the cause of parkinsonism remains unknown, its symptoms clearly follow from a deficiency in the numbers and function of dopamine-secreting neurons located in the basal ganglia of the brain. The clinical disease emerges when dopamine is depleted to about 20 percent of normal. In other words, the disease results when about 80 to 90 percent of dopamine neurons are lost. (Recall from Chapter 17 that the antipsychotic efficacy of neuroleptic drugs occurs when about 80 percent of dopamine$_2$ receptors were blocked.) The clinical syndrome of parkinsonism comprises four cardinal features:[2] (1) bradykinesia (slowness and poverty of movement); (2) muscle rigidity (especially a "cogwheel" rigidity); (3) resting tremor, which usually abates during voluntary movement; and (4) an impairment of postural balance leading to disturbances of gait and falling. These and the frequently seen secondary manifestations of Parkinson's disease are listed in Table 18.1.

The availability of effective treatments for the symptoms of parkinsonism has radically altered the prognosis of this disease. In most cases, good functional mobility can be maintained for many years and the life expectancy of an affected individual has been greatly expanded. Replacement of the dopamine or the administration of either dopaminergic agonists or inhibitors of dopamine breakdown can restore function and ameliorate much of the symptomatology. These three approaches— dopamine replacement therapy, administration of a dopaminergic agonist, and administration of dopamine-breakdown inhibitors)—underlie the present-day treatment of the disease. Table 18.2 lists the medications and the dosages used for the treatment of parkinsonism.

Levodopa (L-dopa)

Levodopa continues to be the mainstay of therapy for Parkinson's disease. Because a loss of dopamine is the primary problem in patients who have Parkinson's disease, replacement of the dopamine would be expected to ameliorate the symptoms of the disease. It does, but not by itself, because dopamine does not cross the blood-brain barrier from plasma into the CNS. In an intuitive step, the precursor compound in the biosynthesis of dopamine from the amino acid tyramine, a substance called *dihydroxyphenylalanine* or *DOPA* (Figure 18.1), crosses the blood-brain barrier and in the CNS is converted into dopamine, replacing the dopamine that is absent. Therefore, today, levodopa (the *levo* isomer being more active than the *dextro* isomer) is the most effective treatment for parkinsonian motor disability, and many practitioners consider an initial beneficial response an important diagnostic criterion for the diagnosis of parkinsonism.[3]

Mechanism of Action

Levodopa is itself largely inert; its therapeutic as well as its adverse effects result from its conversion to dopamine.[1] Administered orally, levodopa is rapidly absorbed into the bloodstream, where most of it (about 95 percent) is converted to dopamine in the plasma. Although only a small amount (about 1 to 5 percent) of levodopa crosses the blood-brain barrier and is converted to dopamine in the brain, it is enough to alleviate the symptoms of parkinsonism. In the CNS, levodopa is converted to dopamine by decarboxylation, primarily within the presynaptic terminals of dopaminergic neurons in the basal ganglia.[1]

TABLE 18.1 Clinical features of Parkinson's disease

CARDINAL MANIFESTATIONS
  Resting tremor
  Bradykinesia (akinesia, hypokinesia)
  Cogwheel rigidity
  Postural reflex impairment

SECONDARY MANIFESTATIONS

  Cognitive
    Dementia
    Bradyphrenia
    Visuospatial deficits, impaired
      attention and executive function

  Psychiatric
    Depression
    Anxiety
    Sleep disturbances
    Sexual dysfunction

  Craniofacial
    Masked facies
    Decreased eye blinking
    Blurred vision (impaired
      accommodation)
    Olfactory hypofunction
    Dysarthria (soft, palilalic speech)
    Dysphagia
    Sialorrhea

  Autonomic
    Orthostatic hypotension
    Impaired gastrointestinal motility
      Constipation, dysphagia,
        sensation of fullness
    Urinary bladder dysfunction
      Urgency, frequency, loss of control
    Abnormal thermoregulation,
      increased sweating

  Sensory
    Cramps
    Paresthesia
    Pain
    Numbness, tingling

  Musculoskeletal
    Scoliosis
    Wrist and foot dystonia
    Peripheral edema

  Skin
    Seborrhea

  Other
    Micrographia
    Weight loss

From Colcher and Simuni.[2]

TABLE 18.2 Drugs for Parkinson's disease

Agent	Trade name	Daily dose— useful range	Comments
Carbidopa/levodopa	Sinemet	200–1,200 mg levodopa	Half-life 1–3 hours
Carbidopa/levodopa, sustained release	Sinemet CR	200–1,200 mg levodopa	Bioavailability 75% of standard form
Pergolide	Permax	0.75–5.0 mg	Titrate slowly
Bromocriptine	Parlodel	3.75–40 mg	Titrate slowly
Selegiline	1-Deprenyl, Eldepryl	2.5–10 mg	Titrate slowly
Tolcapone	Tasmar	300–600 mg	May alter liver function
Entacapone	Comtan	200–800 mg	Half-life 2–3 hours
Pramipexole	Mirapex	1.5–4.5 mg	Half-life 8–12 hours
Ropinirole	Requip	3–12 mg	Half-life 6 hours

One problem with this therapy, however, is that, when levodopa is administered by itself, large amounts are destroyed by enzymes located both in the intestine and in plasma, so that little drug is available to cross the blood-brain barrier. In addition, the levodopa in the peripheral circulation is converted to dopamine in the body, resulting in undesirable side effects, such as nausea.

Back to basic pharmacology. One approach to solving the problem is to reduce the high levels of dopamine in the systemic circulation while maintaining sufficient quantities in the brain. To do this, the biosynthetic pathway that leads to dopamine (Figure 18.1) must be examined. Since the enzyme *dopa decarboxylase* is responsible for converting dopa to dopamine, by inhibiting this enzyme in the systemic circulation but not in the brain, systemic biotransformation of the drug should be reduced, with a concomitant reduction in blood levels of dopamine and therefore in side effects. The drug would need a unique characteristic: it would have to be active in the body but not cross the blood-brain barrier into the brain.

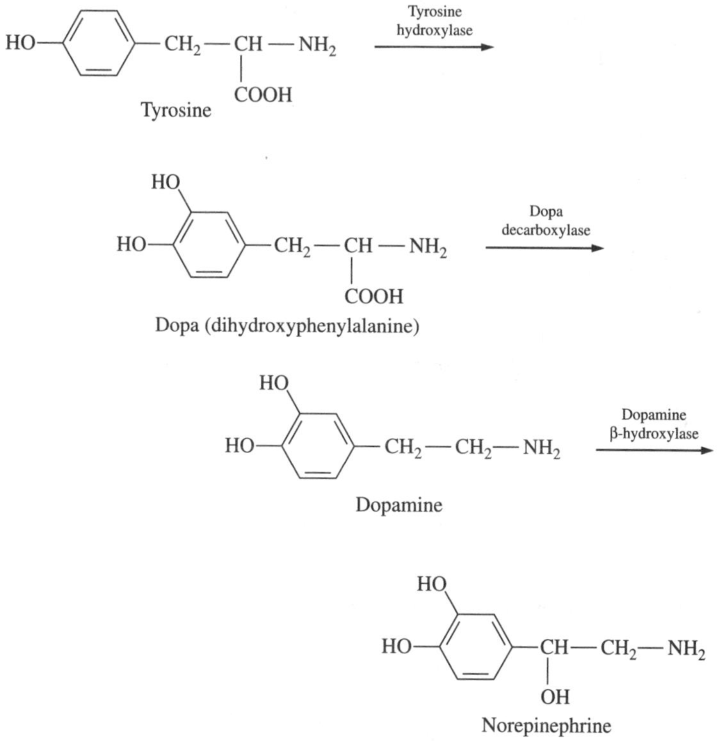

FIGURE 18.1 Synthesis of dopamine from tyrosine.

Thus, the metabolic conversion would occur in the CNS but not in the periphery.

An example of such a drug is *carbidopa,* which is available in combination with levodopa (the combination is marketed as Sinemet). By combining carbidopa with levodopa, the effective dose of levodopa is reduced by 75 percent, with a concomitant reduction in side effects and no loss of CNS therapeutic effect. The current treatment of parkinsonism relies heavily on the use of Sinemet (Table 18.2), and it is the standard of current symptomatic treatment for Parkinson's disease.[4] It provides the greatest antiparkinsonian benefit with the fewest side effects.[4]

Recently, a new advance has been made to this therapeutic regimen. Even with the Sinemet combination, much of an oral dose of levodopa is wasted.[5] The enzyme *catechol-o-methyltransferase* (COMT) in the vasculature of the gastrointestinal tract and liver converts levodopa to a metabolic by-product (3-ortho-methyl-dopa) with no clinical benefit.[5] The half-life and clinical effects of Sinemet can be increased with the addition of a COMT-inhibitory drug. In 1998, the first of these—*talcapone*

(Tasmar)—was introduced; it blocks the COMT enzyme, increasing the half-life of l-dopa and prolonging its effect. Unfortunately, tolcapone has caused a few cases of serious liver toxicity and was withdrawn from the market in Canada, but it is still available in the United States.[7] A second COMT-inhibitor, *entacapone*, became available in 2000 and is not yet associated with liver toxicity.[6-8]

Both tolcapone and entacapone inhibit peripheral COMT; they do not alter central COMT. Inhibition of peripheral degradation of levodopa increases central levodopa and, therefore, central dopamine concentrations:

> Coadministration of entacapone (or tolcapone) with levodopa plus a decarboxylase inhibitor potentiates the effects of levodopa in patients with Parkinson's disease and reduces the "wearing-off" phenomenon.[8]

The half-life of oral entacapone is about two to three hours, which is similar to the half-life of levodopa (about two hours).

Limitations to Levodopa Therapy

While levodopa therapy has a dramatic effect on the symptoms of parkinsonism, as time goes on, the drug becomes less effective and the patient's symptoms fluctuate dramatically between doses. Eventually, this develops into what is called an "off-and-on" or "wearing-off" phenomenon.[1,3] Part of the phenomenon is due to the short half-life of levodopa and can be minimized by increasing the dose, by decreasing the interval between doses, and by adding a COMT inhibitor. This adjustment, however, risks the development of levodopa-induced movement disorders (e.g., dyskinesias), which can be as uncomfortable and disabling as the rigidity and akinesia of parkinsonism.[1] A sustained-release preparation of levodopa/carbidopa (Sinemet CR) can be used to help provide a more stable blood level of the drug and, it is hoped, reduce the dyskinesias.

Another unanswered question with levodopa therapy is whether or not this drug adversely accelerates the course of parkinsonism.[4] One theory of the disease is that the metabolism of dopamine produces free radicals that contribute to the death of the dopamine-releasing neurons. Oxidative stress may therefore be an important precipitating mechanism, and neuroprotective drugs might eventually be of more fundamental use in prevention of the disease rather than therapy. Simon and Standaert[9] discuss possible therapeutic strategies that might eventually be used to reduce or eliminate oxidative stress. For the present, however, there is continuing concern that ameliorating symptoms may be aggravating the disease. Thus, initiation of levodopa therapy is often delayed until the symptoms of parkinsonism actually cause an unacceptable degree of functional impairment. It leaves the clinician in a quandary about how to treat early stages of parkinsonism.[4]

Dopamine Receptor Agonists

Between one and five years after the start of levodopa therapy, most patients gradually become less responsive. This development may be related to a progressive inability of dopamine neurons to synthesize and store dopamine. To relieve this problem, attempts have been made to identify drugs that will directly stimulate postsynaptic dopamine receptors in the basal ganglia. These drugs do not depend on the ability of existing dopaminergic neurons to enzymatically convert the drug to an active compound (i.e., levodopa to dopamine). In addition, if the free radical theory described in the previous paragraph is accepted, these drugs would avoid the biotransformation into potentially neurotoxic metabolites. These drugs might be effective in the late stages of parkinsonism, when dopamine neurons are largely absent or nonfunctional. In addition, they are increasingly being advocated for use in early stages of parkinsonism, especially in patients younger than about 65 years.

Four dopamine receptor agonists are currently available for the treatment of parkinsonism (Figure 18.2): *bromocriptine* (Parlodel), *pergolide* (Permax), *pramipexole* (Mirapex), and *ropinirole* (Requip).[10] Bromocriptine has been available since 1978; pergolide since 1989. Both were derived from the ergot alkaloid lysergic acid, and both have structures that closely resemble that of dopamine (Figure 18.2). They are considered to be only marginally effective, and they have a number of bothersome side effects.[10]

Pramipexole and ropinirole were marketed in 1997; neither was derived from ergot. They have less affinity for dopamine$_2$ receptors than the older drugs; their affinity for dopamine$_3$ receptors is greater. The significance of the dopamine$_3$ receptor specificity is unclear. Also unlike the older two drugs, pramipexole and ropinirole are indicated for use in early-onset parkinsonism: their efficacy and safety profile is much improved over the two older drugs.[10,11] Both can increase one's quality of life in the early stages of the disease by improving motor features and decreasing fluctuations in response to levodopa.[12] Their long half-lives may at least partially explain the reduction in the off-and-on or wearing-off phenomenon seen with levodopa therapy. There is also some evidence that they may possess the desirable "neuroprotective" properties.[10]

Side effects of dopamine agonists include somnolence, dizziness, nausea, hallucinations, and insomnia. Frucht and co-workers[13] describe eight patients on these newer dopamine agonists who experienced sudden attacks of falling asleep at the wheel while taking the drug and driving. Sleep attacks also occurred during other activities. The mechanism underlying the attacks is unknown. The attacks ceased when the drugs were stopped. In reviewing the topic of dopamine agonists, Factor concluded:

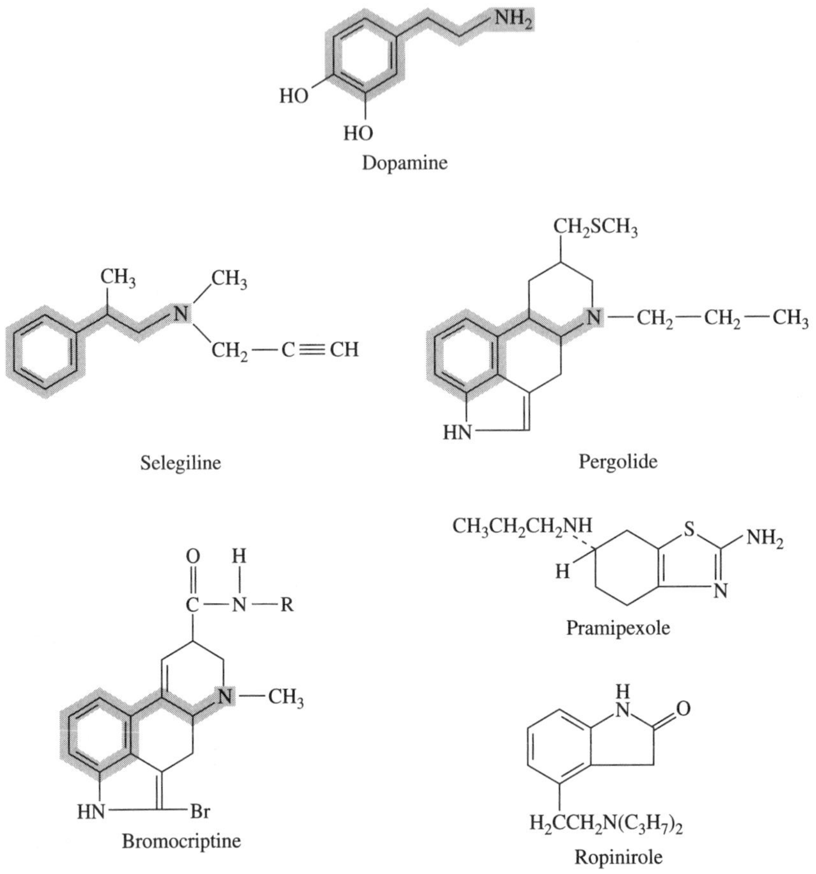

FIGURE 18.2 Structures of dopamine, selegiline and four dopamine receptor agonists that are used to treat parkinsonism. The shaded portions, which are shared by selegiline, bromocriptine, and pergolide, resemble dopamine. The two newer dopamine receptor agonists are structurally unique and have greater affinity for dopamine$_3$ receptors than do older dopamine receptor agonists (which stimulate dopamine$_2$ receptors).

There is much talk about what properties are essential to an ideal antiparkinson drug. Such a drug has a central site of action, mimics dopamine, activates postsynaptic receptors, lacks potency for presynaptic receptors on dying cell terminals, and has no requirements for metabolic conversion. Dopamine agonists fulfill many of these requirements but still lack the potency of l-dopa, which for all its faults is still the best antiparkinson drug available today. Therefore, there is no ideal drug, but there is an acceptable standard of treatment, which currently is a combination of l-dopa and the dopamine agonists. As dopamine agonists are refined and improved, the medical community will move closer to providing patients with a still higher standard of care and an enhanced quality of life.[10]

Selegiline

Selegiline (l-Deprenyl, Eldepryl) effectively ameliorates the symptoms of parkinsonism through a unique mechanism. Chapter 15 discussed two different types of the enzyme monoamine oxidase (MAO) and the emerging use of a selective MAO-A inhibitor (moclobemide) as a clinical antidepressant. In contrast to MAO-A (which is more closely involved with norepinephrine and serotonin nerve terminals), MAO-B has preferential affinity for dopamine neurons. MAO-B is selectively inhibited by selegiline. Selegiline also inhibits the local breakdown of dopamine, thus preserving the small amounts of dopamine that are present. Both actions enhance the therapeutic effect of levodopa. Some[6,14,15] feel that selegiline may provide neuroprotection action.

Selegiline is being used increasingly in the treatment of newly diagnosed, younger patients who have Parkinson's disease, because it appears to slow down the early progression of the disease and delays the need for initiating levodopa therapy.[5,6] Interestingly, selegiline is metabolized to several by-products, including amphetamine and methamphetamine. These metabolic by-products may account for some of the side effects associated with the use of selegiline. Attempts are underway to find routes of delivery for selegiline that bypass intestinal absorption and first-pass metabolism; an example is inhalation through the lungs.

On the positive side, metabolism to amphetamine-related by-products provides three mechanisms that may help to alleviate dopamine deficiency:

1. Inhibition of MAO-B

2. Inhibition of the breakdown of dopamine

3. Metabolism into the active intermediates amphetamine and methamphetamine (which augment dopamine neurotransmission)

Selegiline should be used with caution. A 1995 report from the United Kingdom stated that, in combination with levodopa, selegiline may be associated with a significant increase in morbidity after five years of use. A more recent analysis of these data showed that, while mortality is increased with selegiline use, the increase is only about half as large as originally thought.[16] These data are currently quite controversial. The reason for a possible increase in mortality remains unclear. Ben-Shlomo and colleagues[16] offer some possible explanations.

Muscarinic Receptor Antagonists

Although widely used before the introduction of levodopa, certain anticholinergic agents (muscarinic antagonists) are now used much less and are considered second-tier agents for the treatment of symptoms of parkinsonism. Their use was originally postulated on the basis of an unopposed cholinergic system after death of the dopaminergic neurons.

Occasionally, anticholinergic drugs are used as an adjunct to levodopa in patients with difficult-to-control tremors. Anticholinergic drugs relieve tremor in about 50 percent of patients, but they do not reduce rigidity or bradykinesia. Cognitive dysfunction limits their use, especially in the elderly. Representative agents include *trihexyphenidyl* (Artane), *procyclidine* (Kemadrin), *biperiden* (Akineton), *ethopropazine* (Parsidol), and *benzotropine* (Cogentin).

Nonpharmacologic Treatments

The drugs described have numerous limitations, not the least of which is reduced drug effect after about 10 years of treatment. Thus, alternatives to drug therapy are worth investigating. Arle and Alterman[17] discuss a variety of surgical options, including neuroablative techniques and implantation of deep-brain-stimulating electrodes. Gene-transfer techniques of the future are discussed by Freese.[18]

Last, but not least, nonsurgical, nonpharmacologic management strategies for Parkinson's disease should focus on educating the patient and the family, empowering them to take control over the disease through physical, occupational, and speech therapy, exercise, and good nutrition. "An educated understanding of psychosocial resources will enable the patient and family to develop strategies to cope with lifestyle changes encountered in the successful management of Parkinson's disease."[19] Mendis and colleagues[20] review the overall management of parkinsonism and present both treatment options and algorithms for the management of the early stages of the disease.

STUDY QUESTIONS

1. What is Parkinson's disease?

2. What does it share in common with traditional neuroleptic drugs? Why?

3. List the various ways that dopaminergic action in the brain might be augmented or potentiated.

4. Explain how carbidopa potentiates the action of levodopa.

5. Explain how a COMT inhibitor potentiates the action of levodopa.

6. Differentiate the newer from the older dopamine receptor agonists.

7. How does selegiline work in the treatment of Parkinson's disease?

8. Besides drugs, how might parkinsonism be managed? List the nonpharmacologic options.

REFERENCES

1. D. G. Standaert and A. B. Young, "Treatment of Central Nervous System Degenerative Disorders," in J. G. Hardman, L. E. Limbird, P. B. Molinoff, R. W. Ruddon, and A. G. Gilman, eds., *Goodman and Gilman's The Pharmacological Basis of Therapeutics*, 9th ed. (New York: McGraw-Hill, 1996), 503–513.
2. A. Colcher and T. Simuni, "Clinical Manifestations of Parkinson's Disease," *Medical Clinics of North America* 83 (1999): 327–347.
3. A. J. Hughes, "Drug Treatment of Parkinson's Disease in the 1990s: Achievements and Future Possibilities," *Drugs* 53 (1997): 195–205.
4. R. A. Hauser and T. A. Zesiewicz, "Management of Early Parkinson's Disease," *Medical Clinics of North America* 83 (1999): 393–414.
5. J. P. Hubble, "Novel Drugs for Parkinson's Disease," *Medical Clinics of North America* 83 (1999): 525–536.
6. A. Siderowf and R. Kurlan, "Monoamine Oxidase and Catechol-O-Methyltransferase Inhibitors," *Medical Clinics of North America* 83 (1999): 445–467.
7. "Entacapone for Parkinson's Disease," *Medical Letter on Drugs and Therapeutics* 42 (January 24, 2000): 7–8.
8. K. J. Holm and C. M. Spencer, "Entacapone: A Review of Its Use in Parkinson's Disease," *Drugs* 58 (1999): 159–177.
9. D. K. Simon and D. G. Standaert, "Neuroprotective Therapies," *Medical Clinics of North America* 83 (1999): 509–523.
10. S. A. Factor, "Dopamine Agonists," *Medical Clinics of North America* 83 (1999): 415–443.
11. I. F. Tulloch, "Pharmacologic Profile of Ropinirole: A Nonergoline Dopamine Agonist," *Neurology* 49, Suppl. 1 (1997): S58–S62.
12. M. Dooley and A. Markham, "Pramipexole: A Review of Its Use in the Management of Early and Advanced Parkinson's Disease," *Drugs and Aging* 12 (1998): 495–514.
13. S. Frucht et al., "Falling Asleep at the Wheel: Motor Vehicle Mishaps in Persons Taking Pramipexole and Ropinirole," *Neurology* 52 (1999): 1908–1910.
14. M. B. Stern, "Contemporary Approaches to the Pharmacotherapeutic Management of Parkinson's Disease: An Overview," *Neurology* 49, Suppl. 1 (1997): S2–S9.
15. C. W. Olanow, "Attempts to Obtain Neuroprotection in Parkinson's Disease," *Neurology* 49, Suppl. 1 (1997): S26–S33.

16. Y. Ben-Shlomo et al., "Investigation by Parkinson's Disease Research Group of United Kingdom into Excess Mortality Seen with Combined Levodopa and Selegiline Treatment in Patients with Early, Mild Parkinson's Disease: Further Results of Randomized Trial and Confidential Inquiry," *British Medical Journal* 316 (1998): 1191–1196.

17. J. E. Arle and R. L. Alterman, "Surgical Options in Parkinson's Disease," *Medical Clinics of North America* 83 (1999): 483–498.

18. A. Freese, "Restorative Gene Therapy Approaches to Parkinson's Disease," *Medical Clinics of North America* 83 (1999): 537–548.

19. J. C. Wright, "Nonpharmacologic Management Strategies," *Medical Clinics of North America* 83 (1999): 499–508.

20. T. Mendis, O. Suchowersky, A. Lang, and S. Gauthier, "Management of Parkinson's Disease: A Review of Current and New Therapies," *Canadian Journal of Neurological Sciences* 26 (1999): 89–103.

Integration of Drugs and Psychological Therapies in Treating Mental and Behavior Disorders

Robert M. Julien and Donald E. Lange

Psychological illness rarely occurs in a vacuum. Therefore, psychoactive medications should rarely be prescribed as the sole treatment, although they too often are. In many psychological illnesses, combinations of drug therapy and psychological therapies provide more effective treatment than the use of either alone.[1–3] This chapter explores the complex interaction between pharmacotherapies and psychological therapies in the treatment of several widespread psychological disorders that are thought to be undertreated in medical practice.

Undertreatment of Mental and Psychological Disorders

In December 1999 the Surgeon General of the United States released a report that criticized the state of mental health treatment.[4] The report began with definitions of mental health and mental illness:

Mental health is a state of successful performance of mental function, resulting in productive activities, fulfilling relationships with other people, and the ability to adapt to change and to cope with adversity.

Mental illness is the term that refers collectively to all diagnosable mental disorders. Mental disorders are health conditions that are characterized by alterations in thinking, mood, or behavior (or some combination thereof) associated with distress and/or impaired functioning.

Alzheimer's disease exemplifies a mental disorder largely marked by alterations in thinking (especially forgetting). Depression exemplifies a mental disorder largely marked by alterations in mood. Attention-deficit/hyperactivity disorder exemplifies a mental disorder largely marked by alterations in behavior (overactivity) and/or thinking (inability to concentrate). Alterations in thinking, mood, or behavior contribute to a host of problems—patient distress, impaired functioning, heightened risk of death, pain, and disability, substance abuse/dependence, or personal loss of freedom.

A few facts the Surgeon General's report put forth follow.

- The mental health field is plagued by disparities in the availability of and access to its services.

- A key disparity often hinges on a person's financial status: formidable financial barriers block off needed mental health care from too many people, from those who have health insurance with inadequate mental health benefits to the 44 million Americans who have no insurance at all.

- About one in five Americans experiences a mental disorder over the course of a year.

- Mental illness represents more than 15 percent of the overall burden of disease from all causes and slightly more than the burden associated with all forms of cancer.

- Mental illness, including suicide, ranks second in the burden of disease, second only to cardiovascular disease.

- Depression ranks second only to ischemic coronary artery (heart) disease in the magnitude of disease burden. Schizophrenia, bipolar disorder, obsessive-compulsive disorder, panic disorder, and post-traumatic stress disorder also contribute significantly to the burden represented by mental illness.

- Stigmatism is the most formidable obstacle to future progress in the arena of mental illness and health.

- Nearly two-thirds of all people with diagnosable mental conditions do not seek treatment, although mental disorders can be effectively treated in about 75 percent of cases.

- About 20 percent of American adults are afflicted with a mental or psychological disorder at one point or another in their lifetime.

Depression

Up to a third of patients sitting in a physician's office have a diagnosable psychiatric disorder that largely goes undiagnosed and untreated, and 75 percent are anxiety or depressive disorders.[5] Cognitive, emotional, and behavioral symptoms not part of a diagnosable disorder are also common; the modal psychiatric condition most often seen in general medical practice settings is the DSM-IV category of *mixed anxiety-depression* (Table 19.1).[5] Distressed high users of medical care have even higher rates of psychopathology.

Undertreatment of Depression

Attention to the undertreatment of depression was emphasized in 1993 with publication by the U.S. government of a clinical practice guideline titled "Depression in Primary Care Clinical Practice" (discussed later). In the same year, the American Psychiatric Association published a guideline titled "Practice Guideline for Major Depressive Disorder in Adults."[6] This 1993 guideline was revised and updated in April, 2000. In 1998, the American Academy of Child and Adolescent Psychiatry published a guideline titled "Practice Parameters for the Assessment and Treatment of Children and Adolescents with Depressive Disorders" (discussed

TABLE 19.1 Mixed anxiety-depressive disorder

Persistent or recurrent dysphoric mood lasting at least 1 month
Dysphoric mood is accompanied by at least 1 month of ≥4 of the following symptoms:
    Difficulty concentrating or mind going blank
    Sleep disturbance (difficulty falling or staying asleep or restless unsatisfying sleep)
    Fatigue or low energy
    Irritability
    Worry
    Being easily moved to tears
    Hypervigilance
    Anticipating the worst
    Hopelessness (pervasive pessimism about the future)
    Low self-esteem or feelings of worthlessness
Symptoms caused clinically significant distress or impairment in social, occupational, or other important areas of functioning

later). That the recommendations in these three guidelines have not been implemented has been reported regularly over the past few years.[7-9] Lack of compliance exists despite demonstrated reductions in depression when the guidelines are followed.[10-12] Depression affects an estimated 11 million Americans, or about 6 percent of the population, each year. The associated costs that include everything from treatment costs to loss of workplace productivity are estimated at $44 billion a year. Particularly undertreated are depressed individuals in ethnic minority communities.[13]

Treatment of Depression

There is now general consensus that depression can be best treated by a combination of pharmacotherapy and psychological interventions (Figure 19.1). To understand the reason, it is necessary to tie together the etiology of anxiety and depression, the pharmacotherapy of each, and the neurobiological basis of the psychological or behavioral therapies of each.

Chapter 15 proposed that the effect of antidepressant drugs was an up-regulation of a trophic factor located in hippocampal neurons. Stress and anxiety result in elevated adrenal steroids; this, in turn, reduces the levels of a nuclear protein called *brain-derived neurotrophic factor, or BDNF*. BDNF reductions result in hippocampal neuronal injury; the end result is neuronal dysfunction and a clinical state of depression. The slow onset of action of antidepressant drugs results from the need to increase BDNF by increasing the expression of this protein by increasing its messenger RNA (mRNA) levels. Increased

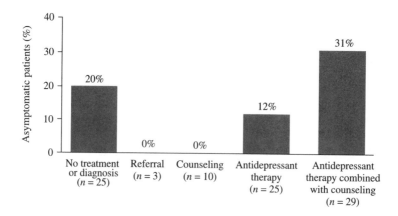

FIGURE 19.1 Percentages of patients who were treated with usual care and who were judged to be asymptomatic at month 8 in relation to the primary treatment pattern during the preceding months. [From Schulberg et al.,[8] with permission.]

BDNF levels result in a trophic repair of neuronal injury.[14,15] Neuronal injury has also been postulated to be involved in the cognitive impairments seen in depression and in their improvement with antidepressant medication.[16]

Thus, depression is associated with hippocampal neuronal dysfunction, stress, and altered cognitive dysfunction. Conversely, increased stress, anxiety, and glucocorticoids cause hippocampal damage, can induce depression, and can produce memory and cognitive impairments. In other words, elevated adrenal steroids and increases in stress, anxiety, and depression are all interrelated.

Antidepressant drugs are extremely effective in reducing anxiety disorders and stress (see Chapter 15). Russo-Neustadt and co-workers[17] demonstrated that a positive, synergistic interaction exists between two distinct interventions, a pharmacologic agent and a behavioral change; this interaction leads to a potentiation of BDNF expression (Figure 19.2). Extending this work, Fujimaki and co-workers[18] demonstrated that coadministration of an antidepressant with an inhibitor of cyclic adenosine monophosphate (cAMP) phosphodiesterase leads to an up-regulation of hippocampal BDNF mRNA (Figure 19.3), indicating again that interventions that "increase expression of BDNF contribute to the neural adaptations that underlie the action of antidepressant treatment."

Therefore, treating anxiety and/or depression (with either medication or psychotherapeutic interventions) acutely increases synaptic concentrations of neurotransmitters and reduces stress and anxiety. The acute change leads to increased expression of BDNF mRNA, increasing BDNF within the neuron. This ultimately improves neuronal trophism, promotes repair of injured hippocampal neurons, and leads to improved neuronal function with relief of both anxiety and depression and with improvements in memory and cognitive functioning. Taken in total, this treatment is a pathogenic model explaining the synergistic effects of combined pharmacotherapy and psychotherapy in relieving the distress of affective disorders such as depression and anxiety.

Role of Drugs as Cotherapy

In addition to treating the acute symptoms associated with a mental disorder, medications serve a *prophylactic function*, altering brain chemistry to prevent the onset of a symptom complex (e.g., reducing the frequency of recurrence of symptomatology). Thus, drugs can be used both to ameliorate debilitating symptoms of illness and to prevent the development of additional symptoms, allowing the introduction of behavioral or psychological interventions.

Illustrating this statement are the new generation of antipsychotic drugs (Chapter 17), which can effectively ameliorate both the positive

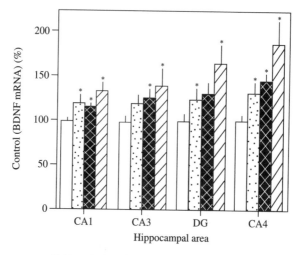

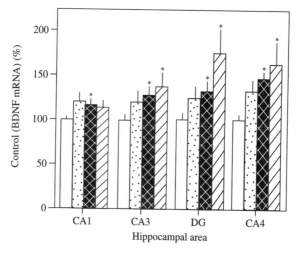

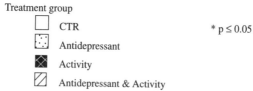

FIGURE 19.2 Quantification of antidepressant- and activity-induced increases in BDNF mRNA in the rat hippocampus. **A.** Treatment with tranylcypromine (a MAO inhibitor) alone caused significant increases in BDNF mRNA in several hippocampal cell fields (CA, CA3, DG, CA4). Additive increases were observed when drug treatment and activity were combined. **B.** Treatment with imipramine (a TCA) alone did not significantly increase hippocampal BDNF mRNA. The combination of imipramine treatment with activity led to significant increases in BDNF mRNA levels compared to controls and also appeared to potentiate BDNF mRNA levels above those observed with activity alone. [From Russo-Neustadt et al.,[17] with permission.]

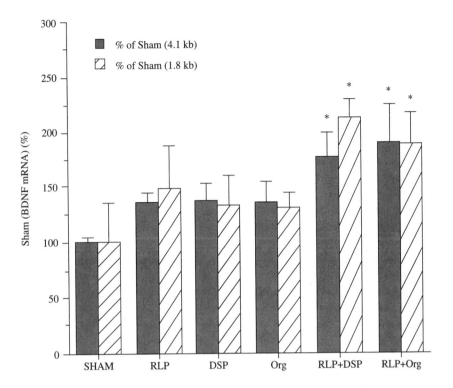

FIGURE 19.3 Influence of 21 days administration of rolipram (RLP, an inhibitor of the enzyme phosphodiesterase) with desipramine (DSP, a TCA-type antidepressant) or organon 4428 (Org, a NE-type reuptake inhibitor antidepressant) on BDNF mRNA in rat hippocampus. Data are presented as percentage of sham (vehicle) treatment and are the mean +/– S.E.M. of 5 to 6 rats for each treatment group. * = p<.05 compared with vehicle control. Combination of a phosphodiesterase inhibitor with either antidepressant significantly increased BDNF mRNA expression. [From Fujimaki et al.,[18] with permission.]

and the negative symptomatology of schizophrenia, permitting the introduction of psychosocial interventions that can assist with the integration of the patient into society and improve his or her functional level therein. These psychosocial interventions provide long-term changes that can persist long after drug therapy is discontinued, if this is the chosen and appropriate course of therapy.

The prescription of a psychotherapeutic medication is only the first step in treatment. Following control of symptoms, introduction of psychological interventions optimizes therapy.[13] In some instances, such as the treatment of anxiety disorders or depression, there is little statistical difference between the effectiveness of antidepressant drugs and psychotherapeutic interventions when either treatment is used alone. Thus, either can be chosen as first-line treatment and the other added as appropriate. In other disorders (such as bipolar disorder and schizophrenia), drug therapy is essential as primary therapy and psychological therapies are introduced following control of symptomatology.

Role of Psychotherapy as Cotherapy

Prior to the 1950s, there was little evidence that psychotherapy was superior to placebo or that prolonged psychotherapy was superior to merely waiting for the patient to spontaneously recover. Over the past 50 years, multiple studies have demonstrated that psychotherapy* is indeed superior to placebo or waiting for spontaneous recovery.[19] Today, research is attempting to do several things:

- Tailor specific psychotherapeutic interventions to specific psychiatric conditions and specific patients
- Determine the appropriate duration, intensity, and complexity of effective therapies
- Assess the interaction between psychotherapeutic interventions with drug therapy

Some conclusions are becoming evident:

- In the treatment of panic disorder, agoraphobia, simple phobias, and, to a lesser extent, social phobias, behavioral and cognitive-behavioral therapies have traditionally been thought to have more consistent and longer-lasting effects than medications.
- Psychotherapy, specifically panic-focused cognitive-behavioral therapy, and medications (SSRIs, TCAs, benzodiazepines, and MAO inhibitors) are equally effective in the acute treatment for panic disorder.[20]
- Combining cognitive-behavioral therapy and medication in the treatment of panic disorder has not yet been convincingly shown to be superior to cognitive-behavioral therapy alone, but additional studies may lead to modification of this statement.[20,21]
- Medications and behavioral techniques are equally effective in the treatment of obsessive-compulsive disorder, posttraumatic stress disorder, and generalized anxiety disorder.

---

*As used in this chapter, the term *psychotherapy* covers a wide range of treatment modalities from education and supportive counseling to insight-oriented, dynamically based therapy.

- In the treatment of major depressive disorder, antidepressant medications and cognitive-behavioral therapy are equally effective and display additional efficacy when used in combination.[22]

- Individuals who respond to cognitive-behavioral therapy for the treatment of depression "tend to be less severely impaired than those who do not respond."[23]

- At the very least, cognitive-behavioral therapy added to pharmacological management of depression "reduces relapse rates for acute major depression and persistent severe residual symptoms."[24]

- In the treatment of eating disorders such as bulimia nervosa, "cognitive-behavioral therapy is the psychological treatment of choice . . . and . . . medication with fluoxetine (an SSRI) adds modestly to the benefit of psychological treatment."[25]

- The positive effects of cognitive-behavioral therapy in treating depression in adults are also seen in adolescents, and treatment gains in adolescents are maintained over time.[26]

- In patients with cigarette dependence and comorbid history of depression, cognitive-behavioral therapy was more effective than an antidepressant (nortriptyline).[27] However, nortriptyline allayed the negative affect that occurs in the days following smoking cessation. Discouragingly, long-term (64 weeks) follow-up indicated that most individuals (depressed or not) had resumed smoking.[27] A three-way trial of cognitive-behavioral therapy, antidepressant medication, and nicotine-replacement therapy has not been reported.

Role of the Treatment Team

No one individual should be a sole caregiver for the patient with mental or psychological illness. A team of caregivers, with members from several disciplines, should collaborate in treatment. One team member is usually a clinician with prescription privileges (a physician or, increasingly, a psychiatric or mental health nurse practitioner). Other clinicians who do not prescribe medication may have responsibility for psychotherapeutic interventions. Other caregivers may include nurses, pharmacists, counselors, vocational rehabilitation counselors, physical or occupational therapists, dieticians, spiritual counselors, family members, and psychiatric, occupational, or recreational assistants. Miller and Keitner[28] review the team approach, suggesting a "sequential" or "cascading" model when providing combined treatment. This is similar to the stepped, collaborative treatment program discussed earlier for treating depression.[12] Various treatments (medication or psychotherapy) are administered in a sequential fashion based on the patient's response or lack of response to a previous treatment. If the patient responds to one treatment, no other may be needed; if there is no response, then a second treatment is added to the first. Continued nonresponse may lead to additional or substitute types of treatments.

Because the prescribing clinician has traditionally acted alone, one might reasonably ask whether the treatment team concept is overly expensive or can deliver a higher quality of care with a better quality of life for the patient at a manageable cost to society. Several articles[29–32] have addressed this issue, especially as it relates to the treatment of depression. In essence, research concludes that a treatment team relieves the prescribing physician of responsibility for handling psychological interventions, reduces hospitalizations, and provides longer, more intensive, more cost-effective case management.

> In the psychiatrist/primary care model, a psychiatrist alternated visits with a primary care physician to assist in the education and pharmacologic treatment of the patient. In the psychiatrist/psychologist team model, the psychiatrist worked with a team of psychologists to improve adherence to and effectiveness of antidepressant treatment, with psychologists also providing brief behavioral treatment in the primary care clinic. It was found that the collaborative model was associated with improved adherence to treatment, increased patient satisfaction with depression care, and improved depression outcome compared with usual care by primary care physicians alone.[33]

How might a treatment team function? Certainly nonprescribing members of the team should be familiar with the pharmacology, uses, limitations, and side effects of the drugs being used by their clients. They need to know which drugs their clients are taking and which therapeutic effects and side effects should be expected. They should also know about alternative medications that may provide equal or superior effectiveness with a more reasonable spectrum of side effects for the particular client. These clinicians must be able to professionally converse with the prescribing physician, monitor drug therapy, and institute psychological therapies appropriate to the condition under treatment. All should monitor for both positive and negative effects and be sensitive to the meaning medications have to their clients, for effective psychotherapy depends on the ability of patients to comply with treatment requirements.[34]

Regardless of their individual roles, all team members share certain basic functions. Most important is that of ongoing assessment, the purpose of which is to obtain an objective report of the patient's signs and symptoms and, as much as possible, to relate them to possible causes. Assessment may include a formal diagnosis, or it may be a description of the development of the client's behavior. Either type of assessment should address both the strengths and the weaknesses of the patient. Most beneficial is an assessment that includes the likely etiology of the problem.

The clinician may list the possible explanations for the observed behaviors in a comprehensive format called the *differential diagnosis,* from which the causes may be determined. Frequently, further assessment is necessary to rule out some of the possible causes. Less plausible causes usually can be readily eliminated. The differential diagnosis then guides further assessment and treatment. Possible causal factors in the differential diagnosis often have markedly different treatments. Consequently, an accurate assessment and diagnosis of the causes of the patient's behavior must precede any treatment planning or therapeutic intervention. Evaluation by mental health professionals is often formalized into a standard diagnostic format. Most often used is the diagnostic system of the fourth edition of the *Diagnostic and Statistical Manual of Mental Disorders,* or DSM-IV.[35]

DSM-IV Classification of Mental Disorders

Diagnosis is the practice of distinguishing one disease from another. In clinical psychology, diagnosis is based on the signs and symptoms of a mental disorder, regardless of the morbid changes producing them. The DSM-IV classification provides a shorthand description of the patterns of behavior that can be expected with each disorder.

> DSM-IV is a categorical classification that divides mental disorders into types based on criteria sets with defining features. . . . In DSM-IV there is no assumption that each category of mental disorder is a complete discrete entity with absolute boundaries dividing it from other mental disorders or from no mental disorder. There is also no assumption that all individuals described as having the same mental disorder are alike in all important ways. This outlook allows more flexibility in the use of the system, encourages more specific attention to boundary cases, and emphasizes the need to capture additional clinical information that goes beyond diagnosis.[35]

In the DSM-IV classification system, each individual being diagnosed is not merely assigned a single diagnostic category (for example, bipolar disorder). Instead, he or she is characterized by clinically relevant factors that are grouped into five "axes":

- Axis I: primary classification (diagnosis) of the major problem requiring attention (for example, alcohol dependence)
- Axis II: mental retardation and personality disorders generally believed to begin in childhood or adolescence and persisting into adult life
- Axis III: any physical disorder that seems relevant to a case and that may have implications for present treatment (for example, asthma that is exacerbated by psychological factors)

- Axis IV: psychosocial and environmental problems that may affect the diagnosis, treatment, and prognosis of the mental disorders listed under Axes I and II (for example, illiteracy or unemployment)

- Axis V: global assessment of psychological functioning, social relationships, and occupational activities (including ratings of both the current level of functioning and the highest level of functioning during the past year)

In emergencies, a preliminary classification is made, even though much information is lacking. In such situations, any assessment is considered tentative and subject to revision as additional medical, psychological, and psychosocial assessments are made.

The first three axes constitute official diagnostic categories of the American Psychiatric Association. Axes IV and V are regarded as supplementary categories for use in clinical and research settings. It is common practice, however, to describe a case using all five axes. The major categories of Axis I classification are listed in Table 19.2. Following is a consideration of 4 of the 16 Axis I categories—mood (or affective) disorders, schizophrenia, anxiety disorders, and eating disorders. These four were chosen because of their prevalence and because they are the disorders most frequently treated with a combination of medication and psychotherapy.

Mood Disorders

The term *mood* refers to a perceptual bias that alters how one views the world. Mood disorders may include major depressive, manic, or hypomanic episodes, dysthymia, or alternating recurrences of one or more such moods. The DSM-IV groups mood disorders into *depressive disorders, bipolar disorders, substance-induced mood disorders*, and *mood disorders due to general medical conditions*. One of these, depression, was discussed earlier in this chapter.

All of us experience mood shifts, such as mild anxiety, depression, sadness, and grief, in response to difficult life events. These responses are natural and certainly do not constitute a mood disorder. The DSM-IV classification pertains to distinct, severe processes that interfere with daily activities. These dysfunctional processes are, however, amenable to treatment. A normal course of bereavement due to environmental factors (for example, death of a loved one) is not classified as a mood disorder, even though it may temporarily incapacitate the individual.

In general, mood disorders are subclassified by type and duration of the mood episode. For example, two weeks of severely depressed mood (as indicated by a specific set of four additionally related symptoms) is required for a diagnosis of a major depressive episode. Two

TABLE 19.2 DSM-IV Axis I categories

Category	Examples
Disorders usually first diagnosed in infancy, childhood, or adolescence	Attention deficit and disruptive behavior disorders, learning disorders, certain eating disorders
Delirium, dementia, and amnestic and other cognitive disorders	Transient or permanent brain dysfunction attributable to such factors as aging, dementia due to head trauma or Alzheimer's, and amnestic disorders (memory loss)
Substance-related disorders	Disorders related to alcohol, all chemical withdrawal syndromes, and some disorders related to or caused by substances such as substance-induced psychotic disorders
Schizophrenia and other psychotic disorders	Chronic disorganized behavior and thought of psychotic proportions (delusions, hallucinations), incoherence, and social isolation; disorders that are well-organized systems of delusions without the incoherence, bizarreness, and other social isolation seen in schizophrenia
Mood disorders	Depression and bipolar disorder
Anxiety disorders	Anxiety, tension, and worry without psychotic features (delusions, hallucinations); post-traumatic (reactive, stress caused) disorders, whether brief or chronic
Somatoform disorders	Physical symptoms for which no medical causes can be found (symptoms apparently not under voluntary control and linked to psychological factors or conflicts)
Factitious disorders	Physical or behavioral symptoms that are voluntarily produced by the individual, apparently in order to play the role of patient and often involving chronic, blatant lying
Dissociative disorders	Sudden, temporary change in the normal functions of consciousness (for example, loss of memory, sleepwalking)
Sexual and gender identity disorders	Deviant sexual thoughts and behavior that are either personally anxiety provoking or socially maladaptive

TABLE 19.2 DSM-IV Axis I categories *(continued)*

Category	Examples
Eating disorders	Disorders of eating such as anorexia nervosa
Sleep disorders	Insomnia or difficulty in going to sleep or staying asleep, excessive daytime sleeping, complaints of sleep disturbance without objective evidence, impairment of respiration during sleep, disturbance of sleeping schedule, sleepwalking, sleep terrors
Impulse control disorders, not classified elsewhere	Maladaptations characterized by failure to resist impulses (for example, pathological gambling, chronic stealing of desired objects, habitual fire setting)
Adjustment disorders	Maladaptive reactions to identifiable life events or circumstances that are expected to lessen and cease when the stressor ceases; reaction may be dominated by depressed mood, anxiety, withdrawal, conduct disorder such as truancy, or a lessening in work or job performance
Mental disorders due to general medical condition, not classified elsewhere	Disorders that may be due to a medical condition, such as a psychotic disorder that emerges in response to renal failure
Other conditions that may be a focus of clinical attention	Includes such things as medication-induced movement disorders such as tardive dyskinesia or partner or parent/child relational problems

Abstracted from DSM-IV, pp. 13–24.

years of mildly depressed mood and the presence of two related symptoms is required for diagnosis of dysthymic disorder.

Assessment and Diagnosis

Careful assessment of psychological disorders is the initial step in effective treatment planning, whether the planned treatment is pharmacological, psychological, or a combination of both. Thorough assessment is helpful in distinguishing between functional and organic causes. In other words, not only is a DSM-IV classification of symptom-based behavioral dysfunction developed, a differential diagnosis of all possible causative factors for the observed behaviors is made. This list is then narrowed to one or perhaps a few possibilities so that the likely cause can be identified and effectively treated.

A thorough assessment also includes an investigation of social and psychological factors that may contribute to pathology. Other sociopsychological conditions may exacerbate existing physical or psychological problems. For example, cessation of cigarette smoking can be accompanied by the emergence or exacerbation of major depressive episodes.[36] Hall and co-workers[27] discuss this scenario.

Treatment

The biological, psychological, and social factors in mood disorders must be addressed in a comprehensive treatment plan. As stated, pharmacotherapy and psychotherapy effectively treat depression, and combining the two further improves efficacy and reduces the probability of relapse.[37] Even reactive (exogenous) depression, adjustment mood disorders, and dysthymia have biological components that require intervention with pharmacological agents along with psychotherapy.[38–40]

An individual's basic perceptual beliefs, cognitive and intellectual processing, and experiences affect that person's interaction with the environment and with other individuals. Eventually a person develops a sense of how self interacts with others. Individuals suffering from a mood disorder learn a pattern of behavior that may cause their problems to become worse and make the disorder resistant to treatment and intervention. Psychological therapies can change the pattern of behavior. There are many techniques, from simple education to supportive counseling to insight-oriented, dynamically based therapy. Cognitive therapy, behavioral therapy, brief psychodynamic psychotherapy, group therapies, and others are frequently used and are effective interventions.

Children and adolescents are being increasingly diagnosed with mood disorders, including major depressive disorder and bipolar disorder.[41] This probably reflects an increased recognition of the disorders rather than an actual increase in their incidence. In either case, practice standards for treating these and other mental and psychological disorders in children and adolescents are available.[42] Pharmacologically, in children and adolescents, tricyclic antidepressants have both questionable efficacy and significant toxicity.[43] The SSRI-type antidepressants are potentially useful and widely prescribed, despite little data to support their efficacy;[44] the SSRIs are only slightly more effective than is placebo in treating depression in children and adolescents, with 35 to 50 percent responding positively to either placebo or active medication (see Chapter 15). Behavioral therapies and family interventions are perhaps preferred over pharmacologic interventions, at least for early intervention in less severe cases.

Bipolar disorder in children and adolescents is being increasingly diagnosed and treated. Approximately 20 percent of all bipolar patients have their first episode during adolescence, 12 percent are hospitalized during this period of their life, and the peak age of onset is between 15 and 19 years of age. Lithium, valproic acid, and (increasingly) gabapentin (Chapter 16) are the mainstays of therapy.[45] The American Academy of Child and Adolescent Psychiatry has published practice parameters for the assessment and treatment of children and adolescents with bipolar disorder.[46] These parameters delineate both the pharmacologic and the psychosocial interventions useful in the treatment of this disorder.

Schizophrenia

The formal DSM-IV definition of schizophrenia is presented in Table 19.3. Symptoms of schizophrenia include hallucinations, delusions, disorganized speech, and bizarre behavior. These are often referred to as the positive symptoms of schizophrenia. Negative symptoms include impaired social interactions, impoverished and blunted affect, an absence of motivation, and significant social withdrawal. The disorder often begins in adolescence or young adulthood, frequently followed by a progressively deteriorating course; few patients make a complete recovery.

Antipsychotic Medication

The drugs used to reduce the symptomatology of schizophrenia are discussed in Chapter 17. Advances in this area occurred rapidly through the 1990s and are continuing into the twenty-first century. In the early 1990s it was stated:

All of the symptoms associated with schizophrenia are affected to some degree by neuroleptics. Positive symptoms, including hallucinations, delusions, and disorganized thoughts, are more responsive to drug treatment than are negative symptoms, such as blunted affect, emotional withdrawal, and lack of social interest. . . . A substantial proportion of schizophrenic patients—about 10 to 20 percent—fail to demonstrate substantial improvement when they are treated with neuroleptics. This subgroup of treatment-refractory schizophrenic patients often requires long-term institutionalization in state hospitals and similar facilities. Clozapine and other atypical antipsychotic drugs may be particularly effective for these patients.[47]

Clozapine and some new-generation antipsychotic drugs are effective in at least 30 percent of patients who are severely disabled by

---

TABLE 19.3 DSM-IV categories of schizophrenia and related disorders

Schizophrenia is a disturbance that lasts for at least 6 months and includes at least 1 month of active-phase symptoms (i.e., two [or more] of the following: delusions, hallucinations, disorganized speech, grossly disorganized or catatonic behavior, negative symptoms). Definitions for Schizophrenia subtypes (Paranoid, Disorganized, Catatonic, Undifferentiated, and Residual) are also included in this section.

Schizophreniform Disorder is characterized by a symptomatic presentation that is equivalent to Schizophrenia except for its duration (i.e., the disturbance lasts from 1 to 6 months) and the absence of a requirement that there be a decline in functioning.

Schizoaffective Disorder is a disturbance in which a mood episode and the active-phase symptoms of Schizophrenia occur together and were preceded or are followed by at least 2 weeks of delusions or hallucinations without prominent mood symptoms.

Delusional Disorder is characterized by at least 1 month of nonbizarre delusions without other active-phase symptoms of Schizophrenia.

Brief Psychotic Disorder is a psychotic disturbance that lasts more than 1 day and remits by 1 month.

Shared Psychotic Disorder is a disturbance that develops in an individual who is influenced by someone else who has an established delusion with similar content.

In **Psychotic Disorder Due to a General Medical Condition,** the psychotic symptoms are judged to be a direct physiological consequence of a general medical condition.

In **Substance-Induced Psychotic Disorder,** the psychotic symptoms are judged to be a direct physiological consequence of a drug of abuse, a medication, or toxin exposure.

Psychotic Disorder Not Otherwise Specified is included for classifying psychotic presentations that do not meet criteria for any of the specific Psychotic Disorders defined in this section or psychotic symptomatology about which there is inadequate or contradictory information.

Reproduced with permission from DSM-IV, pp. 273–274.

negative symptoms. In addition, these new drugs are rapidly becoming accepted as first-line agents because of their effectiveness and their lack of extrapyramidal side effects. By relieving negative symptomatology, they make the patient "reachable" and more amenable to psychosocial interventions in efforts to improve their social functioning and their integration into society.[48]

Psychotherapy and Rehabilitation

The availability of the new-generation antipsychotic drugs has markedly increased the usefulness of psychotherapy in treating mental disorders. These new medications have made it possible for psychotherapy and other interventions to be effective, particularly in the outpatient setting.

> Having established the primary role of antipsychotics, there is evidence that psychosocial therapies, when administered with these agents, improve long-term prognosis. Because chronically psychotic patients have difficulties with social adjustment, reason dictates that they and their families could benefit from such interventions. Regardless of theoretical orientation, it is clear that practitioners should provide psychosocial therapy as part of a comprehensive treatment strategy.[47]

In general, most cost-benefit studies find that the addition of psychological therapies in an outpatient setting encourages drug compliance. Therapeutic interventions improve social skills and assist in the rehabilitation of cognitive functions. Psychological therapy in conjunction with drug therapy also extends relapse time and reduces the intensity of relapse episodes. Typically, the most beneficial strategy is a sociopsychological therapy emphasizing self-esteem, social skills, and cognitive rehabilitation. This emphasis addresses the interaction between the client's symptoms and their social and psychological consequences. These strategies develop and rehabilitate cognitive functions, resulting in a more positive self-image and more effective social and cognitive functioning. Norman and Townsend[49] discuss the role of cognitive-behavioral interventions in reducing psychosis. Sensky and co-workers[50] studied 90 patients with schizophrenia with medication-resistant symptoms, comparing cognitive-behavioral therapy (nine months of therapy) with a nonspecific befriending control intervention. Both therapies were effective in the short term, reducing both positive and negative symptoms. Cognitive-behavioral therapy produced longer-lasting results; continuing improvement was observed even nine months after treatment was stopped. Cognitive-behavioral interventions were thought to be cost-effective, with an average of 24 hours of therapist time spent per clinically successful outcome.

Medication addresses the biophysical component of the disorder. Social therapy, with structured or supported living, teaches and reinforces social skills. Psychological therapy addresses the intrapsychic and psychodynamic issues. Vocational rehabilitation is important in developing self-esteem and establishing financial independence.

Functions of the Treatment Team

The treatment team should teach the client the positive and negative effects of any prescribed drugs; it also answers any questions and relieves any doubts a patient has about any medication. Helping the client remain drug compliant is important in reducing the rate of relapse. In addition, monitoring of drug levels in plasma can provide important information, improve drug effectiveness, and reduce unwanted side effects.[47] The client should also understand the limitations of his or her medication. A team member should help the client understand that motivation, medication, and psychological therapy are all important in stabilization and recovery.

Schizophrenia is relatively uncommon in children and adolescents, and practice parameters for its treatment have only recently been published.[51] Research in this area is, to date, only modest. Campbell, Rapoport, and Simpson[52] discuss the situation, point out the limitations of what is known, and present the untoward side effects of newer drugs (e.g., weight gain). They conclude:

> The atypical antipsychotics should be critically assessed and compared with psychosocial interventions; if effective, the combination of both types of treatments should be evaluated.

Anxiety Disorders

Symptoms of anxiety are normal and serve as an early warning system that helps a person avoid potentially dangerous situations. Excessive anxiety, however, may be a source of significant suffering and require intervention. Anxiety is subtle and pervasive; it accompanies almost every psychiatric disorder. Because anxiety touches everyone, it becomes a disorder only when it is objectively uncomfortable or is perceived to be out of control; the usual feelings of anxiety increase and interfere with normal functioning. Severe symptoms of anxiety require assessment and treatment. Understanding the underlying causes and formulating a differential diagnosis help the clinician determine which drugs and which psychological interventions will be the most effective.[53]

The chronicity of anxiety disorders is similar to that of mood disorders, more enduring than that of substance abuse disorders, but less deep-seated than that of the schizophrenias. Only about 30 percent of individuals with anxiety disorders receive treatment, a percentage that is even lower if generalized anxiety disorder is included. Thus, a high percentage of mental health and addictive disorders are actually anxiety disorders or have a high component of comorbid anxiety. Often, these disorders go untreated or are not treated by behavioral health specialists.

Characteristic of anxiety disorders are the symptoms of anxiety and avoidance behavior. Anxiety is a complex response that includes subjective feelings of dread, apprehension, fear, tension, and related psychomotor responses. The last may include motor tension, increases in autonomic responses (heart rate, blood pressure), vigilance, and scanning. DSM-IV lists several subcategories of the anxiety disorders, which are presented in Table 19.4.

Using drugs to treat anxiety disorders (in both adults and children) is controversial; the controversy arises from diagnostic difficulties, from the chronic nature of many anxieties, and from the addictive potential associated with some of the drugs used in therapy. In the 1960s and 1970s, the benzodiazepine anxiolytics appeared to treat anxiety disorders quickly, effectively, and safely and replaced the barbiturate therapies of the 1950s. Over time, however, the potential addictiveness of benzodiazepine therapy became evident. Similarly, sedative-type anxiolytics, which reduced the outward symptoms of anxiety, could be counterproductive in some cases, producing depression and suppressing cognitive function. With the advent of the antidepressants and the observation that these drugs (especially those of the SSRI type) effectively treat many of the anxieties, sophistication in diagnosing and treating the anxieties similarly expanded. In 1999, one of the SSRIs was FDA approved for use in the treatment of generalized anxiety disorder. Again, it is imperative for both prescribing and nonprescribing clinicians to become knowledgeable about the pharmacology of these drugs, their clinical indications, dosages, and duration of usage. Most important, their limitations must receive as much attention as their assets.

Accurate assessment and diagnosis is especially vital in planning the appropriate treatment for anxiety disorders. Generally, more diffuse and severe anxiety symptoms require some initial pharmacological intervention. Less severe, more circumscribed symptoms of phobias may be more responsive to cognitive and behavioral therapy; in such cases, it is often unnecessary to resort to pharmacotherapy.

Panic Disorder

Panic disorder is one of the most common and most disabling anxiety disorders. Barloon and Noyes[54] discuss Charles Darwin, describing how disabling this disorder was in his life. Panic disorder is considered a chronic condition that requires ongoing maintenance therapy[55] (pharmacologic[56,57] and psychological[58,59]). The prevalence of panic disorder in the general community is about 1.6 percent to 3.2 percent in women and 0.4 percent to 1.7 percent in men. Further, patients with panic disorder account for more than 20 percent of emergency room visits and are 12 times more likely to visit the emergency room than the general population. Patients with panic attacks average 19 medical visits per year, a rate 7 times above normal; they also account for 15 percent of total medical visits. The use of medical services and the health care costs associated with panic disorder are therefore enormous. Added to those are disability costs and unemployment expenses (25 percent of panic disorder patients are fully unemployed). Appropriate treatment is presumed to reduce these disabilities and expenditures.

TABLE 19.4 DSM-IV categories of anxiety disorders

A **Panic Attack** is a discrete period in which there is the sudden onset of intense apprehension, fearfulness, or terror, often associated with feelings of impending doom. During these attacks symptoms such as shortness of breath, palpitations, chest pain or discomfort, choking or smothering sensations, and fear of "going crazy" or losing control are present.

Agoraphobia is anxiety about, or avoidance of, places or situations from which escape might be difficult (or embarrassing) or in which help may not be available in the event of having a Panic Attack or panic-like symptoms.

Panic Disorder without Agoraphobia is characterized by recurrent unexpected Panic Attacks about which there is persistent concern.

Panic Disorder with Agoraphobia is characterized by both recurrent unexpected Panic Attacks and Agoraphobia.

Agoraphobia without History of Panic Disorder is characterized by the presence of Agoraphobia and panic-like symptoms without a history of unexpected Panic Attacks.

Specific Phobia is characterized by clinically significant anxiety provoked by exposure to a specific feared object or situation, often leading to avoidance behavior.

Social Phobia is characterized by clinically significant anxiety provoked by exposure to certain types of social or performance situations, often leading to avoidance behavior.

Obsessive-Compulsive Disorder is characterized by obsessions (which cause marked anxiety or distress) and/or by compulsions (which serve to neutralize anxiety).

Posttraumatic Stress Disorder is characterized by the reexperiencing of an extremely traumatic event accompanied by symptoms of increased arousal and by avoidance of stimuli associated with the trauma.

Acute Stress Disorder is characterized by symptoms similar to those of Post-Traumatic Stress Disorder that occur immediately in the aftermath of an extremely traumatic event.

Generalized Anxiety Disorder is characterized by at least 6 months of persistent and excessive anxiety and worry.

Anxiety Disorder Due to a General Medical Condition is characterized by prominent symptoms of anxiety that are judged to be a direct physiological consequence of a general medical condition.

Substance-Induced Anxiety Disorder is characterized by prominent symptoms of anxiety that are judged to be a direct physiological consequence of a drug of abuse, a medication, or toxic exposure.

Anxiety Disorder Not Otherwise Specified is included for coding disorders with prominent anxiety or phobic avoidance that do not meet criteria for any of the specific Anxiety Disorders defined in this section (or anxiety symptoms about which there is inadequate or contradictory information).

Because Separation Anxiety Disorder (characterized by anxiety related to separation from parental figures) usually develops in childhood, it is included in the "Disorders Usually First Diagnosed in Infancy, Childhood, or Adolescence" section. Phobic avoidance that is limited to genital sexual contact with a sexual partner is classified as Sexual Aversion Disorder and is included in the "Sexual and Gender Identity Disorders" section.

Reproduced with permission from DSM-IV, pp. 393–394.

Comprehensive therapy reduces the severity of the course of panic disorder and enhances outcome. Pharmacologically, the SSRI-type antidepressants are the drugs of choice, except for patients also experiencing severe agitation. For those patients, a benzodiazepine anxiolytic is more effective on a short-term basis, until the anxiety and/or agitation resolves.

An estimated 50 percent of patients with panic disorder experience an episode of major depression,[60] an added impetus for the use of antidepressant medications over alternative agents. Psychological therapies must also address this comorbidity of panic disorder and depression.

Pollack[61] reviewed the psychopharmacology for panic disorder, stating that, with the use of SSRIs, it is important to start low to minimize the increased anxiety associated with the initiation of treatment. According to Pollack, buproprion and trazodone are unique among antidepressants in their relative lack of efficacy in treating panic disorder and other anxiety conditions in contrast to most other antidepressants.

Of the benzodiazepines, alprazolam (Xanax) is the most widely studied for treating panic disorder. Other benzodiazepines that have been studied include lorazepam (Ativan) and clonazepam (Klonopin).[57] The benzodiazepines have a favorable profile of side effects; they lack the anticholinergic side effects of the TCAs and the increased anxiety of the SSRIs. Concomitant use (benzodiazepine plus SSRI) provides rapid anxiolysis and more comprehensive relief of panic and depressive symptoms. Monoamine oxidase (MAO) inhibitors can be effective, but they are seldom used.

For all antidepressant medications, treatment may need to be continued indefinitely, because there is a high rate of relapse with medication discontinuation. Cognitive-behavioral therapeutic (CBT) interventions are also indicated in the treatment of panic disorder. These interventions should target avoidance behaviors that patients have learned over time to reduce the frequency of panic attacks. One part of the CBT approach is teaching the patient specific relaxation and stress management techniques.

Otto[62] reviewed the integrated treatment of panic disorder; CBT techniques were more effective than drug therapy. CBT usually includes

> informational intervention; somatic management skills, including breathing retraining and relaxation skills, and of more importance, cognitive restructuring, which helps patients change their catastrophic responses and fears concerning the somatic sensations; interoceptive exposure (for example, exposing patients to rapid heartbeat, numbness and tingling, and showing them that these sensations do not have to drive them toward a panic attack); and situational exposure, to help agoraphobic patients overcome their fear of having panic attacks in certain situations or settings. . . . Interoceptive exposure . . . is the most important component.

Regarding combinations of CBT and medications, some studies report improvements, while others note that adding medications to CBT provides short-term gains but may reduce the long-term benefits of CBT. Certainly CBT must be reinstituted at or before the time of medication discontinuation.[62] Spiegel and Bruce[63] review the combined use of CBT with benzodiazapine therapy for panic disorder.

Generalized Anxiety Disorder

Although considerable attention focused on anxiety disorder in the 1990s, less attention was devoted to the investigation of generalized anxiety disorder (GAD):

> The emerging picture is that GAD is a common and chronic disorder, affecting primarily women, and one that leads to significant distress and impairment. Subjects with GAD frequently utilize health care services and require medication treatment.[64]

Formerly called anxiety neurosis, GAD occurs at a rate that equals or exceeds the other anxiety disorders. GAD is also comorbid with other psychological disorders, especially depression and dysthymia:[65]

> GAD is associated with disability, medically unexplained symptoms, and overutilization of medical resources. Two-thirds of individuals with current GAD had an additional current psychiatric diagnosis (usually major depression or dysthymia), and 98 percent of those with lifetime GAD had another lifetime psychiatric diagnosis. GAD may be a crucial factor in modifying the presentation, course, and outcome of major depression.

Patients with GAD have a moderate amount of disability and impairment in quality of life. GAD is especially common in the elderly.[66] Treatment of GAD is at an elementary stage. One mainstay of the self-medication (or self-prescription) for GAD is alcohol, which effectively produces a short-term anxiolytic action. Until the mid- to late 1990s, benzodiazepines were the prescribed agents of choice, but their use is associated with significant "emergent anxiety and/or withdrawal-related symptomatology":[67]

> Twenty-five percent of patients treated with lorazepam showed rebound anxiety, and 40 percent of them utilized reserve medication because they found drug discontinuation to be intolerable.

In the mid-1990s, buspirone (BuSpar) was demonstrated to effectively reduce symptomatology with efficacy superior to placebo and equal to lorazepam.[68] At that time, buspirone was considered to be the drug of choice for GAD in situations where a slow onset of action and a "subtle" effect was acceptable.[69] By 1997, buspirone was widely used for persistent anxiety without panic attacks, the latter often requiring therapy with an SSRI-type antidepressant. As stated in 1997:

> Buspirone does not impair memory or motor coordination, is not associated with abuse or dependence, is not cross-tolerant with alcohol, and does not produce a withdrawal reaction. In addition, buspirone has a progressive onset of action and produces few adverse drug reactions when combined with other agents. If the patient does not respond to buspirone, we encourage nefazodone, a $5\text{-}HT_2$ antagonist, or one of the serotonin selective reuptake inhibitors.[68]

As was discussed in Chapter 1, buspirone is rapidly metabolized as it is being absorbed; when given with grapefruit juice, its bioavailability is markedly increased. This discovery is likely to encourage its administration with grapefruit juice, a practice that will likely increase its clinical efficacy.

In 1999, reflecting the usefulness of SSRI-type antidepressants as anxiolytics, an extended release dosage form of one of them (Effexor-XR) was FDA approved for clinical use in the treatment of GAD. Head-to-head comparison of Effexor-XR and buspirone (taken with grapefruit juice) in the treatment of GAD has not been reported.

Regarding psychotherapies, cognitive-behavioral therapies, which teach clients to examine how their unrealistic thoughts and ruminations affect their behavioral functioning, have proven efficacy.[71] Relaxation therapy, biofeedback, and stress management are used to teach patients how to relax even under stress. Many anxious people worry about being unable to cope. They fear losing control, "going crazy," or being publicly embarrassed. As a consequence, the fears increase the anxiety in a vicious circle. Anxious thoughts increase anxiety symptoms, which, in turn, generate even more anxious thoughts. Cognitive-behavioral techniques help patients break this circle by allowing them to deal appropriately with anxious thoughts and their related behavioral expressions.

Because GAD is a chronic, relapsing, and debilitating disorder, both acute efficacy and long-term prevention of relapse must be considered when choosing both drug and psychotherapeutic interventions. Ideally, cognitive-behavioral therapies should accompany pharmacologic treatment.[71] Psychotherapeutic intervention should certainly begin before medication is discontinued in order to minimize the likelihood of relapse.

Specific Phobia and Social Phobia

The phobias are characterized by extreme anxiety about a specific object (specific phobia) or a generalized or discrete social situation (social phobia). Patients with social phobias are at high risk for developing mood or anxiety disorders and schizophrenia. According to learning theory, individuals select the behavior that moves them from a state of stress to a state in which the stress is reduced. Thus, if a conditioned stimulus is repeatedly presented in a manner that does not produce a conditioned emotional response, the original association is extinguished. Systematic desensitization (targeted exposure therapy) pairs fear-evoking incidents with relaxation training in a sequence that finally leads to the presentation of the original fear-inducing or anxiety-arousing stimulus.

When the patient with a phobia displays severe anxiety symptoms, anxiolytics may be administered to treat acute symptoms. For longer-term pharmacological management, antidepressant agents are indicated, especially those with anxiolytic properties. Alprazolam (Xanax) can be quite effective, as are serotonin-specific antidepressants.[72]

Obsessive-Compulsive Disorder

Obsessive-compulsive disorder (OCD) is characterized by recurrent and disturbing thoughts (obsessions) and/or repetitive behaviors (compulsions) that the individual feels driven to perform but recognizes as irrational or excessive. Once thought to be a rare condition, it is now estimated to be present in about 2 percent of the general population, making it the fourth most common psychiatric disorder.[73]

> Although traditionally viewed as resistant to a variety of therapeutic interventions, recent advances have been made in the psychopharmacologic and behavioral therapy of OCD. In particular, the clear efficacy of serotonin reuptake inhibitors, such as clomipramine, fluvoxamine, fluoxetine, and sertraline, has been established in double-blind studies in patients with OCD. Consistent with these drug response data are the hypotheses that changes in serotonin function are critical to the treatment of OCD and perhaps involved in the pathophysiology of at least some patients with the disorder.[73]

SSRIs are commonly used for treating OCD; they are effective in approximately 40 to 60 percent of OCD patients. Furthermore, current research indicates that a combination of medication and behavioral therapies is more effective than the use of either drugs or psychological interventions alone. Simpson and co-workers[74] studied cognitive-behavioral therapy (using exposure and ritual prevention) as an adjunct to SSRIs in an open trial in six patients who remained symptomatic despite SSRI treatment. In all six patients, there was a further reduction in OCD symptoms. It therefore appears that because significant OCD symptoms often remain or recur, even when there is substantial improvement with SSRI therapy, a combined drug-CBT approach may be an appropriate strategy.

March and Leonard[75] review OCD in children and adolescents, noting that 1 in 200 young persons suffers from the disorder:

> OCD-specific cognitive-behavioral psychotherapy and pharmacotherapy with a serotonin reuptake inhibitor define the psychotherapeutic and pharmacotherapeutic treatments of choice, respectively.

In 1998, practice parameters for the assessment and treatment of children and adolescents with OCD were published.[76] That document concluded:

> Two modalities have been systematically assessed and empirically shown to ameliorate core symptoms: cognitive-behavioral therapy (primarily exposure/response prevention) and serotonin reuptake inhibitor medication. . . . Because OCD frequently occurs in the context of other psychopathology and adaptive difficulties, additional individual and family psychotherapeutic, pharmacological, and educational interventions often are necessary.

Posttraumatic Stress Disorder

It is generally accepted that transient and long-lasting neurological alterations may underlie acute and long-term neuronal responses to traumatic stress. Comorbidity is frequent; individuals with posttraumatic stress disorder (PTSD) experience a high incidence of GAD, phobias, depression, and substance abuse. Thus, the treatment of PTSD must be comprehensive and individualized, utilizing carefully balanced pharmacotherapeutic and psychotherapeutic interventions that address both the PTSD and any comorbid disorder. According to Vargas and Davidson:[77]

> Symptom relief provided by pharmacotherapy enables the patient to participate more thoroughly in individual, behavioral, or group therapy.

Most drugs that are effective for PTSD are also useful for treating major depression and panic disorder. Thus, numerous drugs have been tried, including TCAs, MAO inhibitors, trazodone, the SSRIs, clonidine, guanfacin, brofaromine, valproate, carbamazepine, benzodiazepines, and others.[78–80] No one drug or class of drugs is universally effective in treating the disorder, although some feel that a serotonergic action is necessary for good clinical effect in PTSD, analogous to the situation with OCD.[77] Some clinicians advocate the use of hypnotic techniques to facilitate working through the traumatic events. This approach is based on the frequently observed interrelationship between dissociative reactions and physical trauma.

Eating Disorders

Only in recent years have eating disorders (bulimia nervosa and anorexia nervosa) been considered amenable to pharmacologic treatment. For bulimia nervosa, in particular, the role of medication has expanded with double-blind, placebo-controlled studies demonstrating significant decrease in the frequency of binge-eating behavior in response to antidepressant medications.[81–82] While various classes of antidepressant medications have been tried, a revised practice guideline for the treatment of patients with eating disorders[83] states:

> The SSRIs are currently considered to be the safest antidepressants and may be especially helpful for patients with significant symptoms of depression, anxiety, obsessions, or certain impulse disorder symptoms or for those patients who have had a suboptimal response to previous attempts at appropriate psychosocial therapy.

Even short-term psychotherapies (e.g., CBT or interpersonal therapies) reduce binge frequency equal to or exceeding the effects of medication treatment. Thus, it seems reasonable to expect that combination therapy would provide additive effects. Combining medication and psychotherapy may improve the outcome in selected patients.[84]

Most authors concur that to initiate treatment of bulimia nervosa, nonpharmacologic approaches should be attempted first and medication added for either the unresponsive patient or one in whom depression or an anxiety disorder is diagnosed as a comorbid disorder. Major depression is the most common comorbid disorder; others include anxiety disorders, substance abuse, and a past history of anorexia nervosa.

Medication failure can result from poor compliance, from vomiting the medication, or from other causes. Blood level analysis may be necessary before concluding that the drug attempt was a failure. Numerous other agents have been tried, but none has been effective when subjected to carefully controlled trials. The course of bulimia may require long-term antidepressant therapy with careful monitoring of side effects and compliance.

In anorexia nervosa, pharmacologic treatment has a very limited role; psychiatric therapy is more important. Psychotherapy, often with CBT components, group therapy, family therapy, nutrition counseling, and so on are all necessary. Drug therapy is primarily aimed at treating comorbid depression following weight gain.[83] However, double-blind studies of antidepressants (versus placebo) show little improvement in weight (weight gain), mood, or body perception. Certainly, however, a trial of antidepressant therapy is warranted in patients who do not respond to psychotherapeutic interventions.

Practice Standards

As the 1990s began, it became apparent that numerous psychophar-macologic interventions and psychotherapeutic treatments of various psychological disorders were being conducted with minimal evalua-tion for either therapeutic efficacy or cost effectiveness. Therefore, three associations—the American Psychiatric Association (APA), the U.S. Agency for Health Care Policy and Research (AHCPR), and the American Academy of Child and Adolescent Psychiatry (AACAP)—began publishing on a regular basis practice guidelines that are, in essence, comprehensive reviews of patient care strategies to assist clinicians in making clinical decisions regarding the treatment of specific patients. The APA and AHCPR guidelines were directed to-ward mental health disorders in adults; the AACAP guidelines were directed specifically toward mental health disorders in children and adolescents.

The goal of these clinical practice guidelines is to improve the care of patients. The guidelines are not intended to serve as standards of care for medical, psychological, or legal purposes. They do, however, present a consensus of expert opinion regarding disorders, their diag-noses, and the efficacy of various treatments. It is our opinion that all behavioral health professionals should be familiar with these practice guidelines, have them available for reference, and keep up with new or revised guidelines as they are released.

In several instances there was overlap between the guidelines de-veloped by the APA and those developed by AHCPR. For example, in 1996 both groups published guidelines for the treatment of nicotine dependence. As a result of this overlap, in 1997 the AHCPR ceased this activity; AHCPR now provides support services for other organi-zations developing practice guidelines. AHCPR has chosen to be a repository for the practice guidelines of many professional organiza-tions and topics (today, more than 600 different clinical guidelines for all areas of medicine). A recent article by Gillespie[85] reviews the use of the AHCPR on-line clearinghouse for access to these guide-lines. The Web site of this national guideline clearinghouse is www.guideline.gov.

This introduction to the topic of clinical practice guidelines presents only those published by the APA and the AACAP. Several guidelines have already been cited, but because of their importance, all are listed here.

APA Practice Guidelines

In 1991 the APA embarked on a process of developing practice guide-lines, which have been periodically published in its journal, the *American Journal of Psychiatry*. In 1996, the APA collected and reprinted in book form the first five sets of guidelines:[86]

- Psychiatric Evaluation of Adults
- Eating Disorders
- Major Depressive Disorder in Adults
- Treatment of Patients with Bipolar Disorder
- Treatment of Patients with Substance Abuse Disorders: Alcohol, Cocaine, Opioids

A sixth guideline was published in 1996: "Practice Guideline for the Treatment of Patients with Nicotine Dependence."[87] In 1997, the APA published "Practice Guideline for the Treatment of Patients with Schizophrenia,"[88] followed by its eighth guideline, "Practice Guideline for Treatment of Patients with Alzheimer's Disease and Other Dementias of Late Life." In May 1998, the APA published "Practice Guideline for the Treatment of Patients with Panic Disorder."[20] These were followed in May 1999 by "Practice Guideline for the Treatment of Patients with Delirium" and in January 2000 with its first revised guideline, "Practice Guideline for the Treatment of Patients with Eating Disorders (Revision)."[83] As noted earlier, the revised guideline for treating depression appeared in April 2000.[6]

As they are developed, each guideline is published as a supplement in the *American Journal of Psychiatry*. As with the revised guideline for eating disorders and depression, completed guidelines are scheduled for periodic revision.

AACAP Practice Parameters

In 1997 the Council of the AACAP published practice parameters for the assessment and treatment of children and adolescents with bipolar disorder[46] and depression,[42] a first for these populations of patients. Additional practice parameters were collated and published as special supplements to the *Journal of the American Academy of Child and Adolescent Psychiatry* in October 1997,[89] October 1998,[90] and December 1999.[91] Because of their importance, we list all the topics for which standards for children and adolescents have been published to date (see the review by Bernet[92]).

The 1997 supplement contained practice parameters on the following topics:

- Psychiatric assessment of children and adolescents
- Psychiatric assessment of infants and toddlers
- Forensic evaluation of children and adolescents who may have been physically or sexually abused
- Child custody evaluation

- Anxiety disorders
- Attention-deficit/hyperactivity disorder
- Conduct disorder
- Substance abuse disorders
- Bipolar disorder
- Schizophrenia

The 1998 supplement contained practice parameters on the following topics:

- Posttraumatic stress disorder
- Obsessive-compulsive disorder
- Depressive disorders

The 1999 supplement contained practice parameters on the following topics:

- Mental retardation
- Autism and pervasive developmental disorders
- Children and adolescents who are sexually abusive of others

Currently, the Workgroup on Quality Issues of the American Academy of Child and Adolescent Psychiatry component that develops practice parameters has identified about 50 additional topics to consider for future practice parameters. Bernet[92] discusses the workings of the process in more detail.

Zito and co-workers[93] reviewed prescription records from the years 1991 through 1995 for psychotropic medications for 2- to 4-year-old preschoolers. Dramatic increases over this time period were noted. In 1995, the most prescribed psychotropic medications were stimulants (12.3 per 1000 preschoolers, 90 percent of which were methylphenidate), and antidepressants (3.2 per 1000 preschoolers). In total, in 1995, about 1.5 percent of all children 2 to 4 years old were receiving stimulants or antidepressants. Today, this number is probably considerably larger, the more so with the addition of prescriptions for both the new-generation antipsychotic drugs and the anticonvulsant-antimanic drugs that have become popular. Coyle,[94] in discussing the Zito report, states that the prescription explosion is occurring without empirical evidence to support either efficacy or safety of the drugs in this age group. Coyle concludes:

> It appears that behaviorally disturbed children are now increasingly subjected to quick and inexpensive pharmacologic fixes as opposed to

informed, multimodal therapy associated with optimal outcomes. These disturbing prescription practices suggest a growing crisis in mental health services to children and demand more thorough investigation.

Finally, in the year 2000, *Psychiatric Clinics of North America* is publishing comprehensive reviews on the diagnosis and treatment of Borderline Personality Disorder (March), Obsessive-Compulsive Disorder (June), and Depression (December).

REFERENCES

1. J. B. Persons, M. E. Thase, and P. Crits-Christoph, "The Role of Psychotherapy in the Treatment of Depression," *Archives of General Psychiatry* 53 (1996): 283–290 (with four additional commentaries).
2. M. E. Thase et al., "Treatment of Major Depression with Psychotherapy or Psychotherapy-pharmacotherapy Combinations," *Archives of General Psychiatry* 54 (1997): 1009–1015.
3. C. F. Reynolds, "Nortriptyline and Interpersonal Psychotherapy as Maintenance Therapies for Recurrent Major Depression: A Randomized Controlled Trial in Patients Older Than 59 Years," *Journal of the American Medical Association* 281 (1999): 39–45.
4. U.S. Department of Health and Human Services, *Mental Health: A Report of the Surgeon General*. Rockville, Md.: U.S. Department of Health and Human Services, Substance Abuse and Mental Health Services Administration, Center for Mental Health Services, National Institutes of Health, National Institute of Mental Health, December, 1999.
5. J. B. Frank, K. Weihs, E. Minerva, and D. Z. Lieberman, "Women's Mental Health in Primary Care," *Medical Clinics of North America* 82 (1998): 359–383.
6. American Psychiatric Association, "Practice Guideline for the Treatment of Patients with Major Depressive Disorder (Revision)," *American Journal of Psychiatry* 157, Number 4 (April, 2000): 1–45.
7. R. M. A. Hirschfeld et al., "The National Depressive and Manic-depressive Association Consensus Statement on the Undertreatment of Depression," *Journal of the American Medical Association* 277 (1997): 333–340.
8. H. C. Schulberg et al., "The Usual Care of Major Depression in Primary Care Practice," *Archives of Family Medicine* 6 (1997): 334–339.
9. M. D. Cabana et al., "Why Don't Physicians Follow Clinical Practice Guidelines? A Framework for Improvement," *Journal of the American Medical Association* 282 (1999): 1458–1465.
10. C. A. Melfi et al., "The Effects of Adherence to Antidepressant Treatment Guidelines on Relapse and Recurrence of Depression," *Archives of General Psychiatry* 55 (1998): 1128–1132.
11. W. Katon et al., "Stepped Collaborative Care for Primary Care Patients with Persistent Symptoms of Depression," *Archives of General Psychiatry* 56 (1999): 1109–1115.

12. K. B. Wells et al., "Impact of Disseminating Quality Improvement Programs for Depression in Managed Primary Care: A Randomized Controlled Trial," *Journal of the American Medical Association* 283 (2000): 212–220.

13. D. A. Sclar, L. M. Robison, T. L. Skaer, and R. S. Galin, "What Factors Influence the Prescribing of Antidepressant Pharmacotherapy? An Assessment of National Office-based Encounters," *International Journal of Psychiatry in Medicine* 28 (1998): 407–419.

14. E. S. Brown, A. J. Rush, and B. S. McEwen, "Hippocampal Remodeling and Damage by Corticosteroids: Implications for Mood Disorders," *Neuropsychopharmacology* 21 (1999): 474–484.

15. S. E. Lindley, T. G. Bengoechea, A. F. Schatzberg, and D. L. Wong, "Glucocorticoid Effects on Mesotelencephalic Dopamine Neurotransmission," *Neuropsychopharmacology* 21 (1999): 399–407.

16. S. C. Heinrichs, "Stress-axis, Coping and Dementia: Gene-Manipulation Studies," *Trends in Pharmacological Sciences* 20 (1999): 311–315.

17. A. Russo-Neustadt, R. C. Beard, and C. W. Cotman, "Exercise, Antidepressant Medications, and Enhanced Brain-derived Neurotrophic Factor Expression," *Neuropsychopharmacology* 21 (1999): 679–682.

18. K. Fujimaki, S. Morinobu, and R. S. Duman, "Administration of a cAMP-phosphodiesterase-4-inhibitor Enhances Antidepressant Induction of BDNF mRNA in Rat Hippocampus," *Neuropsychopharmacology* 22 (2000): 42–51.

19. S. J. Kingsbury, "Where Does Research on the Effectiveness of Psychotherapy Stand Today?" *The Harvard Mental Health Letter* (September 1995): 8.

20. Work Group on Panic Disorder, "Practice Guideline for the Treatment of Patients with Panic Disorder," *American Journal of Psychiatry* 155, Suppl. (May 1998): 2–3.

21. M. G. Gelder, "Combined Pharmacotherapy and Cognitive Behavior Therapy in the Treatment of Panic Disorder," *Journal of Clinical Psychopharmacology* 18 (Supplement 2, 1998): 2S–5S.

22. R. J. DeRubeis, L. A. Gelfand, T. Z. Tang, and A. D. Simons, "Medications Versus Cognitive Behavior Therapy for Severely Depressed Outpatients: Mega-analysis of Four Randomized Comparisons," *American Journal of Psychiatry* 156 (1999): 1007–1013.

23. D. Jayson et al., "Which Depressed Patients Respond to Cognitive-behavioral Treatment?" *Journal of the American Academy of Child and Adolescent Psychiatry* 37 (1998): 35–39.

24. E. S. Paykel et al., "Prevention of Relapse in Residual Depression by Cognitive Therapy," *Archives of General Psychiatry* 56 (1999): 829–835.

25. B. T. Walsh et al., "Medication and Psychotherapy in the Treatment of Bulimia Nervosa," *American Journal of Psychiatry* 154 (1997): 523–531.

26. M. A. Reinecke, N. E. Ryan, and D. L. DuBois, "Cognitive-behavioral Therapy of Depression and Depressive Symptoms During Adolescence: A Review and Meta-analysis," *Journal of the American Academy of Child and Adolescent Psychiatry* 37 (1998): 26–34.

27. S. M. Hall et al., "Nortriptyline and Cognitive-behavioral Therapy in the Treatment of Cigarette Smoking," *Archives of General Psychiatry* 55 (1998): 683–690.

28. I. W. Miller and G. I. Keitner, "Combined Medication and Psychotherapy in the Treatment of Chronic Mood Disorders," *Psychiatric Clinics of North America* 19 (1996): 151–170.

29. H. J. Henk et al., "Medical Costs Attributed to Depression Among Patients with a History of High Medical Expenses in a Health Maintenance Organization," *Archives of General Psychiatry* 53 (1996): 899–904.

30. L. S. Meredith, K. B. Wells, S. H. Kaplan, and R. M. Mazel, "Counseling Typically Provided for Depression," *Archives of General Psychiatry* 53 (1996): 905–912.

31. W. Katon et al., "A Multifaceted Intervention to Improve Treatment of Depression in Primary Care," *Archives of General Psychiatry* 53 (1996): 924–932.

32. K. B. Wells, "Caring for Depression in Primary Care: Defining and Illustrating the Policy Context," *Journal of Clinical Psychiatry* 58, Suppl. 1 (1997): 24–27.

33. W. Katon et al., "Collaborative Management to Achieve Treatment Depression Guidelines," *Journal of Clinical Psychiatry* 58, Suppl. 1 (1997): 20–23.

34. D. L. Sprenger and A. M. Josephson, "Integration of Pharmacotherapy and Family Therapy in the Treatment of Children and Adolescents," *Journal of the American Academy of Child and Adolescent Psychiatry* 37 (1998): 887–889.

35. American Psychiatric Association, *Diagnostic and Statistical Manual of Mental Disorders*, 4th ed. (Washington, D.C.: American Psychiatric Association, 1994).

36. K. B. Stage, A. H. Glassman, and L. S. Covey, "Depression After Smoking Cessation: Case Reports," *Journal of Clinical Psychiatry* 57 (1996): 467–469.

37. E. Frank et al., "Interpersonal Psychotherapy and Antidepressant Medication: Evaluation of a Sequential Treatment Strategy in Women with Recurrent Major Depression," *Journal of Clinical Psychiatry* 61 (2000): 51–57.

38. R. A. Friedman and J. H. Kocis, "Pharmacotherapy for Chronic Depression," *Psychiatric Clinics of North America* 19 (1996): 121–132.

39. J. H. Kocis et al., "Maintenance Therapy for Chronic Depression," *Archives of General Psychiatry* 53 (1996): 769–774.

40. M. E. Thase et al., "A Placebo-controlled, Randomized Clinical Trial Comparing Sertraline and Imipramine for the Treatment of Dysthymia," *Archives of General Psychiatry* 53 (1996): 777–784.

41. C. Z. Garrison et al., "Incidence of Major Depressive Disorder and Dysthymia in Young Adolescents," *Journal of the American Academy of Child and Adolescent Psychiatry* 36 (1997): 458–465.

42. American Academy of Child and Adolescent Psychiatry, "Practice Parameters for the Assessment and Treatment of Children and Adolescents with Depressive Disorders," *Journal of the American Academy of Child and Adolescent Psychiatry* 37, Suppl. (October 1997): 63S–83S.

43 B. Geller et al., "Critical Review of Tricyclic Antidepressant Use in Children and Adolescents," *Journal of the American Academy of Child and Adolescent Psychiatry* 38 (1999): 513–516.

44. G. J. Emslie, J. T. Walkup, S. R. Pliszka, and M. Ernst, "Nontricyclic Antidepressants in Children and Adolescents," *Journal of the American Academy of Child and Adolescent Psychiatry* 38 (1999): 517–528.

45. N. D. Ryan, V. Bhatara, and J. M. Perel, "Mood Stabilizers in Children and Adolescents," *Journal of the American Academy of Child and Adolescent Psychiatry* 38 (1999): 529–536.

46. J. McClellan and J. Werry, principal authors, "Practice Parameters for the Assessment and Treatment of Children and Adolescents with Bipolar Disorder," *Journal of the American Academy of Child and Adolescent Psychiatry* 36 (1997): 138–157.

47. S. R. Marder, A. Ames, W. C. Wirshing, and T. Van Putten, "Schizophrenia," *Psychiatric Clinics of North America* 16 (1993): 567–588.

48. O. Blin, "A Comparative Review of New Antipsychotics," *Canadian Journal of Psychiatry* 44 (1999): 235–244.

49. R. Norman and L. A. Townsend, "Cognitive-behavioral Therapy for Psychosis: A Status Report," *Canadian Journal of Psychiatry* 44 (1999): 245–252.

50. T. Sensky et al., "A Randomized Controlled Trial of Cognitive-behavioral Therapy for Persistent Symptoms in Schizophrenia Resistant to Medication," *Archives of General Psychiatry* 57 (2000): 165–172.

51. American Academy of Child and Adolescent Psychiatry, "Practice Parameters for Assessment and Treatment of Children and Adolescents with Schizophrenia," *Journal of the American Academy of Child and Adolescent Psychiatry* 36, Suppl. (October 1997): 177S–193S.

52. M. Campbell, J. L. Rapoport, and G. M. Simpson, "Antipsychotics in Children and Adolescents," *Journal of the American Academy of Child and Adolescent Psychiatry* 38 (1999): 537–545.

53. O. Brawman-Mintzer and R. B. Lydiard, "Biological Basis of Generalized Anxiety Disorder," *Journal of Clinical Psychiatry* 58, Suppl. 3 (1997): 16–25.

54. T. J. Barloon and R. Noyes, "Charles Darwin and Panic Disorder," *Journal of the American Medical Association* 277(1997): 138–141.

55. M. H. Pollack and M. W. Otto, "Long-term Course and Outcome of Panic Disorder," *Journal of Clinical Psychiatry* 58, Suppl. 2 (1997): 57–60.

56. J. W. Jefferson, "Antidepressants in Panic Disorder," *Journal of Clinical Psychiatry* 58, Suppl. 2 (1997): 20–24.

57. J. R. T. Davidson, "Use of Benzodiazepines in Panic Disorder," *Journal of Clinical Psychiatry* 58, Suppl. 2 (1997): 26–28.

58. M. K. Shear and K. Weiner, "Psychotherapy for Panic Disorder," *Journal of Clinical Psychiatry* 58, Suppl. 2 (1997): 38–43.

59. D. H. Barlow, "Cognitive-behavioral Therapy for Panic Disorder: Current Status," *Journal of Clinical Psychiatry* 58, Suppl. 2 (1997): 32–36.

60. J. M. Gorman and J. D. Coplan, "Comorbidity of Depression and Panic Disorder," *Journal of Clinical Psychiatry* 57, Suppl. 10 (1996): 34–43.

61. M. H. Pollack, "Psychopharmacology Update," *Journal of Clinical Psychiatry* 58 (1997): 38–40.

62. M. W. Otto, "Integrated Treatment of Panic Disorder," *Journal of Clinical Psychiatry* 58 (1997): 40–42.

63. D. A. Spiegel and T. J. Bruce, "Benzodiazepines and Exposure-based Cognitive Behavioral Therapies for Panic Disorder: Conclusions from Combined Treatment Trials," *American Journal of Psychiatry* 154 (1997): 773–781.

64. O. Brawman-Mintzer and R. B. Lydiard, "Generalized Anxiety Disorder: Issues in Epidemiology," *Journal of Clinical Psychiatry* 57, Suppl. 7 (1996): 3–8.

65. P. P. Roy-Byrns and W. Katon, "Generalized Anxiety Disorder in Primary Care: The Precursor/Modifier Pathway to Increased Health Care Utilization," *Journal of Clinical Psychiatry* 58, Suppl. 3 (1997): 34–38.

66. E. J. Lenze et al., "Comorbid Anxiety Disorders in Depressed Elderly Patients," *American Journal of Psychiatry* 175 (2000): 722–728.

67. L. A. Mandos et al., "Placebo-controlled Comparison of the Clinical Effects of Rapid Discontinuation of Ipsapirone and Lorazepam After Eight Weeks of Treatment for Generalized Anxiety Disorder," *International Clinical Psychopharmacology* 10 (1995): 251–256.

68. J. J. Sramek et al., "Efficacy of Buspirone in Generalized Anxiety Disorder with Coexisting Mild Depressive Symptoms," *Journal of Clinical Psychiatry* 57 (1996): 287–291.

69. E. Schweizer and K. Rickels, "Strategies for Treatment of Generalized Anxiety in the Primary Care Setting," *Journal of Clinical Psychiatry* 58, Suppl. 3 (1997): 27–31.

70. R. E. Hales, D. A. Hilty, and M. G. Wise, "A Treatment Algorithm for the Management of Anxiety in Primary Care Practice," *Journal of Clinical Psychiatry* 58, Suppl. 3 (1997): 76–80.

71. A. G. Harvey and R. M. Rapee, "Cognitive-behavioral Therapy for Generalized Anxiety Disorder," *Psychiatric Clinics of North America* 18 (1995): 859–870.

72. B. Black, T. W. Uhde, and M. E. Taylor, "Fluoxetine for the Treatment of Social Phobia," *Journal of Clinical Psychopharmacology* 12 (1992): 293–295.

73. Symposium, "New Frontiers on OCD Spectrum Research for Psychiatry and Primary Care," *Journal of Clinical Psychiatry* 57, Suppl. 8 (1996).

74. H. B. Simpson, K. S. Gorfinkle, and M. R. Liebowitz, "Cognitive-behavioral Therapy as an Adjunct to Serotonin Reuptake Inhibitors in Obsessive-compulsive Disorder: An Open Trial," *Journal of Clinical Psychiatry* 60 (1999): 584–590.

75. J. S. March and H. L. Leonard, "Obsessive-compulsive Disorder in Children and Adolescents: A Review of the Past Ten Years," *Journal of the American Academy of Child and Adolescent Psychiatry* 34 (1996): 1265–1273.

76. American Academy of Child and Adolescent Psychiatry, "Practice Parameters for the Assessment and Treatment of Children and Adolescents with Obsessive-compulsive Disorder," *Journal of the American Academy of Child and Adolescent Psychiatry* 37, Suppl. (October 1998): 27S–45S.

77. M. A. Vargas and J. Davidson, "Post-traumatic Stress Disorder," *Psychiatric Clinics of North America* 16 (1993): 745.

78. L. Katz, W. Fleisher, K. Kjernisted, and P. Milanese, "A Review of the Psychobiology and Pharmacotherapy of Posttraumatic Stress Disorder," *Canadian Journal of Psychiatry* 41 (1996): 233–238.

79. M. A. Hertzberg, M. E. Feldman, J. C. Beckham, and J. R. Davidson, "Trial of Trazodone for Posttraumatic Stress Disorder Using a Multiple Baseline Group Design," *Journal of Clinical Psychopharmacology* 16 (1996): 294–298.

80. C. R. Marmar et al., "Open Trial of Fluvoxamine Treatment for Combat-related Posttraumatic Stress Disorder," *Journal of Clinical Psychiatry* 57, Suppl. 8 (1996): 66–70.

81. S. J. Crow and J. E. Mitchell, "Integrating Cognitive Therapy and Medications in Treating Bulimia Nervosa," *Psychiatric Clinics of North America* 19 (1996): 755–760.

82. J. Yager, ed., "Eating Disorders, *Psychiatric Clinics of North America* 19, no. 4 (December 1996).

83. American Psychiatric Association, "Practice Guideline for the Treatment of Patients with Eating Disorders (Revision)," *American Journal of Psychiatry* 157, Suppl. (January 2000).

84. D. M. Garner and P. E. Garfinkel, eds, *Handbook of Treatment for Eating Disorders*, 2nd ed. (New York: Guilford, 1997).

85. G. Gillespie, "On-line Clinical Guidelines Help Trim Costs," *Health Data Management* 8 (2000): 38–45.

86. American Psychiatric Association, *Practice Guidelines* (Washington D.C.: American Psychiatric Association, 1996).

87. American Psychiatric Association, "Practice Guidelines for the Treatment of Patients with Nicotine Dependence," *American Journal of Psychiatry* 153, no. 10, suppl. (October 1996): 1–31.

88. American Psychiatric Association, "Practice Guideline for the Treatment of Patients with Schizophrenia," *American Journal of Psychiatry* 154, no. 4, suppl. (April 1997): 1–63.

89. *Journal of the American Academy of Child and Adolescent Psychiatry* 36, no. 10, suppl. (October 1997).

90. *Journal of the American Academy of Child and Adolescent Psychiatry* 37, no. 10, suppl. (October 1998).

91. *Journal of the American Academy of Child and Adolescent Psychiatry* 38, no. 12, suppl. (December 1999).

92. W. Bernet, "Introduction, Practice Parameters for the 21st Century," *Journal of the American Academy of Child and Adolescent Psychiatry* 38, no. 12, suppl. (December 1999), 1S–4S.

93. J. M. Zito et al., "Trends in the Prescribing of Psychotrophic Medications to Preschoolers," *Journal of the American Medical Association,* 283 (2000): 1025–1030.

94. J. T. Coyle, "Psychotropic Drug Use in Very Young Children," *Journal of the American Medical Association,* 283 (2000): 1059–1060.

Chapter 20

Herbal Medicines Used in the Treatment of Psychological Disorders

Writing a review of the pharmacology of herbal medicines presents a daunting challenge. On the one hand, some people feel that, because they are found in nature, herbals are, by definition, safe, effective, and nontoxic. Is this true? Are they efficacious? Are they "safe"? Should they be freely available for purchase and use? What is their potential for causing toxic reactions or producing compulsive abuse? Should these compounds be regulated by the government? The approach here is to describe what is known about the pharmacokinetics, pharmacodynamics, side effects, toxicities, and drug interactions for each of the herbal compounds commonly used in the treatment of psychological disorders or that might have significant CNS actions.

Many drugs derived from natural herbal sources have already been covered in this text, including caffeine, nicotine, cocaine, morphine, codeine, tetrahydrocannabinol, scopolamine, myristicin, elemicin, and mescaline (Table 20.1). Certainly no reasonable person would advocate the free availability of cocaine, morphine, or psychedelics. Regulatory control is essential and has already been implemented for many of these "herbal" drugs.

Covered here are agents and herbals with presumed CNS actions that have not already been covered in this test. Often, their actions are not clearly delineated and their efficacy debated. Nonetheless, they are heavily promoted and used for the treatment of various psychological

TABLE 20.1 Some of the naturally occurring psychoactive drugs already covered in this book

Drug	Chapter	Used in therapeutics	Drug of abuse
Cocaine	7	Rarely	Yes
Caffeine	8	Occasionally	Probably
Nicotine	8	No	Yes
Lithium	16	Yes	No
Morphine	9	Yes	Yes
Codeine	9	Yes	Yes
Tetrahydrocannabinol	11	Rarely	Yes
Scopolamine	12	Occasionally	Occasionally
Mescaline	12	No	Yes
Myristicin/Elemicin	12	No	Yes
Psilocybin/Psilocin	12	No	Yes
Dimethyltryptamine	12	No	Yes
Bufotenine	12	No	Yes
Ololiuqui	12	No	Yes
Harmine	12	No	Yes
DHEA	15	Possibly	Possibly
Omega-3 fatty acids	16	Possibly	No

disorders. In some cases, such promotion may be warranted. In other cases, regulation is either currently needed (e.g., ephedrine) or perhaps will be needed should widespread use become a societal problem (e.g., kava).

In the late twentieth and early twenty-first centuries, herbal medications have attracted enormous interest, almost as if they were something new. Of course, herbal medicines are ancient; they've been with us for thousands of years. Since the isolation of morphine from crude opium extract in the 1860s, scientists called *pharmacognosists* have sought to identify pharmacologically active ingredients in natural materials. The term applied to this area of study is called *pharmacognosy*.

In this chapter the focus is primarily on herbal medicines that are used to treat psychiatric symptoms or disorders, that produce changes in mood, thinking, or behavior as a side effect, or that interact with psychiatric medications.[1] A newly published edition of the *Physician's Desk Reference* is devoted to herbal medicines, although it does not contain critical analysis of potential or claimed efficacy.[2]

Each of the herbs discussed in this chapter presumably contains an active ingredient that accounts for its clinical use. In many cases, the presumed active ingredient has not yet been identified, so discussion is oriented to the plant material and the safety, side effects, drug interactions, and efficacy in treating symptoms or diagnoses (Table 20.2).

The use of many herbal medications still is a bit of a lottery, due to incomplete knowledge of active ingredients, absence of standardization, different purities, and so on.[3] The final composition of a plant product varies according to what part of the plant is used, where it was grown, what time of year it was grown or harvested, the reputation of the grower, processor, packager, marketer, promoter, and so on. Regulation of the herbal medicine industry is needed to ensure that people receive what they purchase. Certainly people have a right to know what they are taking.

It is somewhat unclear how this era of widespread, largely unregulated availability and promotion of herbal products came about. While herbals have been used from the time of Hippocrates and patent medicines were widely promoted in the United States until the early part of the twentieth century, federal regulations in the 1920s severely restricted the sale and nonprescription use of such products, most of which contained large amounts of alcohol as well as "natural" drugs such as cocaine and opium. But then the passage of the Dietary Supplement Health Education Act of 1994 severely restricted the Food and Drug Administration's ability to exert control over herbal products (Congress passed the act under heavy lobby pressure). Thus, since 1994, any product could be labeled a "supplement" as long as the product made no claim to affect a "disease." Thus, a manufacturer cannot claim that a product "alleviates depression;" rather, it "promotes emotional balance." An herbal product cannot be claimed to alleviate the signs and symptoms of Alzheimer's disease; rather, it enhances "mental sharpness." Neither safety nor efficacy must be demonstrated.[3] Promotion of many herbs addresses the fact that fatigue, headache, insomnia, depression, and anxiety are the most common reasons patients cite for seeking treatment from alternative practitioners. These are also the symptoms and complaints most often underappreciated and untreated by medical doctors.

St. John's Wort

St. John's wort is the common name for the flowering plant *Hypericum perforatum*. It is named after St. John the Baptist because it blooms around his feast day (June 24) and exudes a red color symbolic of his blood.[4] It has many constituents with biological activity, including naphthodianthrones, flavinoids, and xanthones. *Hypericin* (Figure 20.1), a naphthodianthrone (and possibly *pseudohypericin* and/or hyperforin), is generally considered to be the active ingredient, and dosage of the herb is based on its presumed hypericin content. The term

TABLE 20.2 Herbal remedies commonly used to treat psychiatric symptoms*

Herb	Common usage	Quality of evidence category[†]	Adverse effects	Cautions/ contraindications	Drug interactions
Black cohosh	Menopause symptoms	I	GI upset (rare), headaches, CV depression	Pregnancy, lactation	Hormonal treatments (theoretical)
	PMS	II			
	Dysmenorrhea	III			
German chamomile	Insomnia	III	Allergy (rare)	Allergy to sunflower family of plants	None reported
	Anxiety	III			
Evening primrose	Schizophrenia	IV	None reported	Mania, epilepsy	Phenothiazines, NSAIDs, corticosteroids., ß-blockers, anticoagulants
	ADHD	IV			
	Dementia	IV			
Ginkgo	"Cerebrovascular insufficiency" symptoms	I	Headache, GI upset	Pregnancy, lactation, potential bleeding (e.g., PUD)	Anticoagulants
	Dementia	I			
Hops	Insomnia	III	Allergy, menstrual irregularity	Depression, pregnancy, lactation	Sedative-hypnotics, alcohol (both theoretical)
Kava	Insomnia	III	Scaling of skin on extremities	Pregnancy, lactation	Benzodiazepines, alcohol
	Anxiety	III			
	Seizures	IV			
Lemon balm	Insomnia	IV	None reported	Thyroid disease, pregnancy, lactation	CNS depressants, thyroid medications
	Anxiety	III			

TABLE 20.2 Herbal remedies commonly used to treat psychiatric symptoms* *(continued)*

Herb	Common usage	Quality of evidence category†	Adverse effects	Cautions/ contraindications	Drug interactions
Passion flower	Insomnia Anxiety	III] III]	Hypersensitivity vasculitis, sedation	Pregnancy, lactation	Insufficient data
Skullcap	Insomnia Anxiety	IV] IV]	Sedation, confusion, seizures	Pregnancy, lactation	Insufficient data
St. John's wort	Depression	I	Photosensitivity, GI upset, sedation, anticholinergic	CV disease, pregnancy. lactation, pheochromocytoma	Drugs that interact with MAOIs
Valerian	Insomnia Anxiety	III] III]	Sedation	Pregnancy, lactation	CNS depressants

From Wong, Smith, and Boon.[1]

*PMS = premenstrual syndrome; GI = gastrointestinal; CV = cardiovascular; ADHD = attention deficit with hyperactivity disorder; NSAIDs = nonsteroidal anti-inflammatory drugs; PUD = peptic ulcer disease; CNS = central nervous system; MAOIs = monoamine oxidase inhibitors.
†Quality of evidence: I = evidence from at least two properly randomized controlled trials; II = evidence from well-designed trials without randomization; III = opinions of respected authorities based on clinical experience, descriptive studies, or reports of expert committees; IV = insufficient evidence to warrant conclusions about efficacy or safety.

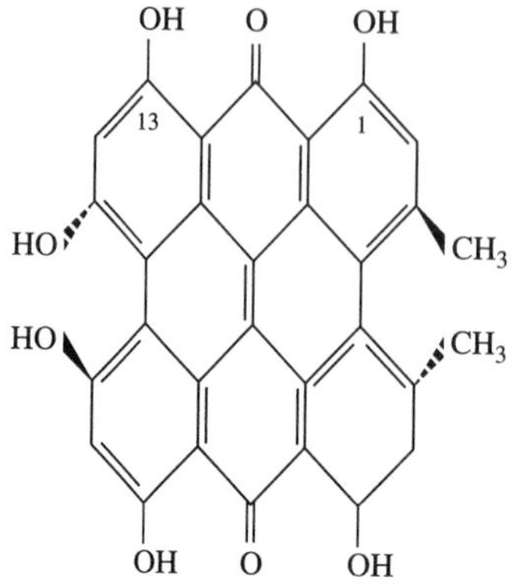

FIGURE 20.1 Structural formulas of hypericin and pseudohypericin.

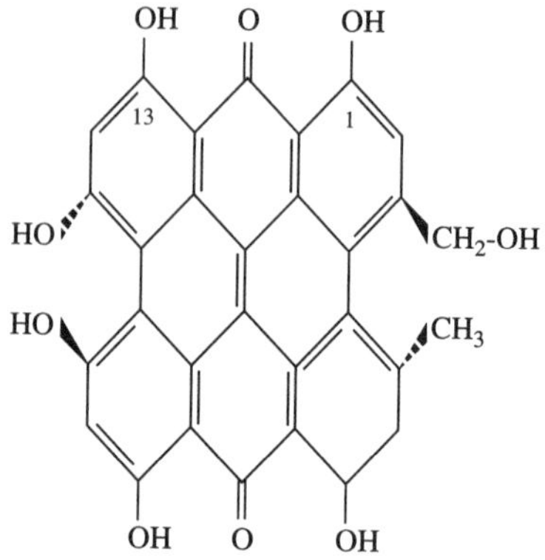

hypericin is from the Greek *hyper* and *eikon*, which mean "to overcome an apparition"; the ancients believed in its ability to ward off evil spirits.[4] The amount of hypericin varies widely in different parts of the plant, under different growth conditions, and at different times of the year.

Indications

St. John's wort is licensed in Germany for the treatment of anxiety, depression, and insomnia. In the United States, of course, no claims of effectiveness in treating these disorders may be made; it is legally sold only as a dietary supplement, perhaps promoting emotional balance. Despite this, the herbal is widely used for its presumed efficacy as a mild antidepressant.

Pharmacokinetics

Hypericins in St. John's wort are absorbed following oral administration with peak blood levels achieved in about 5 hours (Figure 20.2). Hypericin has an elimination half-life of about 25 hours; it thus achieves steady-state concentrations in the brain in about 4 to 6 days (Figure 20.3).[5] Only about 15 to 20 percent of the administered hypericin reaches the central circulation and is available systemically. A hypericin-containing skin patch is now available, but comparative adsorption data is not available.* Whether hypericin is metabolized, how it is metabolized, metabolites, and routes of excretion are unknown.

---

*Called St. John's Transdermal Patch, it is a "dietary supplement" that cannot be eaten, an interesting twist on current political and regulatory standards.

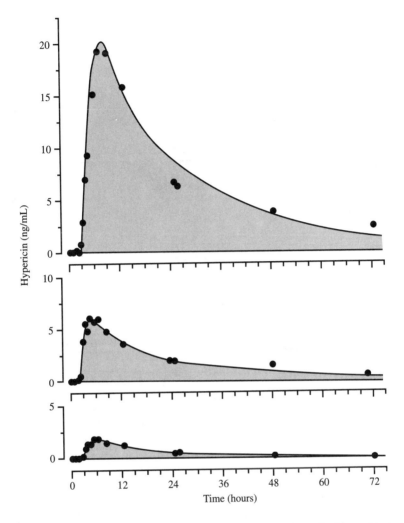

FIGURE 20.2 Time course of concentration of hypericin in plasma in three subjects after receiving a single dose of 300-mg (lower graph), 900-mg (middle graph), or 1800-mg (upper graph). [From Staffeldt et al.[5]]

St. John's wort contains bioflavinoids, one of which is *quercitin.* Quercitin inhibits the drug-metabolizing enzyme CYP1A2. It theoretically could interact with numerous other drugs, affecting their own bioavailability. For example, it may reduce the effectiveness of codeine (blocking conversion to morphine) and increase the blood levels of caffeine and several psychoactive medications, including tricyclic antidepressants and antipsychotic drugs. Further research on the clinical significance of quercitin-induced CYP1A2 inhibition appears needed.

A. Hypericin

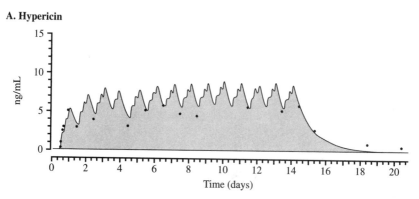

B. Pseudohypericin

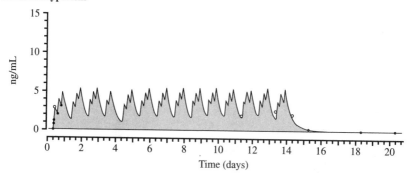

FIGURE 20.3 Time course of concentrations of (**A**) hypericin and (**B**) pseudohypericin in a subject taking one 300-mg tablet of hypericum extract three times daily for 14 days. [From Staffeldt et al.[5]]

Pharmacodynamics

The mechanism of action of hypericin and hypericum extracts is unclear. Initially, it was thought that inhibition of monoamine oxidase (Chapter 15) would account for its antidepressant action. However, while MAO inhibition can be demonstrated in vitro at high concentrations, the effect is too weak to account for clinical efficacy.[6] In a brief report, Muller and Rossol[7] reported that hypericum extract reduced, in vitro, the expression of serotonin receptors. They stated:

> Unlike classic antidepressants, which block the neurotransmitter, hypericum extract might "block" the entry point, leading to an increased level of neurotransmitters and, therefore, an antidepressant effect.

More recent reports hypothesize a hypericin-induced blockade of the presynaptic reuptake of serotonin, norepinephrine, and dopamine.[1] Other reported effects of hypericin include binding to GABA receptors, benzodiazepine receptors, and glutaminergic NMDA-type receptors.[1] Rats treated for 6 months with hypericum extract showed a 50 percent increase in serotonin 1A and 2A receptors without changes in receptor affinity.[8]

Thus, since MAO inhibition is not responsible for hypericin's antidepressant action, the mechanism may involve blockade of neurotransmitter reuptake; it may involve increases or decreases at a transcriptional level involving receptor expression; or it may involve another as yet unrecognized and perhaps unique action. Gambarana and co-workers[9] reported that, in rats, *Hypericum perforatum* extract

> acutely protected animals from the sequelae of unavoidable stress; . . . *H. perforatum* reverted the escape deficit maintained by repeated stressors and preserved the animal's capacity to learn to operate for earning a positive reinforcer. It was concluded that *H. perforatum* contains some active principle(s) endowed with antidepressant activity.

Clinical Efficacy

Linde and co-workers[10] conducted a meta-analysis of the clinical efficacy of St. John's wort for depression. They concluded that, over a period of 2 to 4 weeks of treatment, hypericum extract was superior to placebo. Commenting on this review, DeSmet and Nolen[11] stated:

> Although promising, these studies are not sufficient to accept the use of hypericum extract in major depression . . . [S]pecific studies in severely depressed patients are still missing, as are longer-term studies to assess the risk of relapse and the possibility of late side effects. Of the four trials that have compared a hypericum monopreparation with a synthetic antidepressant, none lasted longer than six weeks. All tested the comparator drug . . . at the lower end of the usual dose range, and none of the reports described a homogenous patient group with major depression defined by the criteria of the *Diagnostic and Statistical Manual of Mental Disorders*.

Similarly, Wong, Smith, and Boon[1] state:

> Overall, there are inadequate data regarding long-term use and efficacy in severe depression. There are concerns regarding the standardization and quality control of commercial preparations. Clearly, more research is needed to address these shortcomings in the literature.

Kim and co-workers[12] conducted a similar meta-analysis. From a total of 651 patients, they concluded that *"Hypericum perforatum* was more effective than placebo and similar in effectiveness to low-dose tricyclic antidepressants in the short-term treatment of mild to moderately severe depression." However, they were careful to state that "serious questions remain regarding the research design of the studies analyzed."

Philipp, Kohnen and Hiller[13] reported that hypericum extract (1 gram/day) was comparable in efficacy to imipramine (100 mg/day), and superior to placebo. Commenting on this study, Linde and Berner[14] noted that this "confirms the existing evidence that hypericum extract is more effective than placebo in mild and moderately severe depression." Linde and Berner added, however, that the dose of hypericum was high, the dose of imipramine was low, and the superiority of both drug treatments over placebo was "not impressive," with placebo responses being quite robust.

All these authors agree that "there is good evidence for the efficacy of St. John's wort for the treatment of depression." In late 1998, the United States Office of Complementary and Alternative Medicine of the National Institutes of Health began a large three-year, multicenter clinical trial comparing St John's wort with both placebo and fluoxetine. Results should be available in the year 2003. Until then,

> Existing data on the therapeutic effects of St. John's wort are provocative. However, well-designed clinical trials are needed to determine long-term safety and therapeutic guidelines for its use for different depressive disorders. Prior to the availability of such information, patients who choose to use St. John's wort should use the regimen shown to be effective in (limited, short-term) clinical trials: 300 mg 3 times a day of the extract standardized to 0.3% hypericin. St. John's wort is generally well tolerated, but can cause photosensitivity, especially in fair-skinned persons taking large doses. It should not be used during pregnancy or with other psychoactive agents.[4]

Side Effects

Side effects of St. John's wort are few. There are rare reports of photodermatitis, precipitation of a hypomanic state, and possible nerve toxicity (demyelination). More commonly, dry mouth, GI upset, dizziness, sedation, and constipation are reported. Combined with SSSRs, a serotonin syndrome can be precipitated.

Conclusions

> There is evidence that extracts of hypericum are more effective than placebo for the treatment of mild to moderately severe depressive disorders. Further studies comparing extracts with standard antidepressants

in well-defined groups of patients and comparing different extracts and doses are needed.[10]

An overview of 23 clinical studies in Europe found that it may be useful in cases of mild to moderate depression and caused far fewer side effects than standard drugs did. Eventually, consumers should know more: The federal government is funding a three-year study that will compare the herb with a prescription antidepressant and a placebo. Side effects: dizziness, dry mouth, increased sensitivity to sunlight.[3]

Ginkgo

The ginkgo tree (*Ginkgo biloba*) is one of the oldest deciduous tree species on earth.[1] The extract of ginkgo is referred to as EGb-760 and is one of the most popular plant extracts used in Europe to alleviate symptoms associated with a range of cognitive disorders, including dementia. In the United States, in order to avoid FDA regulations, it is promoted not to treat cognitive dysfunctions but, for example, to provide "mental sharpness," provide antioxidant protection, maintain healthy circulatory perfusion, and so on. Published medical indications include dementia, chronic cerebrovascular insufficiency (insufficient blood flow to the brain), and brain protection secondary to cerebral or head trauma.

The active ingredients in ginkgo extracts are not completely known. The standardized commercial preparation contains 24 percent ginkgo flavinoids and 6 percent terpenoids. As noted in the discussion of St. John's wort, flavinoids inhibit CYP1A2 and create drug interactions through this mechanism.

Flavinoids and terpenoids are antioxidants that "scavenge" free radicals that have been implicated as the mediators of the cellular damage observed in Alzheimer's disease. Ginkgolide B (a terpenoid) inhibits a platelet-activating factor, interfering with platelet aggregation and slowing blood clotting (as does aspirin). This antiplatelet action by itself could provide therapeutic effectiveness by limiting abnormal clot formation in small arteries (as aspirin does). Adversely, it may increase the tendency to bleed and it may well interact with other blood thinners (again, as does aspirin). Presumed antioxidant effects have not been convincingly demonstrated to correlate well with efficacy in treating cognitive dysfunction.

Pharmacokinetics

Taken orally, *Ginkgo biloba* extracts appear to be readily absorbed, although blood levels of any of the substances found in the extract have not been reported. Plasma concentrations of ginkgo flavinoids peak in plasma at two to three hours after ingestion. The mechanisms of elimination of these substances from the body is not known. It is also not known whether any of these flavinoids or terpenoids are metabolized before excretion. Kleijnen and Knipschild[15] reported that portions of the extract are excreted in the urine and feces and through the lungs. The half-life is thought to be about 5 hours.

Pharmacodynamics

The EGb-761 extract of ginkgo contains multiple compounds that are thought by some individuals to act on unidentified processes involved in the homeostasis of inflammation and oxidative stress, presumably providing membrane protection and neurotransmission modulation.[16] EEG studies[17] demonstrate an activating effect with increased alpha-wave activity, indicative of increased alertness and perhaps of improved cognitive performance (perhaps similar to the effects of caffeine on the EEG).

Clinical Results

Most early studies on ginkgo extract were too poorly conducted to merit conclusions. Kleijnen and Knipschild[15] reviewed these studies, noting a general conclusion that ginkgo produced significant improvement in symptoms such as memory loss, concentration difficulties, fatigue, anxiety, and depression. Improvements were observed in patients severely affected with Alzheimer's disease; there was no significant improvement in individuals with mild to no memory impairment (presumably these individuals had normal blood circulation to the CNS). LeBars and co-workers[16] conducted a 52-week double-blind, placebo-controlled study of EGb-761 in 309 patients with mild to severe Alzheimer's disease or multi-infarct dementia. At 26 and 52 weeks of treatment, extract-treated patients, compared with nonmedicated controls, exhibited modest improvements in both objective testing of cognitive performance and in the caregiver's evaluation of social functioning. A "clinician's global impression of change" was unaffected. These data were in general agreement with those reported by Kanowski and colleagues[18] in 1996. O'Hara and co-workers[4] state: "While statistically significant, such modest effects are of uncertain clinical benefit."

Oken and co-workers[19] reviewed 50 studies on *Ginkgo biloba* for neurological disorders and concluded that patients function slightly better than those taking placebo. Wong, Smith, and Boon[1] reviewed the uses of ginkgo extract and concluded that there is no clear evidence of efficacy in the treatment of depression, impotence (including antidepressant-induced sexual dysfunction) or brain injury.

Side Effects and Precautions

Side effects of ginkgo include headache and GI upset, but they are mild and infrequent. Headache is most common and can be minimized by starting with a low dose and increasing it gradually. There is concern about increased bleeding and the potential for interaction with aspirin and other anticoagulants.[20] Safety in pregnancy and during lactation has not been established. As stated earlier, drug interactions may occur secondary to CYP1A2 inhibition.

Kava

Preparations made from the roots of kava (*Piper methysticin*) have been used for ceremonial and social purposes by the peoples of the South Pacific for thousands of years. Captain James Cook first described kava in the account of his voyage in 1768. Further scientific study was not made until the early days of pharmacology and pharmacognosy in 1886.

Kava is used by the Oceanic peoples as an antianxiety drug, similar to our use of ethyl alcohol. Kava induces relaxation, improves social interaction, promotes sleep, and plays an important role in the sociocultural life of the islanders of the South Pacific. At higher doses, Kava produces sleep and stupor, again like alcohol. Standardized extracts of kava are used for the therapy of anxiety, tension, and restlessness.

Chemistry

There are multiple agents with pharmacological activity in kava. Most interest centers on the alpha-pyrones commonly referred to as kava lactones, found in the fat-soluble portions of the plant root.[21] Other compounds in kava contribute to efficacy, and the sedative activity of a crude preparation exceeds that of extracted kava lactones. However, as the kava lactone content of the root varies from 3 percent to 20 percent, preparations standardized for kava lactone content are preferred to crude preparations.[21]

Pharmacokinetics

When taken as the extract, kava lactones appear to be well absorbed; much less absorbed when the isolated substances are taken (why this is so is unknown). Little is known about the distribution, metabolism, and excretion of the ingredients.

Pharmacodynamics

The mechanism of action of ingredients in kava is poorly elucidated.[1] Kava pyrones appear to bind to various GABA receptors or to the benzodiazepine-binding site. A kava lactone has been shown to block sodium channels, an anesthetic-like effect. Kava has been shown in animals to be anticonvulsant, muscle relaxant, and neuroprotective (much as are benzodiazepines and barbiturates). The EEG alterations induced by kava resemble those induced by benzodiazepines. Uebelhack and colleagues[22] reported that kava, either in extract form or as pure kava lactones, was a reversible inhibitor of monoamine oxidase-B (MAO-B). The significance of this is unknown, since the antidepressant effect of MAO inhibitors results from MAO-A inhibition (Chapter 15), while the food interactions result from MAO-B inhibition. The Uebelhack group states, however: "The inhibition of MAO-B by kava pyrone-enriched extracts might be an important mechanism for their psychotropic activity."[22] Therefore, tentatively, one can hypothesize that kava's action should closely resemble that of the traditional sedative-hypnotic compounds.

Clinical Results

At a dose of up to 70 mg of kava lactone, an anxiolytic effect is noted. At higher doses (125 to 210 mg), sedation is produced. In Oceanic cultures, doses of 250 mg are consumed several times, and inebriation is quite rapidly induced. Pittler and Ernst[23] reviewed kava studies and concluded that "data imply that kava extract is superior to placebo as a symptomatic treatment for anxiety." However, "important caveats exist, which prevent firm conclusions."

Side Effects and Complications

Side effects include drowsiness, nausea, muscle weakness, blurred vision, and (with chronic use) yellow skin discoloration. Kava probably should not be combined with alcohol, benzodiazepines, barbiturates, THC, or other CNS depressants.[20] Kava should probably not be taken before driving or operating machinery.

If kava is an intoxicant, as it appears to be, it is interesting that barbiturates and benzodiazepines are restricted to prescription use, alcohol has age restrictions, marijuana is illegal, but kava is available without restriction.

Ephedrine (Ma-huang)

Ephedrine is the naturally occurring psychoactive drug found in *Ephedra sinica*, also called Ma-huang. The medicinal parts are the young canes collected in autumn and the dried rhizome with roots.[2] Ephedrine is a potent psychostimulant that acts by releasing the body's own stores of the catecholamine neurotransmitters, epinephrine (adrenalin), norepinephrine, and dopamine.

Pharmacologically, ephedrine closely resembles the amphetamines, although the duration of action of ephedrine is considerably shorter. Because of this, ephedrine-containing products (e.g., Metabolife 356 and many others) should not be considered as metabolic supplements, dietary supplements, or any other such nondrug-implying designation. Ephedrine is a potent psychostimulant that should be under regulation of the FDA.

Deaths from ephedrine are not infrequent. The adrenalin and other catecholamines released by ephedrine increase blood pressure, heart rate, the force of cardiac contraction, and cardiac output of blood. Cardiac arrhythmias can be serious and potentially devastating. As with any adrenalin-releasing drug, it relieves bronchoconstriction and therefore provides relief from mild asthma, although tolerance rapidly develops. Like amphetamines, ephedrine temporarily reduces appetite, is a cardiovascular stimulant, and is a psychostimulant. Its disadvantages, however, far outweigh any therapeutic utility. In athletics, ephedrine is a "doping" substance. Numerous drug interactions occur and many are serious and potentially fatal. Several herbal preparations contain both ephedrine and caffeine: this is a combination that should be avoided because caffeine increases the cardiovascular toxicity of ephedrine.

Other Herbals with CNS Activity

A variety of other herbals have been used to treat signs and symptoms of CNS dysfunction. Here, we briefly list a few. Complete descriptions may be found in the *PDR for Herbal Medicines*[2] and in the review by Wong, Smith, and Boon.[1]

Valerian (*Valeriana officalis*) has a long history of use as a mild sedative and as an anxiolytic as well as an antidepressant. The mechanism behind this action is obscure; some data indicate that it may affect GABA receptors, thus acting as a type of mild benzodiazepine. Indeed, GABA itself is a component of valerian, leading some to state that valerian is a source of naturally occurring GABA, which it is. The problem with this is that GABA only very poorly crosses the blood-brain barrier, and it is unlikely that this source of GABA affects the CNS. Other postulated actions include as a 5-HT$_A$ agonist and as a monoamine oxidase inhibitor. They are reviewed by Wong, Smith, and Boon[1] and by Yager, Siegfreid, and DiMatteo.[24] Reported side effects of valerian include liver toxicity, headache, excitability, and uneasiness. There are potential drug interactions between valerian and SSRI-type antidepressants, perhaps precipitating a serotonin syndrome (Chapter 15).[24] Nevertheless, it is generally concluded that valerian can produce anxiolysis and CNS depression similar to that produced by benzodiazepines.[20] There is no evidence to indicate that valerian is superior to existing sedative-hypnotic agents for the treatment of insomnia.[1] The safety of valerian during pregnancy has not been clearly described, so valerian probably should not be used by pregnant women.[4] It would be expected that valerian would potentiate the effects of other CNS depressants, such as ethyl alcohol, and caution is warranted. Valerian should not be taken before driving or in other situations when alertness is required. The usual precautions applying to other sedatives apply as well to valerian. As does St. John's wort, valerian contains quercitin; this substance inhibits the drug-metabolizing enzyme CYP1A2 and can possibly result in clinically significant drug interactions.

German chamomile (*Matricaria recutita*) is used to treat mild insomnia and anxiety (it also has a multitude of non-CNS uses).[4] The herb contains flavinoids that are postulated to have affinity for the benzodiazepine receptor and perhaps for a histamine receptor, either perhaps inducing a sedative effect. No controlled clinical trials have investigated these properties.

Evening primrose (*Oenothera biennis*) has been promoted for the treatment of schizophrenia and ADHD, but little scientific evidence or cultural tradition backs up these claims. Primrose contains a variety of fatty acids, and these substances are postulated to be deficient in both schizophrenia and ADHD. If omega-3 fatty acids have therapeutic usefulness in the treatment of bipolar disorder (Chapter 16), evening primrose may be a productive area for future research. Primrose may exacerbate epilepsy and has been reported to cause drug interactions with a variety of other compounds.

Hops (*Humulus lupulus*) are used in the brewing industry as a component in beer. Hops also have a long history of use as a mild sedative-hypnotic agent. No clinical studies support use of hops as a single agent to treat either insomnia or anxiety.[1] Used as a sedative, drug interactions occur, especially potentiation of the effects of other sedatives such as alcohol and benzodiazepines. Use of hops should be avoided in depression, in pregnancy, and during lactation.[1]

Lemon balm (*Melissa officinalis*), *passion flower* (*Passiflora incarnata*), and *skullcap* (*Scutellaria laterifolia*) are all thought to possess CNS sedative properties and are promoted for use as sedatives and anxiolytics. Data of efficacy are lacking, as is information on active ingredients and mechanisms of action. As sedatives, the usual precautions apply, including those concerning drug interactions and both cognitive and motor impairments.

Conclusions

In an objective summary, Wong, Smith, and Boon[1] made the following concluding statements:

- With the exception of St. John's wort for depression and ginkgo for dementia, there is insufficient evidence to recommend the use of herbal medicines in the treatment of psychiatric illness.

- None of these herbal remedies is clearly superior to current conventional treatments.

- Because these products are widely available and often used by the general public, more clinical research is needed to establish safety and efficacy.

- The advances of modern medicine . . . are greater than at any other time in history. . . . However, the experience and healing traditions of other cultures, whether in less developed countries or in history, should not be ignored.

- Contemporary medical research may finally allow us to separate the traditional remedies that can effectively treat disease from those that are superstition and myth.

- In addition, research . . . may uncover novel treatments for psychiatric illness or yield fresh insights into basic disease mechanisms.

Miller[25] and Fugh-Berman[26] discuss some of the drug-herb interactions associated with the use of herbal medications. Over the next few years we will undoubtedly see many studies relating to the safety, efficacy, and drug interactions associated with these substances. Until then, caution is warranted: patients should tell prescribing physicians of their use of herbal medications, and most herbals should probably be avoided in pregnancy until they can be proven safe.

Although significant numbers of children and adolescents are receiving one or more herbal medications, studies of these compounds in this age population are unavailable. In some cases, youths may purchase the drugs themselves, as the drugs are easily available, relatively inexpensive, and widely advertised or endorsed by their peers. In other cases, the young people may be dosed by their parents in attempts to medicate such disorders as ADHD, depression, anxiety, or insomnia. Jurgens[26] and Murphy[27] address this issue, and both authors conclude that currently, no data exist to support the use of herbals in the treatment of psychiatric disorders in children. Until such evidence becomes available, these agents probably should not be administered to children, especially for prolonged periods of time or in the presence of other medications.[27]

STUDY QUESTIONS

1. Describe the recent legislation changing the herbal industry. How has it helped society? How has it hurt?

2. List some of the herbals discussed in other chapters in this book. Which of them should be more freely available? Defend your answer.

3. What is hypericin? Describe its pharmacokinetics. What is the evidence for its efficacy?

4. What is ginkgo? What are its claimed actions? What evidence is there for efficacy to improve memory? For other uses?

5. What is kava? Does it have therapeutic potential? Does it have abuse potential? What drug does it appear to most resemble? Should there be legal restrictions on its use? Defend your answer.

6. What is Ma-huang? What is its active ingredient? Does it have a potential for abuse? Might it induce toxicity? Should its use be regulated? Defend your answer.

7. What in valerian might result in drug interactions?

8. Are there any unaddressed concerns about the use of herbals in pregnancy or in women who might become pregnant? What about in breast-feeding females?

REFERENCES

1. A. H. C. Wong, M. Smith, and H. S. Boon, "Herbal Remedies in Psychiatric Practice," *Archives of General Psychiatry* 55 (1998): 1033–1044.
2. *PDR for Herbal Medicines* (Montvale, N.J.: Medical Economics Company, 1998, 2nd edition, 2000).
3. Consumers Union, "Herbal Rx: The Promises and Pitfalls," *Consumer Reports* 64 (March 1999): 44–48.
4. M. A. O'Hara, D. Kiefer, K. Farrell, and K. Kemper, "A Review of Twelve Commonly Used Medicinal Herbs," *Archives of Family Medicine* 7 (1998): 523–536.
5. B. Staffeldt et al., "Pharmacokinetics of Hypericin and Pseudohypericin after Oral Intake of the Hypericum Perforatum Extract LI 160 in Healthy Volunteers," *Journal of Geriatric Psychiatry and Neurology* 7, Suppl. 1 (1994): S47–S53.
6. H.-M. Thiede and A. Walper, "Inhibition of MAO and COMT by Hypericum Extracts and Hypericin," *Journal of Geriatric Psychiatry and Neurology* 7, Suppl. 1 (1994): S54–S56.
7. W. E. G. Muller and R. Rossol, "Effects of Hypericum Extract on the Expression of Serotonin Receptors," *Journal of Geriatric Psychiatry and Neurology* 7, Suppl. 1 (1994): S63–S64.
8. R. Teufel-Mayer and J. Gleitz, "Effects of Long-term Administration of Hypericum Extracts on the Affinity and Density of the Central Serotoninergic 5-HT$_{1A}$ and 5-HT$_{2A}$ Receptors," *Pharmacopsychiatry* 30 (1997): 113–116.

9. C. Gambarana et al., "Efficacy of an *Hypericum Perforatum* (St. John's Wort) Extract in Preventing and Reverting a Condition of Escape Deficit in Rats," *Neuropsychopharmacology* 21 (1999): 247–257.

10. K. Linde et al., "St. John's Wort for Depression—An Overview and Meta-analysis of Randomized Clinical Trials," *British Medical Journal* 313 (1996): 253–258.

11. P. DeSmet and W. A. Nolen, "St. John's Wort as an Antidepressant," *British Medical Journal* 313 (1996): 241–242.

12. H. L. Kim, J. Streltzer, and D. Goebert, "St. John's Wort for Depression," *Journal of Nervous and Mental Disease* 187 (1999): 532–539.

13. M. Philipp, R. Kohnen and K.-O. Hiller, "Hypericum Extract versus Imipramine or Placebo in Patients with Moderate Depression: Randomized Multicentre Study of Treatment for Eight Weeks," *British Medical Journal* 319 (2000): 1534–1539.

14. K. Linde and M. Berner, "Commentary: Has Hypericum Found Its Place in Antidepressant Treatment?" *British Medical Journal* 319 (2000): 1534–1539.

15. J. Kleijnen and P. Knipschild, "*Ginkgo biloba*," *Lancet* 340 (1992): 1136–1139.

16. P. L. LeBars et al., "A Placebo-controlled, Double-blind, Randomized Trial of an Extract of Ginkgo Biloba for Dementia," *Journal of the American Medical Association* 278 (1997): 1327–1332.

17. T. M. Itil et al., "Central Nervous System Effects of *Ginkgo biloba*, a Plant Extract," *American Journal of Therapeutics* 3 (1996): 63–73.

18. S. Kanowski et al., "Proof of Efficacy of the *Ginkgo biloba* Special Extract EGb 761 in Outpatients Suffering from Mild to Moderate Primary Degenerative Dementia of the Alzheimer type or Multi-infart Dementia," *Pharmacopsychiatry* 29 (1996): 47–56.

19. B. S. Oken, D. M. Storzbach, and J. A. Kaye, "The Efficacy of *Ginkgo biloba* on Cognitive Function in Alzheimer's Disease," *Archives of Neurology* 55 (1998): 1409–1415.

20. J. A. Leak, "Herbal Medicine: Is It an Alternative or an Unknown? A Brief Review of Popular Herbals Used by Patients in a Pain and Symptom Management Practice Setting," *Current Review of Pain* 3 (1999): 226–236.

21. Botanical Report, "Kava: Nature's Answer to Anxiety," *Health Counselor* 6 (1995): 33–35.

22. R. Uebelhack, L. Franke, and H.-J. Schewe, "Inhibition of Platelet MAO-B by Kava Pyrone-enriched Extract from *Piper methysticum forester* (Kava-Kava)," *Pharmacopsychiatry* 31 (1998): 187–192.

23. M. H. Pittler and E. Ernst, "Efficacy of Kava Extract for Treating Anxiety: Systematic Review and Meta-Analysis," *Journal of Clinical Psychopharmacology* 20 (2000): 84–89.

24. J. Yager, S. L. Siegfried, and T. L. DiMatteo, "Use of Aternative Remedies by Psychiatric Patients: Illustrative Vignettes and a Discussion of the Issues," *American Journal of Psychiatry* 156 (1999): 1432–1438.

25. L. C. Miller, "Herbal Medicinals: Selected Clinical Considerations Focusing on Known or Potential Drug-Herb Interactions," *Archives of Internal Medicine* 158 (1998): 2200–2211.

26. A. Fugh-Berman, "Herb-Drug Interactions," *The Lancet* 355 (2000): 134–138.

27. S. P. Kutcher, editor, "Focus on Herbal Medicine," *Child & Adolescent Psychopharmacology News* 4 (December, 1999): 1–6.

GLOSSARY

Abstinence syndrome   State of altered behavior that follows cessation of drug administration.

Acetylcholine   Neurotransmitter in the central and peripheral nervous systems.

Additive effect   Increased effect that occurs when two drugs that have similar biological actions are administered. The net effect is the sum of the independent effects exerted by the drugs.

Adenosine   Chemical neuromodulator in the CNS, primarily at inhibitory synapses.

Adenylate cyclase   Intracellular enzyme that catalyzes the conversion of cyclic AMP to adenosine monophosphate.

Affective disorder   Type of mental disorder characterized by recurrent episodes of mania, depression, or both.

Agonist   Drug that attaches to a receptor and produces actions that mimic or potentiate those of an endogenous transmitter.

Aldehyde dehydrogenase   Enzyme that carries out a specific step in alcohol metabolism: the metabolism of acetaldehyde to acetate. This enzyme may be blocked by the drug disulfiram (Antabuse).

Alzheimer's disease   Progressive neurological disease that occurs primarily in the elderly. It is characterized by a loss of short-term memory and intellectual functioning. It is associated with a loss of function of acetylcholine neurons.

Amphetamine   A behavioral stimulant.

Anabolic-androgenic steroid   Testosterone-like drug that acts to increase muscle mass and produces other masculinizing effects.

Anandamide   Endogenous chemical compound that attaches to cannabinoid receptors in the CNS and to specific components of the lymphatic system.

Anandamide receptor   Receptor to which anandamide and tetrahydrocannabinol bind.

Anesthetic drugs   Sedative-hypnotic compounds used primarily in doses capable of inducing a state of general anesthesia that involves both loss of sensation and loss of consciousness.

Antagonist   Drug that attaches to a receptor and blocks the action of either an endogenous transmitter or an agonist drug.

Anticonvulsant   Drug that blocks or prevents epileptic convulsions. Some anticonvulsants (e.g., carbamazepine, valproic acid) are also used to treat certain nonepileptic psychiatric disorders.

Antidepressant   Drug that is useful in treating mental depression in depressed patients but does not produce stimulant effects in nondepressed persons. Subdivided into seven classes or categories.

Antipsychotic drugs   Drugs that have the ability to calm psychotic states and make the psychotic patient more manageable. Two classes are defined: classical and new generation.

Anxiolytic   Drug used to relieve the symptoms associated with defined states of anxiety. Classically, refers to the benzodiazepines and related drugs.

Attention-deficit/hyperactivity disorder (ADHD)   Learning and behavioral disability characterized by reduced attention span and hyperactivity.

Autonomic nervous system   Portion of the peripheral nervous system that controls or regulates the visceral, or automatic, functions of the body, such as heart rate and blood pressure.

Barbiturates   Class of chemically related sedative-hypnotic compounds that share a characteristic six-membered ring structure.

Basal ganglia   Part of the brain that contains vast numbers of dopamine-containing synapses. Forms part of the extrapyramidal system. Parkinson's disease follows dopamine loss in this structure.

Benzodiazepines   Class of chemically related sedative-hypnotic agents of which chlordiazepoxide (Librium) and diazepam (Valium) are examples.

Bipolar disorder   Affective disorder characterized by alternating bouts of mania and depression. Also referred to as *manic-depressive illness.*

Blackout   Period of time during which one may be awake but memory is not imprinted. It frequently occurs in persons who have consumed excessive alcohol or to whom have been administered (or who have taken) large doses of sedative drugs.

Brain syndrome, organic   Pattern of behavior induced when neurons are either reversibly depressed or irreversibly destroyed. Behavior is characterized by clouded sensorium, disorientation, shallow and labile affect, and impaired memory, intellectual function, insight, and judgment.

Brand name   Unique name licensed to one manufacturer of a drug. Contrasts with **generic name,** the name under which any manufacturer may sell a drug.

Caffeine   Behavioral and general cellular stimulant found in coffee, tea, cola drinks, and chocolate.

Caffeinism   Habitual use of large amounts of caffeine.

Cannabis sativa   Hemp plant; contains marijuana.

Carbidopa   Drug that inhibits the enzyme dopa decarboxylase, allowing increased availability of dopa within the brain. Contained in Sinemet.

Central nervous system (CNS)   Brain and spinal cord.

Cirrhosis   Serious, usually irreversible liver disease. Usually associated with chronic excessive alcohol consumption.

Clonidine (Catapres) Antihypertensive useful in ameliorating the symptoms of narcotic withdrawal.

Cocaine A behavioral stimulant.

Codeine Sedative and pain-relieving agent found in opium. Structurally related to morphine but less potent; constitutes approximately 0.5 percent of the opium extract.

Comorbid disorder Psychiatric disorder that coexists with a second psychiatric disorder (e.g., multisubstance abuse in a patient with a major depressive disorder).

Convulsant Drug that produces convulsions by blocking inhibitory neurotransmission.

COX inhibitors Aspirin-like analgesic drugs that produce their actions by inhibiting the enzyme cyclooxygenase. Two variants of the enzyme occur: COX-1 and COX-2. Some drugs are specific for COX-2; others are nonspecific inhibitors.

Crack Street name for a smokable form of potent, concentrated cocaine.

Cross-dependence Condition in which one drug can prevent the withdrawal symptoms associated with physical dependence on a different drug.

Cross-tolerance Condition in which tolerance of one drug results in a lessened response to another drug.

Delirium tremens (DTs, "rum fits") Syndrome of tremulousness with hallucinations, psychomotor agitation, confusion and disorientation, sleep disorders, and other associated discomforts, lasting several days after alcohol withdrawal.

Dementia General designation for nonspecific mental deterioration.

Detoxification Process of allowing time for the body to metabolize and/or excrete accumulations of drug. Usually a first step in drug abuse evaluation and treatment.

Differential diagnosis Listing of all possible causes that might explain a given set of symptoms.

Dimethyltryptamine (DMT) Psychedelic drug found in many South American snuffs.

Disinhibition Physiological state of the central nervous system characterized by decreased activity of inhibitory synapses, which results in a net excess of excitatory activity.

Dopamine transporter Presynaptic protein that binds synaptic dopamine and transports the neurotransmitter back into the presynaptic nerve terminal.

Dose-response relation Relation between drug doses and the response elicited at each dose level.

Drug Chemical substance used for its effects on bodily processes.

Drug absorption Mechanism by which a drug reaches the bloodstream from the skin, lungs, stomach, intestinal tract, or muscle.

Drug administration Procedures through which a drug enters the body (oral administration of tablets or liquids, inhalation of powders, injection of sterile liquids, and so on).

Drug dependence   State in which the use of a drug is necessary for either physical or psychological well-being.

Drug interaction   Modification of the action of one drug by the concurrent or prior administration of another drug.

Drug misuse   Use of any drug (legal or illegal) for a medical or recreational purpose when other alternatives are available, practical, or warranted, or when drug use endangers either the user or others with whom he or she may interact.

Drug receptor   Specific molecular substance in the body with which a given drug interacts to produce its effect.

Drug tolerance   State of progressively decreasing responsiveness to a drug.

DSM-IV   *Diagnostic and Statistical Manual of Mental Disorders*, Fourth Edition (1994), a publication of the American Psychiatric Association.

Electroconvulsive therapy (ECT)   Nonpharmacological treatment used for major depression.

Endorphin   Naturally occurring protein that causes endogenous morphine-like activity.

Enkephalin   Naturally occurring protein that causes morphine-like activity.

Enzyme   Large organic molecule that mediates a specific biochemical reaction in the body.

Enzyme induction   Increased production of drug-metabolizing enzymes in the liver, stimulated by certain drugs that increase the rate at which the body can metabolize them. It is one mechanism by which pharmacological tolerance is produced.

Epilepsy   Neurological disorder characterized by an occasional, sudden, and uncontrolled discharge of neurons.

Fetal alcohol syndrome   Symptom complex of congenital anomalies, seen in newborns of women who ingested high doses of alcohol during critical periods of pregnancy.

G-protein   Specific intraneuronal protein that links transmitter-induced receptor alterations with intracellular second-messenger proteins or with adjacent ion channels.

Gamma-aminobutyric acid (GABA)   Inhibitory amino acid neurotransmitter in the brain.

Generic name   Name that identifies a specific chemical entity (without specifically describing the chemical). Often marketed under different brand names by multiple manufacturers.

Glutamic acid   An excitatory amino acid neurotransmitter.

Hallucinogen   Psychedelic drug that produces profound distortions in perception.

Harmine   Psychedelic agent obtained from the seeds of *Peganum harmala*.

Hashish   Extract of the hemp plant (*Cannabis sativa*) that has a higher concentration of THC than does marijuana.

Heroin Semisynthetic opiate produced by a chemical modification of morphine.

Hypothalamus Structure located at the base of the brain, above the pituitary gland.

Hypoxia State of relative lack of oxygen in the tissues of the body and the brain.

ICE Street name for a smokable, free-base form of potent, concentrated methamphetamine.

Levodopa Precursor substance to the transmitter dopamine, useful in ameliorating the symptoms of Parkinson's disease.

Limbic system Group of brain structures involved in emotional responses and emotional expression.

Lithium Alkali metal effective in the treatment of mania and depression.

Lysergic acid diethylamide (LSD) Semisynthetic psychedelic drug.

Major tranquilizer Drug used in the treatment of psychotic states.

Mania Mental disorder characterized by an expansive emotional state, elation, hyperirritability, excessive talkativeness, flights of ideas, and increased behavioral activity.

MAO inhibitor (MAOI) Drug that inhibits the activity of the enzyme monoamine oxidase.

Marijuana Mixture of the crushed leaves, flowers, and small branches of both the male and female hemp plant (*Cannabis sativa*).

Mescaline Psychedelic drug extracted from the peyote cactus.

Minor tranquilizer Sedative-hypnotic drug promoted primarily for use in the treatment of anxiety.

Mixed agonist–antagonist Drug that attaches to a receptor, producing weak agonist effects but displacing more potent agonists, precipitating withdrawal in drug-dependent persons.

Monoamine oxidase (MAO) Enzyme capable of metabolizing norepinephrine, dopamine, and serotonin to inactive products.

Monoamine oxidase inhibitor (MAOI) See **MAO inhibitor**.

Morphine Major sedative and pain-relieving drug found in opium, comprising approximately 10 percent of the crude opium exudate.

Muscarine Drug extracted from the mushroom *Amanita muscaria* that directly stimulates acetylcholine receptors.

Myristin Psychedelic agent obtained from nutmeg and mace.

Neurotransmitter Endogenous chemical released by one neuron that alters the electrical activity of another neuron.

Nicotine Behavioral stimulant found in tobacco.

Ololiuqui Psychedelic drug obtained from the seeds of the morning glory plant.

Opioid Natural or synthetic drug that exerts actions on the body similar to those induced by morphine, the major pain-relieving agent obtained from the opium poppy (*Papaver somniferum*).

Opium   Crude resinous exudate from the opium poppy.

Parkinson's disease   Disorder of the motor system characterized by involuntary movements, tremor, and weakness.

Partial agonist   A drug that binds to a receptor and exerts only part of the action exerted by the endogenous neurotransmitter or that produces a submaximal receptor response.

Peptide   Chemical composed of a chain-link sequence of amino acids.

Peyote   Cactus that contains mescaline.

Pharmacodynamics   Study of the interactions of a drug and the receptors responsible for the action of the drug in the body.

Pharmacokinetics   Study of the factors that influence the absorption, distribution, metabolism, and excretion of a drug.

Pharmacology   Branch of science that deals with the study of drugs and their actions on living systems.

Phencyclidine (Sernyl, PCP)   Psychedelic surgical anesthetic. Acts by binding to and inhibiting ion transport through the NMDA-glutamate receptors.

Phenothiazine   Class of chemically related compounds useful in the treatment of psychosis.

Physical dependence   State in which the use of a drug is required for a person to function normally. Such a state is revealed by withdrawing the drug and noting the occurrence of withdrawal symptoms (abstinence syndrome). Characteristically, withdrawal symptoms can be terminated by readministration of the drug.

Placebo   Pharmacologically inert substance that may elicit a significant reaction largely because of the mental set of the patient or the physical setting in which the drug is taken.

Potency   Measure of drug activity expressed in terms of the amount required to produce an effect of given intensity. Potency varies inversely with the amount of drug required to produce this effect—the more potent the drug, the lower the amount required to produce the effect.

Psilocybin   Psychedelic drug obtained from the mushroom *Psilocybe mexicana*.

Psychedelic drug   Drug that can alter sensory perception.

Psychoactive drug   Chemical substance that alters mood or behavior as a result of alterations in the functioning of the brain.

Psychological dependence   Compulsion to use a drug for its pleasurable effects. Such dependence may lead to a compulsion to misuse a drug.

Psychopharmacology   Branch of pharmacology that deals with the effects of drugs on the nervous system and behavior.

Psychopharmacotherapy   Clinical treatment of psychiatric disorders with drugs.

Psychotherapy   Nonpharmacological treatment of psychiatric disorders utilizing a wide range of modalities, from simple education and supportive counseling to insight-oriented, dynamically based therapy.

Receptor   Location in the nervous system at which a neurotransmitter or drug binds to exert its characteristic effect. Most receptors are members of genetically encoded families of specialized proteins.

Reye's syndrome Rare CNS disorder that occurs in children; associated with aspirin ingestion.

Risk-to-benefit ratio Arbitrary assessment of the risks and benefits that may accrue from administration of a drug.

Scopolamine Anticholinergic drug that crosses the blood-brain barrier to produce sedation and amnesia.

Second messenger Intraneuronal protein that, when activated by an excitatory G-protein, initiates the neuronal response to the initial neurotransmitter attachment to an extracellular receptor.

Sedative-hypnotic drugs Chemical substances that exert a nonselective general depressant action on the nervous system.

Serotonin (5-hydroxytryptamine, 5-HT) Synaptic transmitter in both the brain and the peripheral nervous system.

Serotonin-specific reuptake inhibitor (SSRI) Second-generation antidepressant drug.

Serotonin syndrome Clinical syndrome resulting from excessive amounts of serotonin in the brain. Can follow use of excessive doses of SSRIs. Characterized by extreme anxiety, confusion and disorientation.

Serotonin withdrawal syndrome Clinical syndrome that can follow withdrawal or cessation of SSRI therapy. Characterized by mental status alterations, severe flu-like symptoms, and feeling of tingling or electrical shock sensations in the extremities.

Side effect Drug-induced effect that accompanies the primary effect for which the drug is administered.

Tardive dyskinesia Movement disorder that appears after months or years of treatment with neuroleptic (antipsychotic) drugs. It usually worsens with drug discontinuation. Symptoms are often masked by the drugs that cause the disorder.

Teratogen Chemical substance that induces abnormalities of fetal development.

Testosterone Hormone secreted from the testes that is responsible for the distinguishing characteristics of the male.

Tetrahydrocannabinol (THC) Major psychoactive agent in marijuana, hashish, and other preparations of hemp (*Cannabis sativa*).

Therapeutic drug monitoring (TDM) Process of correlating the plasma level of drugs with therapeutic response.

Tolerance Clinical state of reduced responsiveness to a drug. Can be produced by a variety of mechanisms, all of which require increased doses of drug to produce an effect once achieved by lower doses.

Toxic effect Drug-induced effect either temporarily or permanently deleterious to any organ or system of an animal or person. Drug toxicity includes both the relatively minor side effects that invariably accompany drug administration and the more serious and unexpected manifestations that occur in only a small percentage of patients who take a drug.

INDEX

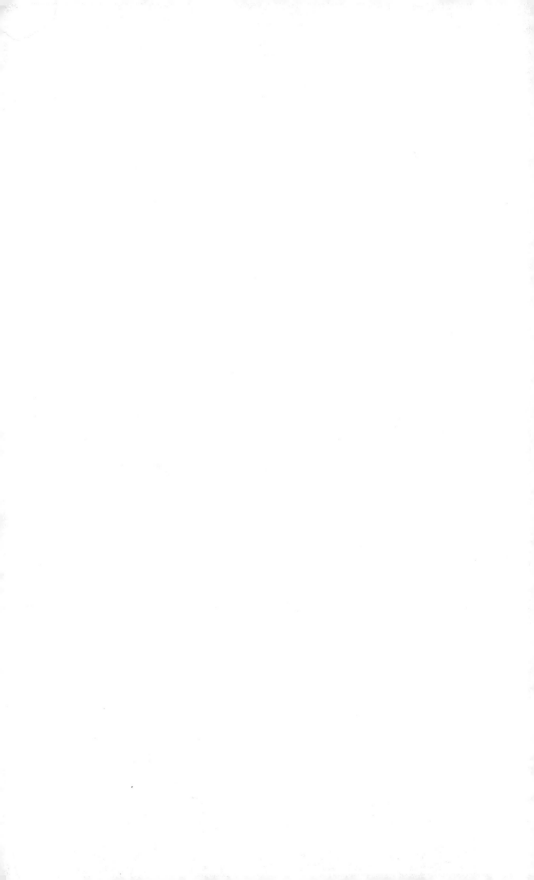